Principles and Practice of
Travel Medicine

Principles and Practice of
Travel Medicine

Edited by
Jane N. Zuckerman

Academic Centre for Travel Medicine and Vaccines,
Royal Free and University College Medical School, London, UK

JOHN WILEY & SONS, LTD

Chichester • New York • Weinheim • Brisbane • Singapore • Toronto

Other Wiley Editorial Offices

John Wiley & Sons, Inc., 605 Third Avenue,
New York, NY 10158-0012, USA

WILEY-VCH Verlag GmbH, Pappelallee 3,
D-69469 Weinheim, Germany

John Wiley & Sons Australia, Ltd, 33 Park Road, Milton,
Queensland 4064, Australia

John Wiley & Sons (Asia) Pte, Ltd., Clementi Loop #02-01,
Jin Xing Distripark, Singapore 129809

John Wiley & Sons (Canada), Ltd., 22 Worcester Road,
Rexdale, Ontario M9W 1L1, Canada

Library of Congress Cataloging-in-Publication Data

    Principles and practice of travel medicine / edited by Jane N. Zuckerman
        p.   cm.
    Includes bibliographical references and index.
    ISBN 0-471-49079-2 (cased : alk. paper)
    1. Travel—Health aspects.   I. Zuckerman, Jane N.
    [DNLM: 1. Travel.   2. Communicable Diseases.   3. Preventive Medicine—methods. QT
250 P957 20001]
    RA783.5.P75   2001

                                       2001026216

British Library Cataloguing in Publication Data

A catalogue record for this book is available from the British Library

ISBN 0-471-49079-2

Typeset in 9/10pt Times from the author's disks by Vision Typesetting, Manchester
Printed and bound in Great Britain by Antony Rowe Ltd, Chippenham, Wiltshire
This book is printed on acid-free paper responsibly manufactured from sustainable forestry,
in which at least two trees are planted for each one used for paper production.

Contents

Contributors

Susan Anderson *Clinical Assistant and Professor of Medicine, Office of Medical Education, Stanford University School of Medicine, 251 Campus Drive, MSOB X-365, Stanford, CA 94305-5490, USA*

Michael Bagshaw *Head of Medical Services, British Airways Health Services, Waterside, PO Box 365 (HMAG), Harmondsworth UB7 0GB, UK*

Indran Balakrishnan *Clinical Lecturer, Department of Medical Microbiology, Royal Free and University College Medical School, Rowland Hill Street, London NW3 2PF, UK*

Nicholas J. Beeching *Senior Lecturer in Infectious Diseases, Liverpool School of Tropical Medicine, Pembroke Place, Liverpool L3 5QA, UK*

Norman T. Begg *Head of Medical Affairs, GlaxoSmithKline, Stockley Park West, Uxbridge, Middlesex UB11 1BT, UK*

Peter J. Benton *Surgeon Commander, Institute of Naval Medicine, Alverstoke, Gosport, Hampshire PO12 2DL, UK*

Frank J. Bia *Professor of Medicine and Laboratory Medicine, Yale University School of Medicine, 333 Cedar Street, New Haven, CT 06520-8030, USA*

Verity Blackwell *Specialist Registrar in Dermatology, The Middlesex Hospital, 1st Floor, Arthur Stanley House, Tottenham Street, London W1P 6PG, UK*

Robert Bor *Professor, Psychology Department, London Guildhall University, Calcutta House, 1 Old Castle Street, London E1 7NT, UK*

Eric Caumes *Consultant Dermatologist, Department of Infectious Diseases, Hôpital Pitié Salpétrière, 47–83 Boulevard de L'Hôpital, 75651 Paris, Cedex 13, France*

Ann L. N. Chapman *Specialist Registrar, Department of Infection and Tropical Medicine, Birmingham Heartlands Hospital, Bordesley Green East, Birmingham B9 5SS, UK*

Claire Davey *Consultant Ophthalmologist, Royal Free Hampstead NHS Trust, Pond Street, London NW3 2QJ, UK*

Alex T. Dewhurst *Research Registrar in Anaesthesia and Transport Medicine, Academic Department of Anaesthetics, 1st Floor Crosspiece, The Middlesex Hospital, Mortimer Street, London W1N 8AA*

Christopher J. Ellis *Consultant Physician, Department of Infection and Tropical Medicine, Birmingham Heartlands Hospital, Bordesley Green East, Birmingham B9 5SS, UK*

Charles D. Ericsson *Professor of Medicine, Head, Clinical Infectious Diseases and Director, Travel Medicine Clinic, Division of Infectious Diseases, Department of Internal Medicine, University of Texas Houston Medical School, 6431 Fannin Street, JFB, 1.728, Houston, TX 77030, USA*

Philip R. Fischer *Professor of Pediatrics, Mayo Medical School, Mayo Clinic, 2000 First Street SW, Rochester, MN 55905, USA*

Kenneth L. Gamble *Executive Director, Missionary Health Institute, Toronto General Hospital, 200 Elizabeth Street, Eng-212, Toronto, ON M5G 2C4, Canada*

J. Simon R. Gibbs *Consultant Cardiologist, National Heart and Lung Institute, Imperial College of Science, Technology and Medicine, Department of Cardiology, Charing Cross Hospital, London W6 8RF, UK*

Stephen H. Gillespie *Professor of Medical Microbiology, Royal Free and University College Medical School, Rowland Hill Street, London NW3 2PF, UK*

John C. Goldstone *Consultant Anaesthetist, Academic Department of Anaesthetics, 1st Floor Crosspiece, The Middlesex Hospital, Mortimer Street, London W1N 8AA, UK*

Robert Grenfell *Public Health Physician, Grenfell Health Consulting Pty Ltd, 126 Barnes Boulevard, Horsham, Victoria 3400, Australia*

Elaine C. Jong *Clinical Professor of Medicine, University of Washington, Seattle, and Co-Director, Travel and Tropical Medicine Service, Hall Health Travel Clinic, Box 35-4410 Seattle, WA 98195-4410, USA*

Jay S. Keystone *Professor of Medicine, University of Toronto, Tropical Disease Unit, Toronto General Hospital, 200 Elizabeth Street, Eng-212, Toronto, ON M5G 2C4, Canada*

David G. Lalloo *Senior Clinical Lecturer in Tropical Medicine, Alistair Reid Venom Research Unit and WHO Collaborating Centre for the Control of Antivenoms, Liverpool School of Tropical Medicine, Pembroke Place, Liverpool L3 5QA, UK*

Ted Lankester   *Director, InterHealth, 157 Waterloo Road, London SE1 8US, UK*

Robert J. Ligthelm   *Consultant Physician, Havenziekenhuis and Instituut voor Scheeps en Tropenziekten, Haringvliet 2, 3002 TD Rotterdam, The Netherlands*

Louis Loutan   *Head of Unit and Senior Consultant, Travel and Migration Medicine Unit, Department of Community Medicine, University Hospital of Geneva, Rue Micheli-du-Crest 25, 1211 Geneva 14, Switzerland*

Debbie Lovell   *Research Clinical Psychologist, Oxford University Psychiatry Department, Warneford Hospital, Oxford OX3 7JX, UK*

Maria D. Mileno   *Assistant Professor of Medicine, Department of Medicine, Brown University School of Medicine, and Director of The Travel Medicine Service, The Miriam Hospital, Providence, RI, USA*

David R. Murdoch   *Clinical Microbiologist, Canterbury Health Laboratories, P.O. Box 151, Christchurch, New Zealand*

Virginia Murray   *Deputy Medical Director, Medical Toxicology Unit, Avonley Road, London SE14 5ER, UK*

Hans D. Nothdurft   *Director, University Travel Clinic, Department of Infectious Diseases and Tropical Medicine, University of Munich, Leopoldstrasse 5, 80802 Munich, Germany*

Luis Ostrosky-Zeichner   *Clinical Fellow, Division of Infectious Diseases, Department of Internal Medicine, Univesity of Texas Houston Medical School, 6431 Fannin Street JFB 1.728, Houston, TX 77030, USA*

Linda Papadopoulos   *Senior Lecturer, Psychology Department, London Guildhall University, Calcutta House, 1 Old Castle Street, London E1 7NT, UK*

Justin Parker   *Lecturer, Psychology Department, London Guildhall University, Calcutta House, 1 Old Castle Street, London E1 7NT, UK*

Andrew J. Pollard   *Pediatric Infectious Disease Society Clinical Fellow, BC Research Institute for Children's and Women's Health, Room 375, 950 West 28th Avenue, Vancouver, BC V5Z 4H4, Canada*

Theresa Richardson   *Specialist Registrar, Department of Ophthalmology, Royal Free Hampstead NHS Trust, Pond Street, London NW3 2QJ, UK*

Kathryn N. Suh   *Consultant in Infectious Diseases, Department of Medicine, Division of Infectious Diseases, Queen's University, Kingston, Ontario, Canada*

Dominique Tessier   *Medical Director, Medisys Travel Health Clinic, 500 Sherbrooke St West, 11th Floor, Montreal, Quebec H3E 1X5, Canada*

R. David G. Theakston   *Professor of Medical Biology, Alistair Reid Venom Research Unit and WHO Collaborating Centre for the Control of Antivenoms, Liverpool School of Tropical Medicine, Pembroke Place, Liverpool L3 5QA, UK*

Thomas L. Treadwell   *Chief, Infectious Disease, Metrowest Medical Center, Framingham Union Campus, 115 Lincoln Street, Framingham, MA 01702, USA*

Pieter-Paul A. M. van Thiel   *Consultant Physician, Department of Infectious Diseases, Tropical Medicine and Aids, Academic Medical Centre, University of Amsterdam, Meibergdreef 9, 1105 AZ Amsterdam, The Netherlands*

Francisco Vega-López   *Consultant Dermatologist, The Middlesex Hospital, 1st Floor, Arthur Stanley House, Tottenham Street, London W1P 6PG, UK*

Sharon B. Welby   *Clinical Lecturer in Travel Medicine, Liverpool School of Tropical Medicine, Pembroke Place, Liverpool L3 5QA, UK*

Robert E. Wheeler   *President, Voyager Medical Seminars, 9 Corduroy Road, Amherst, NH 03031-2724, USA*

Arie J. Zuckerman   *Professor of Medical Microbiology, Royal Free and University College Medical School, Rowland Hill Street, London NW3 2PF, UK*

Jane N. Zuckerman   *Medical Director of Academic Centre for Travel Medicine and Vaccines and Royal Free Travel Health Centre, Royal Free and University College Medical School, Rowland Hill Street, London NW3 2PF, UK*

Foreword

Travel medicine is one of the newer and important areas of medicine requiring specialist knowledge, academic centres and dedicated clinical services to meet the health and medical needs of the increasing number of leisure and business travellers, and also to cater for the medical aspects of population movements related to economic, political and social factors.

Health, preventive medicine, environmental factors and safety are essential considerations, not only for the traveller but also for the host country and for the country of residence on return. The hundreds of millions of people who travel between countries each year influence profoundly the epidemiology of disease, particularly infections, the environment, facilities and natural resources, and they also have a marked impact on economic, demographic, technological and cultural factors.

Disease knows no frontiers and almost any place in the world can be reached within 24–36 hours, which is less than the incubation period of most infectious diseases. Health care professionals must be able to prevent, identify and treat all known infectious diseases irrespective of geographical and climatic limitations. They must be well versed in the development of new and improved vaccines and the rapid advances in the development of new drugs and treatments.

While the discipline of travel medicine evolved initially from infectious diseases, tropical medicine and preventive medicine, and historically from quarantine and international health regulations, the subject encompasses the whole range of clinical and preventive medicine; this includes care of the traveller with special needs, such as children, the elderly, pregnant women and the disabled, and travellers with cardiovascular, respiratory, metabolic, renal, gastrointestinal, neurological and malignant diseases, and other conditions, including behavioural disorders. Important components of travel medicine include not only vaccinations and prophylaxis against malaria but also advice on accident prevention, sexual health and guidance on contraception, safety of food and water, and hygienic and other precautions.

It is well known that medical students, nurses, doctors and other health care professionals, particularly in the industrialised and developed countries, receive little training in tropical medicine and in diseases and hazards outside their own environment. Yet many infectious diseases largely ignore temperature gradients. This has now been recognised by a number of universities and medical schools in North America, Europe, Australia and the Far East, which have established academic departments in travel and geographical medicine.

The opportunity to advance the subject of travel medicine arose when Jane Zuckerman proposed the establishment of an academic centre at the Royal Free Hospital School of Medicine of the University of London. The concept and the need for such a centre was approved by the Research and Development Committee, by the Education Committee and subsequently by the Council of the School, and the Centre for Travel Medicine and Vaccines was opened in 1995. The Royal Free Hampstead NHS Hospital Trust supported the School's initiative and, later, the proposal for a dedicated travel clinic to serve the staff, students and patients and the travelling public.

On a more personal note, my wife and I are proud of the achievements of our daughter, Jane, and of her dedication to the advancement of her subject, and we are confident that this volume on the principles and practice of travel medicine will meet with the success it so clearly deserves.

Arie J. Zuckerman
Professor of Medical Microbiology in the University of London
Principal and Dean of the Royal Free Hospital School of Medicine and of the Royal Free and University College Medical School, 1989–1999

Preface

The specialty of travel medicine has evolved rapidly as a result of the massive increase in international travel facilitated by the introduction of economical and fast air transport across the world, the construction of transcontinental road and rail connections, giant ship cruisers, travel to and exploration of regions and areas that were previously inaccessible or remote, and the explosive increase in tourism. The World Tourism Organisation, for example, has predicted that international travel, currently in excess of 500 million people each year, will increase by 80% between 1995 and 2010. This also means exposure of travellers to genes, bacteria, viruses, fungi and parasites and other health hazards in the new environment, and the transfer of genes and microorganisms across continents to the host population.

Travel medicine extends well beyond diseases of warm climate and the exigencies of travel and tropical life. It includes exposure to new environments and new cultures, and new hazards ranging from high-altitude and deep-sea environments to medical problems of cosmic radiation and space travel; emerging and re-emerging infections; safe food, safe water, safe clothing; natural and accidental disasters; and issues such as jet lag, fear of flying, air rage and tourist risk of violence. Extensive knowledge of current and new vaccines and of prophylactic and therapeutic drugs is essential. The re-emergence of infections such as diphtheria and syphilis in parts of eastern Europe, the HIV pandemic, increasing numbers of cases of legionella infection in travellers, the epidemiology of drug-resistant malaria, extensive outbreaks of dengue fever and antigenic shifts of influenza A are examples of the imperative need for rapid access to accurate information an internationally recognised epidemiological database.

Travellers with special needs must be evaluated with care and advised accordingly. They include the diabetic traveller, the immunocompromised, those with cardiovascular, renal, neurological, gastrointestinal, malignant and other disorders, psychological and psychiatric illnesses, pregnant women, children and the elderly.

Knowledge of all these aspects of travel health and medicine are, therefore, an essential requirement for the many health care professionals providing advice to and clinical care of the traveller. This volume of *Principles and Practice of Travel Medicine* is addressed to practising physicians and nurses in primary care, occupational health and hospital settings, and to public health physicians, pharmacists and administrators, and, as a source textbook, to undergraduate and postgraduate students. A welcome recent development has been the implementation of teaching of the discipline of travel health and medicine in the form of postgraduate diploma and degree courses as well as study days. Teaching of the subject in the undergraduate curriculum is a feature in medical schools, and it has been introduced successfully at the Royal Free and University College Medical School, including the provision of a special study module. We hope that this book will serve the students well.

I am grateful to my many friends and colleagues who have contributed so willingly and enthusiastically to this book, through which we hope to stimulate health care professionals to consider issues in travel medicine as part of their clinical practice. I also hope that this text may enhance the profile of travel medicine and contribute to its development as a distinct specialty, which may subsequently be recognised as a component of training in infectious disease and tropical medicine as well as part of the undergraduate curriculum.

I would also like to express my gratitude to the editorial and production staff of John Wiley & Sons, in particular Charlotte Brabants and Suzanne Kriston, for their patience and unwavering support.

Finally, I am particularly indebted to my parents for their continued support and encouragement and without whom the inspiration for and concept of this book would never been realised.

Jane N. Zuckerman
London

Section I

Travel Medicine

Trends in Travel

Thomas L. Treadwell

Metrowest Medical Center, Framingham, Massachusetts, USA

INTRODUCTION

One of the great social phenomena of recent history is the increasing mobility of the human population. Since the early nineteenth century, massive human migration has occurred in response to economic hardship, war, famine, and social injustice. These international movements have included five major waves of migration between 1815 and 1914 (60 million out of Europe alone), massive displacements of populations around two World Wars, and ongoing worker migrations to industrialized countries. The health problems of international migration for both traveler and the country of destination are well known and include epidemics of infectious diseases, malnutrition, physical and psychological trauma, and the introduction of disease into new populations. As recent events in central Africa and the Balkans illustrate, forced human migration is still a reality and is associated with particularly poor health outcomes.

Fortunately, human international wanderings do not occur only out of hardship or economic necessity. As Robert Louis Stevenson wrote in *Travels with a Donkey* (1878), 'For my part, I travel not to go anywhere, but to go. I travel for travel's sake. The great affair is to move'. This is, in part, tourism, which also emerged as a major economic and social force in the twentieth century. As opposed to the migrant, the tourist is a short-term visitor traveling to a locality outside his or her usual environment. Most tourism is domestic, but this chapter will focus only on trends in international tourism. The growth and economic importance of international tourism, although only a tiny fraction of total human movement, should not be underestimated. As McKay (1981) wrote 20 years ago, 'Never in history have so many people traveled, have people traveled so far or have they traveled so fast'.

THE RAPID GROWTH IN TOURISM

Fifty years ago, international tourism was relatively uncommon and highly concentrated in a handful of industrialized countries. In 1950, there were an estimated 25 million international arrivals, and roughly a dozen destination countries accounted for more than 95% of total international tourism (Handszuh and Waters, 1997). By 1970, there were in excess of 150 million arrivals per year, with the increase largely due to the arrival of jet travel. By 1993 there were an estimated 500 million international arrivals, and it is estimated that 660 million international arrivals will have occurred by the end of 2000 (Figure 1.1). Even conservative estimates suggest that there may be nearly one billion international tourist arrivals by the year 2010 (WTO, 2000). The expansion of tourism has exceeded 7% per year for the past four decades, and continues, in many parts of the world, to be the fastest growing segment of the economy.

The rapid rise in international tourism has many causes:

- Improvement in world economies, especially in developing countries.
- Relative decrease in the cost of transportation.
- Development of tourist economies and infrastructure, and expansion to developing countries.
- Increase in leisure time and disposable income, particularly in an aging population in developing countries.
- Economic globalization, with more international business travel.
- Increasing trend of students studying and visiting abroad.
- Increased wealth and mobility of immigrants returning to their native countries to visit.
- Local improvements in political stability in some parts of the world.
- Heightened awareness and interest in foreign culture and ecologies.
- Improved marketing of travel, including the Internet.

Principles and Practice of Travel Medicine. Edited by Jane N. Zuckerman.

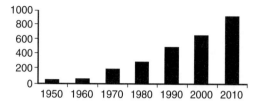

Figure 1.1 International tourist arrivals (millions). (Modified from WTO, 2000)

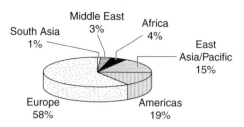

Figure 1.2 International tourist arrivals: market share. (Modified from WTO, 2000)

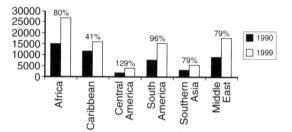

Figure 1.3 Tourist arrivals (thousands): 10 year growth rate (%) and total arrivals in selected regions. (From WTO, 2000)

- Increases in publication (books and magazines) about travel and adventure.

Although there has been a steady rise in tourism for the past several decades, both global and local influences may also serve to reduce tourist arrivals in some years and regions. Rising fuel/transportation costs, political instability, and conflicts are obvious causes of focal declines in tourism (e.g. falling tourism recently in the former Yugoslavia and Mexico).

DESTINATIONS

All travel, and in particular long-distance travel, has associated health risks. Even the European business tourist staying in a five-star hotel in North America is more likely to be unwell than if he or she had remained back at the office. Although the majority of international tourism is between developing countries, a major trend in international travel is the increase in exotic destinations. From the travel medicine standpoint, the increase in travel to developing countries has the most important implications.

Europe has always dominated as the leading destination for tourists, with a 60% market share and nearly 400 million tourist arrivals in 1999 (Figure 1.2). Reasons for this domination include the proximity of European countries to one another, the ease of air, rail, and car transportation among the European countries, the advanced structure of the European tourist industry, and Europe's popularity as a destination, particularly for European and American tourists. The Americas are a distant second in tourist arrivals, with approximately 20% of the total international arrivals in 1999 (123 million). In fact, all of the top 15 tourist destinations except for China (a recent arrival to this list) are in Europe or America. Twenty-five years ago, the top 15 tourist destinations controlled more than 95% of the market. While these regions have continued to dominate the tourist industry and to enjoy growth, their share has dipped to less than two-thirds. In the years 1995 to 1998, international tourism grew at 4% per annum (the United States 2.3% and Europe 4.3%). In contrast, more impressive growth rates are being seen in many developing areas. The most rapidly growing tourist areas are East Asia/Pacific, the Middle East, and Africa.

Many developing countries are currently enjoying double-digit annual growth rates in tourism. For example, in the years 1995–1998, Central America had nearly a 10% annual growth rate, and Cuba grew at a rate of nearly 25% per year. Several countries in Africa, even countries with poor economic conditions and affected by political turmoil, have enjoyed recent growth rates in excess of 20% per year. Figure 1.3 depicts the 10-year growth of selected regions of particular interest to travel clinics.

ECONOMICS OF INTERNATIONAL TOURISM

Tourism is currently the fastest growing major economy in the world. In the past five decades, there has been approximately 7% annual growth in international travel, and it was estimated that four and a half trillion dollars would be spent on international tourism in the year 2000 (WTO, 2000). Tourism receipts are the leading export item in the world, now leading automotive products, food, and oil. One in nine workers worldwide is employed in this industry, and for nearly 40% of countries tourism is the major source of currency (Wilson, 1995).

In tourist receipts, the United States leads all other countries, receiving nearly 75 billion dollars in 1999. Not surprisingly, Europe has more than half of total tourist receipts: the list of the world's top 15 tourism earners includes nine European countries. However, in parallel with the increases in tourist destinations to less-developed regions, other areas of the world are garnering an increased share of the tourist market. The most rapid

Table 1.1 World's top international tourism spenders (1998)

Country	Spend ($US billions)
1. United States	56.1
2. Germany	46.9
3. Japan	32.3
4. United Kingdom	28.8
5. France	17.8
6. Italy	17.7
7. Netherlands	11.0
8. Canada	10.8
9. China	9.5
10. Austria	9.2

From WTO (2000).

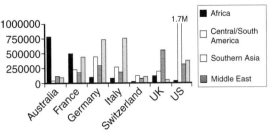

Figure 1.4 International arrivals in selected developing areas (1999). (From WTO, 2000)

economic growth in tourism has been in East Africa and the Pacific, which had 15% of the market share in tourist receipts in 1998. The World Tourism Organization (WTO) has estimated that the market share of this region will grow from 3% in 1970 to more than 20% in 2010. Although regions such as the Middle East, Southern Asia and Central America, and Africa command less than 10% of total tourist receipts, better than average growth is expected in these developing areas. The implications for the economies of these needy areas and for travel medicine are obvious.

Not surprisingly, the major industrial powers spend the most money on international tourism, with the top four countries accounting for more than one-third of total international tourism expenditures (Table 1.1).

OUTBOUND TOURISM

Like politics, most international travel is local. More than half international travel originates in Europe, with most of these travelers bound to major destinations in other localities in Europe or North America; for example, almost 90% of international travelers from the United Kingdom are bound for Europe or North America (WTO, 2000). Approximately 20% of international travelers originate in the United States, but more than half go to Canada or Mexico. Currently, 15% of international travel originates in East Asia, which is the most rapidly expanding source of international tourism.

Obviously, most patients who use travel clinics are planning visits to less-developed regions in the world. If we examine selected 'high-risk' destinations, distinct differences among North America, Europe, and Australian tourists emerge. These differences arise in part because of the proximity of Europe to Africa and the Middle East, shared languages/cultures, and in some cases, former colonial relationships. For example:

• Most 'north–south' international travel from the United States is to Mexico and the Caribbean. In 1999, only 3% of US tourists visited Central/South America,

compared with 8% visiting lower risk areas in the Caribbean.
• Nearly 5% of French international tourists visit Africa, compared with 0.25% from the United States. Ten times more tourists from France visit East Africa than from the United States.
• More visitors from Switzerland arrive in East Africa yearly than from North America.
• The United Kingdom sends twice as many visitors to South Asia as does the United States.
• Exotic travel from Australia is particularly common, with 9% of tourists visiting Africa and 13% Southern Asia.

Figure 1.4 depicts tourist arrivals to selected developing areas from Australia, the United States and Europe.

TOURISM TYPES

The major determinants of travel risk include not only the destination and underlying age and health of the traveler, but also the type of travel. Most international tourism is for pleasure (Figure 1.5). Although good statistics regarding the actual types of pleasure tourism are lacking, the vast majority of international tourists on holiday will visit industrialized countries. Most of the tourists on pleasure trips to less-developed regions stay at resorts or go on organized tours. Just as in North American national parks, where most visitors seldom stray more than a few steps from their automobile, most travelers to developing areas stay within sight of the beach, shopping areas, or the tour bus. Particular attention should be paid to the increasing numbers of travelers interested in more adventurous trips, not only students studying or vacationing in out-of-the-way places, but also older tourists. Interest in ecotourism, trekking, and exposure to indigenous populations, although but a fraction of the total tourism in developing areas, will probably become more popular and will warrant expert pretravel advice. In the next two decades, we will also need to face the challenge of providing health care to many more elderly international travelers.

Business and conference travel is also on the rise, currently nearly 20% of the total. Although of lower risk

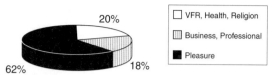

Figure 1.5 International tourism: type of travel (1998). VFR = visiting friends/relatives. (From WTO, 2000)

than other types of tourism, the adverse health problems of this type of travel have been well documented (Kemmerer *et al.*, 1998). Economic globalization and expansion of foreign markets in developing regions will increase business travel to higher risk areas.

One-fifth of international tourism is for visiting friends/relatives, for health reasons, or for religious pilgrimage. A particularly common type of tourism from industrialized regions is the immigrant family visiting their native country. Very often, family groups include children born in Europe or North America traveling to less-developed regions for lengthy stays with relatives. This type of tourism carries a particularly high risk for the travelers and is a challenge for the travel clinic and physicians preparing them for their trip. All of the cases of typhoid fever and most of the malaria seen in our travel clinic during the past 15 years have been associated with family travel to developing areas. As immigrant populations from Africa, Southern Asia, and developing parts of the Americas mature, this type of tourism will undoubtedly increase.

SUMMARY

'The vagabond, when rich, is a tourist' (Paul Richard, *The Scourge of Christ*, 1929). People's psychological need to travel, in the setting of global economic expansion and improved transportation, has resulted in the rapid growth of international tourism. Health care workers interested in emporiatrics should pay particular attention to increased numbers of elderly travelers and to increases in tourism to developing regions of the world.

REFERENCES

Handszuh H and Waters S (1997) Travel and tourism patterns. In *Textbook of Travel Medicine and Health* (eds Dupont H and Steffen R), pp 20–26. Decker, Hamilton, Ontario.

Kemmerer T, Celtron M, Harper L and Kozarsky P (1998) Health problems of corporate travelers: risk factors and management. *Journal of Travel Medicine*, **5**, 184–187.

Mackay D (1981) The British citizen abroad. The present state of tropical medicine in the United Kingdom. *Transactions of the Royal Society of Tropical Medicine and Hygiene*, **75** (suppl.), 45–47.

Wilson M (1995) Travel and the emergence of infectious diseases. *Emerging Infectious Diseases*, **1**, 39–46.

WTO (2000) *World Tourism Highlights*, 2nd edn. World Tourism Organization, Madrid. www.world-tourism.org

2

Epidemiology of Health Risks and Travel

Hans D. Nothdurft

University of Munich, Munich, Germany

Eric Caumes

Hôpital Pitié Salpétrière, Paris, France

GLOBAL BURDEN AND SIGNIFICANCE OF INFECTIOUS DISEASES

Infectious and parasitic diseases are causing considerable morbidity and mortality worldwide. They are by far the leading cause of death in developing countries (Figure 2.1), where infections are the major reason for the enormous loss of life years as a result of disability and premature death (WHO, 1999), especially during childhood.

In industrialised countries, many infectious diseases were controlled successfully during the twentieth century by improvements in hygiene and nutrition as well as by the availability of anti-infective chemotherapy and preventive measures (e.g. vaccines). As a consequence, the importance of infectious diseases has been regarded as becoming very small, and probably vanishing completely, at least in the developed world. However, during the last two decades infectious diseases have regained considerable significance and interest even in high-income countries. The reasons for this are varied:

- Medical advances for the treatment of malignancies and chronic diseases have resulted in a growing population of immunocompromised patients susceptible to opportunistic infections that may limit severely the success of modern therapies (e.g. transplantation).
- New and old pathogens have been determined to either cause or contribute to cancers (e.g. hepatocellular carcinoma) or other diseases not considered to be associated in the past with infection (e.g. peptic ulcer disease).
- Changes in modern life styles (e.g. travel, outdoor activities, drug abuse) have created new risks of acquiring certain infections.
- Emerging and re-emerging infectious diseases (Table 2.1) as well as emerging resistance against anti-infective drugs (Table 2.2) have clearly shown their potential for global spread.

BURDEN AND SIGNIFICANCE OF TROPICAL INFECTIOUS DISEASES

Tropical infectious diseases in a classical sense are limited geographically to areas where specific conditions of tropical climate and ecology must be present as a *conditio sine qua non* for the transmission and spread of the pathogen responsible (specific diseases of the tropics). Typically, these diseases are transmitted by specific vectors (e.g. malaria, arbovirus infection, leishmaniasis, trypanosomiasis, filariasis), or require special intermediate hosts (e.g. schistomiasis and other trematode infections), specific reservoirs (e.g. Lassa fever, monkeypox) or micro-ecological conditions (e.g. stronglyoidiasis).

Of all infectious diseases specific to the tropics, malaria is the main cause of death (WHO, 1998). Other tropical diseases, such as schistosomiasis and filariasis, are responsible for chronic morbidity and severe limitation of activity in very large populations (Table 2.3).

There are many other infectious diseases (e.g. cholera, leprosy, geohelminthic infections) that may be transmitted principally worldwide but nowadays are confined mainly or exclusively to developing countries in the tropics (Table 2.3). This is usually due to socioeconomic conditions and is largely independent of a tropical climate or other specific conditions associated with a tropical environment. Nevertheless, these infections are often regarded as tropical infectious diseases in a broader sense (typical diseases of the tropics).

In addition to specific and typical tropical infectious diseases, developing countries also carry the main burden of the most important infectious diseases occurring worldwide (Table 2.4). Last but not least, developing countries are usually more affected by emerging and re-emerging diseases (Table 2.1), as appropriate actions are usually severely limited by lack of resources and weak health system structures. Often, this also applies to the

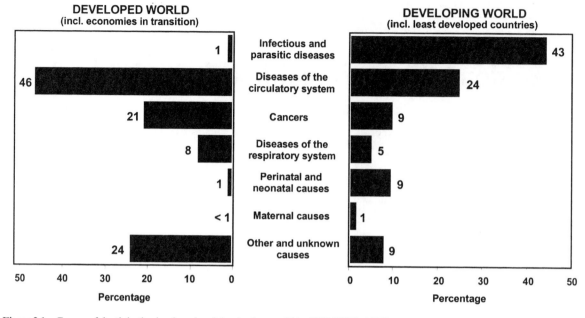

Figure 2.1   Causes of death in the developed and developing world in 1997 (WHO, 1998)

Table 2.1   Important examples of emerging and re-emerging infectious diseases

Emerging	Re-emerging
HIV/AIDS	Tuberculosis
Lyme disease	Malaria
Haemolytic uraemic syndrome	Cholera
EHEC	Dengue fever
Hanta pulmonary syndrome	Rift valley fever
Japanese encephalitis	African trypanosomiasis
Cyclosporiasis	Plague
Ebola haemorrhagic fever	West Nile fever
Lassa fever	
Ross River fever	
Nipah virus disease	

EHEC = enterohaemorrhagic *Escherichia coli*.

emergence of resistance against available drugs in major pathogens (Table 2.2).

DIMENSIONS OF INTERNATIONAL TRAVEL AND MIGRATION

During recent decades, global migration has expanded tremendously (Figure 2.2). In 1997, the figures for worldwide travel exceeded 600 million international arrivals, and it is estimated that there will be more than 1 billion travellers per annum before the year 2015 (WTO, 1998). The reasons for international travel are mainly tourism,

Table 2.2   Important examples of emerging resistance

Methicillin-resistant *Staphylococcus aureus* (MRSA)
Glycopeptide-resistant enterococci and staphylococci
Gram-negative enterobacteria
Streptococcus pneumoniae and *Neisseria* spp.
Salmonella and other bacteria causing diarrhoeal disease
Tuberculosis
Malaria (*Plasmodium falciparum*)
HIV

business and education; however, in some regions of the world, migrant workers and refugees contribute substantially to international migration (Table 2.5).

In 1996, Germany was ranked as the world's top spender on international tourism (Table 2.6), with 77.7 million international departures, including more than 4 million destinations to developing countries in tropical and subtropical regions. On the other hand, more than 9% of the population registered in Germany during 1997 were foreign nationals, with 75% originating from countries outside the European Union, and an increasing number of foreigners originating from tropical countries. The main reasons for nontourist immigration to Germany, as is the case in the whole of Europe, are work, family reunification, education and political reasons (refugees, asylum seekers). There is a considerable fluctuation of this population, with both immigration and emigration rates of approximately 10% per annum (Statistisches Bundesamt, 1998).

Table 2.3 Global burden of tropical infectious diseases (thousands, WHO estimates in 1997)

| Disease | Deaths | Cases | | Persons with severe limitation of activity |
		New (incidence)	All (prevalence)	
Malaria[a]	1500–2700	300 000	—	—
Dengue fever[a]	140	3100	—	—
Noma/cancrum oris	110	140	770	30
African trypanosomiasis	100	150	400	200
Leishmaniasis[a]	80	2000	12 000	—
Amoebiasis	70	48 000	—	—
Hookworm disease	65	—	15 000	—
Ascariasis	60	—	250 000	—
Onchocerciasis[a]	45	—	18 000	770
Chagas disease[a]	45	300	18 000	—
Yellow fever[a]	30	200	—	—
Schistosomiasis[a]	20	—	200 000	120 000
Japanese encephalitis	10	45	—	—
Cholera (reported in 1996)	10	145	—	3000
Leprosy	2	570	1150	—
Lymphatic filariasis[a]	—	—	120 000	120 000

[a]Diseases specific to tropical and subtropical climates.

Table 2.4 Global epidemiology of the most important infectious diseases (millions, WHO estimates for 1997)

	No. of deaths	No. of cases	No. of infected persons
Respiratory infections	3.7	—	—
Infectious diarrhoea	2.5	—	—
Tuberculosis	2.9	70–80	1700
Malaria	1.5–2.7	300	—
HIV/AIDS	2.3	3	30.6
Total	12.9–14.1		
Global no. of deaths in 1997	52.2		
Deaths due to infections in 1997	17.3 (33%)		

From WHO (1998).

TROPICAL INFECTIOUS DISEASES AND MIGRATION

Historically, the spread of tropical infectious diseases has been linked closely to migration. *Schistosoma mansoni* infection and onchocerciasis have been introduced most probably to South and Central America by the importation of Africans as slaves. Malaria has always travelled with military troops and decided the outcomes of many battles and wars. In addition, the spread of tropical infectious diseases is typically favoured by political crises that are accompanied by large population movements (e.g. refugees) and breakdown of control measures. Recent examples are the re-emergence of African trypanosomiasis in southern Sudan and the spread of schistosomiasis in Somalia.

Today, pathogens can travel at high speed and are able to reach all parts of the world within 24 hours. Highly contagious agents, such as influenza viruses, may cause epidemics in distant foci within a short time; however, most infections specific to the tropics need certain environmental conditions for autochthonous spread. Single cases may be exported worldwide, but further dissemination is limited to areas where suitable vectors, intermediate hosts, reservoirs, or ecological conditions are present (Table 2.7). Nevertheless, some infections originating in tropical countries have shown the potential for global spread. *Human immunodeficiency virus* (HIV) is a formidable example of such a pathogen. Occasionally, even tropical 'high-risk' pathogens (e.g. *Lassa virus*, *Ebola virus*, *Marburg virus*) may be exported to nonendemic areas (Table 2.8). However, the risk of further spread as a consequence of migration seems to be low at the moment because the known or presumed zoonotic reservoirs are probably restricted geographically and human-to-human transmission seems to be limited to close contacts and to nosocomial spread under poor hygienic conditions (Table 2.7). Nevertheless, the future emergence of new pathogens combining high pathogenicity and high infectivity and/or resistance against available drugs cannot be excluded.

Sometimes the conditions for successful spread of a tropical pathogen are exported well in advance of the pathogen establishing itself. For example, reinfestation

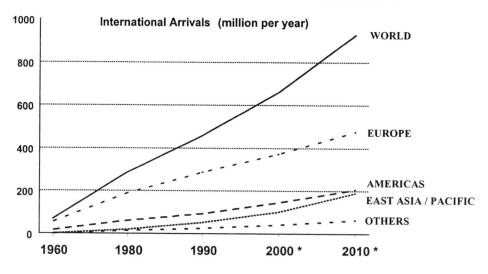

Figure 2.2   Development of international travel (WHO, 1998; OECD, 1998). Asterisk indicates projected figures

Table 2.5   International migration in 1997

Category	Millions
International arrivals	612[a]
Migrant workers	25–30[b]
Refugees	23[c]
Internally and externally displaced people	Approximately 50[c]

[a]WTO.
[b]UNDP.
[c]UNHCR.

Table 2.6   German travellers in 1996

International travellers: 77.7 million
Intercontinental travellers: 7.6 million
Travellers to tropical and subtropical destinations: 4.9 million
DM expenses for international travel: 75.7 billion

From WTO (1998).

Table 2.7   Risk of importation and dissemination of some infections with epidemic potential in developed countries

Infection	Importation	Secondary cases	Epidemic spread
Ebola fever, Lassa fever	+	(+)	−
Yellow fever	+	−	−
Plague	+	(+)	−
Cholera	+ +	(+)	−
HIV infection	+ + +	+ + +	+ + +
Multiresistant tuberculosis	+ +	+ +	+ +
Malaria	+ + +	−	−
Dengue fever	+ + +	−	−

with *Aedes aegypti* in South America and the export of the Asian 'tiger mosquito' *A. albopictus* by scrap vehicle tyres to the USA and southern Europe have provided the environment for the autochthonous spread of dengue viruses (Perez *et al.*, 1998). In addition, global warming and short-term climatic fluctuations (e.g. El-Niño) may facilitate the spread of vectors and pathogens of tropical infectious diseases (e.g. malaria, dengue fever) to more temperate climates (Maskell *et al.*, 1993).

Migration also contributes to the biological interplay between pathogens and their hosts as well as between different infective agents. Genetic exchange between different strains or species (e.g. influenza viruses, HIV, enterobacteria, schistosomes) within the same host or between human and zoonotic reservoirs may result in the emergence of pathogens with altered virulence, immunogenicity or sensitivity to drugs.

More than ever before, migration is the major driving force for the dissemination of new and old infectious diseases and associated problems (e.g. resistance). As an important consequence of these effects of globalisation, the health problems of tropical countries are gaining more worldwide significance and attention today.

HEALTH RISKS TO TRAVELLERS

Data about the morbidity and mortality of travel-related health risks are still sparse and not comprehensive. The most valuable data have been obtained in epidemiological studies based on questionnaires. These provide a general approach to the problem, regardless of the

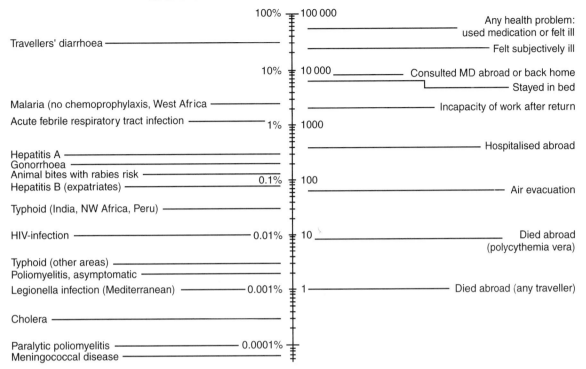

Figure 2.3 Health problems during a stay in developing countries: incidence rate per month (Steffen and Dupont, 1994)

Table 2.8 Imported cases of viral haemorrhagic fever that may be transmitted directly from human to human in developed countries, since 1967

Year	Virus	Imported to
1967	Marburg	Germany and Yugoslavia
1971	Lassa	USA
1974	Lassa	Germany
1975	Marburg	South Africa
1976	Ebola-Zaire	UK
1976	Lassa	USA
1989	Ebola-Reston	USA
1992	Ebola-Reston	Italy
1994	Ebola-Ivory Coast	Switzerland
1995	Ebola-Zaire	Italy
1996	Ebola-Reston	USA
1996	Ebola-Zaire	South Africa
2000	Lassa	Germany and UK

destination. Field studies carried out by local physicians show that the frequency of the different diseases varies according to the region visited. Studies of travellers on return to their country of origin generally focus on diseases such as malaria, viral hepatitis, dengue fever, leptospirosis, schistosomiasis, cutaneous larva migrans and leishmaniasis; more general studies do not provide a clearer picture of travel-associated diseases, either because the study populations are too small, or because the

data are incomplete. Studies based on data collated by health insurance and assistance companies based overseas are also biased. One important source of bias is that the different reasons for travel (tourism, business, residence, immigration, etc.) are rarely taken into account. And even the apparently uniform group represented by 'tourists' comprises backpackers, trekkers, subaqua divers, organised groups, and so on. These studies have formed the basis for an incidence scale of the main diseases and conditions contract-ed while travelling (Figure 2.3) (Steffen and Dupont, 1994).

Some large studies have been based on questionnaires in which travellers describe health problems arising during the trip (Kendrick, 1972; Reid et al., 1980; Peltola et al., 1983; Steffen et al., 1987). The response rate to such questionnaires is about 75%.

The proportion of travellers who fall ill varies from 15 to 43%: 1209 (15%) of 7886 Swiss travellers (Steffen et al., 1987), 5644 (21%) of 26 119 American travellers (Kendrick, 1972), 868 (33%) of 2665 Finnish travellers (Peltola et al., 1983) and 950 (43%) of 2211 British travellers (Reid et al., 1980). Among the Swiss travellers, 1.6% consulted a specialist in tropical medicine on their return, while 4.2% saw a family doctor (Steffen et al., 1987); 5.4% of the American travellers saw a doctor on their return (Kendrick, 1972). Five per thousand travellers in both studies were admitted to hospital.

Most physicians agree that diarrhoea represents half to two-thirds of health problems; upper respiratory tract infections are in second place (14–31%) followed by fever (12–15%). Skin conditions affected 12% of Swiss travellers in one study, making this the fifth most frequent health problem (Steffen et al., 1987).

Sexually transmitted diseases are also a frequent cause of morbidity. Genital discharges and ulcerations were reported by 0.6% and 0.1%, respectively, of 7886 Swiss travellers (Steffen et al., 1987). In a cohort of 2665 Finnish travellers, 39% of round-the-world travellers and 30% of tourists to Thailand reported 'at-risk' sexual behaviour (Peltola et al., 1983).

These studies show differences according to the destination and type of travel. In the cohort of Swiss travellers, health problems were significantly more frequent among young adults, travellers to West Africa, backpackers, those travelling for long periods, people working abroad and travellers staying with local residents; malaria was most frequent on return from Africa (Steffen et al., 1987). Sunburn and insect bites were most frequent in Finnish tourists having stayed in Thailand (Peltola et al., 1983). Tourists fall ill especially with respiratory and gastrointestinal diseases, more often than people who travel on business (Reid et al., 1980).

Studies carried out in the field by local doctors provide useful information on travel-associated diseases. Two such studies have been conducted in Nepal. Among the 12 437 French tourists who stayed in Nepal in 1984, 838 (6.7%) consulted the doctor at the French Embassy; they had a total of 860 health problems, including 255 cases of diarrhoea (29.6%), 151 ear, nose and throat (ENT) infections (17.7%), 107 skin conditions (12.4%), 69 cases of fever (8%) and 36 sexually transmitted diseases (4%). Ten travellers (0.08%) were admitted to hospital, nine (0.07%) were evacuated, 15 (0.12%) were repatriated, two underwent surgery locally, and one died (Caumes et al., 1991a). The 151 ENT infections comprised 28 cases of otitis (3.2%), 34 of pharyngitis (3.9%), 40 of sinusitis (4.6%), 45 of bronchitis (5.2%), and four of pneumonia (0.4%), one of which was fatal. The 107 skin conditions consisted of bacterial (4.3%) or fungal skin infections (1.8%), scabies (2%) and allergies (1.5%). Only three cases of fever were due to malaria (Nepal is not a major endemic zone for malaria), whereas 11 were due to typhoid. The other study carried out in Kathmandu involved 19 616 travellers of all nationalities presenting to a private clinic (Shlim, 1992). The main illnesses were gastrointestinal infections (31%), respiratory tract infections (21%) and skin conditions (10%); the frequency of diarrhoea (shigellosis and giardiasis) was higher during the hot season preceding the monsoon.

Travellers to the Maldives and Fiji appear to have a different pattern of illnesses. In the Maldives, ear infections (often otitis externa), superficial injuries (often due to coral and shellfish) and solar allergies represented, respectively, 24%, 14% and 13% of presenting illnesses (Plentz, 1992). In Fiji, ear problems, injuries (some contracted in the marine environment) and skin rashes (often related to sun exposure) each accunted for 10% of visits to a doctor, while skin infections accounted for 13% and

gastrointestinal disorders for 20% (Raju et al., 1992). In both these studies (carried out in islands particularly popular with tourists), diarrhoea, upper airway infections (excluding otitis) and fever were less-frequent presenting illnesses than in Nepal.

It is thus clear that travel diseases vary according to the country visited: diarrhoea and upper airway infections are prevalent in colder, mountainous regions such as Nepal, while skin conditions and superficial injuries are more common in coastal areas.

In a German study of 17 042 travellers who sought medical advice on their return, the main presenting symptoms were diarrhoea ($n = 11 795$; 69%), fever ($n = 3408$; 19%) and skin conditions ($n = 1875$; 11%) (Nothdurft and Löscher, 1993). In a French study involving 926 travellers, the main presenting illnesses were fever ($n = 406$; 43%), due to malaria in 272 cases (66%); gastrointestinal infections ($n = 119$; 12%); skin infections ($n = 73$; 7%); and sexually transmitted diseases ($n = 23$; 2%) (Cuzin-Ferrand et al., 1993). In the tropical medicine department in Paris the main reasons for consultation were skin conditions (33.9%), gastrointestinal disorders (24.8%) and fever (28.4%) (Caumes et al., 1991b). Five patients (4.6%) had two conditions, giving a total of 114 problems in 109 patients. No firm diagnosis could be made in 31 cases; most of these patients had diarrhoea (19 cases) of fever (eight cases) which resolved spontaneously.

Annually, there are approximately 10 000 reported cases of imported malaria in Europe (Legros and Danis, 1998). Malaria is the main cause of fever on return to France, accounting for 45% and 66% of cases in the two French studies (Caumes et al., 1991b; Cuzin-Ferrand et al., 1993). In the German study, malaria accounted for only 6% of fevers on return (Nothdurft et al., 1992; Nothdurft and Löscher, 1993), explained by the different selection criteria of the population studied.

Estimates of the risk of individual malaria infection have so far largely been based upon infection rates in the local population. Assumptions based on the completely different risk behaviour of travellers and locals in endemic areas are naturally only inaccurate approximations, accepted, however, in the absence of better methods of calculation (Muehlberger et al., 1998). Thus, the worldwide highest risk of malaria has been calculated as being in West Africa (approximately 2% of all unprotected travellers), followed by the more frequently visited East Africa (Steffen et al., 1990).

A more realistic assessment of the risk of malaria infection in travellers can be made from the evidence of specific antibodies against the immunodominant surface protein of the sporozoites, the circumsporozoite protein (CSP). Several studies of nonimmune travellers demonstrated that the risk of transmission is quantifiable geographically by the evidence of CSP antibodies. In one study, the seroconversion rate of CSP antibodies in travellers to Kenya was as high as 4.9% after return, indicating a high exposure risk in that country (Jelinek et al., 1998) (Table 2.9).

Dengue fever is probably also common as an imported

Table 2.9 Antibody reactions to circumsporozoite (CS) antigen of *Plasmodium falciparum* among international travellers: distribution and geometric mean titres (Jelinek *et al.*, 1998)

Geographical area	All travellers ($n = 2131$)	Positive[a] travellers ($n = 104$)	Seropositive travellers/ all travellers to area (%)	Risk ratio[b]
Central America	311	13	4.2	0.86
South America	290	7	2.4	0.49
East Asia	120	4	3.3	0.68
Indian subcontinent	412	9	2.2	0.45
West Asia	90	1	1.1	0.24
Southeast Asia	686	23	3.4	0.69
East Africa	124	27	21.8	4.5
West Africa	72	16	22.2	4.5
Southern Africa	26	4	15.4	3.2

[a]Defined as CS-antibody titre > 6.25 IEU (international ELISA units).
[b]Risk ratio (RR) calculated as risk of becoming seropositive at a certain location over risk for the total population (RR $= 1.0$: average risk for seropositivity for all travellers).

Table 2.10 Causes of death among 2463 American tourists (Hargarten *et al.*, 1991)

Cause of death	Percentage (%)
Cardiovascular	49
Road accidents	7
Drowning	4
Other accidents	12
Infectious diseases	1
Other/Unknown	25

disease; however, in common with many other infectious diseases that are not notifiable, no valid data are available. A prospective study in travellers with febrile disease compatible with dengue fever after returning from dengue-endemic areas revealed dengue fever confirmed by diagnostic tests in 6.9% (Jelinek *et al.*, 1997). From this study and others, the incidence of dengue fever imported to Germany may be estimated as 300–500 cases per 100 000 travellers per year.

In 1989, Hargarten assessed the causes of death in 2463 American tourists in 1975 and 1984 (Hargarten *et al.*, 1991). The main causes were cardiovascular conditions (49%), road accidents (7%), drowning (4%), and other accidents (12%); in 25% of cases the cause of death was unidentified, while infectious diseases only accounted for 1% of fatalities (Table 2.10). Two Swiss studies conducted in 1987, involving 247 and 68 travellers, confirmed the major role of road accidents (13% and 12%), drowning (4% and 9%), and cardiovascular disease (14% and 15%); the cause was unidentified in a large proportion of cases (29% and 58%), and infections were rarely the cause of death (3%) (Lustenberger, 1988).

The frequency and severity of road accidents in tropical countries explains why they are the main reason for medical evacuation. Over a 2 year period (1992 and 1993), a French health insurance and assistance company carried out 1263 medical evacuations, of which 494 (39%) were for trauma (43% of cases were due to road accidents, 36% to falls, 10% to sports accidents, 5% to drowning, and 3% to criminal attack); the other causes were cardiovascular, psychiatric and surgical (De Courcy and Gauterau, 1994).

With regard to traffic accidents, those involving motorcycles are especially common among tourists. In Bermuda, one study showed that motorcycle accidents accounted for 92% of all traffic injuries among tourists, as compared with 71% among residents. The rates of motorcycle-related injuries were respectively 94 per 1000 person-years among tourists and 16 per 1000 person-years among residents (relative risk for tourists: 5.6). The highest rate among tourists was found in the 50–59 year age group. According to the authors, the significantly higher rate of motorcycle accidents among tourists may be related to the use of unfamiliar vehicles in unknown surroundings, inexperience, and the requirements to drive on the unfamiliar side of the road in Bermuda (Carey, 1996).

REFERENCES

Carey MJ and Aitken ME (1996) Motorbike injuries in Bermudas: a risk for tourists. *Annals of Emergency Medicine*, **28**, 424–429.

Caumes E, Brücker G, Brousse G *et al.* (1991a) Travel-associated illness in 838 French tourists in Nepal in 1984. *Travel Medicine International*, **9**, 72–76.

Caumes E, Bellanger F, Brücker G *et al.* (1991b) Pathologie observée au retour de voyage en dehors d'Europe: 109 cas. *Presse Medicale*, **20**, 1483–1486.

Cuzin-Ferrand L, Bequet L and Armengaud M (1993) Have a nice trip, see you later . . . In *Programme and Abstracts of the 3rd Conference on International Travel Medicine*, Paris, p. 89 (abstract 45).

De Courcy A and Gauterau T (1994) Approche du risque traumatologique en voyage. In *Programme et Abstracts de la*

Premiere Journée Francaise de Médicine de Voyage, Paris, p. 32 (abstract 2).

Hargarten SW, Baker TD and Guptil K (1991) Overseas fatalities of United States citizen travelers: an analysis of deaths related to international travel. *Annals of Emergency Medicine*, **20**, 622–626.

Jelinek T, Dobler G, Hölscher M *et al.* (1997) Prevalence of infection with Dengue virus among international travellers. *Archives of Internal Medicine*, **157**, 2367–2370.

Jelinek T, Blüml A, Löscher T *et al.* (1998) Assessing the incidence of infection with *Plasmodium falciparum* among international travelers. *American Journal of Tropical Medicine and Hygiene*, **59**, 35–37.

Kendrick MA (1972) Study of illness among Americans returning from international travel. *Journal of Infectious Diseases*, **126**, 684–685.

Legros F and Danis M (1998) Surveillance of malaria in European Union countries. *Eurosurveillance*, **3**, 45–47.

Lustenberger I (1988) Todesfälle von Schweizern in Ausland. Thesis, University of Zurich.

Maskell K, Mintzer IM and Callander BA (1993) Health and climate change: basic science of climate change. *Lancet*, **324**, 1027–1031.

Muehlberger N, Jelinek T, Schlipkoeter U *et al.* (1998) Effectiveness of chemoprophylaxis and other determinants of malaria in travellers to Kenya. *Tropical Medicine and International Health*, **3**, 357–363.

Nothdurft HD and Löscher T (1993) Imported infections in German travelers returning from tropical countries. In *Programme and Abstracts of the 3rd Conference on International Travel Medicine*, Paris, p. 86 (abstract 39).

Nothdurft HD, von Sonnenburg F and Löscher T *et al.* (1992) Importierte Infektionen bei Tropenreisenden. *Mitteilungen der Osterreichischen Gesellschaft für Tropenmedizin und Parasitologie*, **14**, 233–230.

Peltola H, Kirönseppä H and Hölsä P (1983) Trips to the south—a health hazard. Morbidity of Finnish travelers. *Scandinavian Journal of Infectious Diseases*, **15**, 375–381.

Perez JG, Clark GG, Gubler DJ *et al.* (1998) Dengue and dengue haemorrhagic fever. *Lancet*, **352**, 971–977.

Plentz K (1992) Nontropical and noninfectious diseases among travelers in a tropical area during a five-year period (1986–1990). In *Travel Medicine 2*, Proceedings of the 2nd Conference on International Travel Medicine, Atlanta, 1991, (eds HO Lobel, R Steffen and PE Kozarsky), p. 77.

Raju R, Smal N and Sorokin M (1991) Incidence of minor and major disorders among visitors to Fiji. In *Travel Medicine 2*, Proceedings of the 2nd Conference on International Travel Medicine, Atlanta, 1991 (eds HO Lobel, R Steffen and PE Kozarsky), p. 62.

Reid D, Dewar RD, Fallon RJ *et al.* (1980) Infection and travel: the experience of package tourists and other travellers. *Journal of Infection*, **2**, 365–370.

Shlim DR (1992) Learning from experience: travel medicine in Kathmandu. In *Travel Medicine 2*, Proceedings of the 2nd Conference on International Travel Medicine, Atlanta, 1991 (eds HO Lobel, R Steffen and PE Kozarsky), pp 40–42.

Statistisches Bundesamt (1998) *Statistisches Jahrbuch für die Bundesrepublik Deutschland*. Metzler-Poeschel, Stuttgart.

Steffen R and Dupont HL (1994) Travel medicine: what's that? *Journal of Travel Medicine*, **1**, 1–3.

Steffen R, Rickenbach M, Wilhelm U *et al.* (1987) Health problems after travel to developing countries. *Journal of Infectious Diseases*, **156**, 84–91.

Steffen R, Heusser R and Machler R (1990) Malaria chemoprophylaxis among European tourists in tropical Africa: use, adverse reactions and efficacy. *Bulletin of the World Health Organization*, **68**, 313–322.

WHO (1998) *The World Health Report 1998*. World Health Organization, Geneva.

WHO (1999) *Report: Removing Obstacles to Healthy Development*. World Health Organization, Geneva.

WTO (1998) *Yearbook of Tourism Statistics 1998*. World Tourism Organization, Madrid.

3

Fitness to Travel

Dominique Tessier

Medisys Travel Health Clinic, Montreal, Canada

INTRODUCTION

Maintaining good health of travellers is the major purpose of travel medicine. It is important to individualise counselling regarding the possibility of illnesses like malaria abroad, the individual's health, including allergies, the need for Medic-Alert signs and adrenaline (epinephrine) to be carried, the requirements for first-aid kits, prevention of sexually transmitted disease and HIV infection, food intake and even the common cold.

Very few travellers will come to a travel medicine specialist asking if they are 'fit to travel'. Most have already taken a decision before coming to a consultation, even with very serious health conditions. It may be because of a lack of knowledge, as the potential risks of going to different environments and climates are not necessarily known by the average person. Often it is because the traveller feels that the trip cannot be postponed or the itinerary changed for any of a number of reasons: a relative at risk of dying; a chronic disease putting the traveller's own life at risk; a special religious gathering; or the magnificent reputation of a site that someone wants to see before dying. Whatever the reason, many will travel to places one would prefer them not to go to. A simplistic approach would be to deny 'a licence to travel'. It seems more reasonable, however, to try to inform the traveller of the potential risks, to know how to evaluate their 'fitness to travel' and how to avoid some of the risks, and diminish the impact of those that are inevitable. The health care provider must keep in mind that the purpose of the consultation is not to discourage travelling but rather to provide travellers with the best counselling possible in accordance with their health status and the type of travel planned.

All consultation should begin with the gathering of basic information concerning the trip planned. To advise travellers correctly, it is important to ask about all countries to be visited, with questions regarding stay, particularly at night, in rural areas. It is also important to know the exact period and duration of the travel, with special attention given to season, which may influence the risk of acquisition of malaria and other infectious diseases. Travellers returning to their native country to visit family will often venture to more remote areas and take fewer precautions concerning food hygiene.

DIABETES

The initial evaluation of a diabetic traveller should include the individual's understanding of his or her own disease and what to do in case of complications while abroad, the availability of health care in the areas visited, the availability and understanding of glycaemia (usually capillary), the possibility of carrying insulin for the whole trip or the need to make adjustment with local products (insulin preparations vary quite significantly from one country to another), the understanding of the importance of foot care, and of the role of the sun on a more rapid absorption of insulin, the adjustment needed for jet lag, and the need to carry syringes and a letter of authorisation.

Diabetic patients should be prepared for travel like most other travellers. They can be given all the vaccines indicated. Special attention should be taken to ensure that influenza and pneumococcal immunisations are up to date. Hepatitis B vaccination is strongly recommended as diabetics are at greatest risk of receiving health care and injections abroad. They should carry their own needles, even if they are not taking insulin. For all travellers carrying needles and syringes, a letter on official stationary and signed by the attending physician, should be provided. An example of such letter is shown in Figure 3.1. A Medic-Alert bracelet (engraved with the wearer's allergies or other medical conditions) is also recommended. Malaria prophylaxis should be used when recommended.

Diabetic patients need to be ultracautious when travelling, and always be prepared for long delays. This means carrying extra food, medications and glucagon. These should be in 'carry-on bags' and not in luggage that is not

Principles and Practice of Travel Medicine. Edited by Jane N. Zuckerman.
© 2001 John Wiley & Sons Ltd.

Traveller's Health Center
Complete address

Date: _____, 200__

Mr/Mrs

I, _____, MD, certify that _____ carries
with him/her a medical kit that includes prescribed medications, syringes and needles to be used by a
doctor, during his/her trip in case of emergency. These are recommended for personal use only to avoid
the risk of accidental transmission of infectious diseases. They are not to be sold.

_____
Medical Director
Travellers' Clinic

Figure 3.1   Letter of authorisation

accessible during the journey. They should know that special meals can easily be ordered on most flights or cruises if requested, ideally 1 week in advance. Insulin is stable at room temperature for about 1 week but extremely hot temperatures should be avoided. It can thus be transported easily in the carry-on bags. As it may freeze during long trips, it should not be placed in luggage carried in the hold.

Information on countries to be visited and services for diabetic patients can be obtained from the International Diabetes Federation, who can also provide a card with blood glucose equivalents for different countries (see Additional Resources).

Susceptibility to Hypoglycaemia

Diabetic patients should take all necessary precautions to avoid hypoglycaemia. Fast sugars and snacks should be carried as well as glucagon. When travelling alone, a person in charge (flight attendant, tour guide) should be informed of the treatment to be given in case of suspected hypoglycaemia. To decrease the risks, doses of insulin may be omitted on long trips with many time zones being crossed. With severe jet lag, hyperglycaemia would be preferred over hypoglycaemia. Never overlap two insulin injections.

Susceptibility to Infection

Vaccines

There is no specific contraindication to any of the travel vaccines or drugs. Malaria prophylaxis should be used when needed. The first-aid kit should include antibiotics with instructions on how and when to use them.

Diarrhoea

Prophylactic antimicrobial agents are not generally recommended for diabetic travellers. The use of fluoroquinolones such as ciprofloxacin is considered the first choice. As an alternative for the self-treatment of travellers' diarrhoea, co-trimoxazole, azithromycin or clarithromycin might be offered. Bismuth subsalicylate (Pepto-Bismol) should be used with moderation.

Susceptibility to Complications

Foot hygiene is extremely important for any diabetic patient. Special care needs to be taken to avoid injuries during long travel. Blister dressings are useful for decreasing friction on a foot sore and decreasing the risk of ulceration. Sensible shoes are essential if walking is planned.

CARDIORESPIRATORY PROBLEMS

Cardiopulmonary conditions that are not stable can result in major travel problems, especially during overseas flights or when staying in places at high altitude.

High altitude increases the work of the heart during the first days of acclimatisation. Patients who have symptomatic heart disease risk a deterioration of their symptoms at high altitude. A person who cannot walk at a fast pace or go up one single flight of stairs without shortness of breath at sea level will be likely to be in trouble at high altitude, including during air travel. Oxygen can be provided during the journey on most commercial flights, with no problem. Arrangements need to be made by an experienced physician at least 1 week in advance. A nasal cannula, when available, is often more comfortable than a mask. The level of 8000 feet (2400 m) should not be exceeded by patients with congestive heart failure.

FOOD ALLERGIES

Allergies and anaphylaxis are potentially severe, life-threatening problems for the traveller. Allergies to egg protein and some antibiotics are contraindications to some vaccines, such as yellow fever. Severe food allergy, in a country where travellers can hardly make themselves understood, is a life-threatening condition. Carrying pictures of the ingredients or food to be avoided could help, but will not guarantee the safety of meals. In such circumstances, it is advisable to carry adrenaline (epinephrine) and a Medic-Alert bracelet or card.

PREGNANCY

Pregnancy needs more than passing attention. It is not *per se* a contraindication to any travel, except air travel, as commercial airlines may limit travel near the expected time of delivery. Certain precautions need to be taken to protect the developing fetus and the mother in specific situations.

Pretravel Visit

Before any trip far from home or involving difficult living conditions without ready access to health care, a pregnant woman should consult her obstetrician and have a careful assessment. An ultrasound should be carried out to eliminate an extrauterine pregnancy or a placenta praevia. The pregnant traveller and her companion should be informed of signs of possible labour or complications and of the basic emergency procedures to be performed if needed. A placental cord clamp can be carried.

Pregnancy increases the risk of thrombophebitis, as does a long trip at high altitude. A pregnant woman with varicose veins or an increased risk of vein thrombosis should follow carefully the following recommendations: drink a lot of water; request an aisle seat to enable leg stretching; walk a few steps every hour; do not cross your legs; and do not use sleeping pills or a muscle relaxant which might increase blood stasis. In the presence of severe anaemia (haemoglobin less than 8.5 g%), oxygen should be provided during air travel. Arrangements need to be made by an experienced physician at least 1 week in advance.

Susceptibility to Infection

Vaccines

Live vaccines are to be avoided whenever possible for pregnant women, especially during the first trimester. Most obstetricians would advise vaccination to be given after the first trimester. In most situations, however, the risk of a serious infection far outweighs the minimal known risk or the theoretical risk of vaccination. Risk–benefit needs to be carefully assessed in each case.

Malaria

Malaria is a common and serious infectious disease, transmitted by mosquito bites from dusk to dawn. Personal protective measures are very effective in reducing the risk of acquiring malaria. All pregnant travellers to endemic areas should be counselled about the use of insect repellent containing 35% or less of DEET on their exposed skin, the use of bed nets and to wear clothing that reduces the area of exposed skin. Insecticides such as permethrin or deltamethrin on clothes and bed nets are very safe and can contribute to reducing the risk further.

In many endemic areas, a medication to reduce the risk significantly (but never completely) should be taken. Some drugs are contraindicated during certain stages of a pregnancy, but in most cases an acceptable alternative is available. This is especially important when a woman will inevitably be exposed to malaria.

Diarrhoea

Prophylactic antimicrobial agents are not generally recommended for pregnant travellers. The use of fluoroquinolones such as ciprofloxacin is contraindicated. As an alternative for the self-treatment of travellers' diarrhoea, co-trimoxazole, azithromycin or clarithromycin may be offered. Bismuth subsalicylate (Pepto-Bismol) should be avoided.

Travel Insurance

Travel insurance can and should be obtained before departure. After the 24th week of pregnancy, this insurance should include coverage for the newborn baby, in case of premature labour.

THE ELDERLY TRAVELLER

There is no age limit for travel. Health conditions, including cognitive fitness, are the only aspects that should be evaluated. All aged travellers should remember that they will usually have a decreased resistance to long trips and strenuous effort. Luggage should be sensible, using porters when available, or the new form of luggage on wheels.

THE IMMUNOCOMPROMISED TRAVELLER

Immunocompromised persons, including HIV-infected

individuals travel extensively. They do so for pleasure, business, family reasons or religious considerations. To tell a severely immunosuppressed person not to travel is unrealistic and does not take into consideration his or her own priorities. Health care providers need to be aware of the most important risks, the preventive measures available and how to inform the potential traveller about risks and options. Preparing an immunocompromised individual for international travel requires attention to a number of important issues that, for the most part, are similar to those faced by any traveller with a chronic condition. These considerations include: (1) restrictions on crossing international borders; (2) vaccination requirements and their effectiveness and safety; (3) susceptibility to infections present at the destination; and (4) accessibility of health care overseas and the possible need for medical evacuation home (Health Canada, 1994).

Vaccines

There is a very large and increasing number of vaccines available worldwide. Although most are safe for immunocompromised persons, some precautions are necessary with live attenuated vaccines (Tables 3.1 and 3.2). These include the yellow fever vaccine, the Bacille Calmette–Guérin (BCG, against tuberculosis) vaccine, the oral polio (Sabin) vaccine, measles, mumps and rubella (MMR) vaccine, oral typhoid vaccine, oral cholera vaccine and the new varicella vaccine. All inactivated or component vaccines can be offered to immunocompromised individuals if exposed. Among those, some are recommended strongly for them, such as influenza and pneumococcal vaccines. These vaccines represent no risk for HIV or persons with AIDS. Some severely immunocompromised individuals may respond poorly to immunisation. Other strategies may thus be needed to protect them, such as passive immunisation with specific immunoglobulins or preventive medication or rapid treatment. All immunisations should be given by personnel with special training and a good understanding of the principles and risks.

Severe complications have been reported after immunisation with live vaccines in immunosuppressed hosts.

Yellow Fever and Oral Cholera Vaccines

These vaccines are only indicated for travellers to certain specific destinations in some countries. The consultation should thus ascertain the exact itinerary and the eventual indications. These vaccines are contraindicated in severely immunocompromised individuals. Such travellers to an area for endemic yellow fever should be recommended to change the itinerary or to follow strictly physical mosquito precautions if the trip is unavoidable. When yellow fever vaccine is required to cross a border but no portion of the trip would be in an infected area, a certificate

Table 3.1 Vaccines generally to be avoided in immunocompromised individuals

Vaccine	Administration
BCG	No exception
MMR	If no immunosuppression
Oral cholera	Not recommended
Varicella	Immunise close contacts
Yellow fever	If strongly indicated
Vivotif (typhoid)	Use injectable vaccine
Oral polio	Use injectable vaccine
	Avoid for close contacts

Table 3.2 Vaccines safe for use in immunocompromised individuals

Vaccine	Notes
Diphtheria	—
Hepatitis A, B and A, B	—
Hib	—
Influenza	—
Japanese encephalitis	Rare indications
Lymerix	Probably safe
Meningococcal	—
Pertussis	Prefer acellular
Polio, inactivated	—
Pneumococcal	—
Rabies	Pre- or postexposure
Tetanus	—

indicating a contraindication for the vaccine can be considered. This certificate can only be delivered by an authorised yellow fever centre. The list of these clinics is available on the Web at the LCDC site, Health Canada (see Additional Resources). The traveller should be aware that, in the face of an epidemic, he or she could be denied entry in some countries if not immunised.

Bacille Calmette–Guérin (BCG) Vaccine

The administration of BCG vaccine to immunocompromised persons is contraindicated because of its potential to cause disseminated disease (USPHS/IDSA, 1999).

Measles, Mumps and Rubella (MMR) Vaccine

Six deaths have been linked with measles vaccine virus infection in immunocompromised individuals. Because of the severity of the disease, the vaccine should be administered to HIV-positive persons not severely immunosuppressed.

Oral Polio (Sabin) Vaccine (OPV)

OPV should never be given to any immunosuppressed individual, regardless of the level of immunosuppression, their household members or their close contacts. The risk of vaccine-associated paralytic poliomyelitis is increased by immunosuppression.

Varicella Vaccine and Varicella Zoster Immune Globulin (VZIG)

Very little data regarding the safety and efficacy of varicella vaccine in immunocompromised adults are available, and no recommendation for use can be made for this population.

Hepatitis A Vaccine

Several inactivated and attenuated hepatitis A vaccines have been developed and evaluated in human clinical trials and in nonhuman primate models of hepatitis A virus infection (D'Hondt, 1992); however, only inactivated vaccines have been evaluated for efficacy in controlled clinical trials (Innis *et al.*, 1994). The vaccines licensed currently are Havrix (SmithKline Beecham Biologicals), Vaqta (Merck and Co., Inc.), Avaxim (Pasteur Merieux Connaught) and Epaxal (Berna Products). All four are inactivated vaccines.

Environmental Risks

Food and Water

The risk of infection from food and water among immunocompromised persons is increased during travel to developing countries. Persons who travel to such countries should intensify food and water precautions (Table 3.3). They should be advised that ice made with tap water, unpasteurised milk and dairy products (common), and items sold by street vendors are usually unsafe. Foods and beverages that are generally safe include steaming-hot food, fruit peeled by the traveller, bottled (especially carbonated) beverages, hot coffee and tea, beer, wine, and water brought to a rolling boil for 1 min. Treatment of water with iodine or chlorine might not be as effective as boiling but can be used when boiling is not practical (USPHS/IDSA, 1999). Water purifiers can be of some value.

Persons from developed countries who travel to developing countries are at substantial risk of hepatitis A infection (Steffen *et al.*, 1994). All hepatitis A seronegative individuals should be offered the vaccine or, if severely immunosuppressed, immunoglobulin.

Immunocompromised persons should be educated and advised about the many ways that *Cryptosporidium* can be transmitted. Modes of transmission include direct con-

Table 3.3 Precautions to be taken by immunocompromised individuals to avoid infection from potentially contaminated food or drink

- Cook meat and poultry to 73.8 °C
- Wash fruit and vegetables thoroughly and carefully
- Reheat ready-to-eat foods until steaming hot
- Use treated, boiled or bottled water
- Avoid:
  Raw or undercooked eggs
  Foods containing raw eggs
  Raw or undercooked (pink) poultry, meat or seafood
  Unpasteurised dairy products
  Soft cheeses
  Fountain beverages
  Ice cubes, if the source is unclear
  Raw oysters
- Avoid crosscontamination of foods

tact with infected adults, children in nappies, and infected animals; drinking contaminated water; coming into contact with contaminated water during recreational activities; and eating contaminated food (USPHS/IDSA, 1999).

Health care providers should advise immunocompromised persons not to eat raw or undercooked eggs (including foods that might contain raw eggs, e.g. some preparations of Hollandaise sauce, Caesar and other salad dressings, and mayonnaise); raw or undercooked poultry, meat or seafood; or unpasteurised dairy products. Poultry and meat should be well cooked and should not be pink in the middle (internal temperature more than 73.8 °C). Produce should be washed thoroughly before being eaten (USPHS/IDSA, 1999).

Cryptosporidium can also be transmitted by drinking contaminated water, ice made from contaminated tap water, fountain beverages served in restaurants, bars, theatres, and eating contaminated food (USPHS/IDSA, 1999). Nationally distributed brands of bottled or canned carbonated soft drinks are safe to drink. Commercially packaged noncarbonated soft drinks and fruit juices that do not require refrigeration until after they are opened (i.e. those that can be stored unrefrigerated on grocery shelves) are also safe (Health Canada, 1994). Immunocompromised persons should avoid eating raw oysters because cryptosporidial oocysts can survive in oysters for more than 2 months and have been found in oysters taken from some commercial oyster beds.

Special Topics

Restrictions on Crossing International Borders

Before scheduling a trip to a foreign country, HIV-infected individuals should be made aware that a number of countries screen for evidence of HIV infection and can deny entry to seropositive individuals. In Canada, an unofficial list of entry requirements for crossing international borders may be obtained from the Laboratory Centre for Disease Control (see Additional Resources). Such requirements may change without notification and verification with consulates or embassies is advisable.

Susceptibility to Infection

Many infections encountered by travellers are associated with increased morbidity and mortality in immunocompromised persons. These individuals are more likely to have adverse reactions to drugs used to treat infection (Health Canada, 1994).

Malaria. Malaria is a common and serious infectious disease, transmitted by mosquito bites from dusk to dawn. Personal protective measures are very effective in reducing the risk of acquiring malaria. All travellers to endemic areas should be counselled about the use of insect repellent containing DEET on exposed skin, the use of bed nets and to wear clothing that reduces the amount of exposed skin. An insecticide such as permethrin or deltamethrin on clothes and bed nets can reduce the risk further.

In many endemic areas, a medication to reduce the risk significantly, but never completely, should be taken. Some of these medications are metabolised at the cytochrome P_{450}. Mefloquine is a good example. Drug interaction should thus be a concern. Other drugs may contain a medication the HIV-infected person is already taking, at a different dose. For example, Malarone contains atovaquone. Other medications could be used with acceptable efficacy for individuals with an already complicated therapy or those who have experienced severe side-effects with previous changes in regimens. Azithromycin, rarely used in practice because of limited efficacy, and primarily cost, is an example. Doxycycline, increasingly used for chloroquine-resistant areas, can increase the risk of photosensitivity or of a recurrence of candidiasis.

Malaria can kill any healthy individual in just 3 days. Because HIV-infected persons are more likely to experience fever as a symptom of opportunistic infection, malaria could go unrecognised and lead to death or severe complications. *Travellers and health care providers alike must consider the diagnosis of malaria in any febrile illness that occurs during or after travel to a malaria-endemic area* (Health Canada, 1997).

Diarrhoea. Prophylactic antimicrobial agents are not generally recommended for travellers; however, for immunocompromised travellers, antimicrobial prophylaxis may be considered, depending on the level of immunosuppression and the region and duration of travel. The use of fluoroquinolones such as ciprofloxacin (500 mg per day), can be considered when prophylaxis is deemed necessary. As an alternative (e.g. for children, pregnant women and persons already taking co-trimoxazole for *Pneumocystis carinii* pneumonia prophy-

laxis), co-trimoxazole might offer some protection against travellers' diarrhoea. The risk of toxicity should be considered before treatment with co-trimoxazole is initiated solely because of travel.

Antimicrobial agents such as fluoroquinolones should be given to all patients before their departure, to be taken empirically (e.g. 1 g stat. followed, if diarrhoea persists, by 500 mg of ciprofloxacin twice a day for 3 days) should travellers' diarrhoea develop. Fluoroquinolones should be avoided for children aged less than 18 years and pregnant women, and alternative antibiotics should be considered. Travellers should consult a physician if the diarrhoea is severe and does not respond to empirical therapy, if their stools contain blood, if fever is accompanied by shaking chills, or if dehydration develops. Antiperistaltic agents (e.g. diphenoxylate and loperamide) can be used to treat mild diarrhoea. They can also supplement the antibiotic treatment if needed (a plane to catch for example). These agents should not be administered to patients who have a high fever or who have blood in the stool.

Some experts recommend that HIV-infected persons who have *Salmonella* gastroenteritis should be given antimicrobial therapy to prevent extraintestinal spread of the pathogen. However, no controlled study has demonstrated a beneficial effect of such treatment, and some studies of immunocompetent persons have suggested that antimicrobial therapy can lengthen the shedding period. The fluoroquinolones, primarily ciprofloxacin (750 mg twice a day for 14 days), can be used when antimicrobial therapy is chosen (USPHS/IDSA, 1999). Fluoroquinolones should not be used during pregnancy.

SPECIAL SITUATIONS

Persons with physical impairments, including mobility, hearing, seeing or cognitive problems need more attention. They should be informed of special services available for them in most hotels, airplanes or cruises. They should also know that they might not be accepted for some journeys; for example, severe vision problems could mean that a traveller would not be accepted alone on a cruise ship.

Contagious Diseases

Infectious diseases that are airborne or easily transmissible by contact are contraindications to travel. They may require the intervention of Public Health Officers. In cases of doubt, always consult the Public Health authorities for clearance before departure.

INSURANCE

Most travellers should obtain health insurance for travel

before leaving home. A signed contract is highly preferable to the glossy pamphlet of the cover offered to all carriers of a specific credit card. Pre-existing medical conditions do not preclude insurance cover: a higher premium can be offered, or the pre-existing condition would not be covered but accidents and other problems would be.

A booklet produced by the International Association for Medical Assistance to Travellers (IAMAT) is a good resource for finding English-speaking physicians.

CONCLUSION

Fitness to travel is an abstract concept that is greatly influenced by the mental predisposition of the traveller. With very few exceptions, provided that good preparation and counselling is offered and understood, any traveller can undertake a journey safely.

REFERENCES

D'Hondt E (1992) Possible approaches to develop vaccines against hepatitis A. *Vaccine*, **10**(suppl. 1), S48–52.

Health Canada (1994) Statement on travellers and HIV/AIDS. *Canadian Medical Association Journal*, **152**, 379–380.

Health Canada (1997) Canadian recommendation for the prevention and treatment of malaria among international travellers. *Canada Communicable Disease Report*, **23**, S5.

Innis BL, Snitbhan R, Kunasol P *et al.* (1994) Protection against hepatitis A by an inactivated vaccine. *JAMA*, **271**, 28–34.

Steffen R, Kane MA, Shapiro CN *et al.* (1994) Epidemiology and prevention of hepatitis A in travelers. *JAMA*, **272**, 885–889.

USPHS/IDSA (1999) *Guidelines for the Prevention of Opportunistic Infections in Persons Infected with Human Immunodeficiency Virus*, 48(RR10), pp. 1–59. US Public Health Service and Infectious Disease Society of America, Washington DC.

ADDITIONAL RESOURCES

International Diabetes Federation
1 reu Defacqz
B-1000 Brussels, Belgium
www.idf.org

Tropical Health and Quarantine
Population and Public Health Branch
Health Canada
Tel 613 954 3236
Fax 613 954 5414
http://www.hc-sc.gc.ca/pphb-dgspsp/tmp-pmv/prof_e.html

4

Management of a Travel Clinic

Elaine C. Jong

University of Washington, Seattle, Washington, USA

INTRODUCTION

The travel clinics of today have their roots in the public health and military medicine service clinics of the past, where preventive medicine strategies such as immunizations against vaccine preventable diseases, and precautions, prophylaxis and treatments for malaria, diarrhea, and sexually transmitted diseases were applied towards protecting the health of specific populations. During the decades following World War II, modern transportation and communication systems fostered a phenomenal growth in international travel for tourism, business and relief missions. The health concerns of increasingly large numbers of travelers gradually created the impetus to adapt traditional public health principles to meet the health needs of individual travelers. In many venues today, travel medicine goes beyond the traditional public health focus on hygiene and communicable diseases, to encompass other aspects of health during travel: from jet lag, high altitude illness and snakebites, to personal safety, crosscultural psychosocial issues, accidental and motor vehicle injuries, and emergency medical evacuations. Since behavioral changes are often necessary in addition to medical interventions to prevent many of the health hazards associated with travel, a large component of travel medicine practice today focuses on health education for the individual traveler.

TRAVEL CLINIC MODELS

Given the many variations in health services available for travelers at diverse local, national, and international locations, a consistent system for travel clinic nomenclature helps clients and colleagues easily distinguish among organizational models. In the descriptions that follow, travel clinic types are named on the basis of the level of services provided (Table 4.1). The services range from administration of travel immunizations only (travel immunization clinics), to clinics where immunizations are

accompanied by comprehensive trip health risk assessment, prescription of medications, and extensive travel health advice (travel health clinics). Other travel clinics provide the services listed above, plus perform pretravel physical examinations and diagnostic tests that are often necessary for expatriate assignments, foreign work permits, or fitness certifications for special activities, such as scuba diving or mountain climbing (travel medicine clinics). Such clinics also advise special travelers, such as those with impaired immunity or who have chronic health conditions or illnesses. The fourth kind of clinic is staffed by clinicians with special expertise in the diagnosis and treatment of tropical and exotic diseases, who provide consultation for travelers returning from travel abroad with serious or persistent medical problems (travel and tropical medicine clinics).

The clinical environment suitable for a travel clinic is determined by the anticipated scope of practice. Travel health services can be provided as an added feature in many settings, including public health clinics, private medical practices, occupational health clinics, student health centers, and emergency departments, or can be organized as a dedicated travel clinic. Dedicated travel clinics may be operated as freestanding entities located in independent offices, multispecialty clinic buildings, medical centers, and shopping centers, or even at international airports.

TRAVEL CLINIC STAFF

Travel medicine embraces a wide variety of medical specialties: experienced and knowledgeable practitioners are to be found among the physicians, nurses, and other clinical providers of internal medicine, family practice, pediatrics, emergency medicine, occupational medicine, infectious diseases, tropical medicine, military medicine, and refugee/migration medicine. Other health care workers, health educators, mental health professionals, and medical social workers who have international work

Principles and Practice of Travel Medicine. Edited by Jane N. Zuckerman.
© 2001 John Wiley & Sons Ltd.

Table 4.1 Travel clinic categories according to level of service

Travel clinic type	Services provided	Clinical providers[a]
Travel immunizations clinic	Travel immunizations (immunization protocols)	RN
Travel health clinic	Travel immunizations (immunization protocols)	RN
	Travel health advice	RN/ ARNP/ PA/ MD/ DO
	Prescription of travel medications	ARNP/ PA/ MD/ DO
	Letters and travel documents	ARNP/ PA/ MD/ DO
Travel medicine clinic	Travel immunizations	RN
	Travel health advice	RN/ ARNP/ PA/ MD/ DO
	Prescription of travel medications	ARNP/ PA/ MD/ DO
	Letters and travel documents	ARNP/ PA/ MD/ DO
	Counsel patients with special needs	ARNP/ PA/ MD/ DO
	Physical examinations and forms	ARNP/ PA/ MD/ DO
Travel and tropical medicine clinic	(All services in categories above)	ARNP/ PA/ MD/ DO
	Diagnosis and Treatment of illness in returned travelers, immigrants, and refugees	

RN = Registered Nurse; ARNP = Advanced Registered Nurse Practitioner; PA = Physician Assistant; MD = Doctor of Medicine; DO = Doctor of Osteopathy.
[a]Clinical Providers licensed in the USA are used as example.

experience in public sector, private sector, missionary and relief work also contribute significantly to the field. What brings this diverse group of practitioners together is a common interest and dedication towards assuring the mental and physical health of travelers before, during, and after international travel.

The key challenge facing travel medicine as a unique medical specialty is to define the core body of knowledge that transcends the wide spectrum of health perspectives (Jong and Southworth, 1983; Hargarten *et al.*, 1991; Steffen and Lobel, 1995; Hill and Behrens, 1996; Dardick and Baker, 1997; Reid and Keystone, 1997; Ryan and Kain, 2000). The Internet has greatly heightened awareness of global health conditions in real time, and drives the need

for timeliness and coordination of disease surveillance, advice to travelers in response to news of health conditions abroad, access to medical care and pharmaceuticals across national boundaries, and crosscultural communication related to health issues. The clinical group of the American Society of Tropical Medicine and Hygiene (ASTMH) has defined a core body of knowledge that encompasses both travel medicine and clinical tropical medicine, and sponsors a certification examination for physicians. The International Society of Travel Medicine (ISTM) is currently working on similar objectives for travel health providers, which will establish benchmarks for travel nurses and other health care providers involved in the field. The web sites of these two professional societies should be consulted for further details (see Additional Resources).

INFORMATION REQUIREMENTS

The first requirement for a travel clinic of any kind is to establish reliable and up-to-date information sources. The publications of the World Health Organization (WHO) and the Centers for Disease Control and Prevention (CDC) often serve as official references for local standards of practice. Both organizations publish annual or biannual printed versions of their updated recommendations on advice and health information for international travel, but the most recently updated information is available at their web sites (see Additional Resources) in between publishing dates.

The Asia Pacific Travel Health Association (APTHA), the Australian National Health and Medical Research Council (NHMRC), the Canadian Laboratory Centre for Disease Control, the China International Travel Health Association (CITHA), the Public Health Laboratory Service (PHLS) in the United Kingdom, and the Taiwan Travel Health Association are among the other national and regional public health entities that produce advisories relevant to the health of travelers. Local public health departments, and travel clinics affiliated with academic medical centers can also serve as resources for information and guidance.

There is a growing body of journals, periodicals, and books that serve as valuable references in a travel clinic (Jong and McMullen, 1995, 1997; DuPont and Steffen, 1997; Freedman, 1998; Jong, 1999; Bia, 2000). A world map showing countries, major cities, and international time zones, as well as a comprehensive world atlas giving elevations and physical characteristics of land masses within countries are especially valuable for pretrip assessments. Charts showing average maximum and minimum temperatures at destinations throughout the year are also helpful for planning.

In addition, many travel clinics find that some of the software and web-based programs offered by subscription from private vendors provide convenience, efficiency, and summarized information in travel clinics whose patient care operations are extensively computerized. The best ways to become acquainted with these commercial products is to search the Web, consult with or visit travel clinics where these programs are installed or visit vendor demonstrations at professional meetings. In smaller clinic operations where subscriptions to commercial programs are not cost-effective, an excellent level of information can still be provided if the clinic director or designee regularly reviews the postings on the CDC and WHO Web sites, participates in one of the list serve groups open to members of the ISTM and/or the ASTMH (see Additional Resources), and is responsible for updating the rest of the clinic staff.

Travel and tropical medicine clinics providing assessment, diagnosis, and treatment for ill returning travelers will find that participation in the clinical e-mail discussion groups will augment and update the information found in standard textbook references. In addition to the discussion groups for members of the ASTMH and the ISTM organizations, the e-mail postings of ProMED covering disease outbreaks and emerging infections worldwide can be very useful in the evaluation of post-travel patients. The ProMED subscription list is open to any interested party (see Additional Resources).

TRAVEL CLINIC OPERATIONS

Travel medicine services can be provided in almost any clinic space suitable for patient care. If the travel clinic is part of a larger organization, space and support service requirements are less because of shared clinic functions, such as marketing and promotion, telephone and patient reception, appointment scheduling, patient registration, patient waiting room, medical records storage, secretarial and administrative support (including the ordering of clinic supplies and pharmaceuticals, data management, and accounting), patient billing, payer (or insurance) relations, and custodial services.

Vaccine injections at travel immunization clinics may be administered in multipatient or group clinic settings if necessary, as most vaccines are now administered in the upper arm, and privacy screens or curtains may be used for patients receiving injections of immune globulin in the gluteus muscle. However, a private room is necessary for patient interviews to conduct individual trip risk assessment and patient counseling, as sensitive topics may be discussed. Likewise, physical examinations require privacy, an examination table, the usual medical equipment and supplies, and, often, the help of a medical assistant. Thus, the clinical activities of some travel clinics require the use of dedicated patient examination rooms. Depending on a clinic's location, specific standards for licensure of patient care facilities may govern room dimensions, provisions for patient privacy, presence of a sink in the room for hand-washing, sanitation of medical equipment and linens, hazardous waste disposal, and patient access to toilet facilities.

A clinic that administers travel immunizations has to determine the age range to be served (pediatric, adult, or both). Specific tasks for a travel immunization clinic would include:

- Develop the patient health history intake form.
- Adopt age-appropriate vaccine protocols and patient vaccine information sheets.
- Obtain supplies of the WHO form *International Certificates of Vaccination* to serve as the individual traveler's official immunization document.
- Apply for status as an official Yellow Fever Vaccine Center.
- Establish clinic patient immunization records.
- Have age-appropriate vaccine consent forms.
- Train staff in vaccine administration and scheduling of doses.
- Order and store vaccine supplies.
- Provide temperature-monitored refrigerator and freezer equipment for vaccine storage.
- Provide for safe disposal of needles, syringes and vaccine vials.
- Develop protocols for triage and care of patients who experience adverse side-effects associated with immunization.
- Establish on-site capability for emergency medical care of a patient who develops acute anaphylaxis following receipt of a vaccine.

Travel and tropical medicine clinics find that identifying reliable clinical laboratories that can perform advanced parasitic diagnostic tests, and pharmacies that are willing to stock or obtain antiparasitic drugs, is essential for patient care. Often, regional or national public health agencies can assist clinicians practicing outside metropolitan areas in obtaining information about sources for the less common laboratory tests and drugs.

Depending on local requirements for licensure of health care providers and the scope of practice defined for each type of licensure, the travel clinic staff may consist of physicians, nurse practitioners or physician assistants, and/or specially trained registered nurses working with a physician or physician group.

APPROACH TO TRIP RISK ASSESSMENT

The Three Basic Topics

The three basic topics that should be covered during a travel clinic encounter are:

- Immunizations for vaccine-preventable diseases
- Medications for malaria chemoprophylaxis, as appropriate for the planned itinerary
- Instructions for management and treatment of travelers' diarrhea.

The advice given for each of these topics will be determined by the specific geographic destinations and activities planned at each.

All travelers should be requested to bring records of

previous immunizations with them. An old 'Certificates of Immunization' form is ideal for assessing the current vaccine status of repeat travelers. If old immunization records are not available at the initial clinic visit, then a systematic review of the routine (standard), the required, and the recommended travel immunizations, combined with a knowledge of the patient's health status, previous travel, and detailed itinerary (see below) for the new trip, will enable formulation of a travel immunization plan. Serum antibody tests to determine immunity to specific vaccine-preventable diseases can be performed as needed if there is sufficient time before trip departure.

As mentioned earlier, many ailments of travelers are not vaccine-preventable. The health care provider in a travel immunization clinic has an opportunity and an obligation to advise the traveler if further pretravel health measures beyond immunizations are prudent for the planned itinerary—even if this might necessitate an additional pretravel clinic visit with another provider or even at another clinic.

The selection of malaria chemoprophylaxis and the need to employ additional precautions to decrease the risk of malaria infection are determined by the age and health status of the traveler, history of drug allergies or drug intolerance, and anticipated patient compliance with the recommended regimen. Recommendations on the drug of choice for a given malaria risk assessment may vary from country to country and depend somewhat on which drugs are approved, licensed, and marketed in the country where travel advice is being given.

Traveler education on the relative advantages and disadvantages of the various malaria drug regimens and on the compliance issues is often a time-consuming process. The relative risks of adverse drug reactions with a given antimalarial drug regimen must be balanced against the risk of malaria infection when a suboptimal regimen is selected. Traveler acceptance of malaria chemoprophylaxis recommendations will be influenced by dosing interval: weekly (chloroquine, mefloquine) versus daily (doxycycline, primaquine, atovaquone plus proguanil (Malarone)). Other factors include duration of post-travel chemoprophylaxis, i.e. 1 week (primaquine, Malarone) versus 4 weeks (chloroquine, doxycycline, mefloquine) after leaving the endemic area, and last, but not least, the total cost of one drug regimen versus another for the recommended duration of therapy. Travelers also need to understand the importance of not discontinuing or switching regimens while traveling, except as advised by knowledgeable health care professionals, despite well-intentioned warnings and advice from friends and fellow travelers. The emergence of resistant strains of chloroquine-resistant *Plasmodium falciparum* (CRPF) and multidrug-resistant malaria, and widespread publicity in the lay press about adverse side-effects associated with mefloquine (Lariam), one of the highly efficacious drugs that may be used for prevention of CRPF, add to the challenge of giving advice on malaria chemoprophylaxis.

Travelers' diarrhea is a common and well-known scourge of international travel, and a leading motivation for travelers to seek pretravel health advice. Questions about vaccines for diarrheal diseases, preventive therapy with probiotics, prophylaxis with bismuth subsalicylate or antimicrobials, and advice on the safety of food and water at their destination(s) are common. International travelers need clear instructions about how to select and use oral rehydration fluids, bismuth subsalicylate, probiotics, and antimotility drugs such as loperamide alone or combined with single dose or short-term antimicrobial therapy as self-treatment once stricken by travelers' diarrhea. Patient care instructions about signs and symptoms indicating a need for professional medical care are also important.

Emerging drug resistance among enteric pathogens to antimicrobials commonly used in the treatment of travelers' diarrhea (trimethoprim plus sulfamethoxazole, ciprofloxacin, and others) fuels the search for new approaches for prevention and treatment of travelers' diarrhea. Highly efficacious vaccines against common forms of travelers' diarrhea and the potential benefits from alteration of intestinal microecology are two areas of continuing research

Health Status of the Traveler

The travel clinic intake form records age, place of birth, general health status, allergies to medications or other substances, prior residence overseas and or international travel, general health (acute or chronic illness, disability, pregnancy or planned pregnancy, lactation), list of medications taken on a regular basis (both prescribed and over-the-counter), vitamins, herbal preparations, and dietary preferences.

Review of Itinerary

Dates of trip departure and return home, and a list of interim destinations with anticipated dates at each destination, plus the accommodations and activities at each destination should be the first items on the patient intake sheet. These data are needed to determine the time available to do pretravel immunizations and to calculate appropriate supplies of malaria chemoprophylaxis, medications for travelers' diarrhea, and other drugs to be included in the travel medicine kit, and to assess the potential health risks of the given itinerary.

In terms of health risks, multiple destinations add to the complexity of pretravel preparation and planning because of varying health regulations and environmental conditions. Hygiene, sanitation, and insect control are more challenging in a tropical climate compared to a temperate climate. As travelers go from urban to rural to remote locations within a country, access to organized health care, in case of an emergency, and telecommunications, to indicate the need for emergency evacuation, become more and more difficult. When the duration of a trip is prolonged, the chance of a traveler becoming ill while still away from home, with the necessity of consulting unfamiliar medical systems, is more likely than with a shorter trip because many of the common diseases of travelers have short incubation periods (< 3 weeks).

Learning the details about the anticipated style of travel, such as mode of transportation, accommodations, level of contact with local residents, and living conditions, may suggest other topics for advice which might benefit the traveler; for example, hazards of rural travel, vector-borne diseases (besides malaria), animal bites, tuberculosis, sexually transmitted infections, and nutritional concerns. Identifying the purpose of travel, such as tourism, educational or cultural exchange, missionary work, volunteer work, political action, competitive sports, expedition, field work, expatriate assignment, etc., can also highlight special exposures that the traveler can prepare for. Special travel health advice is needed for travel during pregnancy, travel with infants and children, travel with medical conditions, HIV-infected travelers, travel with physical disabilities, senior travel, and adventure and wilderness travelers.

PATIENT INFORMATION BROCHURES

One of the challenges of the travel clinic encounter is to impart the large amount of travel health advice and information applicable to a given trip in a way that can be remembered by the patient within the time allocated for the travel clinic encounter (typically 45–60 minutes). Most travel clinics find that the preparation of patient information brochures, preprinted prescriptions, and printed instructions on what to do for vaccine-associated side-effects will save significant time during the travel clinic appointments. The printed materials enable multiple providers to communicate the advice on each relevant topic and provide prescriptions according to the practice standards determined for the given travel clinic. Health topics that have proven useful in the University of Washington travel clinics over the years include:

- Summary of adverse side-effects of travel immunizations and instructions on when and how to call for help
- Destination country information
- Generic plus brand names of malaria chemoprophylaxis drugs throughout the world
- Insect precautions and repellents
- Food and water precautions
- Travelers' diarrhea management and self-treatment
- Hepatitis A and B
- Sexually transmitted infections
- Sun exposure precautions
- High-altitude illness
- Dengue fever
- Japanese encephalitis
- Schistosomiasis

- Traveling with children
- Medical evacuation insurance
- Travel medicine kits.

CONCLUSION

As international travel becomes more commonplace in the lives of ordinary citizens all over the world, travel clinics are gaining recognition among members of the general public and among other health care institutions for their unique role in promoting the health and safety of travelers. Data from epidemiology and surveillance studies have provided the direction for the content of travel medicine practices to date. As data from evidence-based outcomes studies become available from current and future clinical investigations, it is to be expected that the practice of travel medicine will evolve in response to better understanding the interventions that lead to significant reduction in disease and injury among international travelers.

REFERENCES

Bia F (ed.) (2000) *The Travel Medicine Advisor*. American Health Consultants, Atlanta GA.

Dardick KD and Baker ME (1997) Travel medicine and travel clinics, US and Canada. In *Textbook of Travel Medicine and Health* (eds HL DuPont and R Steffen), pp 34–39. Decker, Hamilton, Ontario.

DuPont HL and Steffen R (eds) (1997) *Textbook of Travel Medicine and Health*. Decker, Hamilton, Ontario.

Freedman D (ed.) (1998) Travel medicine. *Infectious Disease Clinics of North America*, **12**.

Hargarten SW, Baker TD and Guptill K (1991) Overseas fatalities of United States citizen travellers: an analysis of deaths related to international travellers. *Annals of Emergency Medicine*, **20**, 622–626.

Hill D and Behrens R (1996) A survey of travel clinics throughout the world. *Travel Medicine*, **3**, 46–51.

Jong EC (ed.) (1999) Travel medicine. *Medical Clinics of North America*, **83**.

Jong EC and McMullen R (eds) (1995) *The Travel and Tropical Medicine Manual*, 2nd edn. WB Saunders, Philadelphia.

Jong EC and McMullen R (1997) Travel medicine problems encountered in emergency departments. *Emergency Clinics of North America*, **15**, 261–281.

Jong EC and Southworth M (1983) Recommendations for patients traveling. *Western Journal of Medicine*, **138**, 746–775.

Reid D and Keystone JS (1997) Health risks abroad: general considerations. In *Textbook of Travel Medicine and Health* (eds HL DuPont and R Steffen), pp 3–9. Decker, Hamilton, Ontario.

Ryan ET and Kain KC (2000) Health advice and immunizations for travel. *New England Journal of Medicine*, **242**, 1716–1725.

Steffen R and Lobel HO (1995) Epidemiologic basis for the practice of travel medicine. *Journal of Wilderness Medicine*, **5**, 56–66.

ADDITIONAL RESOURCES

Useful Web Sites for Travel Clinics

American Society of Tropical Medicine and Hygiene (ASTMH), 60 Revere Dr., Suite 500, Northbrook, IL 60062.
Reference: Annual Meeting, Certificate Program, and clinical group members e-mail discussion list.
http://www.astmh.org

Centers for Disease Control and Prevention (CDC), Atlanta, GA 30333.
Reference: Travelers' Health section; also, full-text version of *Health Information for International Travel, 2001–2002.*
http://www.cdc.gov

International Society of Travel Medicine (ISTM), P.O. Box 871089, Stone Mountain, GA 30087
Reference: Biannual International Conference and members e-mail discussion list.
http://www.istm.org

ProMED, c/o Federation of American Scientists, 307 Massachusetts Ave. NE, Washington, DC 20002.
http://www.fas.org/promed

World Health Organization (WHO), Avenue Appia 20, 1211 Geneva 27, Switzerland.
Reference: *International Travel and Health Information.*
http://www.who.org

Section II

Infectious Diseases and Travel

5

Epidemiology and Surveillance of Travel-related Diseases

Norman T. Begg

GlaxoSmithKline, Uxbridge, UK

INTRODUCTION

The epidemiology of travel-related disease depends on several factors. Diseases such as cardiovascular illness and respiratory infections, which are common at home, are also common in travellers, irrespective of their destination. In contrast, infectious diseases, which are rare or nonexistent at home, may be common in some destinations. The epidemiology of infectious diseases in travellers reflects global patterns of infectious disease, and as travel destinations become more exotic, the epidemiology of travel-related disease is also changing. Activities that travellers undertake at their destination—food and alcohol consumption, sexual behaviour, sports, sunbathing—all determine the pattern of disease in returning travellers.

OVERVIEW OF THE EPIDEMIOLOGY OF TRAVEL-RELATED DISEASE

Health problems are common in travellers, with about a third experiencing some illness. Most travel-related illness is mild and self-limiting; however, serious infections, such as malaria, and fatal injuries due to road accidents are not uncommon. An overview of the major diseases in travellers is provided below; the detailed epidemiology is covered in the relevant chapters.

Estimates of travel-related morbidity vary according to the method of data collection. Prospective studies provide the best estimate. Figure 5.1 (adapted from Steffen *et al.*, 1987) illustrates the risks of travel-related morbidity for the main travel-associated illnesses. In this study, 15% of travellers reported health problems, 8% consulted a doctor, 1% were admitted to hospital and 3% were unable to work for an average of 15 days. If these figures are applied to the estimated 500 million international air travellers a year (Handszuh and Waters, 1997), there are 75 million cases of travel-related illness a year and 5 million hospital admissions. This burden of disease is inevitably set to rise in the future.

MAJOR DISEASES OF TRAVELLERS

Food- and Water-borne Illness

By far the most common travel-related illness is gastrointestinal infection due to contaminated food and water, better known as travellers' diarrhoea. Travellers' diarrhoea has been estimated to affect about 40% of all travellers from industrialised countries (Peltola and Gorbach, 1997). A wide range of pathogens is responsible, although enterotoxigenic *Escherichia coli* (ETEC), is the commonest cause. Other important agents include *Campylobacter* spp, *Salmonella* spp, *Shigella* spp, *Giardia lamblia*, *Entamoeba histolytica* and several viruses, including rotaviruses, caliciviruses and enteroviruses.

The risk of travellers' diarrhoea varies according to destination, from less than 5% for destinations in western Europe and North America to as high as 75% for some destinations in Africa. Attack rates are highest in young adults.

Although morbidity from travellers' diarrhoea is high, mortality is almost nonexistent. Most people experience a short, self-limiting illness and less than 1% of cases are admitted to hospital.

Respiratory Infections

Respiratory tract infections are common in all countries, in both travellers and nontravellers. Most infections are mild, and (unlike travellers' diarrhoea) do not interfere with daily activity. For this reason it is very difficult to determine the true burden of illness in travellers. One study (Steffen *et al.*, 1987) estimated the incidence of acute

Principles and Practice of Travel Medicine. Edited by Jane N. Zuckerman.
© 2001 John Wiley & Sons Ltd.

Infections   **Other and general**

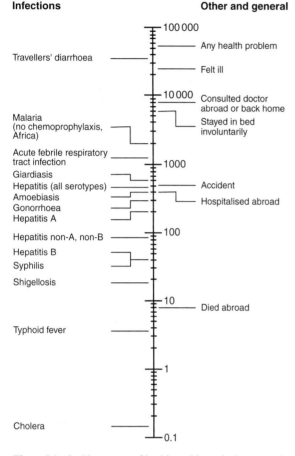

Figure 5.1 Incidence rate of health problems during a stay in developing countries. (Adapted from Steffen *et al.*, 1987)

febrile respiratory tract infection in travellers to be 1261 per 100 000 travellers for a stay of 1 month in a developing country, i.e. an attack rate of 1.26%.

The pathogens causing respiratory infection in travellers are generally speaking the same as those in nontravellers. Three are, however, worthy of special mention: Legionnaires' disease (*Legionella pneumophila*), tuberculosis (*Mycobacterium tuberculosis*) and influenza. Legionnaires' disease causes occasional outbreaks among tourists, often associated with a contaminated hotel water system. During 1999, there were 289 cases of travel-associated Legionnaires' disease in Europe (Public Health Laboratory Service, 2000) and the case fatality rate was significant. Tuberculosis in travellers is uncommon, and most infections occur in those visiting friends and family in endemic countries, or in those working abroad in the long term, such as aid workers. Another risk to travellers is the potential for spread of infection on board aircraft. Transmission of tuberculosis on board aircraft has been described, the risk being greatest for long-haul flights lasting more than 8 h (WHO, 1997).

Influenza outbreaks have been described frequently in travellers on board ships and aircraft, where conditions are ideal for rapid transmission. International travel is important in influenza epidemiology, as this is a major factor in the intercontinental spread of new antigenic variants of influenza viruses. A good example was an outbreak of A/Sydney/05/97 (H3N2) influenza on a cruise ship, which introduced this antigenic variant to both the USA and Canada in 1997 (Centers for Disease Control and Prevention, 1997).

Malaria

The importance of malaria as a disease of travellers lies in the high attack rate, the severity of the disease, and the potential for prevention by chemoprophylaxis and mosquito-avoidance measures. Nearly half of the world's population lives in a malaria-endemic area. The risk to a traveller depends on the country visited, type of area (urban, rural), season, accommodation (e.g. airconditioned or camping), the duration of visit and the effectiveness of prevention measures used. For example, a 1 month visit to west Africa with no chemoprophylaxis carries a risk of 2–3%. Overall an estimated 30 000 travellers from the USA and Europe contract malaria every year; the case fatality is about 2%. The risk to travellers has increased in recent years with the spread of chloroquine-resistant *Plasmodium falciparum* malaria. Malaria epidemiology is described in detail in Chapter 8.

Vaccine-preventable Diseases

There are several infectious diseases in travellers that are potentially preventable by vaccination. By far the most common is hepatitis A. In the USA and Europe, between 30 and 50% of all cases of hepatitis A are travel-associated; imported hepatitis A can also be the source for onward transmission within the community after returning home, especially in children. The relative risk of hepatitis A in travellers, compared with staying at home, was estimated in a UK study to be 20 for travel to eastern Europe, 235 for Africa and 1835 for the Indian subcontinent (Behrens *et al.*, 1995). Another study, in Swiss travellers, expressed the risk as an absolute risk: 300 per 100 000 per month for a stay in a tourist hotel, rising to 2000 per 100 000 per month (i.e. one in 50) for a backpacking trip (Steffen *et al.*, 1994). Hepatitis A is underdiagnosed, particularly in children in whom the infection may be mild or inapparent; thus these studies underestimate the true burden in travellers.

Typhoid fever is common in many countries. There are an estimated 16 million cases worldwide. The risk to travellers is more difficult to assess than for hepatitis A, as typhoid fever is typically an epidemic, rather than an endemic, disease, so the risk for travel to any particular country will depend on whether there is an epidemic at the time of the visit. Steffen (Steffen *et al.*, 1987) estimated the overall risk for travel to a developing country to be 30 per 100 000 per month. An additional risk for travellers is the emergence of antibiotic-resistant strains of *Salmonella typhi* in some countries, especially in Africa and Southeast Asia.

Travellers are also potentially at risk for hepatitis B, with infection occurring through a variety of routes, including sexual intercourse, injecting drug use, blood transfusions and tattooing. The risk in short-term travellers has not been well documented; however, in professionals working abroad it is 80–420 per 100 000 per month of stay (these figures including both symptomatic and asymptomatic disease) (Steffen, 1990).

Meningococcal infection requires close contact for transmission to occur. It is thus rare in most travellers, except in pilgrims (see below) or in travellers living in close proximity to locals in areas where epidemic disease is common, e.g. staying with relatives in the African meningitis belt or in hikers camping in Nepal. Vaccines are available against serogroups A, C, W135 and Y of *Neisseria meningitidis*. In the African meningitis belt, most cases are due to serogroup A and this is also true in Nepal; in other countries, serogroup B, and sometimes serogroup C, strains predominate.

Yellow fever infections are only reported occasionally in travellers. A yellow fever vaccination certificate is required for travel to some countries, although this is mainly to prevent spread of the disease rather than to protect the individual traveller.

Cholera vaccination is no longer mandated or recommended for travellers. The risk of infection in travellers is negligible; it has been estimated to be about 0.2 per 100 000 (Wittlinger *et al.*, 1995).

The risk of poliomyelitis in an unvaccinated traveller during the 1980s was estimated as 2 per 100 000 (Kubli *et al.*, 1987); however, this risk is now declining as a result of the global polio eradication effort (see below). Vaccination is still, however, indicated for travel to many countries. In industrialised countries importations now account for a significant proportion of the few residual polio cases: for example, 5 of 21 cases in England and Wales between 1985 and 1991 were travel-associated; the remainder were vaccine-associated or source unknown (Joce *et al.*, 1992). The greatest risk nowadays is for travellers to the Indian subcontinent, where approximately half of all the world's polio cases are reported.

Diphtheria is also rare in travellers, although a global estimate of risk has not been published. There were only 21 travel-associated cases in England and Wales, a population of 50 million, between 1970 and 1987 (Begg, 1988). The risk has increased in recent years for travellers to the former USSR (see below).

In countries where measles is close to elimination, imported measles now accounts for a significant proportion of the burden of disease. For example, in England and Wales, 24% of sporadic measles cases between 1995 and 1999 were either imported or associated with importation (M. Ramsay, 2000, personal communication). In the USA, measles vaccination is required by some states for

travellers who plan to work or study there, in an effort to prevent importation.

Japanese B encephalitis is also rare in travellers. There have been sporadic reports in the literature; the risk is probably of the order of one per million. Vaccination is only recommended for longer rural stays in endemic countries of Southeast Asia and the Far East.

Another rare vaccine-preventable disease is tick-borne encephalitis. There are no reliable estimates of the number of cases. The risk is confined to forested areas of central and eastern Europe, parts of Scandanavia and Russia, where the tick vector is present.

Bites from potentially rabid animals are common in travellers. Between 0.2% and 0.5% of travellers are bitten per month of travel (Bernard and Fishbein, 1991); however, the risk of rabies is remote, even in the unvaccinated traveller who does not receive postexposure prophylaxis.

Sexually Transmitted Diseases

Travel increases opportunities for casual or commercial sex. Approximately 5% of travellers from Europe to developing countries reported at least one casual sexual encounter while travelling (Laga, 1992). Unprotected sexual activity places the traveller at risk of many sexually transmitted diseases (STDs) (including hepatitis B and human immunodeficiency viral (HIV) infection, both of which are considered elsewhere in this chapter). Most STDs are also common at home; thus in a sexually active traveller it is difficult to determine whether an STD was acquired at home or abroad, particularly if the incubation period is long. This means that reliable data on the incidence of travel-associated STDs are difficult to obtain. In addition, many STDs are asymptomatic, so even if screening is undertaken (and this is unusual) it is usually impossible to determine when and where the infection was acquired. Molecular typing methods have been useful in helping trace the international spread of HIV infection, but they are not yet widely available for other more common STDs. Antibiotic resistance is a useful marker for identifying some travel-associated STDs; for example, penicillinase-producing strains of *Neisseria gonorrhoeae* are much more common in developing countries (especially Southeast Asia) than in Europe or the USA. Steffen (Steffen *et al.*, 1987) found an incidence of gonorrhoea in travellers of 300 per 100 000 per month of travel, which is similar to the risk for hepatitis A.

The age and sex distribution of travel-acquired STDs differs from infections acquired at home. In most developed countries, the highest rates of indigenous STDs are in teenagers and young adults. Travel-associated cases tend to occur more commonly in older adults, particularly adult males.

The vast majority of travel-associated STDs are those which are also common at home: gonorrhoea, chlamydia, trichomoniasis, herpes simplex and genital warts; however, some infections are much commoner in tropical countries and are thus more readily identifiable as travel-

Table 5.1 Causes of death related to international travel
($n = 2463$)

Cause of death	Number (%)
Cardiovascular disease	1207 (49.0)
Other, noninjury deaths	713 (28.9)
Injury deaths	543 (22.0)
Motor vehicle	161
Drowning	97
Air crash	43
Poisoning	39
Burns	22
Other	181

Adapted from Hargarten *et al.* (1991).

associated. Examples include chancroid (*Haemophilus ducreyi*) and donovanosis (*Calymmatobacterium inguinale*).

The incidence of STDs in some countries has increased significantly in recent years. Of particular concern is the rise in syphilis, which has been observed in eastern Europe and countries of the former USSR. The expanding HIV epidemic (see below) has also increased the risks to the sexually active traveller. STDs in returning travellers are likely to become an increasing problem in the future.

Accidents

Most of the burden of less severe illness in travellers is diarrhoea and other infectious diseases. In contrast, accidents are the cause of more serious morbidity and mortality in travellers. Accidents account for less than 2% of all travel-related morbidity (Steffen *et al.*, 1987); however, they are responsible for about 20% of travel-related deaths (Hargarten *et al.*, 1991; Paixo *et al.*, 1991) (Table 5.1); worldwide there are several thousand deaths a year in travellers. The most common cause of death is motor vehicle accidents (accounting for a quarter of all deaths); other causes of accidental deaths in travellers include drowning, air crash, murder, suicide and poisoning (Table 5.1). For nonfatal accidents, the most common causes are motor vehicle accidents, falls and recreational injuries. The age and sex distribution of travel-associated accidents is similar to accidents that occur at home, i.e. with the highest rates in young adult men.

Other Health Problems in Travellers

Cardiovascular disease is common in travellers; indeed, it is the commonest cause of death abroad (Table 5.1), although this is usually because of pre-existing disease and not due to travel. The exception is the risk of venous thrombosis that sometimes accompanies long-haul air travel (Sarvesvaran, 1986), the so-called 'economy-class syndrome'.

Bites and stings are common, although most are harmless or cause only minor distress. Some can be painful (e.g. scorpion bites) but very few require specific treatment, e.g. antivenom. Fatalities due to snake bites or venomous insects are very rare in travellers. The greatest risk from insect bites in travellers is due to malaria, dengue, and other infections for which insects act as vectors.

THE CHANGING EPIDEMIOLOGY OF DISEASE IN TRAVELLERS

As travellers seek increasingly exotic locations, they become exposed to new risks; for example, a rise in imported schistosomiasis has been observed in some countries, following the establishment of Lake Malawi as a popular tourist destination.

The potential for emergence of new infectious diseases and re-emergence of old ones has increased in recent years. Many factors have contributed to this threat, of which the rapid increase in international travel is one. Other factors are the globalisation of the food industry, and social and environmental changes such as deforestation and rapid urbanisation. In addition, the widespread and inappropriate use of antibiotics has led to the emergence of many resistant infectious diseases. At the same time, successful vaccination programmes and other control measures have brought some diseases close to eradication.

While travel has contributed to disease emergence, health problems in travellers can also be a highly sensitive sentinel for changing global disease epidemiology. Illness in a traveller returning to an industrialised country is more likely to be thoroughly investigated than in the country where the illness was acquired, and indeed new infectious agents are often first identified in travellers. This was the case for Lassa fever, which was first identified in 1969 among American missionaries in Nigeria. Similarly, the most sensitive method for monitoring the spread of resistant malaria worldwide is through surveillance of travel-associated disease; for example, chloroquine-resistant *Plasmodium vivax* was first detected in US Army troops returning from Somalia.

Viral Haemorrhagic Fevers

A number of viral haemorrhagic fevers have re-emerged or emerged in recent years. Dengue haemorrhagic fever was almost eradicated in the Americas prior to 1981. The incidence has increased dramatically since then, with epidemics of dengue in Central and South America, the Caribbean and more recently in Southeast Asia. The rising incidence of dengue fever over the past 20 years is mirrored by increasing reports in travellers (for example in the UK) (Table 5.2).

During the last decade there has also been a large increase in the incidence of yellow fever in West Africa,

Table 5.2 Reported cases of dengue fever in UK travellers, 1975–1995

Year	Number of reports
1975–1981	0
1982	6
1983	11
1984	11
1985	1
1986	6
1987	1
1988	6
1989	2
1990	34
1991	12
1992	30
1993	17
1994	22
1995	42

Source: PHLS CDSC.

and recent fatal cases in Swiss, American and German travellers are a reminder of the potential risk in this part of the world. The *Aedes* mosquito is a vector for both dengue and yellow fever. Although yellow fever is confined to South America and Africa, there is concern the infection could spread, via infected travellers, to other continents such as India, where the *Aedes* mosquito is also present. There have also been several outbreaks of Ebola fever in central Africa since the large epidemic in Kiwit, Zaire in 1995, although travellers have not so far been affected.

Nipah virus

In 1999 a previously unrecognised paramyxovirus, now called *Nipah virus*, was identified as the cause of a large outbreak of febrile encephalitic and respiratory illness in Malaysia and Singapore (Centers for Disease Control and Prevention, 1999). The apparent source of infection in humans is exposure to pigs. The method of transmission is not yet known, although human-to-human spread has not been demonstrated. The risk, if any, to travellers is unknown at present.

Diphtheria

Another disease which has re-emerged recently is diphtheria. Diphtheria is rare in travellers, as most people have been vaccinated, and intimate contact with an infectious case is necessary for transmission. During the 1990s however, there was a major resurgence of diphtheria in the former USSR, and importations were reported from several countries including the USA, Italy, Germany, Poland and the UK. This risk is now subsiding as the epidemic in the former USSR has been brought under control.

Meningococcal Disease

Meningococcal disease is usually rare in travellers, with one notable exception—visitors to the annual pilgrimage to Mecca, the Hajj. A large outbreak of serogroup A disease occurred in Mecca in 1987, prompting the requirement by the Saudi authorities for pilgrims to be vaccinated. Another epidemic occurred in the Hajj in 2000, this time due to serogroup W135 infections. Cases were reported in pilgrims returning to the UK, France, The Netherlands, Onman and the USA (WHO, 2000b). This has implications for future vaccination recommendations for travellers. The risk to travellers in sub-Saharan Africa has also increased during the late 1990s, with large epidemics (serogroup A) reported in many countries inside the 'meningitis belt'.

Cholera

Successive cholera pandemics have spread around the globe as a result of international travel. The seventh pandemic started in 1961, and by the early 1990s it had reached South America for the first time in almost a century. It rapidly spread throughout the continent, with devastating consequences: for example, in Peru it caused over 3000 deaths, and the estimated loss to the economy was about £500 million. The eighth pandemic started in Bangladesh in 1992, and was due to an entirely new strain (*Vibrio cholerae* 0139). This new strain has now spread to Africa, where it has caused outbreaks, especially among refugees, in which the case fatality has been as high as 50%.

Acquired Immune Deficiency Syndrome

The AIDS epidemic now affects every country in the world. While the origin of AIDS is still under dispute, the role of travel in its international spread is not. One well-documented route of spread of HIV was travellers returning to Haiti from Africa, and subsequently homosexual male tourists from the USA to Haiti. Within Africa, migrant prostitutes and truck drivers have been particularly important in the spread of HIV. Sex tourists and businessmen have carried the virus from the USA, Europe and Africa to Asia. In many developed countries, the most rapidly increasing category of HIV infections and AIDS cases is heterosexually acquired infections and the majority of these (up to three-quarters) are due to sex with a partner abroad (most commonly in Africa).

Plague

Plague is the classical traveller's disease. The port of

Venice introduced quarantine in the fourteenth century in an effort to halt its spread westwards. In recent years there have been outbreaks of plague in India and Madagascar. Although the impact on travellers was nonexistent in terms of morbidity, the impact on tourism in India was immense, as many countries responded (totally inappropriately) by seeking to prevent trade and travel to and from the affected area. In contrast, the outbreak in Madagascar was almost totally ignored by the international community.

Poliomyelitis

The risk of many vaccine-preventable diseases is now declining, thanks to mass immunisation programmes. Polio is a good example. Because of the substantial efforts to eradicate polio globally, the Americas have been certified as polio-free by WHO since 1993, and eradication is likely to be certified soon in the Western Pacific and in Europe. The disease is still, however, endemic in many countries of Africa and Asia. When global polio eradication is achieved (the current expected date is 2005), polio vaccination for travellers will no longer be needed.

Antibiotic Resistance

Emerging antibiotic resistance is a worldwide problem, particularly in some developing countries where there is indiscriminate use of antibiotics and over-the-counter sales. Incomplete treatment of patients abroad further contributes to the problem. Infections that are of particular concern to the traveller include gonorrhoea, tuberculosis and typhoid fever.

SURVEILLANCE OF DISEASE IN TRAVELLERS

Sources of Data

Passively Acquired Information

In most countries, there is a list of mandatory notifiable infectious disease. This list often includes those that are typically travel-associated, such as malaria, and in some countries there is also a requirement to provide a travel history. Laboratory reports are another valuable source of information on infectious diseases acquired abroad, particularly data from specialist reference laboratories.

For noninfectious disease data, hospital records can provide information about more serious travel-related events such as accidents. Data may also be available on travellers who require repatriation. Death certificates provide information on those who die abroad.

Passively acquired surveillance data have many limitations. Travel histories are poorly recorded on laboratory reports, notification forms, hospital notes and death certificates. Where the history is recorded, it is often vague or inaccurate. Less serious, yet common, events such as travellers' diarrhoea may go totally unreported. Even for more serious infections there is significant underreporting; for example, there were only 22 routine laboratory reports of dengue fever for 1994 in the UK, whereas data from the reference laboratory responsible for confirmation of infections indicated a total of 465 cases during that year (Public Health Laboratory Service, 1995). In addition, there are no routine data available on illnesses acquired abroad when the traveller recovers before returning home. The denominator (number of travellers for each destination) is often incomplete, thus it is not possible to quantify risks accurately. At present these data are obtained from the International Passenger Survey, collected for business purposes and not travel health interests.

Active Surveillance

The most reliable data are those derived from prospective studies in returning travellers, where travel morbidity data are actively sought soon after returning home. Such studies are, by their nature, expensive and difficult to carry out. They are usually undertaken on an *ad hoc* basis, rather than as part of a continuous surveillance scheme. For this reason they cannot usually assess how risks change over time, unless they are repeated at regular intervals using similar study methodology. Serological surveys undertaken before and after travel provide high quality data on travel-related infections.

One of the problems with surveillance of travel-related disease is that there is no clear consensus on who should be responsible for collecting and interpreting the information. WHO and other international organisations such as the International Society for Travel Medicine have an obvious role, but cannot provide information at the individual country level. In some countries, e.g. Switzerland and Scotland, there is a well-developed travel health surveillance function, but in most countries the data are extremely limited; traveller's health is not always seen as a priority by governments, and academic institutions rarely have the considerable resources required to carry out surveillance properly.

Disseminating the Information

Rapid dissemination of accurate and up-to-date information is essential both for the traveller and for those who advise travellers. There are multiple sources of information currently available. Increasingly the information is available electronically (see Additional Resources). WHO publishes regular updates on travel illness in its *Weekly Epidemiological Record* (WER), and a more comprehensive manual of travel advice is published annually by WHO (WHO, 2000a). Public Health organisations and government health departments, e.g. the US Centers for Disease Control, also publish advice and information regularly. There are several books on travel health, aimed at both health professionals and the public (see Further Reading).

There are also numerous phone lines and voice information services which provide information on current risks and recommended vaccines.

The problem with multiple information channels is that inevitably there is conflicting and inconsistent information. Sometimes unsubstantiated information is publicised; this is particularly true when an outbreak has recently been identified and rumours abound. Some information sources are not updated frequently enough, and interpretation of data may vary. Generally speaking, the most reliable information comes from organisations that have access to expert interpretation of data and the resources to ensure that databases are updated in real time.

Surveillance in the Twenty-first Century

Electronic communication is increasingly dominating the capture, interpretation and dissemination of travel health information. This trend will inevitably continue, and linkage of electronic information sources should help improve the consistency of information available. Global information networking is a priority of the WHO and other partners such as the European Union–US Task Force on Emerging Communicable Diseases. There are already some well-established international collaborations on surveillance of travel-related illness. For example, the European Working Group on Legionella Infections (EWGLI) collects data on travel-associated legionnaires' disease from 31 European countries and was first established in 1987; a number of clusters have been detected through the EWGLI scheme that might have been missed in the absence of sharing information between countries. Another example of collaboration at the European level is ENTERNET, a laboratory-based *Salmonella* network comprising countries of the European Union.

Advances in diagnostic methods will improve the speed with which travel-related illnesses can be diagnosed. These tests will increasingly be 'near patient', i.e. will be able to be performed in the physicians' surgery, or even by the patient at home. The challenge here will be to ensure that the information from these tests is captured in a consistent way.

As travel continues to increase, travellers will become increasingly important as a sentinel for global disease surveillance. The International Society for Travel Medicine and the US Centers for Disease Control have recently established a surveillance project, Geosentinel, in 22 travel clinics around the world.

There are a number of ways in which surveillance of travel-related disease could be improved. The travel health industry is starting to become involved in travel health surveillance, albeit somewhat reluctantly. Travel companies are ideally placed to collect information on the health of their customers, and this information should be collected in partnership with travel medicine experts. Travel insurance companies can also provide valuable information, particularly for more serious events that result in insurance claims. Overseas employers and expatriate organisations can provide information on longer-term travellers. Finally, it is important that travel medicine specialists have good communication with the media, both as a source of information and to ensure that messages about risks to travellers are communicated accurately and responsibly.

REFERENCES

Begg NT (1988) Imported diphtheria, England and Wales: 1970–87. In *Travel Medicine*. Proceedings of the First Conference on International Travel Medicine (eds R Steffen, HO Lobel, J Haworth *et al.*). M. Springer-Verlag, London.

Behrens RH, Collins M, Botto B *et al.* (1995) Risk for British travellers of acquiring hepatitis A. *BMJ*, **311**, 193.

Bernard K W and Fishbein DB (1991) Pre-exposure rabies prophylaxis for travellers: are the benefits worth the cost? *Vaccine*, **9**, 833–836.

Centers for Disease Control and Prevention (1997) Update: influenza activity: United States, 1997–98 season. *MMWR. Morbidity and Mortality Weekly Report*, **46**, 1094–1098.

Centers for Disease Control and Prevention (1999) Update: outbreak of Nipah virus—Malaysia and Singapore, 1999. *MMWR. Morbidity and Mortality Weekly Report*, **48**, 335–337.

Handszuh H and Waters SR (1997) Travel and tourism patterns. In *Textbook of Travel Medicine and Health* (eds HL DuPont and R Steffen), p. 20. Decker, Hamilton, Ontario.

Hargarten SW, Baker TD and Guptill K (1991) Overseas fatalities of United States citizen travellers: an analysis of deaths related to international travellers. *Annals of Emergency Medicine*, **20**, 622–626.

Joce R, Wood D, Brown D *et al.* (1992) Paralytic poliomyelitis in England and Wales, 1985–91. *BMJ*, **305**, 79–82.

Kubli D, Steffen R and Schar M (1987) Importation of poliomyelitis to industrialised nations between 1975 and 1984. Evaluation and conclusions for vaccination recommendations. *BMJ*, **295**, 169–171.

Laga M (1992) Risk of infection and other sexually transmitted diseases for travellers. In *Travel Medicine 2. Proceedings of the Second Conference on International Travel Medicine* (eds HO Lobel, R Steffen and PE Kozarsky), pp. 201–203. International Society of Travel Medicine, Atlanta.

Paixo DA, Dewar RD, Cossar JH *et al.* (1991) What do Scots die of when abroad? *Scottish Medical Journal*, **6**, 114–116.

Peltola H and Gorbach SL (1997) Travelers' diarrhea: epidemiology and clinical aspects. In *Textbook of Travel Medicine and Health* (eds HL DuPont and R Steffen), p. 78. Decker, Hamilton, Ontario.

Public Health Laboratory Service (1995) Dengue: current epidemics and risks to travellers. *Communicable Disease Report*, **5**, 14.

Public Health Laboratory Service (2000) Web site www.phls.org.uk.

Sarsvesaran R (1986) Sudden natural deaths associated with commercial air travel. *Medicine, Science and the Law*, **26**, 35–38.

Steffen R (1990) Risks of hepatitis B for travellers. *Vaccine*, **8**, 31–32.

Steffen R, Rickenbach M, Wilhelm U *et al.* (1987) Health problems after travel to developing countries. *Journal of Infectious Diseases* **156**, 84–91.

Steffen R, Kane MA, Shapiro CN *et al.* (1994) Epidemiology and prevention of hepatitis A in travelers. *JAMA*, **272**, 885–889.

WHO (1997) *Tuberculosis and International Air Travel*. World Health Organization, Geneva.

WHO (2000a) *International Travel and Health: Vaccination Requirements and the Health Advice*. World Health Organization, Geneva.

WHO (2000b) Outbreak news. *Weekly Epidemiological Record*, **16** (75), 125–126.

Wittlinger F, Steffen R, Watanabe H *et al.* (1995) Risk of cholera among Western and Japanese travelers. *Journal of Travel Medicine*, **2**, 154–158.

ADDITIONAL RESOURCES

Useful Travel-related Web Site Addresses

British Airways
www.british-airways.com/travel

International Society of Travel Medicine (ISTM)
www.istm.org

ISTM Physicians
www.medicineplanet.com

London School of Hygiene and Tropical Medicine
www.lshtm.ac.uk/itol

Lonely Planet
www.lonelyplanet.com

Scottish Centre for Infection and Environmental Health
(public web site) www.fitfortravel.scot.nhs.co.uk
(health professional web site) www.travax.scot.nhs.uk

Travel Health Online
www.tripprep.com/index/html

Tropical Medicine Bureau in Dublin
www.tmb.ic

UK Department of Health
www.open.gov.uk/traveladvice

UK Foreign and Commonwealth Office
www.fco.gov.uk/travel/

UK Public Health Laboratory Service
www.phls.co.uk

UK Travel Health Site
www.travelhealth.co.uk

US Centers for Disease Control
www.cdc.gov

Weekly Epidemiological Record
www.who.ch/wer/

World Health Organization
www.who.int/ith/english/risks.htm

6

Virus Infections

Arie J. Zuckerman

Royal Free and University College Medical School, London, UK

VIRAL HEPATITIS

Introduction and Definitions

The last three decades have witnessed an explosion in knowledge of viral hepatitis, a major public health problem throughout the world affecting several hundreds of millions of people. Viral hepatitis is an important cause of morbidity and mortality, both from acute infection and chronic sequelae which include, with hepatitis B, hepatitis C and hepatitis D (delta) infection, chronic active hepatitis and cirrhosis, and primary liver cancer with hepatitis B and hepatitis C. The hepatitis viruses include a range of unrelated human pathogens.

Hepatitis A virus (HAV) is a small unenveloped symmetrical RNA virus which shares many of the characteristics of the family *Picornaviridae*. It is the cause of infectious or epidemic hepatitis transmitted by the faecal–oral route. The virus is classified within the genus *Hepatovirus*.

Hepatitis B virus (HBV) is a large double-shelled virus of the hepadnavirus group of double-stranded DNA viruses which replicate by reverse transcription. The virus is endemic in the human population and hyperendemic in many parts of the world; it is estimated to have infected a third of the world's population. It is transmitted by blood-to-blood contact and by the sexual route.

Hepatitis C virus (HCV) is an enveloped single-stranded RNA virus, distantly related to flaviviruses, but not transmitted by arthropod vectors. Seroprevalence studies confirm its wide dissemination in all parts of the world and the importance of the parenteral route of transmission, and transmission by blood and blood products, but in as many as 50% of patients the origin of the infection remains unknown. Several genotypes have been described. Infection is common; it is associated with chronic liver disease and with primary liver cancer.

Hepatitis delta virus (D) (HDV) is an unusual single-stranded circular RNA virus resembling plant viral satellites and viroids. This virus requires hepadnavirus helper functions for propagation in hepatocytes, and is an important cause of acute and severe chronic liver damage in some regions of the world. The modes of transmission are similar to the parenteral transmission of HBV.

Hepatitis E virus (HEV) is an enterically transmitted, nonenveloped, single-stranded RNA virus, which shares many biophysical and biochemical features with caliciviruses. It has caused large epidemics of acute hepatitis in the Indian subcontinent, Central and Southeast Asia, the Middle East, parts of Africa and elsewhere; it is responsible for high mortality during the third trimester of pregnancy. The number of infections with this virus, particularly in developed countries, may be underestimated.

GB viruses and *Hepatitis G virus*. In 1995 two independent viruses, GBV-A and GBV-B, were identified in infectious plasma of tamarin monkeys inoculated with serum from a surgeon (GB) with jaundice. A third virus, GBV-C, was later isolated from a human specimen that was immunoreactive with a GBV-B protein. GBV-C RNA was found in several patients with clinical hepatitis. GBV-A/C, GBV-B and the hepatitis C viruses are members of distinct viral groups whose genomes show regions of sequence identity with flaviviruses. A virus described in 1996 as *Hepatitis G virus* (HGV) is an independent isolate of GBV-C. The role of this virus in viral hepatitis is not established.

TT virus. TT virus stands for the initials of a patient in Japan with post-transfusion hepatitis. TT virus DNA has been detected in up to 97% of the healthy population in some countries. Preliminary evidence indicates that this virus is similar to members of the family *Circoviridae*, viruses which infect plants and farm animals. The pathogenic role, if any, of this virus in human disease remains to be established.

Principles and Practice of Travel Medicine. Edited by Jane N. Zuckerman.

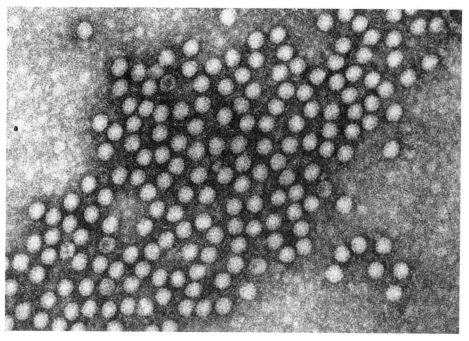

Figure 6.1   Hepatitis A virus: faecal extract from a patient during the incubation period showing the large number of viral particles. × 200 000

HEPATITIS A

Introduction and Definitions

Epidemics of jaundice have been reported for many centuries and the term 'infectious hepatitis' was coined in 1912 to describe these outbreaks. The term 'hepatitis type A' was adopted by the World Health Organization (WHO) in 1973 to describe this form of hepatitis, and the virus was visualised by electron microscopy in human faecal extracts in the same year. *Hepatitis A virus* (HAV) is spread by the faecal–oral route. It remains endemic throughout the world and is hyperendemic in areas with poor standards of sanitation and hygiene. Since the end of World War II in 1945, the seroprevalence of antibodies to HAV has declined in many countries. Infection results most commonly from person-to-person contact, but large epidemics do occur. For example, in 1988, an outbreak of hepatitis A associated with the consumption of raw clams in Shanghai resulted in almost 300 000 cases.

Nature of the Virus

In 1983, HAV was classified in the genus *Enterovirus* of the family *Picornaviridae*, on the basis of its biophysical and biochemical characteristics, including the stability at low pH. This pre-empted the isolation and analysis of complementary DNA clones that led to the determination of the entire nucleotide sequence of the viral genome.

There is limited sequence homology with the enteroviruses and rhinoviruses, although the structure and genome organisation are typical of the picornaviruses. The virus is now classified in the genus *Hepatovirus*. There is only one human serotype of HAV and seven genotypes, but all human HAVs have a single immunodominant epitope which is responsible for generating neutralising antibodies.

Epidemiology and Geographical Distribution

Hepatitis A occurs endemically in all parts of the world, with frequent reports of minor and major outbreaks. The exact incidence is difficult to estimate because of the high proportion of subclinical infections and infections without jaundice, differences in surveillance, and differing patterns of disease. The degree of underreporting is very high.

HAV enters the body by ingestion. The virus then spreads, probably by the bloodstream, to the liver, a target organ, where it replicates in the hepatocytes. Large numbers of virus particles are detectable in faeces during the incubation period (Figure 6.1), beginning as early as 10–14 days after exposure and continuing, in general, until peak elevation of serum aminotransferases. Virus is also detected in faeces early in the acute phase of illness, but relatively infrequently after the onset of clinical jaundice. IgG antibody to HAV that persists is also detectable late in the incubation period, coinciding approximately with the onset of biochemical evidence of liver damage. The virus does not persist and chronic excretion of HAV does not occur. There is no evidence of progression to chronic liver disease.

The mode of transmission of HAV is by the faecal–oral route, most commonly by person-to-person contact in developed countries, and infection occurs readily under conditions of poor sanitation and hygiene and over-crowding. Common source outbreaks are most frequently initiated by faecal contamination of water and food, but waterborne transmission is not a major factor in maintaining this infection in industrialised communities. On the other hand, many foodborne outbreaks have been reported. This can be attributed to the shedding of large quantities of virus in the faeces during the incubation period of the illness in infected food handlers; the source of the outbreak can often be traced to uncooked food or food that has been handled after cooking. Oysters, clams and other shellfish from contaminated water pose a high risk of infection unless heated or steamed thoroughly. There is a similar risk with uncooked vegetables and crops in countries where raw sewage is used as a fertiliser. Although hepatitis A remains endemic and common in the developed countries, the infection occurs mainly in small clusters, often with only a few identified cases.

Hepatitis A is recognised as an important travel-related infection in travellers from low-prevalence areas to endemic countries. As a generalisation, low-prevalence areas include western Europe, the USA and Canada, Australia, New Zealand and Japan. The infection is much more prevalent in other areas of the world, and people travelling to developing countries, including many holiday destinations, are at risk of infection, and are at particularly high risk of infection in rural areas.

Two other sectors of the population are at an increased risk of infection with HAV: those engaging in oral–anal sexual practices and male homosexuality, and injecting drug users. The latter group is at risk because of a combination of poor personal hygiene, faecal contamination of injection equipment which is often shared, the use of water drawn from toilet pans to dissolve drugs, and possible contamination of illicit drugs that are transported in the intestine after swallowing or are carried in the rectum.

Hepatitis A is rarely transmitted by blood transfusion, although transmission by inadequately inactivated and treated blood coagulation products has been reported, as have cases in patients with cancer treated with lymphokine-activated killer cells and interleukin 2 prepared with tissue culture medium supplemented with pooled human serum.

The incubation period of hepatitis A is 3–5 weeks, with a mean of 28 days. Subclinical and anicteric cases are common and, although the disease has in general a low mortality rate, patients may be incapacitated for many weeks. There is no evidence of progression to chronic liver damage.

Reservoir of Infection

The reservoir of HAV is human beings. Rarely hepatitis A may be transmitted to handlers of chimpanzees and other higher nonhuman primates. The source of the infection is usually human.

Pathology

Pathological changes are confined to the liver: marked focal activation of sinusoidal lining cells; accumulations of lymphocytes, and especially histiocytes, in the parenchyma, often replacing hepatocytes lost by cytolytic necrosis, predominantly in the periportal areas; occasional coagulative necrosis resulting in the formation of acidophilic bodies, and focal degeneration. There are no chronic sequelae.

Clinical Features

Inapparent or subclinical infections and infection without jaundice are common with all the different hepatitis viruses, particularly in children under the age of 6 years. The clinical picture ranges from an asymptomatic infection to a mild anicteric illness, to acute disease with jaundice, to severe prolonged jaundice, to fulminant hepatitis.

Differences between the clinical syndromes of acute hepatitis A, acute hepatitis B and other types of viral hepatitis become apparent on analysis of large numbers of well-documented cases, but these differences are not reliable for the diagnosis of individual patients with jaundice.

The following description of the acute illness applies to all types of viral hepatitis. Prodromal nonspecific symptoms, such as fever, chills, headache, fatigue, malaise and aches and pains, are followed a few days later by anorexia, nausea, vomiting and right upper quadrant abdominal pain, followed by the passage of dark urine and clay-coloured stools. Jaundice of the sclera and the skin develop. With the appearance of jaundice, there is usually a rapid subjective improvement of symptoms. The jaundice usually deepens for a few days and persists for 1–2 weeks. The faeces then darken and the jaundice diminishes over a period of about 2 weeks. Convalescence may be prolonged.

In areas of high prevalence, most children are infected with hepatitis A early in life and such infections are generally asymptomatic. Infections acquired later in life are of increasing clinical severity. Less than 10% of cases of acute hepatitis A in children up to the age of 6 are icteric, but this increases to 40–50% in the 6–14 age group and to 70–80% in adults. Of 115 551 cases of hepatitis A in the USA between 1983 and 1987, only 9% of the cases, but more than 70% of the fatalities, were in those aged over 49.

Hepatitis A does not persist in the liver, chronic infection does not occur and there is no evidence of progression to chronic liver disease.

Diagnosis

Diagnosis is based on the detection of specific IgM antibodies by serological tests, usually by enzyme-linked immunosorbent assay (ELISA) or radioimmunoassay. Specific IgA antibody responses may also be measured. Specialised laboratories have developed sensitive immunoassays for detection of hepatitis A antigen in faecal samples, and molecular hybridization can be employed for detection of HAV RNA in faeces. RNA probes have been used for detection of virus in shellfish and in contaminated water.

Management and Treatment

Since faecal shedding of the virus is at its highest during the late incubation period and prodromal phase of the illness, strict isolation of cases is not a useful control measure. Spread of hepatitis A is reduced by simple hygienic measures and the sanitary disposal of excreta.

There is no specific treatment for hepatitis A beyond general supportive measures.

Statutory notification to local health authorities is required in a number of countries.

Passive immunisation with normal human immunoglobulin, or in selected circumstances active immunisation with hepatitis A vaccine, is indicated as soon as possible after exposure and within 2 weeks to all household and sexual contacts, and for those exposed to contaminated food. Immunoglobulin should be given to all classroom contacts in daycare centres (children under 5 years old), and, if there are infants in nappies, immunoglobulin should be given to all potentially exposed children and staff in the centre. Immunoglobulin has been used effectively for controlling outbreaks such as in homes for the mentally handicapped. It is not indicated for contacts in the usual office or factory environment or in schools. Hepatitis A vaccine has, however, been shown to be effective for the control of hepatitis A outbreaks in schools.

Protective Measures and Prevention

General

Strict personal hygiene and good sanitation, with emphasis on thorough handwashing, and sanitary disposal of faeces and urine. Safe and chlorinated water supply. Proper disposal of sewage. Avoid the consumption of raw and inadequately cooked food, including shellfish, in endemic areas.

Passive Immunisation

Normal human immunoglobulin, containing at least 100 international units $(IU)\,ml^{-1}$ of anti-HAV antibody, given intramuscularly before exposure to the virus or early during the incubation period will prevent or attenuate a clinical illness. The dosage should be at least 2 IU of anti-HAV antibody kg^{-1} body weight, but in special cases, such as pregnancy or in patients with liver disease, that dosage may be doubled.

Immunoglobulin does not always prevent infection and excretion of HAV and inapparent or subclinical hepatitis may develop. The efficacy of passive immunisation is based on the presence of HAV antibody in the immunoglobulin and the minimum titre of antibody required for protection is believed to be about $10\,IU\,l^{-1}$.

Immunoglobulin is used most commonly for close personal contacts of patients with hepatitis A and for those exposed to contaminated food. It has also been used effectively for controlling outbreaks in institutions such as homes for the mentally handicapped and in nursery schools. Prophylaxis with immunoglobulin is recommended for persons without HAV antibody visiting highly endemic areas. After a period of 6 months the administration of immunoglobulin for travellers needs to be repeated, unless it has been demonstrated that the recipient had developed HAV antibodies. Active immunisation for travellers is therefore preferred and is strongly recommended.

Active Immunisation

Killed hepatitis A vaccines are prepared from virus grown in tissue culture and inactivated with formalin. The first such vaccine was licensed in 1992 and several preparations are available, including a combined hepatitis A and B vaccine. These vaccines are highly immunogenic and provide long-term protection against infection.

In areas of high prevalence, most children have antibodies to HAV by the age of 3 years and such infections are generally asymptomatic. Infections acquired later in life are of increasing clinical severity. It is important, therefore, to protect those at risk because of personal contact or because of travel to highly endemic areas. Other groups at risk of hepatitis A infection include staff and residents of institutions for the mentally handicapped, daycare centres for children, sexually active male homosexuals, intravenous narcotic drug abusers, food handlers, sewage workers, health care workers, military personnel and members of certain low socioeconomic groups in defined community settings. Patients with blood coagulation defects and patients with chronic liver disease should be immunised against hepatitis A.

In some developing countries, the incidence of clinical hepatitis A is increasing as improvements in socioeconomic conditions result in infection later in life; protection by immunisation would be prudent but strategies are yet to be agreed. Global control of hepatitis A will

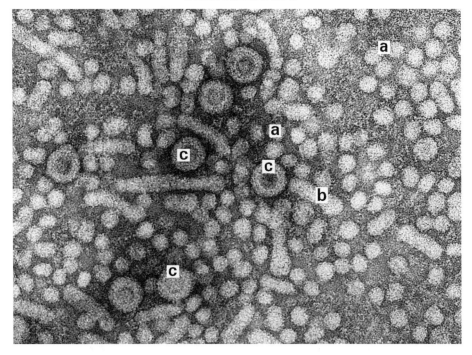

Figure 6.2 Hepatitis B virus: (a) small spherical particles representing excess viral coat protein; (b) tubular structures; (c) double-shelled complete virus. × 400 000

require universal immunisation of infants and will become possible when HAV vaccine is combined in a polyvalent form with other childhood vaccines such as diphtheria, pertussis, tetanus, measles, rubella, mumps and hepatitis B.

HEPATITIS B

Introduction and Definitions

Hepatitis B was referred to originally as 'serum hepatitis'; it is the most common form of parenterally transmitted viral hepatitis, and an important cause of acute and chronic infection of the liver in many countries. More than a third of the world's population had been infected with *hepatitis B virus* (HBV), and WHO estimates that it results in 1–2 million deaths every year.

The clinical features of acute infection resemble those of the other viral hepatitides. The virus persists in approximately 5–10% of immunocompetent adults, and in as many as 90% of infants infected perinatally. Persistent carriage of hepatitis B, defined by the presence of hepatitis B surface antigen (HBsAg) in the serum for more than 6 months, has been estimated to affect about 350 million people worldwide, although not all carriers are infectious. Long-term continuing virus replication may lead to progression to chronic liver disease, cirrhosis and hepatocellular carinoma. Primary liver cancer is one of the 10 most

common cancers worldwide and 80% of such cancers are ascribed to persistent infection with HBV.

Nature of the Virus

The hepatitis B virion is a 42 nm particle comprising an electron-dense nucleocapsid or core (HBcAg) 27 nm in diameter, surrounded by an outer envelope of the surface protein (HBsAg) embedded in membraneous lipid derived from the host cell (Figure 6.2). The surface antigen, originally referred to as Australia antigen, is produced in excess by the infected hepatocytes and is secreted in the form of 22 nm particles and tubular structures of the same diameter.

The nucleocapsid of the virion consists of the viral genome surrounded by the core antigen. The genome, which is approximately 3.2 kilobases in length, has an unusual structure and is composed of two linear strands of DNA held in a circular configuration by base-pairing at the 5′ ends. One of the strands is incomplete and the 3′ end is associated with a DNA polymerase which is able to complete that strand in the presence of deoxynucleoside triphosphates (Figure 6.3).

The genomes of many isolates of HBV have been cloned and the complete nucleotide sequences determined. Analysis of the coding potential of the genome reveals four open reading frames (ORFs) which are conserved between all of these isolates, but there is some

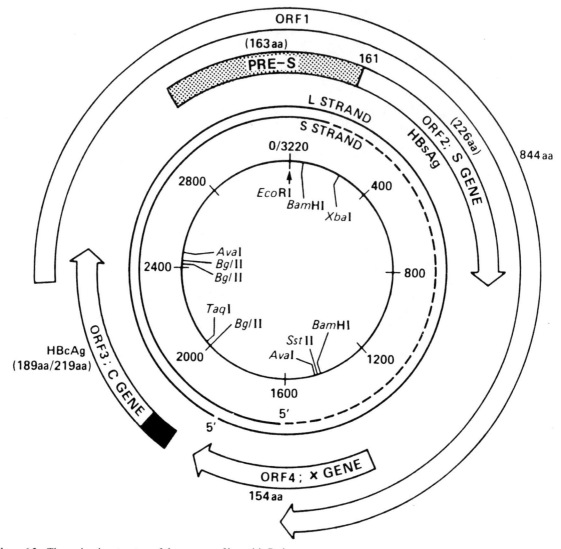

Figure 6.3 The molecular structure of the genome of hepatitis B virus

variation in sequence of up to 12% of nucleotides. The first ORF encodes the various forms of the surface protein. The core ORF has two in-phase initiation codons. The 'precore' region is highly conserved, has the properties of a signal sequence and is responsible for the secretion of HBeAg. The third ORF, which is the largest and overlaps the other three, encodes the viral polymerase. The fourth ORF was designated 'x' because the function of its small gene product was not known initially; however, 'x' has now been demonstrated to be a transcriptional transactivator, and may enhance the expression of other viral proteins.

Surface Antigen Epitopes

There is a variation in the epitopes presented on the surface of the virions and subviral 22 nm particles so that there are several subtypes of HBV which differ in their geographical distribution. All isolates of the virus share a common epitope, a, a domain of the major surface protein which is believed to protrude as a double loop from the surface of the particle. Two other pairs of mutually exclusive antigenic determinants, d or y and w or r, are also present on the major surface protein. These variations have been correlated with single nucleotide changes in the surface ORF which lead to variation in single amino acids in the protein. Four principal subtypes of HBV are recognised: *adw*, *adr*, *ayw* and *ayr*. Subtype *adw* predominates in northern Europe, the Americas and Australasia and also is found in Africa and Asia. Subtype *ayw* is found in the Mediterranean region, eastern Europe, northern and western Africa, the Near East and the Indian subcontinent. In the Far East, *adr* predominates but the rarer *ayr* may occasionally be found in Japan and Papua New Guinea. Other less common variants exist as a result of subdivision of the principal antigenic determinants. More recently, subtyping has been carried out by DNA sequencing of the surface antigen gene, and at least six genotypes, A–F, which differ by more than 8% in the protein sequence, have been identified. Subtyping is mainly of epidemiological or phylogenetic significance.

Surface Antigen mutants

Production of antibodies to the group antigenic determinant *a* mediates crossprotection against all subtypes, as has been demonstrated by challenge with a second subtype of the virus following recovery from an initial experimental infection. The epitope *a* is located in the region of amino acids 124–148 of the major surface protein, and appears to have a double-loop conformation. A monoclonal antibody which recognises a region within this *a* epitope is capable of neutralising the infectivity of HBV for chimpanzees, and competitive inhibition assays using the same monoclonal antibody demonstrate that equivalent antibodies are present in the sera of subjects immunised with either plasma-derived or recombinant hepatitis B vaccine.

During a study of the immunogenicity and efficacy of hepatitis B vaccines in Italy, a number of individuals who had apparently mounted a successful immune response and became anti-surface antibody (anti-HBs)-positive, later became infected with HBV. These cases were characterised by the coexistence of noncomplexed anti-HBs and HBsAg, and there were other markers of hepatitis B infection. Further examination of the antigen using monoclonal antibodies suggested that the *a* epitope was either absent or masked by antibody. Subsequent sequence analysis of the virus from one of these cases revealed a mutation in the nucleotide sequence encoding the *a* epitope, the consequence of which was a substitution of arginine for glycine at amino acid position 145. There is now considerable evidence for a wide geographical distribution of the point mutation in the genome of HBV from guanosine to adenosine at position 587, resulting in an amino acid substitution at position 145 from glycine to arginine in the highly antigenic group determinant *a* of the surface antigen. This is a stable mutation which has been found in viral isolates from children and adults and it has been described in Italy, Singapore, Japan, Brunei, Taiwan, India, USA and elsewhere, and from liver transplant recipients with hepatitis B in the USA, Germany and the UK who had been treated with specific hepatitis B immunoglobulin or humanised hepatitis B monoclonal antibody, and in

patients with chronic hepatitis in Japan and elsewhere.

Other point mutations and substitutions have also been described. The 145 mutation appears to be the most common and to be stable. The region in which this mutation occurs is an important virus epitope to which vaccine-induced neutralising antibody binds, as discussed above, and the mutant virus is not neutralised by antibody to this specificity. The 145 variant virus can replicate as a competent virus, implying that the amino acid substitution does not alter the attachment of the virus to the liver cell. Variants of HBV with altered antigenicity of the envelope protein show that HBV is not as antigenically singular as believed previously and that humoral escape mutation can occur *in vivo*. This finding gives rise to two causes for concern: failure to detect HBsAg may lead to transmission through donated blood or organs, and HBV may infect individuals who are anti-HBs positive after immunisation.

Mathematical modelling suggests that HBV variants may become dominant over the current wild-type virus in 50–100 years.

HBV Precore Mutants

In 1988, a report was published on the nucleotide sequence of the genome of a strain of HBV cloned from the serum of a naturally infected chimpanzee. A surprising feature was a point mutation in the penultimate codon of the precore region to a termination codon. This mutation was found subsequently in some patients with anti-HBe who were positive for HBV DNA in serum by hybridisation. In most cases there was an additional mutation in the preceding codon. Precore variants have been described in many patients with severe chronic liver disease and some failed to respond to treatment with interferon. It has been suggested that the mutants are more pathogenic than the wild-type virus. A precore variant which produces hepatitis B *e* antigen has also been described.

Replication of HBV

HBV and the animal hepadnaviruses are unique among animal DNA viruses in that they replicate through an RNA intermediate.

Epidemiology and Geographical Distribution

Although various body fluids (blood, saliva, menstrual and vaginal discharges, serous exudates, seminal fluid and breast milk) have been implicated in the spread of infection, infectivity appears to be especially related to blood and to body fluids contaminated with blood. The epidemiological propensities of this infection are therefore wide; they include infection by inadequately sterilised syringes and instruments, transmission by unscreened blood transfusion and blood products, by close contact, and by both heterosexual and homosexual contact. Antenatal (rarely) and perinatal (frequently) transmission of hepatitis B infection from mother to child may take place; in some parts of the world (Southeast Asia), perinatal transmission is very common.

It should be noted that transmission of the infection may result from accidental inoculation of minute amounts of blood or fluid contaminated with blood during medical, surgical and dental procedures; immunisation with inadequately sterilised syringes and needles; intravenous and percutaneous drug abuse; tattooing; ear, nose and body piercing; acupuncture; laboratory accidents; and accidental inoculation with razors and similar objects that have been contaminated with blood. Additional factors may be important for the transmission of hepatitis B infection in the tropics; these include traditional tattooing and scarification, blood letting, ritual circumcision and repeated biting by blood-sucking arthropod vectors. Investigation of the role that biting insects may play in the spread of hepatitis B has yielded conflicting results. HBsAg has been detected in several species of mosquitoes and in bed bugs that were either trapped in the wild or fed experimentally on infected blood, but no convincing evidence of replication of the virus in insects has been obtained. Mechanical transmission of the infection, however, is a possibility, but does not appear to be an important route of transmission of HBV.

The incubation period of hepatitis B is 2–6 months. HBsAg first appears during the late stages of the incubation period, 2–8 weeks before the appearance of abnormal liver function tests and jaundice, and is easily detectable by radioimmunoassay or enzyme immunoassay. Enzyme immunoassay is specific and highly sensitive and is used widely in preference to radioisotope methods. The antigen persists during the acute phase of the disease and sharply decreases when antibody to the surface antigen becomes detectable. Antibody of the IgM class to the core antigen is found in the serum after the onset of the clinical symptoms and slowly declines after recovery. Its persistence at high titre suggests continuation of the infection. Core antibody of the IgG class persists for many years and provides evidence of past infection.

During the incubation period and during the acute phase of the illness, surface antigen–antibody complexes may be found in the sera of some patients. Immune complexes have been found by electron microscopy in the sera of all patients with fulminant hepatitis, but are seen only infrequently in nonfulminant infection. Immune complexes also are important in the pathogenesis of other disease syndromes characterised by severe damage of blood vessels, for example, polyarteritis nodosa, some forms of chronic glomerulonephritis, and infantile papular acrodermatitis.

The distribution of infection with HBV varies between geographical regions but it is endemic in all countries and hyperendemic in many parts of the world. Survival of the virus is ensured by the huge reservoir of carriers, estimated conservatively to number in excess of 350 million worldwide, of whom more than 75% are from Southeast Asia and the Western Pacific Region. Other hyperendemic regions include many countries in sub-Saharan Africa. Based on the prevalence of HBsAg among blood donors, a highly selected group, prevalence rates in 1970–1980 extrapolated to the general population were as follows: 0.1% or less in northern Europe, North America and Australasia; up to 5% in southern Europe, the countries bordering the Mediterranean and parts of Central and South America; and 10–20% or more in some parts of Africa, Southeast Asia and the western Pacific.

Reservoir of Infection

The human population. The animal hepadnaviruses do not infect humans and they all have a narrow host range.

Pathology

Pathological changes in the liver include conspicuous focal activation of sinusoidal cells, accumulation of lymphocytes and histiocytes in the parenchyma, often replacing hepatocytes lost by cytolytic necrosis, mainly in the periportal areas, focal degeneration and occasional coagulative necrosis. It has been reported that acute hepatitis B is characterised by more extensive parenchymal abnormalities and inflammatory changes than those found in hepatitis A, whereas portal inflammation and cholestasis are less prominent.

Immune Responses

Antibody and cell-mediated immune responses to various types of antigens are induced during acute infection; however, not all these are protective and, in some instances, may cause autoimmune phenomena that contribute to disease pathogenesis. The immune response to infection with HBV is directed toward at least three antigens: HBsAg, the core antigen, and the e antigen. The view that hepatitis B exerts its damaging effect on hepatocytes by direct cytopathic changes is inconsistent with the persistence of large quantities of the surface antigen in liver cells of many apparently healthy carriers. Additional evidence suggests that the pathogenesis of liver damage in the course of hepatitis B infection is related to the immune response by the host.

Clinical Features and Diagnosis

The clinical features of acute hepatitis B are similar to those of acute hepatitis A and the other hepatitides.

Direct demonstration of virus in serum samples is feasible by visualising the virus particles by electron microscopy, by detecting virus-associated DNA polymerase, and by assay of viral DNA and its amplification by various techniques. All these direct techniques are often impractical in the general diagnostic laboratory, and specific diagnosis must therefore rely on serological tests. Many serological tests, mainly based on ELISA and less commonly used radioimmunoassays, are available for markers of infection with HBV. HBsAg first appears during the late stages of the incubation period and persists during the acute phase, declining rapidly when antibody to the surface antigen (anti-HBs) becomes detectable. Antibody of the IgM class to the core antigen is found in the serum after the onset of clinical symptoms and slowly declines after recovery and is replaced by IgG anticore, which persists for many years. Hepatitis B *e* antigen appears during the acute phase of illness and anti-*e* is detectable with recovery. Molecular techniques are available for HBV DNA polymerase and HBV DNA.

Management and Treatment

There is no specific treatment for acute hepatitis B, but significant developments have been reported with antiviral therapy of chronic infection with interferon α and combination therapy with nucleoside analogues. Lamivudine and famciclovir have been shown to be effective and were licensed recently.

Prevention of Hepatitis B

General measures are based on knowledge of the mode of transmission of hepatitis B and include measures to prevent blood-to-blood contact, the use of sterile syringes, needles and other implements, screening of blood and blood products, protected casual sexual intercourse and other precautions dictated by the propensity for spread of this infection and the huge number of asymptomatic carriers of HBV in the population. The single most effective measure for prevention is active immunisation.

Passive Immunisation with Immunoglobulin

Hepatitis B immunoglobulin is prepared specifically from pooled plasma with high titre of hepatitis B surface antibody and may confer temporary passive immunity under certain defined conditions. The major indication for the administration of hepatitis B immunoglobulin is a single acute exposure to HBV, such as occurs when blood containing surface antigen is inoculated, ingested or splashed on to mucous membranes and the conjunctiva. It should be administered as early as possible after exposure and preferably within 48 h, usually 3 ml (containing $200 IU ml^{-1}$ anti-HBs) in adults. It should not be administered 7 days or more after exposure. It is generally recommended that two doses of hepatitis B immunoglobulin should be given 30 days apart.

Results with the use of hepatitis B immunoglobulin for prophylaxis in neonates at risk of infection with HBV are good if the immunoglobulin is given as soon as possible after birth or within 12 h of birth. Combined passive and active immunisation indicate an efficacy approaching 90%.

Active Immunisation

The major humoral antibody response of recipients of hepatitis B vaccine is to the common *a* epitope, with consequent protection against all subtypes of the virus. First-generation inactivated vaccines were prepared from 22 nm HBsAg particles purified from plasma donations from chronic carriers. These preparations are safe and immunogenic but have been superseded in some countries by recombinant vaccines produced by the expression of HBsAg in yeast cells. The expression plasmid contains only the 3′ portion of the HBV surface ORF and only the major surface protein, without pre-S epitopes, is produced. Vaccines containing pre-S2 and pre-S1 as well as the major surface proteins expressed by recombinant DNA technology are undergoing clinical trial.

In many areas of the world with a high prevalence of HBsAg carriage, such as China and Southeast Asia, the predominant route of transmission is perinatal. Although HBV does not usually cross the placenta, the infants of viraemic mothers have a very high risk of infection at the time of birth, and immunisation protects the infant against perinatal infection.

Immunisation against hepatitis B is now recognised as a high priority in preventive medicine in all countries and strategies for immunisation are being revised. Universal vaccination of infants and adolescents is under examination as the strategy to control the transmission of this infection. More than 90 countries now offer hepatitis B vaccine to all children, including the USA, Canada, Italy, France and most western European countries. However, immunisation against hepatitis B is at present recommended in a number of countries with a low prevalence of hepatitis B only to groups that are at an increased risk of acquiring this infection. These groups include individuals requiring repeated transfusions of blood or blood products, prolonged inpatient treatment, patients who require frequent tissue penetration or need repeated circulatory access, patients with natural or acquired immune deficiency and patients with malignant diseases. Viral hepatitis is an occupational hazard among health care personnel and the staff of institutions for the mentally handicapped, and in some semiclosed institutions. High rates of infection with hepatitis B occur in narcotic drug addicts and intravenous drug abusers, sexually active male homosexuals and prostitutes. Individuals working in areas of high endemicity are also at an increased risk of infections. Women in areas of the world where the carrier state in the group is high are another segment of the population requiring immunisation, in view of the increased risk of transmission of the infection to their offspring. Young infants, children and susceptible persons living in certain tropical and subtropical areas where present socioeconomic conditions are poor and the prevalence of hepatitis B is high should also be immunised.

Hepatitis B and the Traveller

The risk of hepatitis A and hepatitis B to the traveller should not be underestimated. Travellers must take commonsense precautions to reduce the risk of hepatitis B, as outlined above. Great caution is required in any casual intimate or sexual contact, particularly with prostitutes and male homosexuals. All procedures involving penetration of the skin or mucous surfaces must be avoided if possible, including any injections, tattooing, ear and other body piercing, blood transfusion and medical and dental procedures carried out under questionable hygienic conditions.

Immunisation against hepatitis A and hepatitis B is strongly recommended for all travellers to hyperendemic areas, and it is a sensible precaution in case of accidents that require treatment. Combined hepatitis A and B vacines are available, are highly effective and are strongly recommended for all travellers.

HEPATITIS D

Introduction and Definitions

Delta hepatitis was first recognised following the detection of a novel protein, termed delta antigen, by immunofluorescent staining in the nuclei of liver cells in biopsy specimens from patients with chronic active hepatitis B. Later this antigen was found to be a component of a new RNA virus enveloped by the surface antigen of HBV. *Hepatitis delta virus* (HDV) requires a helper function of HBV for its transmission.

Two forms of delta hepatitis infection are known. In the first, a susceptible individual is coinfected with HBV and HDV, often leading to a more severe form of acute hepatitis caused by HBV. In the second, an individual infected chronically with HBV becomes superinfected with HDV. This may cause a second episode of clinical hepatitis and accelerate the course of the chronic liver disease, or cause overt disease in asymptomatic carriers of hepatitis B. HDV is cytopathic and HDAg may be directly cytotoxic.

Delta hepatitis is common in the Mediterranean region, parts of eastern Europe, the Middle East, Africa, South America and some islands in the South Pacific region. It has been estimated that 5% of hepatitis B carriers worldwide (approximately 18 million people) are infected with HDV. In areas of low prevalence of HBV, those at high risk of hepatitis B, particularly intravenous drug abusers, are also at risk of HDV infection.

Nature of the Infectious Agent

HDV is approximately 36 nm in diameter with an RNA genome associated with delta antigen (HDAg) surrounded by an outer lipoprotein coat of HBV, HBsAg. The genome is a closed circular RNA molecule of between 1670 and 1685 nucleotides with some genetic heterogeneity, and resembles those of the satellite viroids and virusoids of plants. Unlike the plant viroids, HDV codes for delta antigen. This is encoded by an ORF in the antigenomic RNA but four other ORFs that are also present in the genome do not appear to be used.

There appear to be three genotypes. Genotype I is the commonest and isolates have been obtained from all parts of the world. Genotype II represent isolates in Taiwan, and this genotype appears to be associated with less severe disease. Genotype III from South America is associated with a fulminant form of hepatitis.

HDV replicates only in hepatocytes and most probably uses the same cell receptors as HBV. Once inside the cells, HDV can replicate in the nuclei in the absence of HBV.

Epidemiology and Geographical Distribution

HDV is bloodborne and is transmitted in the same manner as HBV, essentially by the parenteral route by blood-to-blood contact. The virus is also spread by the sexual route, although less readily than HBV, at a rate of about 10%.

Infection with delta hepatitis has been detected among carriers of HBsAg throughout the world and is referred to as superinfection, but the distribution of HDV is uneven. The infection is endemic in countries bordering the Mediterranean, particularly in southern Italy and in Greece, where as many as 25% of carriers of HBsAg are coinfected. High rates of infection have been found in eastern Europe, particularly in Romania; the former Soviet Union; South America, particularly the Amazon Basin, Venezuela, Columbia (hepatitis de Sierra Nevada de Santa Marta), Brazil (Labrea black fever) and Peru; parts of Africa, particularly West Africa; and some isolated Pacific Islands. In northern Europe, the USA and Australia, HDV infection is relatively uncommon, except among high-risk groups such as intravenous drug abusers and multiply transfused patients such as patients with haemophilia.

Reservoir of Infection

The infection has only been detected in humans.

Pathology

The histological changes are, in general, similar to those of other forms of acute viral hepatitis, with the additional feature of hepatitis delta antigen detected by immunostaining. The histopathological changes in patients with chronic delta hepatitis are those characteristic of chronic hepatitis, except that they tend to be severe.

Clinical Features and Diagnosis

In general, the clinical features of acute coinfection with HDV and HBV are similar to the other forms of hepatitis but tend to be more severe than infection with HBV alone. The picture is complicated, however, and is more severe in some geographical regions, for example South America, and particularly in the case of superinfection with HDV of carriers of hepatitis B with underlying chronic liver disease and active replication of HBV. There is also an association with the genotypes of HDV. Genotype I is predominant throughout the world. Genotype II, which is predominant in Taiwan and in Japan, appears to be less virulent and is associated less frequently with fulminant hepatitis in the acute stage of the disease and in chronic liver disease. Genotype III has so far only been found in northern South America, where hepatitis delta is endemic and acute infections have been associated with severe hepatitis outbreaks with high mortality.

It should be noted that, while generally patients with hepatitis D tend to suffer from a more serious and more often progressive disease than patients with other forms of viral hepatitis, subclinical infections and self-limited infections are common with coinfections of HDV and HBV, in contrast to superinfections with HDV of chronic carriers of HBV.

Diagnosis of hepatitis delta infection is based on a number of tests, including antibodies to delta antigen (anti-HDV), measurements of anti-HDV of the IgM class, detection of delta antigen in serum by immunoassays and in liver biopsies by immunohistochemistry, and detection of HDV RNA by molecular techniques particularly reverse transcriptase polymerase chain reaction (RT-PCR).

Management and Treatment

There is no treatment for acute infection. Interferon α is of limited efficacy in chronic hepatitis D but sustained clearance of HBsAg has been reported in a few patients with short duration of hepatitis D. Other antiviral drugs which have been employed for the treatment of chronic hepatitis B have not been successful. Liver transplantation is a treatment option for end-stage chronic delta liver disease.

Prevention

General protective measures are similar to those recommended for hepatitis B and other bloodborne viral diseases. Prevention of hepatitis D can be achieved by immunisation against hepatitis B in those who are susceptible to hepatitis B. Healthy individuals who are immunised effectively against hepatitis B cannot be coinfected with HDV, as HDV requires a helper function of HBV. A specific HDV vaccine will be required for prevention of superinfection of chronic carriers of HBV, and limited experimental evidence in animals indicates that this approach may be feasible.

HEPATITIS E

Introduction and Definitions

Epidemic hepatitis, which resembles hepatitis A but is caused by a distinct and different virus, has been reported in the Indian subcontinent, Central and Southeast Asia, the Middle East, North and East Africa and Central America. Outbreaks involving tens of thousands of cases have been reported, and *Hepatitis E virus* (HEV) is also a common cause of sporadic acute hepatitis in these countries. Sporadic cases have been seen in other countries and in the highly developed (industrialised) countries in returning travellers from the areas listed above and among migrant labourers. The infection is acute and self-limiting but it is associated with high mortality (10–20%) in pregnant women during the third trimester of pregnancy.

Nature of the Infectious Agent

Morphologically the virus is spherical and unenveloped, measuring 32–34 nm in diameter, with spikes and indentations visible on the surface of the particle. The particles contain a single-stranded positive-sense RNA genome. Physicochemical studies have shown that the virus is very labile and sensitive to freeze–thawing, caesium chloride and pelleting by ultracentrifugation. The genome of the virus is a polyadenylated, positive-sense RNA of about 7200 nucleotides which contains three ORFs. At least seven different genotypes of HEV exist worldwide, and numerous novel strains have been identified from different regions of the world, including the USA, Italy, Greece, Taiwan and China. These novel strains of HEV are distinct from all known strains, such as Burma and Mexico, and from each other. Molecular cloning of the genome of HEV and the expression by recombinant DNA technology of various HEV proteins has led to the development of diagnostic tests, although there are problems of specificity with a number of the assays.

The discovery of a virus, in herds of swine in the USA and Taiwan, that is closely related to HEV is of interest, although it has not yet been established whether this virus can infect humans.

The various properties of HEV suggest that this virus is similar to the caliciviruses; however, HEV resembles most closely the sequences of rubella virus and a plant virus, beet necrotic yellow vein virus. It has therefore been suggested that the three viruses should be placed in separate but related families.

Epidemiology and Geographical Distribution

HEV is spread predominantly by drinking water that is contaminated with human faecal material. Transmission by contaminated food is also likely. The ingestion of contaminated water in regions where HEV is endemic, e.g. in India, Pakistan, Egypt, Burma, China, parts of Russia and the former Soviet Union and parts of Africa and Central America, may result in the infection of thousands of people, predominantly young adults. Sporadic cases are also common in these countries and in returning travellers. Improved serological diagnosis in recent years has led to better understanding of the epidemiology of hepatitis E. For example, seroprevalence studies in Hong Kong indicate that hepatitis E accounts for some 30% of all cases of non-A, non-B, non-C hepatitis, and HEV was found to be a common cause of acute hepatitis in children in Egypt. Sporadic cases in industrialised countries such as western Europe and North America in persons who had not travelled outside their country nor had been in contact with returning travellers are difficult to explain, and the possibility of zoonotic infection, for example by contact with infected swine, needs to be explored.

Reservoir of Infection

Humans are the principal reservoir of infection. A virus similar to HEV has been detected in herds of swine in the USA and Taiwan. It is not known yet whether this virus crosses the species barrier.

Pathology

Histopathological features in the liver are similar to those of other forms of hepatitis, although cholestasis may be more prominent. Ultrastructural changes in the liver, after experimental transmission to nonhuman primates, include the finding of 27–34 nm virus particles during the acute phase of the infection. It is not known whether the virus causes cell injury directly or whether the changes in the liver reflect immune-mediated damage.

Clinical Features and Diagnosis

The average incubation period is a little longer than with hepatitis A, with a mean of 6 weeks. The virus is spread by water and food contaminated by faeces. Secondary cases do not appear to be common. Individual cases cannot be differentiated from other cases of viral hepatitis on the basis of clinical features, although cholestatic features may be more prominent, and fulminant hepatic failure occurs in 10–20% during the third trimester of pregnancy. In epidemics, most clinical cases, which occur predominantly in young adults, will exhibit anorexia, jaundice and hepatomegaly. Serological tests indicate that clinically inapparent cases occur. There is no evi-dence of persistence of the virus in the liver, nor of prolonged excretion in faeces. Chronic liver disease does not occur.

The expression of viral proteins by recombinant DNA technology has led to the development of many diagnostic and research immunoassays. Techniques based on antigenic components of linear peptide epitopes are also available but there is a lack of concordance between many of the assays, particularly with failure to detect hepatitis E antibodies in convalescent sera, and with heterologous strains of the virus. However, considerable improvement of diagnostic reagents has been reported more recently, using other viral proteins and virus-like particles expressed in baculovirus systems. Detection of HEV RNA in serum and faeces by molecular techniques such as Rt-PCR is reliable but limited, at present, to reference laboratories.

Management and Treatment

There is no specific treatment for hepatitis E infection beyond supportive measures.

Prevention

General protective measures are based on strict hygienic precautions and those outlined for hepatitis A in relation to drinking water and consumption of uncooked food. Passive immunisation with immunoglobulin derived from plasma collected in endemic areas does not offer protection against infection with HEV. This reflects the fact that adult populations in endemic regions, who are very likely to have been exposed to HEV in early life, are susceptible to infection with this virus, with high attack rates during epidemics. Vaccines against HEV are under development.

HEPATITIS C

Introduction and Definitions

Specific laboratory diagnosis of hepatitis types A, B and delta revealed an unrecognised form of hepatitis that was clearly unrelated to any of these three types of viruses. Surveys of post-transfusion hepatitis, after the administration of blood and blood products screened for hepatitis B by highly sensitive techniques, provided strong epidemiological evidence of 'guilt by association' of an infection of the liver referred to as non-A, non-B hepatitis.

Attempts to clone the agent of parenterally transmitted non-A, non-B hepatitis were made from a plasma known to contain high titre of the agent by experimental transmission to nonhuman primates. Because it was not known whether the genome was DNA or RNA, a denaturation step was included before the synthesis of complementary DNA so that either DNA or RNA could serve as a template. The resultant cDNA was then inserted into the bacteriophage expression vector λ gt 11 and the libraries screened using serum from a patient with chronic non-A, non-B hepatitis. This led to the detection of a clone that was found to bind to antibodies present in the sera of patients infected with non-A, non-B hepatitis. This clone was used as a probe to detect a larger, overlapping clone in the same library. These sequences hybridised to a positive-sense RNA molecule of about 10 000 nt, which was present in the livers of infected chimpanzees but not in uninfected controls. Homologous sequences were not detected in the chimpanzee or human genomes. By employing a 'walking' technique, the newly detected overlapping clones were used as hybridisation probes to detect further virus-specific clones in the library. Thus, clones covering the entire viral genome were assembled and the completed nucleotide sequence of hepatitis C virus was determined.

Infection with *Hepatitis C virus* (HCV) is prevalent throughout the world, and persistent infection and chronic liver disease are common.

Nature of the Infectious Agent

The amino acid sequence of the nucleocapsid protein is highly conserved among different isolates of HCV. The next domain in the polyprotein also has a signal sequence at its C-terminus and may be processed in a similar fashion. The product is a glycoprotein, which is probably found in the viral envelope and is variably termed E1/S. The third domain may be cleaved by a protease within the viral polyprotein to yield what is probably a second surface glycoprotein, E2/NS1. These proteins are of considerable interest because of their potential use for tests for the direct detection of viral proteins and for the development of HCV vaccines. Nucleotide sequencing reveals that both domains contain hypervariable regions.

The nonstructural region of the HCV genome is divided into regions NS2 to NS5. In the flaviviruses, NS3 has two functional domains, a protease that is involved in cleavage of the nonstructural region of the polyprotein and a helicase that is presumably involved in RNA replication. Motifs within this region of the HCV genome have homology to the appropriate consensus sequences, suggesting similar functions.

The genome of HCV comprises about 10 000 nt of positive-sense RNA, lacks a 3' poly-A tract and has a similar gene organisation to members of the family *Flaviviridae* and is considered the prototype of the genus *Hepacivirus*. All of these genomes contain a single large ORF, which is translated to yield a polyprotein (of around 3000 amino acids in the case of HCV) from which the viral proteins are derived by post-translational cleavage and other modifications.

HCV consists of a family of highly related viruses but nevertheless there are up to 11 distinct genotypes and various subtypes with differing geographical distribution. There is no firm evidence of an association between genotypes and greater pathogenicity. The C, NS3 and NS4 domains are the most highly conserved regions of the genome, and therefore these proteins are the most suitable for use as capture antigens for broadly reactive tests for antibodies to HCV.

The degree of divergence apparent within the viral envelope proteins implies the absence of a broad cross-neutralising antibody response to infection by viruses of different groups. In addition, there is considerable sequence heterogeneity among almost all HCV isolates in the N-terminal region of E2/NS1, suggesting that this region may be under strong immune selection. Sequence changes within this region may occur during the evolution of disease in individual patients and may play an important role in progression to chronicity.

Epidemiology and Geographical Distribution

Infection with HCV occurs throughout the world. Much of the seroprevalence data are based on blood donors, who represent a selected population. The prevalence of antibodies to HCV in blood donors varies from 0.02% to 1.25% in different countries. Higher rates have been found in southern Italy, Spain, central Europe, Japan and parts of the Middle East, with as many as 19% in Egyptian blood donors. Until screening of blood donors was introduced, hepatitis C accounted for the vast majority of non-A, non-B post-transfusion hepatitis. However, it is clear that, while blood transfusion and the transfusion of blood products are efficient routes of transmission of HCV, these represent a small proportion of cases of acute clinical hepatitis in a number of countries (with the exception of patients with haemophilia).

Current data indicate that, in 50% or more of patients in industrialised countries, the source of infection cannot be identified; although transmission by contact with blood and contaminated materials is likely to be important, 35% of patients have a history of intravenous drug misuse. Household contact and sexual exposure do not appear to be major factors in the epidemiology of this common infection, and occupational exposure in the health care setting accounts for about 2% of cases. Transmission of HCV from mother to infant occurs in about 10% of viraemic mothers and the risk appears to be related to the level of viraemia. It should be noted, however, that information on the natural history of hepatitis C is limited because the onset of the infection is often unrecognised and the early course of the disease is indolent and protracted in most patients. Coinfection with HBV is not uncommon.

Reservoir of Infection

The only known reservoir of infection is humans.

Pathology

There is evidence that 50–80% or more of infections with HCV progress to chronic liver disease. Histological examination of liver biopsies from asymptomatic 'healthy' blood donor carriers of HCV show that none has normal liver histology and up to 70% have chronic active hepatitis and/or early cirrhosis. Histological changes at the time of the first biopsy in patients with biochemical chronic hepatitis C also show chronic active hepatitis in the majority. Characteristic histological changes include heavy lymphocytic infiltration in the portal and periportal areas. Progression to cirrhosis is common, and in a number of countries such as Japan, progression to hepatocellular carcinoma is an important feature of chronic hepatitis C. The mechanism underlying carcinogenesis is likely to be associated with the process of fibrosis and regeneration of liver cells, as there is no DNA intermediate in the replication cycle of HCV or integration of viral nucleic acid.

Whether the virus is cytopathic or whether there is an immunopathological element remains unclear, but a combination of factors including gender, excessive alcohol intake and coexisting viral disease (particularly hepatitis B) are important interactive factors.

Clinical Features and Diagnosis

Most acute infections are asymptomatic, fewer than 30% of acute infections have nonspecific symptoms and some develop mild jaundice. Fulminant hepatitis has been described but is uncommon. Extrahepatic manifestations include mixed cryoglobulinaemia, membraneous proliferative glomerulonephritis and porphyria cutanea tarda.

Between 50 and 80% of patients do not clear the virus by 6 months and develop chronic hepatitis. The rate of progression of chronic hepatitis is highly variable. Chronic hepatitis C infection leads to cirrhosis within two decades of the onset of infection in at least 20% of patients. Chronic infection is also associated with an increased risk of hepatocellular carcinoma, which occurs on a background of inflammation and regeneration related to chronic hepatitis over three or more decades. The risk of developing hepatocellular carcinoma is estimated at 1–5% after 20 years, but this varies considerably in different areas of the world. Hepatocellular carcinoma develops more commonly in men than in women.

Current routine diagnostic tests for detection of antibodies to HCV are sensitive and specific and most screening tests are based on enzyme immunoassays, with confirmatory tests based mainly on recombinant immunoblot assays. The presence of antibodies to specific antigenic components of HCV is variable and may or may not reflect viraemia. Detection and monitoring of viraemia are important for management and treatment and sensitive molecular techniques are available for the measurement of HCV RNA.

The identification of specific genotypes is important, with observations suggesting an association between response to antiviral treatment with interferon and particular genotypes.

Management and Treatment

Management of hepatitis C infection is difficult. The patients must be excluded from donating blood and should be advised about the known modes of transmission of the virus, particularly by the parenteral route. Alcohol may act synergistically with HCV in causing liver damage, and alcohol intake must be reduced to the absolute minimum, if any. Consideration of life style risks for other viral infections such as hepatitis B and HIV infection is essential.

Treatment with interferon α has been shown to yield good and sustained responses in 25–40% of selected patients. Studies indicate that younger patients without cirrhosis, with genotype 2 and 3 infection, are more likely to respond to treatment for several months than patients with genotype 1, and better response is obtained in patients with a lower viral load. Combination therapy with ribavirin, a synthetic guanosine nucleoside analogue, indicates that up to 50% of patients who have relapsed after treatment with interferon α have a sustained biochemical and virological response to combined treatment.

Prevention

Vaccines against HCV are not available, despite considerable efforts. Prevention of transmission to contacts is based on measures described for HBV and other blood-borne viruses.

HIV AND AIDS

Introduction and Definitions

The global pandemic of infection with the human immunodeficiency virus (HIV) and the acquired immunodeficiency syndrome (AIDS) has attracted more publicity and political debate than any other infection. The scale of the pandemic is illustrated by the fact that, since the

original description of AIDS in 1981, AIDS has been reported in more than 190 countries, with an estimated number of HIV infections by the beginning of 1998 of more than 30 million people, with over 2.3 million deaths in 1997 alone. The precise incidence of HIV infection in the population is not known but the projected cummulative infections are expected to reach 40 million in the

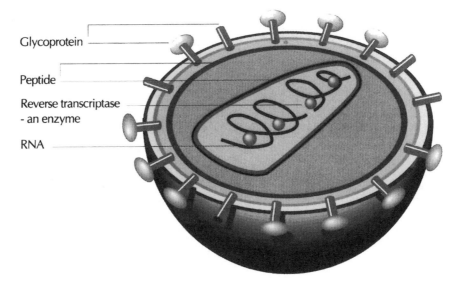

Glycoprotein

Peptide

Reverse transcriptase
- an enzyme

RNA

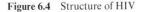

Figure 6.4 Structure of HIV

year 2000. More recently, the pandemic of HIV has evolved into essentially an infection transmitted heterosexually in the developing and poor countries of the world, accounting now for over 75% of all cases of AIDS, and infection of groups defined as at 'high risk' in the industrialised communities. These include young adult homosexual and bisexual males in major cities and their partners, intravenous drug abusers and their sexual partners, and persons who change their sexual partners frequently.

It should be noted that the risk to travellers depends to a large extent on their own behaviour and exposure to risk, and that the epidemic of HIV is not confined by geographical boundaries or to particular regions. There is no evidence of transmission of HIV by purely social and household contact or by leisure activities such as swimming, and there is no evidence of transmission by insects.

Nature of the Infectious Agent

Human retroviruses, as is the case in other vertebrates, exist in two forms: as genetic elements in chromosomal DNA (endogenous retroviruses) and as horizontally-transmitted infectious RNA viruses (exogenous retroviruses). Endogenous retroviruses probably evolved from transposable elements; they are present in most vertebrates and some other life forms as DNA proviruses in the germ line, and most of these are silent or have become pseudogenes.

Exogenous retroviruses are transmissible and three are associated with human disease: *Human T-cell leukaemia virus 1* (HTLV-1) is associated with adult T-cell leukaemia and tropical spastic paraparesis, HTLV-2 is associated with hairy cell leukaemia and HIV is the cause of AIDS.

Retroviruses contain RNA genomes and replication involves transcription of the RNA genome into a double-stranded DNA intermediate by a viral enzyme referred to as reverse transcriptase.

HIV was isolated in 1983. The HIV particle is an icosahedral sphere which is enveloped and has 72 projections consisting of two glycoproteins, gp120 and gp41. Glycoprotein 41 traverses the lipid bilayer. The matrix protein (p17) covers the internal surface of the virus, and p24 constitutes the core shell, which encloses the two copies of the single-stranded HIV RNA (Figure 6.4).

HIV uses the CD4 molecule on the surface of both immature T lymphocytes and mature CD4 + T-helper lymphocytes for initial attachment to cells. This receptor is also present in lower amounts on monocytes, macrophages and antigen-presenting dendritic cells. Other coreceptors are also present to promote the entry of the virus into susceptible cells, where, after uncoating of the virus, reverse transcription, integration and expression of the viral genome occur, followed by viral assembly and release of virus. Infected cells are ultimately destroyed by a direct cytopathic effect, but most of the cells are not killed and may therefore form an important reservoir for persistent infection with virus shedding. There are two major antigenic types of HIV, HIV-1 and HIV-2, which share approximately 40% of genetic homology. While both types cause AIDS, it appears that HIV-2 is less pathogenic; it occurs mainly in West Africa and sporadically elsewhere. Phylogenetic analysis of HIV-1 has revealed at least 10 subtypes, but the more recent identification of highly divergent HIV-1 strains, principally from patients in Cameroon, led to classification of HIV-1 into two groups. The major (M) group corresponds to HIV-1 strains disseminated widely throughout the world, and an outlier group (O) corresponding to the highly divergent

HIV-1 strain, identified originally in Cameroon but found subsequently in Gabon, Europe and the USA.

Epidemiology and Geographical Distribution

The global dissemination of HIV was referred to in the introduction to this section. In industrialised countries most reported cases of AIDS occur in one or more of the following groups:

- Sexually active homosexual or bisexual men (genital–oral, genital–anal and genital–genital sex)
- Intravenous drug abusers
- Patients with haemophilia and others with severe co-agulation disorders who received unheated blood factor concentrates
- Recipients of unscreened blood transfusions (in the past)
- Sexual partners of the above groups
- Children born to mothers infected with HIV.

Since the late 1980s there has been a substantial decrease in HIV prevalence among men who have sex with men, but an increase in heterosexual transmission, with the highest rates in women.

Another epidemiological pattern is emerging in countries of eastern Europe and the former Soviet Union, where infection with HIV has increased dramatically, mainly in association with intravenous drug abuse and unprotected sexual transmission. Nosocomial transmission of HIV accounts for over 50% of children with AIDS in Romania and the Russian Federation. The epidemic in sub-Saharan Africa involves well over 20 million people, and an estimated 4–5 million children. The prevalence rate in the population ranges from 1–15 to 20% or more. About 7500 people are infected daily. Infection is typically the result of heterosexual and perinatal transmission. HIV-2 is found principally in West Africa, with a prevalence of about 10%. The prevalence of HIV and AIDS is increasing dramatically in Asia, with most cases (approaching 90%) occuring in India, Burma and Thailand. Initially most infections were in intravenous drug abusers, spilling rapidly into prostitutes and their clients and into the general population. The predominant mode of spread of HIV in Asia is by heterosexual transmission. The prevalence of infection among pregnant women is increasing rapidly. The pattern of the prevalence of HIV infection and AIDS in the Caribbean and Latin America is similar to that described initially in North America, but with an apparently rapid increase in heterosexual transmission since the late 1980s.

Reservoir of Infection

The reservoir of infection is humans. The origin of HIV is still debated and the distant evolutionary relationship with *Simian immunodeficiency virus* is being examined.

Pathology

Antigen-presenting cells which prime naive T lymphocytes form a complex system of cells referred to as dendritic cells. These cells express class I and class II molecules of the major histocompatibility complex (MHC) and specific chemokines, which act as coreceptors with CD4 molecules. CD4 permits binding of HIV-1 gp120 to cells, but the chemokine coreceptors allow fusion and penetration of the virus into the host cell. Dendritic cells are readily infected by HIV-1 and support viral replication in the presence of activated lymphocytes, and 95% of HIV-1 variants transmitted are macrophage-tropic. The Langerhans cells are either infected by the virus or pick up the virus and then migrate to regional lymph nodes. The virus is disseminated rapidly throughout the lymphoid system and later enters the bloodstream and further replication occurs. After transition to the chronic phase of the disease, virus particles trapped in the follicular dendritic cell network become the dominant form of HIV-1, and the number of circulating virus particles falls. Latent infection of CD4+ T lymphocytes results in the establishment of replication-competent HIV-1 proviral DNA, a reservoir for the virus.

The intrinsic ability of HIV-1 to mutate rapidly allows the virus to escape immune surveillance and specific immune responses so that it is able to continue to infect cells and replicate, representing, together with a stable reservoir of virus, a continuous source for infection of CD4+ T lymphocytes. CD4+ T cells are damaged in several different ways: virus replication can destroy the cell as a result of damage of the cell membrane; viral genetic material may interfere with the metabolism of the cell; and the virus may infect and destroy progenetior lymphoid cells. CD4+ T cells may also be destroyed by autoimmune reactions that kill uninfected cells, and is likely that anti-HIV immune effector cells kill many cells infected with the virus.

The number of circulating CD4+ lymphocytes correlates significantly with the development of bacterial, fungal, parasitic and viral opportunistic infections, including *Mycobacterium tuberculosis*, *M. avium* complex and *Streptococcus pneumoniae* infections, candidiasis, cryptococcosis, histoplasmosis, coccidioidomycosis, toxoplasmosis, enteric helminthic infections, *Pneumocystis carinii* pneumonia, herpes zoster, mucocutaneous herpes, polyomavirus and others. Various tumours are also found in patients with AIDS including non-Hodgkin lymphomas, Kaposi sarcoma, cancer of the central nervous system, invasive cervical cancer and others.

Clinical Features and Diagnosis

Primary HIV infection is often asymptomatic but may present as an acute illness with fever, sweating, myalgia and arthralgia, sore throat, lymphadenopathy, nausea and vomiting, diarrhoea, headache and other neurological symptoms and a rash lasting between 2 and 4 weeks, but symptoms such as fatigue may persist for many weeks or months. Most patients then become asymptomatic, usually for years. The incubation period is 2–4 weeks after infection, with a range of 5–90 days or longer. Following primary infection, there may be a slow and progressive decrease in the number of CD4 + cells and an increase in CD8 + cells.

AIDS is the late manifestation of infection with HIV, characterised by a marked depletion of CD4 + cells, resulting in a reversal of CD4 + : CD8 + cell ratio. The progressive immunodeficiency is accompanied by a wide range of opportunistic infections, neoplasms, and may present with AIDS encephalopathy (AIDS dementia complex) and other neurological complications that may occur in the absence of opportunistic infections. The Centers for Disease Control (Atlanta, USA) definition of AIDS, adopted in the USA in 1992, is helpful. The definition is based on a positive test for HIV and the following:

1. A CD4 + T cell number of less than $200\,mm^{-3}$ (the normal count is $600–1000\,mm^{-3}$) of whole blood, or a CD4 + T cell/total lymphocytes percentage of less than 14%, or
2. A CD4 + T cell number of $200\,mm^{-3}$ or over and any of the following conditions: fungal diseases, including candidiasis, coccidioidomycosis, cryptococcosis, histoplasmosis, isosporiasis; *Pneumocystis carinii* pneumonia; cryptosporidosis, or toxoplasmosis of the brain, bacterial diseases including pulmonary tuberculosis and other *Mycobacterium* species, recurrent *Salmonella* septicaemia; viral diseases, including cytomegalovirus infection, HIV-related encephalopathy, HIV wasting syndrome, chronic ulcer or bronchitis due to herpes simplex, or progressive multifocal leucoencephalopathy; malignant diseases such as invasive cervical carcinoma, Kaposi sarcoma, Burkitt lymphoma, primary lymphoma of the brain, or immunoblastic lymphoma; recurrent pneumonia due to any age.

Laboratory screening tests for HIV-1 and HIV-2 are based mostly on a variety of ELISAs based on antigens consisting of viral lysates or recombinant proteins corresponding to the immunodominant epitopes of HIV-1 (including the group 0 variants) and HIV-2. Rapid and simple laboratory tests are also used in developing countries, based on filtering serum through a membrane coated with recombinant HIV-1 and HIV-2 antigens. Confirmatory assays are generally based on Western blot techniques, but other immunoblot methods are also available. Strain serotyping methods and subtyping techniques are available. Virus isolation is carried out in high security laboratories. PCR and nested-PCR is used for the detection of proviral HIV DNA. The amount of virus in peripheral blood (viral load) is assessed by measurement of plasma RNA. p24 antigenaemia is measured by ELISA. Genotypic drug resistance assays are important for treatment and monitoring antiviral therapy.

Management and Treatment

The management of the patient with HIV is dictated by the level of disease activity that is indicated by the degree of immunodeficiency and viral load; it includes the management of opportunistic infections and other syndromes associated with immunodeficiency and malignancy.

There has been rapid and substantial progress in the development and availability of specific antiviral drugs since 1987. These include nucleoside inhibitors of reverse transcriptase and the more recent introduction of protease inhibitors. The optimal treatment is by a combination of drugs with substantial clinical benefit, and several nucleoside reverse transcriptase inhibitors, nonnucleotide reverse transcriptase inhibitors and protease inhibitors are available. Treatment and virological monitoring should be carried out under the supervision of specialists. Note that HIV resistance to all classes of antiretroviral drugs has now been described and monitoring for genotypic resistance is important. Treatment should be aimed at preventing or delaying the emergence of drug resistance.

Prevention

The key approaches are health education and prevention of infection by immunisation. Travellers are not at increased risk of infection with HIV unless they engage in risk behaviour (see below) or are exposed to unscreened or inadequately screened blood transfusion or inadequately sterilized syringes, needles and medical and surgical instruments. Unsafe sexual practices and intravenous exposure to illicit drugs pose a high risk of infection to travellers. The following explicit recommendations will reduce the risk of infection:

- Avoid mouth contact with the vagina, penis or anus.
- Avoid all sexual practices that could cause tears in the lining of the vagina, anus and rectum, or the penis.
- Avoid sexual activities with partners from high-risk groups: prostitutes (female and male), homosexual men (particularly those who change partners frequently), bisexuals and intravenous drug users (male and female).
- Avoid all other activities that involve the exchange of body fluids.
- If the health status of the partner is not known, a condom must be used for all sexual practices in which the exchange of body fluids occurs (this includes wet kissing, oral sex—either male or female), and obviously vaginal or anal sexual intercourse.

There are enormous hurdles to be surmounted in vaccine development against HIV. These include the considerable genetic heterogeneity of HIV strains and the emergence of new genetic variants; incomplete knowledge of viral–host interactions; and the practical complexity of ensuring the safety of candidate vaccines and mounting clinical trials and later efficacy vaccine studies. Nevertheless, progress is being made and the following are some candidate vaccines undergoing clinical trial:

- Recombinant subunit vaccines: gp160 and gp120
- Recombinant particle vaccines: Ty-p24 virus-like particles
- Recombinant virus vectors: vaccinia-gp160; vaccinia-gp160, gag, pol; canarypox gp160; canarypox gp120TM, gag, protease; canarypox gp120 TM, gag, pol, nef

- Recombinant bacteria: attenuated *Salmonella typhi* gp120
- Synthetic peptides: V3 (envelope); p17 (core); V3 fused with T-cell helper gag epitope; V3 fused with T-helper env epitope; multiple V3 on polylysine backbone
- DNA-based immunisation: gp160 and rev; gag
- Combination of some of the above preparations.

HIV vaccine development is a high priority but progress is likely to be slow, particularly because of the inherent difficulties associated with safety and efficacy.

VIRAL GASTROENTERITIS

Introduction and Definitions

Human gastroenteritis can be caused by bacteria, viruses and parasites, and diarrhoeal illness is second only to respiratory diseases in terms of morbidity and mortality, with very high mortality in children in the developing countries.

Viruses that cause human gastroenteritis belong to different virus families: rotaviruses account for about 70% of gastroenteritis in children; enteric adenoviruses approximately 12%; caliciviruses, including small round structured viruses (SRSVs), 8%; and astroviruses are responsible for 8% of all cases of gastroenteritis in children. Other viruses can also infect the gastrointestinal tract in conditions of immunosuppression but these are not considered in this section.

There are two epidemiological patterns. During childhood, viral diarrhoea occurs as an endemic disease, caused mainly by group A rotaviruses, subgroup F adenoviruses, classical human caliciviruses and astroviruses. The principal mode of transmission is by the faecal–oral route, by close contact and fomites. The second pattern is epidemic, affecting all ages, and caused mainly by SRSVs and at times by group B and C rotaviruses and by astroviruses. Infection is transmitted frequently by contaminated food or water.

Nature of the Infectious Agent

Rotaviruses

These viruses have a genome of 11 segments of double-stranded RNA encoding six structural proteins and five nonstructural proteins within a wheel-like structure, as seen by electron microscopy. Group A rotaviruses, of which there are 10 serotypes, are major pathogens in humans and animals; groups B and C are not important causes of illness in infants and young children.

After neonatal or primary infection a specific serotype humoral immune response develops, but there is also partial protection against subsequent infections by other rotavirus serotypes. Second, third and fourth infections confer progressively greater protection. The immune cor-

relates of protection from rotavirus infection (which can be without symptoms) and disease are not fully understood.

Adenoviruses

Adenoviruses are large icosohedral viruses measuring 70–80 nm in diameter, with a linear double-stranded DNA. There are more than 100 antigenic types, of which 49 distinct serotypes in six different subgroups, A–F, infect humans, causing mainly acute respiratory disease, follicular conjunctivitis, epidemic keratoconjunctivitis, cystitis and, less frequently, gastroenteritis. Adenoviruses associated with gastroenteritis belong to subgroup F, serotypes 40 and 41.

Small Round Structured Viruses (SRSVs)

The first member of this group was recognised by immune electron microscopy, during a large outbreak of acute gastroenteritis in a school in Norwalk in the USA, as a 27–35 nm particle. After cloning and sequencing of *Norwalk virus* it was classified as a calicivirus. The genome consists of a single-stranded RNA, and the name calicivirus describes a particle with cup-shaped depressions on its surface. The subsequent identification of other viruses causing gastroenteritis led to a classification based on the morphology of SRSVs comprising *Norwalk virus* and Norwalk-like viruses with a diameter of 27–35 nm, so-called classical caliciviruses with a diameter of 30–40 nm and astroviruses with a diameter of 28–30 nm. Picornaviruses with a 27 nm diameter and parvoviruses with a diameter of 18–20 nm are included among the 'featureless' small round viruses (SRVs).

Epidemiology, Clinical Features and Geographical Distribution

Viral gastroenteritis occurs throughout the world.

The incubation period of rotavirus gastroenteritis is 1–2 days with a sudden onset of illness with watery diarrhoea lasting 4–7 days, vomiting and rapid dehydration. The spectrum of illness ranges from mild to severe. Virtually all children become infected during the first 3–5 years of life, but severe diarrhoea and dehydration occur primarily in children under the age of 3 years.

Rotavirus is also an important cause of nosocomial gastroenteritis. Rotavirus infection in adults occurs among those caring for children with diarrhoea, in travellers and in the elderly. The virus is transmitted mainly by the faecal–oral route.

The incubation period of SRSVs ranges from 10 to 48 h; diarrhoea, vomiting or both last for 1–2 days. The illness occurs typically in older children and adults, and is uncommon in preschool children. Outbreaks occur in schools, camps and holiday centres, hospitals, cruise ships and so on, and are associated with ingestion of contaminated drinking or recreational water (swimming pools), uncooked shellfish, eggs, cold foods and salads. The faecal–oral route alone does not, however, explain the explosive outbreaks that have been documented. Very large numbers of virus particles are present in vomit and vomiting is often projectile, so aerosol transmission, particularly in enclosed spaces, is likely.

Human astrovirus infections occur in childhood, often without symptoms, and in the elderly, and occasionally as the cause of foodborne outbreaks of diarrhoea. Transmission is by the faecal–oral route, person-to-person contact and possibly fomites. The seasonal incidence is highest during the winter.

Pathology

The pathogenesis of rotavirus infection is based on increasing necrosis of the gut epithelium, leading to loss of villi, loss of digestive enzymes, reduction of absorption and increased osmotic pressure, resulting in diarrhoea. These changes are followed by increased fluid secretion. The onset of dehydration may be rapid. Pathological changes in the ileum resulting from infection with SRSVs include blunting of intestinal villi, crypt hyperplasia and cytoplasmic vacuolation and lymphocytic infiltration of the lamina propria.

Pathological changes observed in animals infected with species-specific astroviruses reveal infection of mature enterocytes at the tip of the villi of the small intestine.

Diagnosis

Specific diagnosis of viral gastroenteritis is relatively easy by electron microscopy and immune electron microscopy of faecal extracts. The principal routine techniques for rotavirus include ELISA and passive particle agglutination. Molecular techniques are also available. Enteric adenoviruses are detected in faecal extracts mainly by ELISA using subgroup F-specific monoclonal antibodies, and by electron microscopy and immune electron micro-scopy. Laboratory diagnosis of SRSVs and astroviruses is by electron microscopy or immune electron microscopy, ELISA and RT-PCR.

Management and Treatment

Oral rehydration with fluids containing sugar and electrolytes is most important, and in severe cases, particularly in children, rapid fluid replacement intravenously is a life-saving measure. If the ability to drink is lost, parenteral administration of fluid is a medical emergency. Oral bismuth subsalicylate has been found to be beneficial in children with acute watery diarrhoea.

Antibiotics have no place in the treatment of viral gastroenteritis and specific antiviral therapy is not available.

In general, travellers' diarrhoea does not require intensive treatment apart from general supportive measures, but blood in the stools and persistent diarrhoea longer than a few days requires urgent medical attention and laboratory investigation.

Protective Measures and Prevention

General food and water hygiene measures and strict personal hygiene are important, as are sensible precautions with the consumption of food and water. Viruses causing gastroenteritis are highly contagious and spread can be rapid. Careful handwashing, personal hygiene, disinfection, and safe disposal of contaminated material and faeces are important. Outbreaks in hospitals, nurseries, holiday centres and cruise ships require meticulous application of these measures.

A rotavirus vaccine, a rhesus-based rotavirus vaccine-tetravelent (RRV-TV), has been licensed in the USA and elsewhere. RRV-TV is a live attenuated oral vaccine which incorporates a rhesus monkey rotavirus strain (with human serotype G3 specificity) and three single-gene human–rhesus reassortants. Immunisation early in life, which mimics the child's first natural infection, will not prevent all subsequent disease but should prevent most cases of severe rotavirus diarrhoea including hospital admission for treatment. The US Advisory Committee on Immunization Practices (1999a) recommends routine immunisation with three oral doses of RRV-TV for infants at the age of 2, 4 and 6 months. This vaccine can be administered together with DPT, Hib vaccine, oral polio vaccine, inactivated polio vaccine and hepatitis B vaccine. RRV-TV is effective but has now been withdrawn owing to a number of adverse events.

Vaccines against other viruses causing gastroenteritis are not available.

POLIOMYELITIS AND OTHER ENTEROVIRUS INFECTIONS

Introduction and Definitions

The enteroviruses belong to the family *Picornaviridae* (small RNA viruses) comprising five genera: enteroviruses, rhinoviruses, hepatoviruses, cardioviruses and aphthoviruses. Most infections with enteroviruses are inapparent, but some may cause serious infection of the central nervous sytem, heart, skeletal muscles, liver and pancreas.

Sixty-six serotypes of enterovirus have been isolated from humans and can replicate in the epithelium of the nasopharynx, gastrointestinal tract, lymphoid tissue, reticuloendothelial system, and, in the case of HAV the liver. The virus may spread to other organs and may cause severe disease—for example, the central nervous system (polioviruses), the myocardium, causing myocarditis (coxsackie viruses), and others. Prevention by immunisation is limited so far to poliomyelitis and hepatitis A. From the point of view of the traveller, poliovirus and HAV are considered to be the most important of the enteroviruses. This section considers, therefore, only poliomyelitis; hepatitis A infection has been discussed earlier in this chapter. It should be noted that two genera of the *Picornaviridae* cause diseases of animals: the cardioviruses cause disease in mice, and the aphthoviruses cause foot-and-mouth disease of cattle.

Nature of Poliovirus

All the picornaviruses have similar morphology, molecular and structural properties and replication strategies. The virion is an icosahedral, unenveloped small particle measuring approximately 27 nm in diameter and containing a single positive strand of RNA of approximately 7500 nucleotides. Picornaviruses multiply in the cytoplasm, and the RNA acts as a messenger to synthesize viral macromolecules. Viral RNA replicates in complexes associated with the cytoplasmic membranes.

There are three serotypes of polioviruses, 1–3. The virus enters the body by mouth and replication occurs in the oropharynx and the cells lining the alimentary tract. A viraemic phase follows. Within the central nervous system the virus spreads along nerves and extensive replication destroys motor neurons, particularly of the anterior horn cells of the spinal cord, leading to paralysis. Virus is shed from the throat and in the faeces. Faecal shedding may continue for several weeks.

Epidemiology and Geographical Distribution

The major route of transmission of poliovirus is faecal–oral where sanitation and standards of hygiene are poor. Pharyngeal spread is relatively more important in areas where sanitation is good and, in the past, during epidemics in industrialised countries.

Poliomyelitis can affect all age groups. In areas with poor sanitation most infants were infected early in life and acquired active immunity while still protected by maternal antibodies. The infection occurred worldwide before the introduction of large-scale immunisation, and the highest incidence of clinical disease was in temperate zones and in the more developed countries, most commonly during summer and autumn. It was expected that poliomyelitis caused by wild-type virus would be eradicated from most (if not all) countries at the beginning of the third millenium, and it is likely that polioviruses found in nature will probably be derived from oral poliovirus vaccine strains.

The incubation period is commonly 7–14 days for paralytic cases, with a reported range of 3–35 days. Cases are most infectious 7–10 days before and after the onset of symptoms, and virus may be shed in the faeces for 6 weeks or longer.

Reservoir of Infection

The reservoir of infection is human, most frequently persons with inapparent infection, especially children.

Clinical Features and Diagnosis

Most infections are asymptomatic or range in severity from nonparalytic fever, headache, nausea and gastrointestinal symptoms to asceptic meningitis and paralysis. Most clinical illnesses resolve without paralysis. The clinical syndrome may be biphasic, with a minor illness followed by remission, but subsequently develops into a major severe illness. Paralysis of respiratory muscles and swallowing usually threatens life. Paralysis is typically asymmetric. Case fatality rates in paralytic cases vary from 2 to 10% in different epidemics and increase dramatically with age.

Differential clinical diagnosis includes postinfectious polyneuritis, Guillain–Barré syndrome and other causes of paralysis. Differential diagnosis of acute nonparalytic poliomyelitis includes asceptic meningitis, bacterial meningitis, brain abscess and encephalitis.

Laboratory diagnosis is based on viral isolation from faecal samples 24–48 h apart, and type identification based on molecular techniques. Faecal samples should also be obtained from household and other close contacts.

It should be noted that other enteroviruses, particularly *Coxsackie virus A7* and *Human enterovirus 71*, occasionally cause poliomyelitis-like illness.

Prevention

Inactivated (Salk) and live attenuated (Sabin) vaccines

VIRUS INFECTIONS

have been used for mass immunisation most successfully, and WHO set a target of global eradication of poliomyelitis by the year 2000. Wild-type poliovirus transmission was eradicated from the Americas in 1991 and has been eradicated from many other industrialised countries. The risk of oral polio vaccine-associated poliomyelitis has been estimated by WHO at between 0.5 and 3.4 cases per million susceptible children. This has re-established a role for the use of inactivated vaccine, and a strategy for immunisation with the Salk vaccine is being established in the USA and elsewhere. In the meantime, routine universal immunisation with the live attenuated oral poliovirus vaccine continues in the majority of countries and no adult should remain unimmunised against poliomyelitis.

Booster (reinforcing) immunisation for adults is recommended for travellers to areas or countries where poliomyelitis is endemic.

INFLUENZA

Introduction and Definitions

Influenza is a highly infectious acute respiratory disease causing epidemics and pandemics throughout the world. While it is usually a self-limiting disease, it can be complicated by bronchitis and secondary bacterial pnuemonia, and in children by otitis media. Primary influenza virus pneumonia is rare but carries a high case fatality rate. Epidemics are generally associated with a large number of excess deaths among the elderly and among those with underlying chronic respiratory and cardiac diseases, renal or metabolic diseases and immunosuppression. Epidemics and pandemics occur at unpredictable intervals.

There are three types of influenza virus, A, B and C. Type A causes widespread epidemics and pandemics, type B is associated with regional and widespread epidemics, and type C is associated with sporadic cases and minor local outbreaks.

Nature of the infectious agent

The influenza viruses are spherical enveloped RNA viruses measuring 80–120 nm in diameter, and filamentous enveloped particles may also occur.

The RNA genome of influenza A and B viruses consists of eight separate segments containing 10 genes, whereas influenza C virus contains only seven RNA segments. The RNA segments are complexed with nucleoprotein to form a nucleocapsid with helical symmetry which is enclosed in an envelope consisting of a lipid bilayer with two surface glycoproteins, the haemagglutinin and the neuraminidase. Influenza C virus has a single surface glycoprotein.

The three influenza viruses are classified on the basis of the nucleoprotein, which is stable and has no serological crossreactivity. The haemagglutinin and neuraminidase undergo genetic variation in influenza A and B viruses as a result of genetic reassortment, whereas the glycoprotein of influenza C virus is stable.

Influenza A subtypes are classified by the antigenic uniqueness of the surface glycoproteins, with the haemagglutinin designated as H and the neuraminidase as N. Fifteen subtypes of haemagglutinin (H1–H15) and nine subtypes of neuraminidase (N1–N9) have been identified, and variants are described by the geographical site of isolation, the culture number and year of isolation, e.g. A/Japan/305/57(H2N2), A/Hong Kong/1/68(H3N2), A/Sydney/5/97(H3N2), and, in the case of influenza B, B/USSR/2/87, B/Beijing/184/93, and so on. Various influenza A subtypes have been isolated from wild and domestic aquatic birds, from pigs, horses, mink, seals and whales. Animal reservoirs are believed to be the sources of new human subtypes, probably by genetic reassortment with human strains facilitated by the segmented viral genome. The emergence of completely new subtypes (referred to as antigenic shift) occurs at irregular and unpredictable intervals and only with influenza A viruses. Completely new subtypes are responsible for pandemics. Minor antigenic variations (antigenic drift) are associated with annual epidemics and regional outbreaks.

Epidemiology and Geographical Distribution

Influenza viruses are transmitted readily by airborne spread by sneezing, coughing or speaking, particularly among crowds in enclosed spaces. A single infected person can transmit the virus to a large number of susceptible individuals. Transmission also occurs by direct contact through droplet spread and also by contact with dried mucus.

The incubation period is short, usually 1–5 days.

In temperate zones, epidemics tend to occur during the winter months (northern hemisphere from November to March, southern hemisphere from April to September), and in the tropics influenza can occur throughout the year but often in the rainy season.

Age-specific attack rates during an epidemic reflect existing immunity from past experience with strains related to the epidemic subtype and the extent of exposure, so that the incidence of infection is often highest in children of school age.

Reservoir of Infection

Humans are the reservoir for human infections, and animal reservoirs (see above) are believed to be the sources of new human influenza A subtypes.

Pathology

Influenza viruses replicate in the columnar epithelium cells of the respiratory tract. The viruses attach to permissive cells through the haemagglutinin subunit, which binds to cell membrane glycoproteins or glycolipids containing the viral receptor N-acetylneuraminic acid. Replication of the virus is completed within about 6 h and kills the host cell, and desquamation of the superficial mucosa occurs. Virus is shed together with desquamated cells through the respiratory tract by mucociliary transport. Virus can be recovered from respiratory secretions for about 3–8 days. Viraemia is rare.

Occasionally, the infection may involve the alveoli, resulting in interstitial viral pneumonia which is associated with a high mortality. In most cases with pneumonia, the pneumonia is caused by secondary bacterial infection.

Clinical Features and Diagnosis

The clinical picture is of abrupt onset of fever, malaise, headache, sore throat, myalgia, coryza and a dry cough lasting 2–5 days. The clinical features in children and in the elderly may differ in some respects and children may present with febrile convulsions, conjunctivitis, croup, otitis media, bronchitis and gastrointestinal symptoms. Diagnosis based on clinical presentation is difficult but more likely if influenza is known to be common in the community.

Specific diagnosis is based on viral isolation by culture, detection of viral antigens in nasopharyngeal cells by immunostaining or in respiratory secretions by ELISA, detection of viral nucleic acid and by antibody tests of paired samples showing a rise in specific antibody by haemagglutination inhibition, ELISA, complement fixation and neuralisation. Rapid bedside diagnostic tests are expected to be introduced shortly.

It should be noted that virus isolation is critical in outbreaks in order to characterise the virus fully and identify antigenic shifts and drifts. Precise characterisation of the virus is essential for the formulation of vaccines for the following year.

Management and Treatment

Management is symptomatic in uncomplicated cases, but specific antiviral drugs are available and are indicated under certain circumstances.

Amantadine and rimantadine have 70–90% efficacy in preventing influenza A if given prophylatically to adults or children during the period of exposure to the virus. These drugs are not free of side-effects and viral resistance may emerge during treatment. Rimantadine has fewer side-effects. These drugs may be given prophylactically for individuals who had not been vaccinated and are in high-risk groups for complications (see below). The drugs may be used therapeutically and will ameliorate the severity and during of illness if given within 48 h of the onset of symptoms.

Newer drugs which inhibit specifically the neuraminidase of both influenza A and B are completing phase III clinical trials and have been licensed in a number of countries (Zanamavir or Relenza, which is administered by inhalation). Zanamavir (Relenza) is effective in preventing influenza in healthy adults, and, when given therapeutically within 36 h of the onset of illness, reduces the duration of illness by 1–2 days. Oseltamivir (Tamiflu) is a similar drug which can be administered orally.

Prevention

Inactivated influenza vaccines have been used for some 40 years; they provide protection against illness in 50–90% in healthy young adults but this may be lower in other groups, such as the elderly. The vaccine strains are grown in eggs (and therefore contraindicated for individuals with egg allergy) and formulated according to the prevailing current strains. In 1999 the recommended trivalent vaccine was influenza A H1N1, influenza A H3N2 and influenza B. The vaccine is given parenterally in one dose.

The risk of influenza during travel varies and depends on the time of the year and destination (see above) and contact with people from different parts of the world where influenza may be prevalent. Influenza can be a severe illness, especially in groups at high risk of developing complications. These include the following:

- Persons 65 years old or older
- Residents of nursing homes and any other long-term care facilities that house persons of any age who have chronic medical conditions
- Adults and children who have chronic disorders of the pulmonary or cardiovascular systems, including children with asthma
- Adults and children who have the following medical conditions:
    Chronic metabolic diseases (e.g. diabetes mellitus)
    Renal dysfunction
    Haemoglobinopathies
    Immunosuppression
- Children and teenagers (aged 6 months–18 years) receiving long-term aspirin therapy
- Women who will be in their second or third trimester of pregnancy during the influenza season.

    Vaccine is also recommended for the following groups:

- Healthcare personnel
- Employees of nursing homes and long-term care facilities who have contact with patients or residents
- Providers of home care to persons at high risk
- Household members (including children) of person in high-risk groups.

The following should also consider vaccination before travel:

- Those travelling to tropical areas at any time of the year if they have not been immunised against influenza during the most recent autumn or winter

- Those travelling in a large organised tourist group (e.g. in cruise ships, long-haul buses) at any time of the year.

Live attenuated, cold-adapted influenza virus vaccines which are administered intranasally are in use in Russia and are under development in Australia, the USA and elsewhere.

GENITAL HERPES

Introduction and Definitions

Herpesviruses are disseminated widely in nature and infect most animal species. Eight herpesviruses have been isolated from humans so far: *Human herpesvirus 1* (HHV-1; *Herpes simplex 1*, HSV-1); HHV-2 (*Herpes simplex 2*, HSV-2); HHV-3 (*Varicella-zoster virus*, VZV); HHV-4 (*Epstein–Barr Virus*, EBV); HHV-5 (*Human cytomegalovirus*); and HHV-6, -7 and -8.

Herpesviruses share a number of biological properties, including the ability to code for a large number of enzymes involved in nucleic acid metabolism, synthesis of viral DNA and capsid assembly take place in the nucleus, and the viral envelope is acquired during migration from the nucleus, production of infectious virus is accompanied by cell destruction, and the herpesviruses establish latent infection in the host.

The herpesviruses affecting humans are probably the viruses that have been studied most extensively. Genital herpes, caused most frequently by HSV-2 but also by HSV-1, is the most relevant to the traveller.

Nature of the Infectious Agent

The herpes simplex viruses belong to a family of large enveloped DNA viruses, measuring 120–300 nm, containing linear double-stranded DNA. HSV-1 and HSV-2 are closely related, with approximately 70% genomic homology.

HSV-1, HSV-2 and VZV form a subfamily named the *Alpha herpesvirinae*, characterised by a very rapid reproductive cycle, rapid destruction of the host cell and ability to multiply in a variety of host tissues. These viruses establish latent infection in the dorsal root ganglia. Reactivation of latent virus is associated with stimuli such as stress, menstruation, and ultraviolet light, in the presence of a fully developed immune response, the production of recurrent infection and virus shedding. Reactivation may occur at intervals throughout life.

Epidemiology and Geographical Distribution

HSV is disseminated throughout the world and is endemic in all the human populations examined. Humans are the only natural host. Transmission of the virus is by direct contact between a susceptible person and an individual shedding the virus. Transfer of the virus occurs by infection of a mucosal surface or by entry through skin abrasions and lesions such as cuts. Replication of the virus occurs at the site of infection, followed by a short period of viraemia. The primary infection is usually asymptomatic.

The site of primary infection for HSV-1 is most frequently the oral cavity and oropharynx, often by kissing, and by early adult life infection rates are in the order of 90–95%. The site of infection for HSV-2 is the genital mucosa and transmission is by intimate sexual contact. However HSV-1 and HSV-2 may infect at either of these sites (between 10 and 40% of primary genital infections may be caused by HSV-1). It should be noted that although infection with HSV-2 is transmitted sexually, seroprevalence rates of about 30–60%, which increase with sexual maturity, do not attain the levels of infection with HSV-1. Seroprevalence of HSV-2 is related to socioeconomic factors but particularly to the number of sexual partners.

Previous infection with HSV-1 does not protect against HSV-2, but those who had been infected with HSV-1 usually experience milder symptoms with HSV-2 compared with those who had not experienced either form of the virus.

Transmission is by direct contact with infected secretions, obviously when genital lesions are present; however, the virus can be excreted asymptomatically and this may occur in 2% of women. The presence of viral DNA, detected by PCR in genital swabs, in the absence of virus from women with a history of recurrent genital herpes suggests persistent viral infection (chronicity) rather than recurrent infection. Nevertheless, about 60% of those infected with HSV-2 will report recurrent infection.

The incubation period is 2–20 days, with an average of about 1 week.

Pathology

Pathological changes in the skin include ballooning of infected cells, cell degeneration, formation of multinucleated giant cells, inflammatory changes and the accumulation of vesicular fluid between the layers of the epidermis and dermis. The vesicular fluid contains large quantities of virus. Scarring after healing is uncommon. Vesicles are less prominent, in general, when mucous membranes are infected. Shallow ulcers are more common as the vesicles rupture rapidly because of the thin layer of protective stratified epithelium. The intensity of the inflammatory response is significantly less marked with recurrent disease.

Clinical Features and Diagnosis of Genital HSV Infection

Primary genital infection is frequently a severe clinical illness lasting 3 weeks or longer. The primary disease is associated with fever, malaise, bilateral inguinal lymphadenopathy and pain, which can be very severe. In women the infection usually involves the vulva, vagina and cervix. The lesions may extend to the perineum, the upper thigh and the buttocks. Women frequently have dysuria and urinary retention due to urethral involvement and cystitis. In men, lesions are found on the glans penis, the prepuce or the penile shaft. Perianal and anal infections are common in homosexual men.

Complications include aseptic meningitis in 10%. Sacral radiculomyelitis with associated neuralgias may occur in both men and women. Resolution of the symptoms of primary infection may extend over several weeks.

Recurrent genital herpes is a milder disease in comparison with primary infection, but it is, nevertheless, distressing. A limited number of vesicles appear and localised irritation is a more prominent feature than pain. The frequency of recurrence varies from patient to patient. It is estimated that approximately 30% have no recurrences, 30% have about three recurrences each year, and the remainder more frequent recurrences.

Diagnosis in the laboratory is by viral isolation by culture, direct or indirect immunofluorescence, immunoperoxidase techniques, enzyme- and radioimmunoassays and nucleic acid detection.

Treatment

The treatment of choice of skin and mucous membrane lesions is with 5% acyclovir triphosphate in an aqueous cream base. Severe orofacial herpes and severe genital herpes are treated with oral acyclovir for 5 days. Prevention of overt recurrent infection is by oral acyclovir given over prolonged periods of months. Systemic infections are treated by slow intravenous infusion of acyclovir.

Prevention

Vaccines for HSV-1 and HSV-2 are under clinical evaluation. Other methods for prevention are those which apply to reducing the risk of contracting sexually transmitted infections, including the frequency of sexual contact, the number of sexual partners, particularly those who change sexual partners frequently (prostitutes, sexually active homosexual men), and safe sex (activities which do not allow exchange of body fluids, including consistent and correct condom use and other mechanical barriers). Medical advice must be sought if symptoms develop.

RABIES

Introduction and Definitions

Rabies is a viral infection which is transmitted in the saliva of infected mammals; it causes an acute encephalomyelitis that is almost always fatal. Human pathogens of medical importance are members of the genus *Lyssavirus* and *Vesiculovirus*. Almost all cases of human rabies, a lyssavirus infection, are caused by a bite of a rabid animal. Although the risk of rabies is highest in countries of most of Asia, Africa and South America and it is rare as a human infection in Western Europe and North America, every year, for example, up to 40 000 people receive postexposure prophylaxis in the USA.

Nature of the Infectious Agent

Rabies virus is a member of the family *Rhabdoviridae*, with a characteristic bullet shape. There are some 80 other bullet-shaped viruses which infect animals (including fish), plants, invertebrates and insects. For practical purposes, only *Rabies virus* is considered below, but other members of the *Lyssavirus* group which include the serologically related *Lagos bat virus, Mokola virus* and *Duvenhage virus* in Africa, and *Duvenhage virus* in Europe (European bat virus) should be noted.

Rabies virus is a negative-sense, non-segmented, single-stranded RNA virus measuring about 75 × 180 nm. The helical nucleocapsid of 30–35 coils is surrounded by an outer lipid bilayer membrane with surface projections about 8 nm in length. The viral genome encodes five proteins, three of which are associated with the ribonucleoprotein complex, which, together with the viral RNA, aggregate in the cytoplasm of infected neurons to form the characteristic Negri bodies. The matrix protein (M) and the glycoprotein (G) are associated with the viral envelope. The glycoprotein is required for virus infectivity and recognises specific cell receptors. It is also the only rabies virus protein known to induce neutralising antibody.

The effect of chemical agents on rabies virus is underlined by the importance of thorough cleansing of the wound with soap or detergent. The virus is destroyed by quaternary ammonium disinfectants, 1% soap solutions, ionic and nonionic detergents, 5% iodine, common organic solvents such as 45% alcohol, ether and chloroform, formalin and β-propriolactone.

Isolates of rabies virus from naturally infected animals, i.e. wild-type virus, are referred to as 'street' virus, and viruses adapted by laboratory passage in animals or cell culture are referred to as 'fixed' virus.

Epidemiology, Geographical Distribution and Reservoir of Infection

Human rabies is almost always caused by a bite or contamination of surface wounds by virus in saliva, but infection through intact mucosa, for example of the mouth or the conjunctiva, can occur. Aerosol transmission has been implicated in human infection in bat-infested caves and in laboratory accidents. Human-to-human transmission has been reported rarely, for example, by transplantation of infected corneas, and in the older literature. Rabies has not been reported in nursing and medical staff, but nevertheless there is a risk of exposure by bite or by contaminated saliva during airway care, and appropriate precautions should be exercised. It should also be noted that definitive animal exposure or incident cannot be identified in a significant number of human cases.

Rabies is primarily a disease of animals and most human cases occur in the developing world. The only areas free of animal rabies include Australia and New Zealand and islands such as the UK and Ireland, and the Pacific Islands. Rabies is most prevalent among wild foxes, wolves and jackals, followed by domestic dogs, skunks, cats, farm animals, bats and others. The principal reservoir in Africa, Central America (including Mexico), South America and Asia is the unvaccinated domestic dog. There is little information about rabies in wildlife in tropical areas. The major reservoir of infection in Europe is the red fox, and rabies has been identified in Central European deer. The major sources in the USA include skunks, bats and racoons.

Pathology

Although rabies virus receptors appear to coincide with the distribution of acetylcholine receptors, the virus can enter the cell independently of these receptors. The virus may access the peripheral nerves directly or it may replicate in the muscle tissue, remaining at or near the site of introduction into the host for most of the incubation period, essentially at motor endplates, replicating in monocytes and later involving the peripheral nerves via the neuromuscular junctions. The virus then moves centripetally to the central nervous system for replication. Subsequently it moves centrifugally to many tissues, including the salivary glands. Pathological changes in the brain are not profound, apart from the pathognomonic Negri bodies. Few neurons are involved, there is limited tissue necrosis and some perivascular cuffing.

Clinical Features and Diagnosis

The incubation period is variable, ranging from a few days to several years, but in most cases the range is 30–90 days. The development of the infection depends on the severity of the exposure, the site of the bite and whether the wounds were inflicted through bare skin, and other factors.

Prodromal symptoms are nonspecific, although behaviour disturbances are often present, including anxiety, depression, hyperactivity, aggression, intolerance to tactile, auditory and visual stimuli, or delirium. Later symptoms of acute encephalitis appear, and clinical features may be confused with tetanus or cerebral malaria, poliomyelitis, botulism, or others. Clinical neurological findings have been classified as either 'furious' or 'paralytic'. Furious rabies is the most common form; it is characterised by spasms in response to external stimuli, which may be tactile, visual, auditory or olfactory and include hydrophobia and aerophobia. Spasms alternate with periods of calm and lucidity, agitation and confusion and dysfunction of the autonomic nervous system. Paralytic rabies involves clinical features ranging from paralysis of one limb to quadriplegia. The disease progresses to severe neurological complications, coma and death. Clinical differential diagnosis of rabies should be considered in every patient with unexplained encephalitits or with neurological signs, particularly where there is a history of animal bite or possible exposure in a country where rabies is endemic.

Diagnosis in the laboratory is established by the detection of rabies antigen, antibody, rabies viral RNA or the isolation of the virus. Rapid diagnosis antemortem is by detection of rabies antigen by direct immunofluorescence in a skin biopsy from the nape of the neck. Other freshly obtained tissues may be used. The virus can be isolated in tissue culture by inoculation of a murine neuroblastoma cell line (NAC 1300) or by inoculation of laboratory rodents. PCR and other molecular tests can be employed. Detection of rabies virus neutralising antibody by a rapid fluorescence focus inhibition test in the serum of unvaccinated persons is also diagnostic, and the presence of antibody in the cerebrospinal fluid confirms the diagnosis. In vaccinated individuals differentiation between antibody due to vaccination or disease is not possible, but vaccination does not produce typically CSF antibody.

Management, Treatment and Prevention

The basic approach to the control of rabies is control of infection of animals where possible, prevention of exposure and immunisation. Treatment of human rabies is based on postexposure management of the wound and prophylaxis.

Methods for the control of rabies in animals are described in a compendium prepared by the National Association of State Public Health Veterinarians of the USA (Compendium of Animal Rabies Control, 1999).

Note that an unprovoked attack by an animal is more likely than a provoked attack to indicate that an animal is rabid and great care must be exercised to avoid contact with stray or unvaccinated dogs, cats and ferrets, particularly in countries where rabies is endemic and vaccination of domestic animals is unlikely.

Treatment of Wounds and Postexposure Immunisation

Attack by a rabid animal constitutes a medical emergency. Immediate and thorough washing of all bite wounds and scratches with soap and water and, if available, a virucidal solution as described above, such as quaternary ammonium disinfectants, ionic and nonionic detergents or 5% iodine, are most important. Avoid closure of the wound surgically unless suture of a large wound is essential because of the size of the wound, the potential for bacterial infection and cosmetic reasons.

Postexposure antirabies immunisation should include the administration of both passive antibody in the form of specific antirabies immunoglobulin and active vaccination with a cell culture vaccine. A desirable postexposure prophylaxis regimen is described in the recommendations of the US Advisory Committee on Immunization Practices (1999b). Briefly, in those not previously vaccinated against rabies, immediate wound cleansing must be followed by:

- Administration of $20 \, IU \, kg^{-1}$ body weight of antirabies immunoglobulin. If feasible anatomically, the full dose should be infiltrated around the wound(s), and any remaining amount should be given intramuscularly but at a distant site from the site of vaccine administration.
- Human diploid cell vaccine, rabies vaccine adsorbed or purified chick embryo cell vaccine should be given intramuscularly into the deltoid muscle—1.0 ml immediately and on days 3, 7, 14 and 28.

In the case of a patient who has been vaccinated previously with any of the above vaccines or with any other type of rabies vaccine, and a documented history of antibody response to the prior vaccination, the following regimen applies after immediate wound cleansing:

- Antirabies immunoglobulin should *not* be given.
- Human diploid cell vaccine, rabies vaccine adsorbed or purified chick embryo cell vaccine should be given intramuscularly into the deltoid muscle immediately (day 0) and on day 3 in a dose of 1.0 ml. The gluteal muscles should never be used because the resulting antibody titres are lower than those achieved by administration into the deltoid muscle.

Primary Vaccination or Pre-exposure Vaccination

Pre-exposure immunisation should be offered to high-risk groups, which include veterinary surgeons and veterinary nurses and assistants, animal handlers, wildlife keepers and handlers, and certain laboratory workers. Pre-exposure immunisation should be considered for other persons who may come into frequent contact with animals potentially infected with rabies or who travel to or reside in areas where animal rabies, particularly dog rabies, is enzootic and immediate access to appropriate medical care is or may be limited.

Primary intramuscular vaccination involves three 1.0 ml injections of one of the vaccines listed above given intramuscularly into the deltoid muscle on days 0, 7, and 21 or 28. Intradermal primary vaccination of three 0.1 ml doses of human diploid cell vaccine, one each on days 0, 7, and 21 or 28 is an alternative schedule.

Note that malaria prophylaxis with chloroquine phosphate (and possibly structurally related compounds, which have not yet been investigated for this effect) decreases the antibody response to antirabies human diploid cell vaccine given concomitantly.

Pre-exposure booster doses of vaccine must be given to laboratory research workers working with rabies virus or those in vaccine production units. Rabies antibody should be measured every 6 months and a booster dose given according to the neutralisation antibody titre.

YELLOW FEVER

Introduction and Definitions

Yellow fever is a disease of antiquity which originated most probably in equatorial Africa and was brought by the slave trade to the great cities of the New World late in the seventeenth century (New York in 1668, Boston in 1691), although it did not reach Europe until the eighteenth century, with extensive epidemics associated with a high mortality of more than 60%. Urban and jungle yellow fever now occur only in parts of Africa and South

America (apart from the rare imported case, e.g. Germany in 1999). Urban yellow fever is an epidemic viral infection of humans transmitted by the *Aedes aegypti* mosquito in the Americas and Africa from infected to susceptible persons. Although *Ae. aegypti* is the important vector in Africa, several other species of mosquito are involved. Jungle yellow fever is an enzootic viral disease transmitted among nonhuman primates (and occasionally humans, e.g. forest workers) by various mosquito vectors.

Yellow fever virus (YFV) is a member of the family

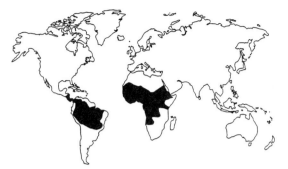

Figure 6.5 Geographical distribution of *Yellow fever virus*

Flaviviridae, genus *Flavivirus*, classified in the past in the togaviruses. The other two genera in this family are *Hepacivirus* and *Pestivirus*, which include important animal pathogens such as *Bovine diarrhoea virus* and *Hog cholera virus*. The medically important flaviviruses are often associated with three major clinical syndromes: haemorrhagic fever with hepatitis (*Yellow fever virus*); encephalitis (*St Louis encephalitis*, *Japanese encephalitis*, *Powassan* and *Tick-borne encephalitis* viruses); febrile illness with rash (*Dengue virus*); and haemorrhagic fever (*Kyasanur Forest disease virus* and sometimes *Dengue virus*).

Nature of the Infectious Agent

Yellow fever virus is the type species of the genus *Flavivirus*. The virus particles are spherical and enveloped with a diameter of 40–50 nm. The nucleic acid consists of a single molecule of positive-sense single-stranded RNA. The virus replicates in the cytoplasm of the cell in association with the rough and smooth endoplasmic reticulum. Viral particles accumulate within lamellae and vesicles and replication is associated with the proliferation of intracellular membranes. The high lipid content of the viral envelope is derived from the host cell membrane.

Epidemiology and Geographical Distribution

Yellow fever occurs in tropical Africa and tropical America between the latitudes of 16°N to 10°S in Africa and 10°N and 40°S in the Americas (Figure 6.5). It has not been seen in Asia or Australasia. Extensive epidemics of yellow fever occurred in recent years in Africa, e.g. Nigeria (1986–1988), Angola (1988), Cameroon (1990) and elsewhere. The largest epidemic recorded took place in Ethiopia (1960–1962) with 30 000 deaths of 100 000 clinical cases. Jungle yellow fever remains endemic in Bolivia, Brazil, Colombia, Ecuador, Peru, Panama, Venezuela and the Guyanas.

The transmission cycles of yellow fever and the interrelationships of its vectors and hosts are complex. YFV in Africa and South America has two distinct epidemiological patterns: jungle (sylvan) yellow fever and urban yellow fever. Jungle yellow fever is maintained among canopy-dwelling monkeys and tree-hole breeding mosquitoes (*Aedes* species in Africa and *Haemagogus* species in South America). The monkey is a transient host because of the short period of viraemia, and the major amplification host is the mosquito, which is infected for life and which is also able to pass the infection transovarially. Human disease occurs sporadically or in small outbreaks and initially only in persons exposed to forest mosquitoes (the enzootic forest cycle).

The jungle yellow fever cycle now represents the most important epidemiological form of yellow fever in relation to human infection. Outbreaks are frequent when forest mosquitoes invade adjacent plantations, forest clearings and villages on the fringes of rain forests and riverine gallery forests. Human-to-human transmission by the highly efficient urban *Ae. aegypti* mosquitoes sustains the epidemics. The expansion of *Ae. aegypti* habitat, particularly in the Americas, raises the possibility of major epidemics, similar to those described in tropical Africa. Note that species other than *Ae. aegypti* may be involved, e.g. *Ae. simpsoni*, *Ae. africanus* and others.

The urban yellow fever cycle is generally maintained by *Ae. aegypti* and reinfestations in towns and villages in South America raise concerns about a resurgence of urban yellow fever, as is the case in towns and rural villages in tropical Africa.

The incubation period of yellow fever is usually 3–6 days but may be longer. Death occurs 7–10 days after the onset of illness, with a fatality rate in indigenous populations in endemic areas generally 5% (but may be considerably higher) and 50% or more in nonindigenous nonimmunised adults.

Reservoir of Infection

The reservoirs of infection in forests are vertebrates, mainly monkeys and possibly marsupials and forest mosquitoes. Transovarian transmission in mosquitoes may contribute to the maintenance of infection. In urban areas, humans and *Ae. aegypti* mosquitoes are the reservoirs.

Pathology

The acute infection both in humans and in animals varies in its severity from a subclinical infection to a rapidly fatal form of the disease. Consequently, description of the pathological lesions is based principally on the findings in fatal cases. The outstanding characteristic lesion of yellow fever is selective necrosis of highly specialised epithelial cells in any affected organ or in myocardial cells. Stromal cells are not involved and there is a striking absence of inflammatory cell response in or around the necrotic lesions.

The hepatic lesion in humans is characteristic. There is diffuse, severe, noninflammatory necrosis of the paren-

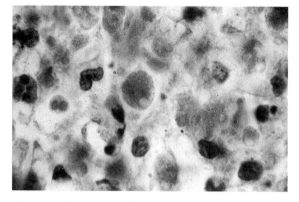

Figure 6.6 Typical Councilman bodies in the liver of a patient with yellow fever. (Courtesy of the World Health Organization)

chymal cells, classically affecting the cells occupying the mid-zones of the lobule. Necrosis, however, may be scattered throughout the liver lobules. Acidophilic masses of necrotic cells are intercalated with surviving cells, and necrotic hyaline cells in the liver have been termed 'Councilman bodies' (Figure 6.6). Fatty changes in the cells tend to be highly variable but they are always present. Haemorrhages in the liver are not usually found. In patients who recover there is complete replacement of necrotic tissue by regeneration. There is no proliferation of connective tissue elements and no permanent scarring of the liver.

The recognition of the diagnostic lesion in the liver led to the development of the viscerotome for the easy and rapid removal of liver tissue from persons who had died from a febrile illness. A viscerotomy service was organised and several hundred thousand specimens were collected and examined. This systematic collection and examination of liver fragments established the epidemiology of yellow fever and resulted in the appreciation of the importance of yellow fever in the populations of endemic regions. Later, it also played an important part in the control of the disease.

The lesions in the kidneys may be as important clinically as those in the liver. The necrotic process involves principally the epithelial cells of the proximal and distal convoluted tubules and there is a variable degree of fatty degeneration affecting, somewhat irregularly, the whole of the renal tubular system. Many hyaline and granular casts are present in the collecting tubules, and calcareous masses containing calcium salts and appreciable amounts of iron are found in the loops of Henle. Vascular congestion is usual but haemorrhages into the glomerular spaces are rare. In the later stages of the disease there may be appreciable bile staining of the tubular epithelium, as well as the formation of bile casts within the tubules.

Examination of the heart reveals a soft and usually yellow-tinged myocardium with some subendocardial haemorrhages and patchy subendocardial fatty changes. Microscopically there is fatty degeneration and fatty infiltration of the cardiac fibres, and necrosis of the nuclei is often found. These changes may also affect the cells of the

sinoauricular node and the bundle of His. Once more, there is a striking absence of any inflammatory cell response.

Encephalitis is not part of the picture of naturally occurring yellow fever in humans, except with neurotropic strains of the virus.

Clinical Features and Diagnosis

The disease is extremely variable in severity and many mild and clinically unrecognisable cases occur. The classical triad of symptoms, namely jaundice, haemorrhages and severe proteinuria, is present only in severe infections.

The disease may be divided into three stages: (1) the initial fever, (2) the 'period of calm', and (3) the period of reaction (in severe cases). The initial fever is usually sudden in onset and lasts from 3 to 4 days with the maximum temperature generally attained within 36 h. Severe headache, often with photophobia, is frequently a prominent feature. Muscle pains are usual in the loin, back and legs, and these may be quite severe. The presence of epigastric pain is almost invariable. As the disease progresses, the Faget sign appears, namely a falling pulse rate with a constant temperature or a slow constant pulse rate with a rising temperature, stressing the lack of correlation between temperature and pulse. During the 'period of calm', which occurs at about the fourth day and may be entirely absent, there is considerable amelioration of the symptoms and complete recovery may follow. In the third stage, the temperature rises again and jaundice appears, first in the sclera, followed by a yellowish tinge of the skin. The gums are swollen and tend to bleed readily on pressure; the tongue is coated but with red edges and tip. The liver is tender but usually not enlarged. The spleen is not palpable. Hiccough may be a very distressing feature, and black vomit, diarrhoea and skin petechiae may occur. Marked bradycardia is characteristic and the blood pressure is low. Haemorrhages may occur in almost any organ. Severe albuminuria is constant, almost from the onset, and oliguria and anuria occur during the terminal stages.

In the malignant form, hyperpyrexia may occur and profuse haemorrhages, black vomit, melaena, purpura, jaundice, disturbances of the central nervous system and anuria may develop by the third day of illness. Delirium and severe toxaemia are present before death.

The overall fatality rate in yellow fever is between 5 and 10% of all diagnosed cases, but it may be higher in a given epidemic and in nonindigenous cases. Relapses are unknown and immunity is usually permanent.

Difficulties in differential diagnosis may be experienced in atypical cases.

Malaria and relapsing fever are usually associated with splenomegaly. Blood smears will reveal malaria parasites or treponemata. Viral hepatitis may present difficulties, but on the whole jaundice is often deeper, proteinuria is uncommon and by the time jaundice appears, the patient is generally afebrile with subjective clinical improvement.

The liver is enlarged and tender. Leptospirosis is differentiated by laboratory tests. Dengue fever may mimic yellow fever closely, but proteinuria is very much less severe and jaundice is very rare. The rash of dengue also distinguishes it from yellow fever. Other haemorrhagic fevers should be considered.

Laboratory diagnosis is based on viral isolation from the blood in the first three days and by serological tests such as ELISA using monoclonal antibodies. Immunofluorescent antibody tests, haemagglutination inhibiting and neutralising antibodies appear within 1 week of onset. Liver biopsy is contraindicated in acute yellow fever. Histopathological changes in postmortem material are no longer regarded as diagnostic.

Management and Treatment

There is no specific treatment. Blood and body fluid precautions are required, and access of mosquitoes is prevented by bed nets and spraying with insecticides. Vaccination of contacts is required. Spraying with insecticides and aerial spraying, where possible, are important; and eliminate, or apply larvicide to, all actual and potential breeding places of *Ae. aegypti* in urban outbreaks.

Prevention

Control of yellow fever has been attained by immunisation and by vector control; however, reinfestation of villages and towns adjacent to forests with *Ae. aegypti* raises concerns about the re-emergence of urban yellow fever.

Yellow fever vaccine is a live attenuated freeze-dried preparation of the 17D strain of YFV grown in leucosis-free chick embryos. The French neurotropic vaccine developed by passage in mouse brain is no longer used. The vaccine should be stored at 2–8 °C and protected from light. The diluent supplied with the vaccine should be stored below 25 °C but not frozen. After reconstitution, the vaccine should be kept cool, protected from light and used within 1 h. Any unused vaccine should be destroyed by disinfection or incineration. A single dose of 0.5 ml is given subcutaneously and provides long-lasting immunity in 99% of recipients. Immunity persists for at least 10 years and probably for life, but international regulations require a booster every 10 years.

Side-effects of immunisation include mild fever, myalgia and headache, which occur in less than 5% of recipients. Hypersensitivity reactions may occur in individuals allergic to egg protein. Encephalitis is extremely rare.

Contraindications include patients undergoing immunosuppressive treatment and with impaired immunological mechanisms, including malignant conditions involving the reticuloendothelial system and lymphoma and leukaemia. Individuals infected with HIV should not be vaccinated. Under these circumstances a letter of exemption is necessary for countries where a yellow fever certificate is required. Infants under 9 months of age should only be immunised if the risk of yellow fever is unavoidable. Pregnancy is a contraindication because of a theoretical risk of fetal damage, but the risk of yellow fever in a high-risk area outweighs any risk of immunisation.

A yellow fever vaccination certificate is now the only certificate that is required for international travel to and from endemic regions.

DENGUE FEVER

Introduction and Definitions

Dengue virus is at present the most important arboviral cause of illness and death in humans. The four serotypes of *Dengue virus*, a subgroup of the genus *Flavivirus*, are distributed widely throughout the tropics and warm climate regions of Africa, Asia, Australia, the Pacific Islands, India, the Caribbean Islands, and the Americas, involving several million people each year. The incidence of the disease corresponds to the distribution of the principal vector, the *Ae. aegypti* mosquito, which maintains the virus in a human–mosquito–human cycle. The incidence of dengue is increasing, with more frequent epidemics and greater severity, and spread to new areas.

Nature of the Infectious Agent

Dengue virus is a distinct antigenic subgroup of the genus *Flavivirus*. There are four serotypes with extensive cross-reactivities and strain variation. After infection, protective immunity is homotypic so that individuals can be infected simultaneously or serially by more than one serotype.

Epidemiology and Geographical Distribution

Reference has been made to the extensive geographical distribution of dengue throughout the tropics and warm climate regions of Africa, Asia, Australia, Oceania, India, the Caribbean Islands and the Americas. Extension to new areas is the result of uncontrolled poor housing settlements, slums and squatter camps on the peripheries of cities, resurgence of infestation with *Aedes* mosquitoes and failure of vector control.

The principal vector is *Ae. aegypti*. Other *Aedes* species of the subgenus *Stegomyia* are also implicated as vectors in Asia and in the Pacific region. Although there are many similarities with the epidemiology of yellow fever, the urban cycle involving domesticated *Aedes* mosquitoes is the most common and most important for both endemic and epidemic dengue. The incubation period is 3–14 days.

Reservoir of Infection

Humans together with the mosquito.

Pathology

All four dengue virus serotypes cause three distinct syndromes: dengue fever, dengue haemorrhagic fever and dengue shock syndrome. The virus replicates in macrophages at the site of the mosquito bite, in the regional lymph nodes and subsequently the reticuloendothelial system. Viraemia is associated with circulating monocytes, and there is often severe leucopenia. A maculopapular rash on the trunk appears on day 3–5 of the illness and spreads to the face and limbs, accompanied frequently by lymphadenopathy, granulocytopenia and thrombocytopenia. Minor mucocutaneous bleeding may occur.

Dengue haemorrhagic fever is the result of increased vascular permeability, unusual bleeding manifestations and involvement of the gut and the liver, with or without encephalopathy, and disseminated intravascular coagulation. In dengue shock syndrome, increased vascular permeability causes decreased plasma volume and clinical shock, which, if uncorrected, may lead to acidosis, hyperkalaemia and death. Most cases of dengue haemorrhagic fever and dengue shock syndrome occur in children and adolescents under the age of 15 years, with a fatality rate of 3–10%.

Dengue haemorrhagic fever and dengue shock syndrome are believed to be the result of 'immune enhancement', whereby homologous and heterologous antibodies binding to the virus, including subprotective levels of maternal dengue antibodies in infants, enhance infection of macrophages via cellular Fc receptors. Another possible explanation is that T cells exacerbate the antibody-enhanced cascade by concomitant release of cytokines by both T cells and damaged macrophages. The alternative hypothesis is that the severe complications of dengue are caused by unusually virulent strains of dengue, particularly serotype 2; however, there is no consistent relationship between strain variation and increased virulence or infectivity.

Clinical Features and Diagnosis

Dengue fever is characterised by sudden fever, headache, vomiting and severe muscle and bone pain of increasing severity. The fever is biphasic, remitting on day 3–5 of the illness, followed by a maculopapular or morbilliform rash, which spreads from the trunk to the limbs and face. This second phase of the illness, which is often accompanied by recurrence of fever, is associated with lymphadenopathy, granulocytopenia and thrombocytopenia. Minor mucocutaneous bleeding may occur. The fever lasts for 3–9 days and is self-limiting.

The clinical features of dengue haemorrhagic fever are characterised by fever, rash and anorexia lasting 3–5 days, followed by hepatomegaly, hypotension and a haemorrhagic diathesis. The dengue shock syndrome is due to decreased plasma volume following increased vascular permeability, and is associated with a significant mortality of up to 10%, but which can be as high as 40–50% if untreated. Diagnosis in returning travellers may be difficult. Serological diagnosis is based on haemagglutination-inhibition and IgM antibody-capture ELISA. Definitive diagnosis is by way of virus isolation and PCR-based techniques.

Treatment is symptomatic and, in case of complications, careful management of clinical shock.

Protective Measures and Prevention

Live attenuated dengue vaccines are undergoing clinical trials. There is no licensed dengue vaccine.

Epidemiological monitoring is important and also provides means of education and control. Vector control is essential, with the aim of eliminating the domesticated *Aedes* mosquitoes. It appears that the results of insecticide and larvicide treatment of stagnant water are temporary, and indeed reinfestations are inevitable. Nevertheless, these are essential tools for control. The traveller should employ the usual measures for the prevention of insect bites.

JAPANESE ENCEPHALITIS, ST LOUIS ENCEPHALITIS, TICK-BORNE ENCEPHALITIS AND OTHER FLAVIVIRUS INFECTIONS

Introduction and Definitions

The flaviviruses may be considered broadly in three major groups according to the associated principal clinical syndromes:

- Those causing haemorrhagic fever, for example, *Yellow fever virus*

- Those associated clinically with fever, rash, myalgia and arthralgia, for example, *Dengue virus*, and
- Those associated primarily with encephalitis, for example, *Japanese encephalitis virus*.

This section is devoted to the flaviviruses associated with encephalitis.

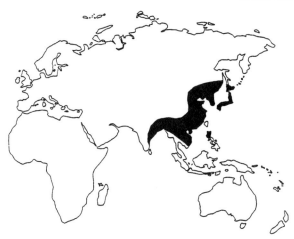

Figure 6.7 Geographical distribution of *Japanese encephalitis virus*

JAPANESE ENCEPHALITIS

Japanese encephalitis virus (JEV) is the commonest cause of arboviral encephalitis in the world.

Nature of the Infectious Agent

JEV can be separated by nucleic acid sequencing into three genotypes with different geographical distribution. The epidemiological significance of this observation is not known. Antigenically, JEV shares some crossreactivity with *St Louis encephalitis virus*.

Epidemiology and Geographical Distribution

JEV occurs in eastern, southeastern and southern Asia including Japan, parts of the former Soviet Union in the Far East, the Western Pacific Islands and India, where it is the major cause of viral encephalitis (Figure 6.7). The vertebrate hosts of the virus are humans and domestic animals, especially pigs, and birds, particularly water birds. The principal vector of the virus is *Culex tritaenorhynchus*, but other species of *Culex, Aedes, Anopheles* and *Mansonia* may be involved.

Japanese encephalitis is endemic in rural areas, especially where pig farming and rice growing coexist. Epidemics occur in both rural and urban areas. The highest transmission rates occur during and immediately after the rainy season. The incubation period is 5–15 days. The virus is not transmitted from person to person. Mosquitoes remain infective for life, and pigs are a major amplifying host of the virus.

Pathology

The target cells for JEV are T cells and peripheral blood mononuclear cells. Strains of virus which invade the central nervous system cause oedema and small haemorrhages in the brain, and lesions include destruction of cerebellar Purkinje cells, neuronal degeneration and necrosis, glial nodules and perivascular inflammation. Pathological lesions in other tissues include hyperplasia of germinal centres of lymph nodes, changes in the spleen, interstitial myocarditis and focal haemorrhages in the kidney. The severity of the lesions varies considerably.

Clinical Features and Diagnosis

Infection may be associated with a nonspecific mild febrile illness or acute meningomyeloencephalitis, occurring at rates which vary from 1 in 20 to 1 in 800 infected persons. Children are affected most commonly in endemic areas, but infection also occurs in older age groups. Mortality rates of those with meningomyeloencephalitis is about 20% in children and up to 50% in those aged over 50 years. Permanent motor and psychological sequelae are common.

Diagnosis is based on serological assays for haemagglutination-inhibition, immunofluorescent and complement-fixing antibodies and IgM-capture ELISA.

Treatment

Treatment is symptomatic and requires excellent nursing care. Anticonvulsant treatment and management of coma may be required.

Prevention and Control

Vector control is difficult and measures to prevent mosquito bites should be deployed. The most important measure of control is active immunisation of humans and domestic animals, especially pigs and horses. Immunisation is recommended for travellers to endemic areas who will be staying for a month or longer, particularly if travel will include rural areas; however, the risks to the traveller are difficult to assess except if there is a high risk of exposure, particularly towards the end of the rainy season.

ST LOUIS ENCEPHALITIS

St Louis encephalitis virus is the principal cause of viral encephalitis in the USA and the outbreak in New York City in 1999 brought viral encephalitis into international prominence once again. The virus is related antigenically to the Japanese encephalitis complex of the flaviviruses. It should be noted that the virus which caused the outbreak

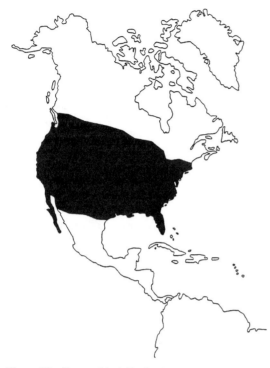

Figure 6.8 Geographical distribution of *St Louis encephalitis virus*

in New York City in 1999 has now been identified as Kunjin/West Nile-like virus.

Epidemiology and Geographical Distribution

The virus is distributed throughout the USA, but it has been found in southern Canada, Central and South America and the Caribbean Islands (Figure 6.8). It is transmitted by the bite of an infected mosquito, and birds, particularly domesticated sparrows, are the principal amplifying hosts. Small mammals such as rodents and domesticated animals may also be infected; however, the virus is maintained in nature in an avian cycle and is transmitted by *Culex* mosquitoes which feed readily on birds.

St Louis encephalitis virus is disseminated widely throughout the USA and causes periodic outbreaks, usually at intervals of several years, in urban settings in California, Texas, the southeast and in the Ohio Mississippi valley.

Clinical Features and Diagnosis

More than 99% of infections with this virus are without symptoms. In clinical cases, the disease is characterised by fever, malaise, nausea and vomiting and headache. Aseptic meningitis or focal encephalitis, and cranial nerve palsies in about 20% of cases, indicate involvement of the central nervous system. Coma may ensue. The case fatality rate is approximately 7% in symptomatic cases but may be higher, particularly in the elderly, when the fatality rate may be 30%.

Rapid diagnosis is based on IgM antibody capture ELISA using serum or cerebrospinal fluid. Immunofluorescence test on cells infected with the virus is also a useful rapid diagnostic technique.

Prevention and Control

A licensed vaccine is not available. The infection is controlled in the USA by vector control, including water drainage and aerial low volume spraying of insecticides in populated areas. Secondary control measures to protect against mosquito bites should be deployed during reported outbreaks.

TICK-BORNE ENCEPHALITIS

Introduction and Definitions

The tick-borne flaviviruses are maintained by tick–mammal cycles and by transovarian transmission in ticks. Humans are infected by virus transmitted by the bite of an infected tick or, less commonly, by drinking unpasteurised milk from infected goats or other mammals. The disease is endemic in forested parts of western, central and eastern Europe and Scandinavia, caused by *Central European encephalitis virus*, and the Far Eastern subtype or *Russian Spring–Summer encephalitis virus*.

Other viruses within the subgroup of tick-borne flaviviruses include *Omsk haemorrhagic fever virus*, *Kyasanur Forest disease virus* (India) and *Powassan virus*, which causes sporadic encephalitis in eastern parts of Canada (Ontario) and the USA. These viruses are not considered further in this text.

Nature of the Infectious Agent

The tick-borne encephalitis viruses are a closely related subgroup of flaviviruses.

Epidemiology and Geographical Distribution

The geographical distribution of the *Central European encephalitis virus* extends to the forested areas of western, central and eastern Europe, Scandinavia, Italy, Yugoslavia and Greece and follows closely the distribution of its arthropod vector, *Ixodes ricinus* (Figure 6.9). *Russian Spring–Summer encephalitis virus* is found in the forest belt and taiga of Russia and Siberia following the distribution of *I. persulcatus* (Figure 6.10). Infection is transmitted by the bite of an infected tick. Domestic animals,

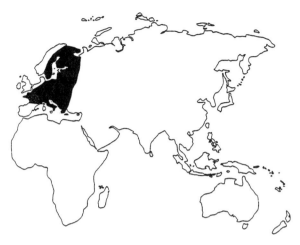

Figure 6.9 Geographical distribution of *Central European encephalitis virus*. Reproduced from Zuckerman *et al.*, 2000

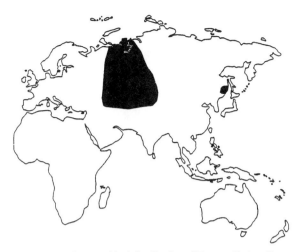

Figure 6.10 Geographical distribution of *Russian Spring–Summer encephalitis virus*. Reproduced from Zuckerman *et al.*, 2000

such as sheep, goats and cows, excrete virus in their milk, and ingestion of unpasteurised milk or unpasteurised milk products may transmit the infection.

The infection is endemic, with increased incidence in the summer months in relation to temperature and humidity which affect tick activity. The infection is common in rural populations, especially in farmers and forest workers, with seroprevalence of 5–20% or even greater.

The incubation period is 8–14 days.

Pathology

The virus replicates in the liver before a significant viraemia occurs. Vascular permeability is altered and the virus crosses the blood–brain barrier. Severe neuronal damage may occur, affecting the cervical segments of the spinal cord, medulla, midbrain and pons. There is glial proliferation and lymphoid proliferation around vessels.

Clinical Features and Diagnosis

The onset of illness is sudden with a nonspecific febrile illness including headache and lassitude. Visual disturbances may occur such as blurring of vision and diplopia. In the majority the illness lasts 4–7 days. A biphasic

illness may follow after a short remission, with fever and signs of meningoencephalitis. Extrapyramidal and cerebellar syndromes may persist for months, and residual paralysis involving the upper limbs and the shoulder girdle is common. Mortality in different outbreaks varies from 1 to 5%.

Serological diagnosis is based on an IgM antibody-capture ELISA on serum or cerebrospinal fluid. Haemagglutination-inhibition or neutralisation tests are useful. Virus can be isolated early after the onset of symptoms.

Prevention and Protective Measures

Forests in some areas of the former Soviet Union are closed to visitors.

Tick repellents are useful on outer clothes and socks, and the arms, legs and ankles must be covered. Travellers who plan to walk, camp or work in late spring and summer in the heavily forested areas listed above, especially where there is heavy undergrowth, should be immunised with a formalin-inactivated vaccine. Two doses of 0.5 ml given intramuscularly 4–12 weeks apart will provide protection for 1 year. An immunoglobulin preparation is also available for postexposure prophylaxis.

VIRAL HAEMORRHAGIC FEVERS

Introduction and Definitions

Yellow fever, which is endemic in Africa and in parts of the Americas, has a long history and is well recognised, and although it may present in severe infections as a

haemorrhagic fever it is considered separately. The term 'exotic viruses' is applied to haemorrhagic viral infections which have been recognised more recently, Marburg vi-

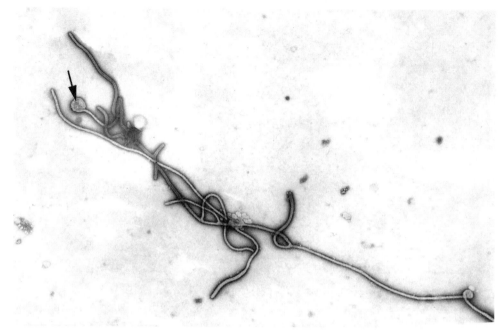

Figure 6.11 Ebola virus (Zaire strain). This electron micrograph illustrates a *single* viral particle with many branches and a torus configuration. Negative stain, × 100 000. (Courtesy of Dr David Ellis, reproduced from *Principles and Practice of Clinical Virology*, 1st edition, 1987)

rus disease (1967), Lassa fever (1969) and Ebola fever (1976). Two other haemorrhagic fevers are discussed in this section, Rift Valley fever and Crimean–Congo haemorrhagic fever; the former because of extensive outbreaks in parts of Africa, including the Nile delta, and the latter because of its sporadic appearance in the Middle East and Pakistan.

Natural Reservoir and Source

Those for *Marburg virus* and *Ebola virus* remain unknown. *Lassa virus* and other arenaviruses are normally transmitted to humans from infected rodents in Africa and South America. *Rift Valley fever virus* is transmitted by mosquitoes. *Crimean–Congo haemorrhagic fever viruses*, common in Africa, Western Asia and parts of the Middle East and in Russia and Republics in the former Soviet Union, are transmitted by tick-bite; human-to-human transmission has only been shown to result from contact with infected blood.

MARBURG VIRUS DISEASE

Marburg virus disease, commonly but incorrectly named 'green monkey' disease, is a severe distinctive haemorrhagic febrile illness of humans, first described in 1967, when 31 cases with seven deaths in Germany and Yugo-

slavia were traced to direct contact with blood, organs or tissue cell cultures from a batch of African green monkeys (*Cercopithicus aethiops*) that had been trapped in Uganda. Several secondary cases occurred in hospital personnel by contact with the blood of patients. One further case was apparently transmitted by sexual intercourse 83 days after the initial illness, and virus was isolated from the semen. The case fatality rate was 29% for the primary cases, but no deaths occurred in the six secondary cases. This previously unrecognised disease was caused by an infectious agent probably new to medical science. Three more cases were reported in Johannesburg in 1975, in two young Australians who crossed central Africa, and a nurse treating them. One of the primary cases died. There have been two other detected recurrences of Marburg virus disease in 1980 and in 1987, all in travellers in rural Africa, and none has led to extensive transmission.

Nature of the Infectious Agent

Marburg virus is classified as a filovirus with two genotypes, Marburg and Ebola. *Marburg virus* has no known subtypes and is antigenically distinct from *Ebola virus*, which has four subtypes. The morphology of these two viruses is unique with a long, but variable, filamentous shape of particles (Figure 6.11). Particles may be branched, circular, U-shaped or resemble a torus (Figure 6.12)

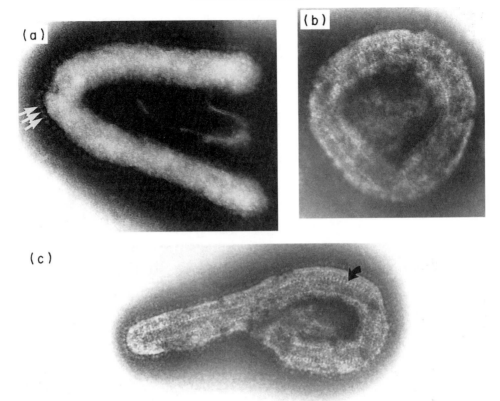

Figure 6.12 (a) Surface spikes on Marburg virus. Negative stain, × 200 000. (b) A torus form of Marburg virus showing the RNA core. Negative stain, × 200 000. (c) A filamentous form of Marburg virus curling up into a torus. The final infective particle is believed to be the torus form. × 200 000. (Courtesy of Dr David Ellis, reproduced from *Principles and Practice of Clinical Virology*, 1st edition, 1987)

and have a diameter of 85 nm. Spikes are present on the surface (Figure 6.12a) and there is an axial channel within the ribonucleoprotein (Figure 6.12c). The genome consists of a single negative-stranded RNA. Molecular analysis of the genome indicates that the filoviruses are the closest relatives to rhabdoviruses and paramyxoviruses.

Epidemiology and Geographical Distribution

The reservoir of the infection remains unknown despite intensive investigation of a host of vertebrates and anthropods. In the case of the Australian traveller who acquired the disease in Zimbabwe, he had often slept outdoors, and once in a house occupied with bats in the attic. He was also stung on the leg while resting at a roadside 6 days before the onset of illness.

The original outbreak resulting from exposure to the blood and tissues of African green monkeys remains unexplained, and since experimental infection of these monkeys invariably results in death, African green monkeys are not the natural host of the virus.

Seroprevalence studies indicate that Marburg virus disease is very rare, and the geographical distribution of primary infection appears to be limited to Central Africa.

The incubation period is 4–16 days. Transmission is by contact with infected blood or tissue and transmission by the sexual route has been described.

Reservoir of the Infection

Not known.

Pathology

There is extensive involvement of the liver, severe renal damage, changes in vascular permeability and activation of the clotting cascade, and disseminated intravascular coagulation with involvement of complex immunological mediators and cytokine release.

Clinical Features and Diagnosis

The illness begins characteristically with sudden onset of fever, malaise, headache and myalgia, followed by nausea, vomiting and watery diarrhoea. A maculopapular rash appears between 5 and 7 days after the onset of illness and is most marked on the buttocks, trunk and lateral aspects of the upper arms. Conjunctivitis is common. A tendency to bleed develops, particularly from the gums and from needle punctures, and severe bleeding into the gastrointestinal tract and elsewhere may occur. There is functional evidence of liver damage but clinical jaundice has not been reported. Renal damage occurs and is manifested by proteinuria, oliguria and viruria.

Laboratory diagnosis includes electron microscopy, indirect immunofluorescence, ELISA and immunoblot techniques. Antigen can be localised in tissues by immunocytochemistry and immunofluorescence, and viral RNA by PCR.

Management and Treatment

Management is essentially supportive. Isolation in a Trexler tent, strict barrier nursing techniques with protective clothing by trained personnel, and careful disposal of patient material and of the deceased are absolutely essential. Laboratory procedures must be carried out in high security level 4 containment facilities.

Protective Measures and Prevention

Epidemiological information, surveillance and health education are important. The natural reservoir of infection remains unknown and vectors have not been identified.

EBOLA VIRUS DISEASE

Ebola virus is the second known filovirus and was first described in 1976. Between August and November 1976, outbreaks of severe and frequently fatal viral haemorrhagic fever occurred in the equatorial provinces of Sudan and Zaire, now the Democratic Republic of Congo, causing widespread international concern. Among the 70 cases in Nzara, Sudan, 33 were fatal. Of the 230 members of the staff in the Maridi hospital, 76 were infected and 41 died. Of the 237 infected persons in Zaire, 211 died. In all, 602 persons were known to have been infected, with an overall fatality rate of 88% in Zaire and 49% in the Sudan. During laboratory investigations carried out to identify the virus, a member of the laboratory staff of the Microbiological Research Establishment, Porton Down in England, contracted the disease but recovered.

Ebola virus reappeared in the Democratic Republic of Congo in 1977: one girl died and her sister had a probable related infection, from which she recovered. A small outbreak occurred in the Sudan in 1979, but the virus was not seen again in Africa until 1994. During 1994–1996, five independent outbreaks were identified: Ivory Coast

(1994), Democratic Republic of Congo (1995) and Gabon (1994, 1995 and 1996). All the sites were in or near tropical forests.

In 1989, *Ebola virus* appeared in cynomolgus monkeys held in a primary quarantine facility in Reston, near Washington DC. Epidemics in cynomolgus monkeys occurred in this facility and others in 1992 and in a primate unit in Italy in 1996. The virus was introduced by monkeys captured in the Phillipines. This strain of *Ebola virus* (Reston) is highly pathogenic for nonhuman primates; it did not cause disease in humans in the USA or the Phillipines, although seroconversions have been detected in several persons in both countries.

There are at least four genetic subtypes of *Ebola virus*: Zaire (EBO-Z), Côte d'Ivoire (EBO-CI), Sudan (EBO-S) and Reston (EBO-R). Human disease has been associated only with EBO-Z, EBO-CI and EBO-S in West and Central Africa (and a laboratory-acquired infection in the UK). The geographical distribution of *Ebola virus*, based on serological surveys, suggests that it may be present in parts of Asia other than the Phillipines and Madagascar.

The source of the virus is not known; however, transmission cycles of the African strains of *Ebola virus* are closely related to the rain forests, although human cases have also occurred in the forest-savannas in the Sudan and Uganda. Nosocomial infections in the medical setting are important, and the epidemic in the city of Kikwit in the Democratic Republic of Congo in 1995, a town of 200 000 people, presented an enormous problem.

The Kikwit outbreak received considerable public attention. A small cluster of cases occurred among the nursing staff of a maternity hospital but was misdiagnosed as epidemic dysentery. Towards the end of the month a similar cluster was identified in the general hospital among the operating staff after a laparotomy on a laboratory technician with suspected typhoid-related abdominal perforation. A viral haemorrhagic fever was diagnosed a few days later. A total of 315 cases were identified, with a case fatality of 81%. The surviving members of 27 households where infection had occurred were interviewed; 16% of 173 household contacts of primary cases developed the infection and all had direct physical contact with the ill person or his or her body fluids. An additional risk was touching a cadaver. The international investigation team concluded that the use of barrier precautions by household members and standard strict universal precautions in hospitals would have prevented the majority of infections, and the introduction of these precautions and other public health measures coincided with the termination of the outbreak. Serological studies indicated a very low rate of subclinical transmission during the outbreak, but it was interesting that there was a significant seroprevalence among the residents of Kikwit and the surrounding villages, thought to represent temporally distant infections.

Experimental Prophylaxis and Treatment

Convalescent serum has not provided protection by passive transfer of putative antibodies; however, hyperimmune anti-Ebola serum produced in horses protected nonhuman primates (baboons) challenged experimentally with *Ebola virus*. Experimental filovirus vaccines are under development. Human monoclonal antibodies against Ebola virus surface protein have been produced from mRNA obtained from bone marrow of survivors. These antibodies may be useful therapeutically. Antiviral drugs are also under development. Carbocyclic 3-deazaadenosine has been shown to cure animals infected experimentally with otherwise lethal Ebola virus infection. Several nucleoside analogue inhibitors of *S*-adenosylhomocysteine hydrolase, an important target for antiviral activity as shown by inhibition of replication of EBO-Z *in vitro*, are being explored.

Protective Measures and Prevention

Although the viral haemorrhagic fevers do not, in general, pose a common hazard to travellers, the incident of the tourist in Zimbabwe in 1975 is notable. The hospital environment at times of outbreaks of infection is a risk to health care personnel and to patients, particularly when universal precautions for contact with blood are not in place and when syringes and needles are not sterilized or are used for more than one patient. Treatment of travellers in hospitals without the highest standards is best avoided at times of outbreaks. Travellers to endemic areas are well advised to carry approved sterile packs containing disposable syringes and needles.

Surveillance and the introduction of strict public health measures, as outlined above, are essential, and the provision of epidemiological information to travel health data bases is important. Since the natural reservoir and vectors of filovirus infection are unknown, sensible precautions are important and include avoidance of quarters infested with bats and vermin, contact with dead animals, particularly chimpanzees, sleeping 'rough' or in the open, and so on.

LASSA FEVER AND ARENAVIRUS INFECTIONS

Introduction and Definitions

In 1969, two missionary nurses in Lassa, in northeast Nigeria, died from a mysterious illness, and a third nurse, who was gravely ill, was evacuated by air for treatment in the USA. This nurse recovered and convalescent plasma from her was used for the treatment of a laboratory worker in the USA who acquired the infection while working with tissue cultures infected with blood from these patients.

Lassa fever received considerable public attention because of the high mortality, which was reported initially among expatriate medical staff and among patients admitted to hospital (20–75%) in West Africa, and the death

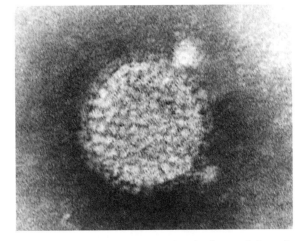

Figure 6.13 Lassa fever virus showing the characteristic sandy grain appearance and surface projections. Negative stain, × 240 000. (Courtesy of Dr David Ellis, reproduced from *Principles and Practice of Clinical Virology*, 1st edition, 1987)

of Dr Jeannette Troup, who first drew attention to the condition and who contracted the infection after carrying out two autopsies while investigating this fever. The virus (Figure 6.13) was isolated and Lassa fever was established as a virus disease of humans.

Nature of the Infectious Agent

Lassa virus is a member of the family *Arenaviridae*, genus *Arenavirus*, and is a pleomorphic enveloped single-stranded RNA particle, usually spherical, varying in size between 80 and 150 nm. The surface is covered by an array of spikes and the virus contains a large number of 20–25 nm granules, believed to be ribosomes of the host cell (Figure 6.13) acquired during the budding of the nucleocapsid from the plasmalemma. Mature infective particles are liberated by budding without destruction of the infected cell. Similar related viruses, grouped together as Mopeia strains, have been found in various areas across Africa from Zaire to Mozambique; some may yet prove to be pathogenic to humans, or may perhaps be useful as a basis for a vaccine.

The genus *Arenavirus* also includes *Lymphocytic choriomeningitis virus*, the *Tacaribe complex viruses* (haemorrhagic fever viruses of South America: *Machupo* and *Junin viruses*) as well as *Lassa virus*, all of which cross-react antigenically. Acute haemorrhagic disease due to *Machupo* and *Junin viruses* represent serious public health problems in Bolivia and Argentina, respectively, and *Guanarito virus* causes Venezuelan haemorrhagic fever. The fifth member of the arenaviruses which causes infection in humans, *Lymphocytic choriomeningitis virus*, is distributed worldwide except in Australia.

The natural reservoir hosts of the arenaviruses are rodents, and these viruses are found predominantly within two families Muridae (for example, mice and rats) and *Cricetidae* (for example, voles, lemmings and gerbils). The natural host of *Lassa virus* is the multimamate rat (*Mastomys natalensis*), which, in common with the host of *Lymphocytic Choriomeningitis virus*, is found in human dwellings and food stores, and is a member of the Muridae. In contrast, all the arenaviruses isolated from South America (with the exception of the *Tacaribe virus*, which was originally isolated from the fruit bat in Trinidad) are associated with cricetid rodents, which are found in open grasslands and forests. Human infection is usually due to contact with rodent excreta, particularly urine, which contaminate food, water and the environment.

Epidemiology and Geographical Distribution

Outbreaks of Lassa fever have occurred in hospitals in Nigeria and Liberia, but an epidemic in Sierra Leone in 1972 occurred in the community. Sporadic cases and outbreaks have been reported from West Africa since the original description of the disease. Many of the outbreaks have been in hospitals, with a high mortality in primary cases reaching 40–45%, but prolonged community outbreaks have also been reported. It should be noted that eight patients were evacuated to Europe or North America, but only one was flown out with full isolation precautions, and the remainder, of whom five were infectious, travelled on scheduled flights as fare-paying passengers. No secondary contact cases resulted.

Mastomys rats are infected at birth and completely asymptomatic peristent infection results. The virus is excreted in urine and other body fluids throughout the life of the rat. Seroconversion rates in the native human population are very high, indicating that the infection is common and usually asymptomatic or mild in endemic areas. Secondary spread occurs from person to person in conditions of overcrowding and in rural hospitals. Medical and nursing attendants or relatives who provide direct personal care are most likely to be infected, with high mortality rates in expatriate staff.

The incubation period is 3–16 days. Contact with contaminated material, aerosol and respiratory spread and cuts and abrasions of the skin are likely portals of infection.

Pathology

The reticuloendothelial system appears to be the major site of viral replication before viraemia. The degree of involvement of organs varies. The major pathogenic pathways appear, in general, to be haemorrhage and an increase in vascular permeability, caused by thrombocytopenia, coagulation defects, varying degrees of disseminated intravascular coagulation resulting from activation of the intrinsic coagulation system, and vasculopathy.

Histologically, the liver is the principal target organ in human Lassa fever virus infection. The degree of inflammatory cell infiltration is slight and is unrelated to the extent of hepatocellular damage. Eosinophilic necroses are scattered throughout the lobules. Coalescence of necrotic foci, which bridge portal-to-portal and portal-to-perivenular areas of the lobule, is a usual feature. Where the damage is more extensive, large portions of individual lobules may be destroyed, but even in these areas the reticulin framework of the liver remains intact. The nonzonal distribution of necrosis distinguishes Lassa fever virus hepatitis from the classic lesion of yellow fever. At necropsy, the extent of necrosis in the liver has been sufficient to implicate liver failure as a major cause of death. Dehydration and haemoconcentration, shock syndrome, haemorrhagic manifestations and cardiovascular collapse herald death.

Clinical Features and Diagnosis

The spectrum of Lassa fever ranges from asymptomatic infection to a fulminating fatal disease. In children the illness is relatively mild.

The onset of illness is usually insidious, with nonspecific febrile features and a sore throat and vomiting. The symptoms suddenly worsen between the third and sixth day of illness, with a high fever and severe prostration out of proportion to the degree of pyrexia. Clinical findings include conjunctivitis, severe pharyngitis and tonsillitis with whitish exudative lesions and small vesicular lesions and ulcerations, lymphadenopathy, occasionally a faint maculopapular rash and later haemorrhagic manifestations. Jaundice has not been reported, although extensive involvement of the liver is a frequent finding. Death is due to shock, anoxia and respiratory and cardiac failure. The differential diagnosis includes malaria, typhoid, yellow fever, influenza and measles.

Laboratory diagnosis is undertaken in maximum security laboratories (category 4) by virus isolation, specific antigen detection by ELISA, specific immunofluorescent staining of acetone-fixed cells, identification of surface glycoproteins and viral neutralisation assays.

Management and Treatment

Supportive measures and passive administration of immune plasma have been succesful, but not always. Intravenous administration of the antiviral drug ribavirin, particularly during the early phase of the illness, has reduced mortality very significantly.

Protective Measures and Prevention

These are essentially as those described above for the other viral haemorrhagic fevers.

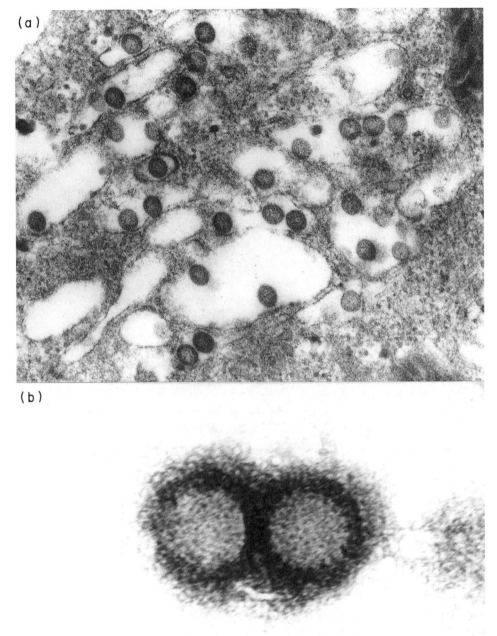

Figure 6.14 (a) Rift Valley Fever virus maturing within host cell vacuoles. × 37 500. (b) Negatively stained Rift Valley Fever virus particles from a patient's serum during the 1977 outbreak in Egypt. × 225 000. (Courtesy of Dr David Ellis, reproduced from *Principles and Practice of Clinical Virology*, 1st edition, 1987).

HAEMORRHAGIC FEVERS OF SOUTH AMERICA

These are described briefly as they do not generally present a hazard to travellers.

Argentinian haemorrhagic fever is caused by *Junin virus*, first isolated in 1958. The virus causes annual out-breaks of severe illness in between 100 and 3500 cases in agricultural workers in the wet pampas, with mortality ranging from 3–15% or more. Outbreaks coincide with the maize harvest between April and July, when the rodent populations reach a peak.

Bolivian haemorrhagic fever is caused by *Machupo virus*, with localised epidemics, which have waned considerably since the 1970s; human infections are now rare. Control of Machupo-infected rodents in households, reducing the opportunity for human contact with contaminated food and soil, accounts for the reduction of reported human infections.

RIFT VALLEY FEVER

Rift Valley fever virus is a member of the family *Bunyaviridae*, genus *Phlebovirus*, and causes an enzootic infection of sheep, cattle, camels and goats in Africa and Madagascar. The virus (Figure 6.14) is transmitted by mosquitoes and the disease is characterised by necrotic hepatitis and a haemorrhagic state, although infections are frequently inapparent or mild. Humans become infected from contact with blood and tissues of domestic livestock or mosquito bite, and the infection is a mild to severe febrile illness with encephalitis, involvement of the eye, and/or haemorrhagic fever in about 1% of cases. Human cases are usually restricted to veterinary surgeons, butchers and others in close contact with the blood of domestic livestock, and there is a potential risk with ritual slaughter.

Specific tests are undertaken in maximum security laboratories and include serology, virus isolation and inoculation of susceptible mice. There is no specific treatment and management is symptomatic.

Prevention and control is based on avoiding contact between a susceptible human or animal and the source of virus, either the infected arthropod or vertebrate. A human formalin-inactivated Rift Valley fever vaccine has been produced in primary green monkey cells and diploid fetal rhesus lung cells for use by veterinary officers, laboratory workers, military personnel and others at risk. When given in three doses it was immunogenic in over 95% of recipients, and Rift Valley fever infection has not been reported in vaccinated persons.

Inactivated tissue culture veterinary vaccines are available for immunization of sheep and cattle. A live attenuated veterinary vaccine has been developed but it is not recommended for use in unaffected enzootic zones.

CRIMEAN–CONGO HAEMORRHAGIC FEVER

A tick-borne haemorrhagic disease was described at the end of World War II in southern Russian and became known as Crimean haemorrhagic fever. Similar diseases were subsequently found in Africa, Pakistan and in the Middle East.

Crimean–Congo haemorrhagic fever virus is a member of the family *Bunyaviridae*, genus *Nairovirus*; like *Rift Valley fever virus*, it is a single-stranded RNA enveloped particle, with an overall diameter of 115–125 nm, which includes a covering of prominent hollow surface spikes that pass out through the viral membrane.

It seems probable that animals such as domestic goats and cattle, together with their ticks, may be a reservoir, particularly in the Middle East, and that humans are infected by contact with these ticks. Infections have also been acquired by staff from contact with the blood of patients in hospitals in Pakistan, Baghdad and Dubai, and there is evidence that infection acquired in this way may carry higher mortality, increasing from 20 to 70%.

The incubation period is about 7 days, followed by a sudden fever, with nausea and vomiting. Like the other haemorrhagic viruses described above, it can cause very extensive bleeding around the mouth, teeth and nose and may sometimes mimic an acute surgical emergency. These, and other severe haemorrhages that can occur into the skin of the upper parts of the body, appear during the following week, when the patient suffers from thrombocytopenia, a reduced white cell count and widespread impairment of liver function, without evidence of any cellular inflammation. There may also be neurological complications. Diagnosis may be confirmed by fluorescence antibody techniques and by direct examination electron microscopy of serum or by infection of suckling mice or BHK cells. Specific treatment is not yet available.

Dugbe, Ganjam, Hazara and *Nairobi sheep disease viruses*, the other members of the genus *Nairovirus*, have all been reported as having caused human infections, although none has proved fatal. There is some evidence of cross-protection among the group.

REFERENCES

Advisory Committee on Immunization Practices (ACIP) (1999a) Rotavirus vacine for the prevention of rotavirus gastroenteritis among children. *Morbidity and Mortality Weekly Report*, **48**, RR-2, 1–23.

Advisory Committee on Immunization Practices (ACIP) (1999b) Human rabies prevention: United States 1999. *Morbidity and Mortality Weekly Report*, **48**, RR-2, 1–23.

Compendium of Animal Rabies Control (1999) *Morbidity and Mortality Weekly Epidemiological Report*, **48**, RR-3, 1–9.

FURTHER READING

Hepatitis A

Catton MG and Locarnini SA (1998) Epidemiology of hepatitis A. In *Viral Hepatitis* (eds AJ Zuckerman and HC Thomas), 2nd edn, pp 29–41. Churchill Livingstone, London.

Koff RS (1998) Hepatitis A. *Lancet*, **351**, 1643–1649.

Lemon SM and Thomas DL (1997) Vaccines to prevent viral hepatitis. *New England Journal of Medicine*, **336**, 196–204.

Steffen R and Gyurech D (1994) Advances in hepatitis A prevention in Travellers. *Journal of Medical Virology*, **44**, 460–462.

Hepatitis B

Chang M-H, Chen C-J, Lai M-S *et al.* (1997) Universal hepatitis B vaccination in Taiwan and the incidence of hepatocellular carcinoma in children. *New England Journal of Medicine*, **336**, 1855–1859.

Harrison TJ, Dusheiko GM and Zuckerman AJ (2000) Hepatitis Viruses. In *Principles and Practice of Clinical Virology* (eds AJ Zuckerman, J Banatvala and JR Pattison, 4th edn, pp. 187–223. Wiley, Chichester.

Van Damme P, Kane M and Mehens A (1997) Integration of hepatitis B vaccination into national immunisation programmes. *BMJ*, **314**, 1033–1036.

Wright TL and Lau JYN (1993) Clinical aspects of hepatitis B virus infection. *Lancet*, **342**, 1340–1344.

Zuckerman JN (1996) Nonresponse to hepatitis B vaccines and the kinetics of anti-HBs production. *Journal of Medical Virology*, **50**, 283–288.

Zuckerman AJ and Zuckerman JN (1999). Molecular epidemiology of hepatitis B virus mutants. *Journal of Medical Virology*, **58**, 193–195.

Hepatitis C

Alter MJ (1997) The epidemiology of acute and chronic hepatitis C. *Clinics in Liver Disease*, **1**, 559–568.

Houghton M (1966) Hepatitis C virus. In *Fields Virology* (eds BN Fields, DM Knipe and PM Howley), 3rd edn, pp 1035–1058. Lippincott-Raven, Philadelphia.

National Institutes of Health Consensus Development Conference (1997) Management of hepatitis C. *Hepatology*, **26** (suppl. 1), 1–155.

Recommendations for Prevention and Control of Hepatitis C Virus (HCV) Infection and HCV-Related Chronic Disease (1998) *Morbidity and Mortality Weekly Report* (suppl.), **47**, 1–39.

Hepatitis D

Di Bisceglie AM (1998) Hepatitis D virus. Epidemiology and diagnosis. In *Viral Hepatitis* (eds AJ Zuckerman and HC Thomas), 2nd edn, pp 371–378. Churchill Livingstone, London.

Hadziyannis SJ (1999) Hepatitis D. *Clinics in Liver Disease*, **3**, 309–325.

Hepatitis E

Bradley DW (1992) Hepatitis E: epidemiology, aetiology and molecular biology. *Reviews in Medical Virology*, **2**, 19–28.

Jameel S, Durgapal H, Habibullah CM *et al.* (1992) Enteric non-A, non-B hepatitis: epidemics, animal transmission and hepatitis E detection by the polymerase chain reaction. *Journal of Medical Virology*, **37**, 263–270.

Mushahwar IK and Dawson GJ (1997) Hepatitis E virus: epidemiology, molecular biology and diagnosis. In *The Molecular Medicine of Viral Hepatitis* (eds TJ Harrison and AJ Zuckerman), pp 33–43. Wiley, Chichester.

Human immunodeficiency virus and AIDS

Armstrong D and Cohen J (eds) (1999) HIV and AIDS (several chapter authors). In *Infectious Diseases*, vol. 2, sect. 5, pp 1.1–28.6. Mosby, London.

Coffin JM (1996) HIV population dynamics *in vivo*: implications for genetic variation, pathogenesis and therapy. *Science*, **271**, 1582–1586.

Starkie J and Dale R (1988) *Understanding AIDS*. Consumers Association and Hodder and Stoughton, London.

Weiss RA, Dalgleish AG and Loveday C (2000) Human retroviruses. In *Principles and Practice of Clinical Virology* (eds AJ Zuckerman, JE Banatvala and JR Pattison), 4th edn, pp 659–693. Wiley, Chichester.

UNAIDS and WHO (1988) *Report on the Global HIV/AIDS Epidemic*. UNAIDS and WHO, Geneva.

Viral Gastroenteritis

Cook SM, Glass RI, LeBaron CW *et al.* (1990) Global seasonality ofrotavirus infections. *Bulletin of the World Health Organization*, **68**, 171–177.

Desselberger U (1998) Viral gastroenteritis. *Current Opinion in Infectious Diseases*, **11**, 565–575.

Desselberger U (2000) Viruses associated with acute diarrhoeal disease. In *Principles and Practice of Clinical Virology* (eds AJ Zuckerman, JE Banatvala and JR Pattison), 4th edn, pp 235–252. Wiley, Chichester.

Vipond IB, Caul EO, Lambden PR *et al.* (1999) 'Hyperemesis hiemis': new light on an old syndrome. *Microbiology Today*, **26**, 110–112.

Polyomyelitis and other Enterovirus Infections

Minor PD, Morgan-Capner M and Muir P (2000) Enteroviruses. In *Principles and Practice of Clinical Virology*, (eds AJ Zuckerman, JE Banatvala and JR Pattison), 4th edn, pp 427–449. Wiley, Chichester.

Salisbury DM and Begg NT (eds) (1996) Poliomyelitis. In *Immunisation against Infectious Disease*, pp 173–182. Stationery Office, London.

Influenza

Centers for Disease Control (1997) Update: influenza activity—United States, 1997–1998 season. *Morbidity and Mortality Weekly Report*, **46**, 1094–1098.

Centers for Disease Control (1998) Update: outbreak of influenza A infection—Alaska and the Yukon Territory, July–August 1998. *Morbidity and Mortality Weekly Report*, **47**, 685–688.

Centers for Disease Control (1998) Prevention and control in influenza: recommendations of the Advisory Committee on Immunisation Practices (ACIP). *Morbidity and Mortality Weekly Report*, no. RR-6.

Cox NJ and Subbarao K (1999) Influenza. *Lancet*, **354**, 1277–1282.

Genital Herpes

Corey L and Spear P (1986) Infections with herpes simplex virus,Part I and II. *New England Journal of Medicine*, **314**, 686–691, 794–757.

Whitley RJ (1996) Herpes simplex viruses. In *Field's Virology* (eds BN Field, DM Knipe and PM Howley), 3rd edn, pp 2297–2342. Raven Press, New York.

Rabies

Nicholson KG (2000) Rabies. In *Principles and Practice of Clinical Virology*, (eds AJ Zuckerman, JE Banatvala and JR Pattison), 4th edn, pp 583–618. Wiley, Chichester.

WHO (1992) Expert Committee on Rabies, 8th report. *World Health Organization Technical Report Series*, **824**.

Yellow Fever

Centers for Disease Control (1990) Yellow fever vaccine: recommendations of the Immunization Practices Advisory Committee (ACIP). *Morbidity and Mortality Weekly Report*, **39**, 1–6.

Schoub BD and Backburn NK (1995) Flaviviruses. In *Principles and Practice of Clinical Virology* (eds AJ Zuckerman, JE Banatvala and JR Pattison), 3rd edn, pp 485–515. Wiley, Chichester.

Stephenson JR (1988) Flavivirus vaccines. *Vaccine*, **6**, 471–482.

Zuckerman AJ (1970) Yellow fever. In *Virus Diseases of the Liver*, pp 110–119. Butterworths, London.

Dengue Fever

Schmaljohn AL and McClain D (1996) Alphaviruses (Togaviridae) and Flaviviruses (Flaviviridae). In *Medical Microbiology* (ed. S Baron), 4th edn, pp 685–700. University of Texas, Galveston.

Schoub BD and Blackburn NK (2000). Flaviviruses. In *Principles and Practice of Clinical Virology* (eds AJ Zuckerman, JE Banatvala and JR Pattison), 4th edn, pp 485–573. Wiley, Chichester.

Japanese Encephalitis, St Louis Encephalitis, Tick-Borne Encephalitis and Other Flavivirus Infections

Salisbury DM and Begg NT (1996) *Immunisation Against Infectious Disease*. Stationery Office, London.

Schmaljohn AL and McClain D (1996) Alphaviruses and flaviviruses. In *Medical Microbiology*, (ed. S Baron), 4th edn, pp 685–700. University of Texas, Galveston.

Schoub DB and Blackburn NK (2000) Japanese encephalitis. Tick-borne encephalitis. In *Principles and Practice of Clinical Virology* (eds AJ Zuckerman, JE Banatvala and JR Pattison), 4th edn, pp 508–510. Wiley, Chichester.

Zuckerman AJ, Banatvala JE, and Pattison JR (eds) (2000) *Principles and Practice of Clinical Virology*, 4th edn. Wiley, Chichester.

Viral Haemorrhagic Fevers

Griffiths PD, Ellis DS and Zuckerman AJ (1990) Other common types of viral hepatitis and exotic infections. *British Medical Bulletin*, **46**, 512–532.

Howard CR (1986). Arenaviruses. In *Perspectives in Medical Virology*, vol. 2 (ed. AJ Zuckerman), pp 1–318. Elsevier, Amsterdam.

Klenk HD (ed.) (1999) Marburg and Ebola viruses. *Current Topics in Microbiology and Immunology*, **235**, 1–217.

Peters CJ and LeDuck J (eds) (1999) Ebola: the virus and the disease. *Journal of Infectious Diseases*, **179** (suppl. 1), S1–S288.

7

Bacterial Infections in Travellers

Christopher J. Ellis and Ann L.N. Chapman

Birmingham Heartlands Hospital, Birmingham, UK

INTRODUCTION

Most practitioners take it for granted that the earlier in the course of a bacterial infection antibacterials are given, the more rapid and certain the patient's recovery; in some conditions, such as leptospirosis and typhoid fever, there is good evidence to support this belief. As the most rapid bacteriological confirmation of diagnosis may take 24 h, a period during which a bacterial population could double in size through as many as 60 generations, it follows that 'therapeutic trials' are good practice in managing patients with acute febrile illness if a bacterial cause is reasonably likely, provided that appropriate samples for laboratory investigations have been taken first, particularly so in the case of those returning from the tropics in whom a firm diagnosis may not be possible before convalescence. Investigations should always include *blood films for malarial parasites* in patients returned from tropical countries, while prudent immediate treatment might include antimalarial therapy in addition to antibacterials that are chosen with a view to covering at least the most rapidly progressive of likely bacterial infections.

The clinical history is crucial to diagnosis and management and will establish not only *where* a returned traveller has been, but exactly *when* (knowledge of incubation periods being invaluable in establishing a differential diagnosis when this includes infections unlikely to be acquired at home), together with answers to specific inquiries into the *traveller's activities* abroad. Sexually transmitted diseases apart, travellers to temperate areas are at particular risk of only one bacterial infection—legionellosis. Although largely a disease of temperate climates, this must also be considered in those returning from the tropics who have 'stopped-over' in air-conditioned hotels on the way back. What the traveller did should include enquiries about sexual activity, walking or working in scrub, any exposure of skin to water in which rats might have urinated, and any ingestion of unpasteurised milk products. Information on immunisation status is generally less important, since the efficacy of

bacterial vaccines other than diphtheria and tetanus toxoid is significantly less than 100%.

One bacterial infection, *tuberculosis*, will not be considered further in this chapter because travel is of little diagnostic relevance, although it is certainly of great epidemiological significance. Most cases of tuberculosis, pulmonary and extrapulmonary, in immigrants from the Indian subcontinent arise within 4 years either of first arrival in the UK or of returning from a visit to the subcontinent lasting several months.

Table 7.1 lists bacterial infections encountered in British returned travellers.

A Note on Urgent Treatment

The two treatable infections most likely to cause rapidly progressive disease in travellers recently returned from the tropics are leptospirosis and falciparum malaria. In both conditions initial diagnostic tests may be negative but treatment with doxycycline or antimalarials should not be delayed if either is possible. The finding of an eschar (which may be mistaken for an infected insect bite) in someone whose activities placed them at risk of typhus should also lead to immediate treatment with doxycycline, although imported typhus fevers are rarely life-threatening.

LEGIONELLOSIS

Definition

Infection with *Legionella pneumophila* may result in one of two distinct diseases: Pontiac fever, a mild nonfocal infection with an incubation period of 1–2 days; and Legionnaires' disease, characterised by pneumonia, with multisystem disease in severe cases, which has an incubation period of between 2 and 10 days, with a median of 6 days.

Principles and Practice of Travel Medicine. Edited by Jane N. Zuckerman.
© 2001 John Wiley & Sons Ltd.

Table 7.1 Bacterial infections in British returned travellers

Infection[a]	Most common features	Incubation (days)	Most rapid diagnosis
Brucellosis (1)	Ingestion of unpasteurised milk products	5–30	Blood culture
Diphtheria (< 1)	Membranous tonsillitis in nonimmune travellers. Indian subcontinent most common source of British imports	2–5	Culture of throat swab = carriage. Membrane + bull neck + toxicity = diphtheria
Typhoid (200)	British Asians visiting Indian subcontinent. Fever usually sustained	7–21	Blood culture
Typhus (10)	Walking in scrub in Africa or Southeast Asia; eschar	Scrub 10–21 Tick 5–7	Serology
Leptospirosis (10)	Exposure to rat-infested water; multisystem; leucocytosis in 80%	4–19	Serology
Endemic relapsing fever (< 1)	Exposed to risk of tick bites; relapsing fever	5–15	Blood film

[a]Values in parentheses are the number of cases currently identified in average years in England and Wales.

Nature of the Infectious Agent

L. pneumophila is a Gram-negative, strictly aerobic bacillus that stains poorly or not at all with standard methods and will not grow on usual bacteriological media. These unusual features explain why it remained unrecognised as a human pathogen until the exceptionally thorough investigation of an outbreak of pneumonia in Philadelphia in 1976.

Epidemiology

L. pneumophila is a saprophyte found in still water where it lives in biofilms in conjunction with a number of other organisms, including environmental amoebae. In order for it to pose a significant threat to human health it must be present in significant numbers, which is only likely with water temperatures of greater than 20 °C, and it must be aerosolised in order that it can be inhaled. Power station cooling towers have given rise to outbreaks but in travellers the major risk appears to be from hotel air conditioning and showers. If plumbing complies with agreed standards then the risk is greatly reduced but new hotels in Mediterranean countries, usually Turkey and Spain, are responsible for a disproportionate number of cases. Sources of infection in travellers from England and Wales in 1998 are listed in Table 7.2 (Joseph *et al.*, 1999):

Reservoir of Infection

See Epidemiology. Infection invariably results from inhalation of bacteria in aerosolised water. Human-to-human transmission has never been described.

Pathology

In most cases of Legionnaires' disease pathological changes are confined to the lung and consist of an acute inflammatory exudate into the alveoli. In severe cases inflammation is generalised and both lungs are involved, but more often part of a single lobe bears the brunt. Panlobar pneumonia is unusual. Organisms are usually found within macrophages in the alveoli but not the bronchi. In severe cases there may be generalised pulmonary oedema and the systemic changes of septic shock.

Clinical Features

Case History 1
A 42-year-old smoker presented 4 days after returning from a 1 week holiday in Turkey. He complained of headaches and feverishness but said his cough was 'no worse than usual'. Clinical examination was normal, other than a temperature of 39 °C. CXR: hazy patch left hilum. Outcome: recovered on clarithromycin therapy. *L. pneumophila* infection was subsequently confirmed serologically. Enquiries revealed that his 62-year-old father-in-law had been on holiday with him and was at home with 'flu'. He was also treated for legionellosis and the diagnosis was subsequently confirmed in him as well.

Legionnaires' disease typically begins as a 'flu-like illness, that is, with aches and pains, headache and malaise. In

Table 7.2 Sources of legionellosis: travellers from England and Wales, 1998

Source	Number
Spain and Spanish islands	37
Turkey	20
France	9
Greece	4
Elsewhere in Europe	9
UK	9
European cruises	3
USA/Canada	5
Caribbean	5
Far East	4
North/East Africa	2
More than one country	8
Total	115

many cases the pneumonic element remains clinically inapparent and any returned traveller exhibiting these symptoms requires a chest X-ray urgently as it may provide a clue to the diagnosis, which would justify immediate administration of appropriate treatment, usually a macrolide antibacterial agent. Most patients have a dry cough but this may not be very noticeable and can be overlooked. Mucopurulent sputum may be produced after 2–3 days of dry cough. The clinician may be put off the diagnostic scent by systemic symptoms such as vomiting, diarrhoea, confusion and delirium, especially in the elderly. Chest radiographs typically show one or more patchy infiltrates, usually involving only one lung, but in severe cases areas of consolidation may be visible in both. Liver function tests characteristically show mild to moderate hepatitis with raised transaminases and slight increase in bilirubin.

Most patients improve after 2–3 days of appropriate therapy but in severe cases—most often in the elderly and those with pre-existing lung disease—the patient may develop respiratory failure and/or shock despite treatment and die within a few days of the onset of symptoms.

The diagnosis must be founded on clinical suspicion as it will not be made by the result of any routine test such as blood culture. The detection of antigen in the urine is the most rapid noninvasive test currently available, giving a positive result within a few days of admission to hospital in 80% of patients with *L. pneumophila* serogroup 1 infection, which causes over 80% of human disease (Plouffe *et al.*, 1995). Direct immunofluorescence of bronchoalveolar washings obtained at bronchoscopy provides the diagnosis in about 50% of cases ultimately proved by culture of sputum in special media containing charcoal, yeast extract, L-cysteine, ferric salts and a pH buffer. The isolation of morphologically characteristic Gram-negative rods in 2–5 days, but not on routine culture media, is presumptive evidence of legionella infection. Serological tests provide retrospective confirmation; however, it is important to recognise that serology may not become

positive for 4–6 weeks after onset of symptoms, and thus an initial negative result taken during the acute phase should not be regarded as excluding legionella infection.

Management

Retrospective analysis of the first outbeak of Legionnaires' disease to be recognised showed that survival rates were higher in patients treated with erythromycin. Subsequently, erythromycin, administered intravenously in ill patients, has become the treatment of choice if the diagnosis of legionellosis is suspected. In severe illness rifampicin is commonly added.

More recently, some of the newer macrolides such as azithromycin have been demonstrated to have superior *in vitro* activity against *L. pneumophila*. Quinolones also have greater *in vitro* activity and may penetrate tissue more effectively than the macrolides, although no prospective controlled *in vivo* trials have been performed (reviewed by Dedicoat and Venkatesan, 1999).

Prevention

There is no vaccine for legionellosis. Enforcement of building regulations to minimise stagnation of warm water that will subsequently be released into the atmosphere substantially reduces the risk of the disease.

In travellers, even a provisional diagnosis of Legionnaires' disease should cause clinicians to enquire about travelling companions who had been exposed to the same environment, in whom immediate treatment at the onset of symptoms would be indicated.

TYPHOID AND PARATYPHOID FEVER

Definition

Systemic infections spread by the faecal–oral route. Unlike the zoonotic salmonellae that cause enteritis, *Salmonella typhi* and *paratyphi* infection is confined to humans and is acquired either from cases or carriers.

Nature of the Infectious Agent

S. typhi are Gram-negative bacilli that possess flagellae, do not ferment lactose in most cases, but do produce hydrogen sulphide from sulphur-containing amino acids.

Epidemiology

The survival of the typhoidal salmonella depends ultimately on deficient sanitation, which ensures transmission to susceptible individuals via food or water that has been contaminated by the faeces or urine of a case or carrier. Cases are infectious from the first week of illness and in most cases bacilli are excreted throughout the remaining illness and for about 1 month thereafter. About 10% of cases excrete bacilli for a further 2 months, while about 2% become permanent carriers. This is most likely in individuals with pre-existing gall bladder disease but *S. typhi* may give rise to a low-grade cholecystis *de novo*. Coexisting *Schistomsoma haematobium* infection of the bladder predisposes to chronic urinary excretion.

Pathology

S. typhi and *paratyphi* typically penetrate the mucosa of the small intestine without giving rise to enterocolitis, but in a minority of cases of typhoid fever there is a history of watery diarrhoea within 1–2 days of the likely time of ingestion of the organism. The bacilli multiply within mononuclear cells in small intestine-associated lymphoid tissue, then pass via lymphatics to continue intracellular multiplication in liver, spleen and bone marrow. About 10 days after ingestion (the incubation period being inversely related to the infecting dose), bacteria enter the bloodstream and symptoms occur. In untreated individuals, inflammation and necrosis continue in lymphoid tissue in the small bowel mucosa until there is considerable mucosal destruction, with resultant intestinal haemorrhage or perforation, typically in the third or fourth weeks of infection.

Clinical Features

Case History 2
A 33-year-old woman was admitted with a 5 day history of fever and headache which began 2 days before she left India, where she had been visiting relatives for 5 weeks. Her temperature was 39 °C but examination was otherwise normal and she did not appear ill. A chest film was clear and no malarial parasites were seen on blood films. The next day Gram-negative bacilli were seen in blood cultures taken on admission and she was prescribed oral ciprofloxacin. The bacilli were identified as *S. typhi* the next day. She remained pyrexial for 5 days but was otherwise well and she made an uncomplicated recovery.

The illness begins insidiously, after an incubation period of between 1 and 3 weeks, with malaise, fever and headache. In most cases the fever gradually increases through the first week and the patient is rarely afebrile. Children, however, often have a swinging fever. At the end of the first week bloodborne spread of the organism may lead to focal symptoms such as cough (and chest X-ray may show areas of consolidation), meningism (occasionally with

lymphocytes in cerebrospinal fluid), constipation or watery diarrhoea (it is as much a myth that diarrhoea is not a feature of typhoid fever as it is that it is usual). Most travellers returning to western countries seek medical advice within a week of onset of fever and therefore the presentation of typhoid fever seen in western Europe and North America is that of a comparatively mild 'flu-like illness with a persistent fever. Provided blood cultures are taken at this point—when the patient is not clinically septicaemic—the diagnosis can be made and the patient treated before becoming significantly ill. By the second and third week of untreated illness the abdomen is likely to become tender and distended and tends to be silent. The liver and spleen are palpably enlarged in at least half of the cases; by the third week of untreated illness complications are likely, the most important being overwhelming septicaemia, severe focal infection such as meningitis or pneumonia and necrosis of the lymphoid follicles (Peyer patches) of the small intestine, leading to ulceration with potentially massive bleeding or perforation. Untreated, mortality from typhoid fever is about 20%, even in previously healthy individuals.

Diagnosis

A 'flu-like illness with documented fever in an individual who has returned from an insanitary region in the previous month should lead to consideration of the diagnosis. Blood cultures should be taken and *S. typhi* will grow in 70–80% of cases in standard media within 2 days. Cultures of bone marrow aspirate have an even higher yield. In a majority of cases cultures remain negative, and a therapeutic trial of an antibacterial agent is justifiable under circumstances that make the diagnosis likely, provided the practitioner bears in mind that the fever typically takes between 3 and 7 days to settle, even when the strain is fully sensitive to the agent used. *S. typhi* serology is unreliable and now rarely used.

TYPHUS FEVERS

Introduction

Imported typhus fevers are generally mild and self-limiting zoonoses that are seen exclusively in travellers who venture on foot into bush and scrub (Table 7.3).

Nature of the Infectious Agent

Rickettsiae are small pleomorphic bacteria that are obligate intracellular parasites and therefore do not grow on standard bacteriological media. Their inability to survive outside the cytoplasm of their host cell results from their dependence on the host for ATP. Outside the host cell they rapidly lose energy and, as a result, their infectivity.

Table 7.3 Rickettsial infection in travellers

Disease (symptoms)	Organism	Geographic distribution	Vector (from rodent reservoir)	Clinical
Rocky Mountain spotted fever	*Rickettsia rickettsii*	June to September in USA (principally eastern) and Canada; Central America	Tick	Prominent rash
Mediterranean spotted fever (boutonneuse fever, tick typhus, South African tick bite fever)	*R. conorii*	Mediterranean coast, Black Sea basin, eastern, central and southern Africa	Tick	Eschar usual
Scrub typhus (tsutsugamushi fever)	*R. tsutsugamushi*	Southwest Pacific, Southeast Asia, Japan	Mite	Eschar usual

Epidemiology

The rickettsiae that cause disease in travellers are zoonoses in the ecology of which humans play an accidental and incidental role, unlike louse-borne typhus, which causes epidemics when people crowd together in refugee camps. Infections in travellers are sporadic and are largely confined to those who wander in woods in North America, bush in Africa and scrub in Southeast Asia. (In Central and North America domestic dogs may act as a reservoir for Rocky Mountain spotted fever (RMSF) rickettsiae so that, in theory, dog ticks could bite people in their homes and thus transmit infection indoors.)

Tick typhus is regularly seen by practitioners working in southern Africa in people who walk in game reserves and similar terrain, and is likely to be seen increasingly in tourists attracted by easier travel between the Republic of South Africa and Zimbabwe. Scrub typhus is found in pockets through much of Southeast Asia and causes sporadic illness in the native population engaged in slash-and-burn subsistence farming. It is comparatively common in the Sylhet region of Bangladesh, the origin of Britain's earliest Indian restauranteurs. On returning to their ethnic homeland, they may help their relatives and become infected in the process.

Pathology

The intracellular multiplication of rickettsiae gives rise to a diffuse lymphocytic vasculitis with endothelial damage. Increased permeability and foci of haemorrhage are the result. Platelet aggregation at sites of vascular injury commonly gives rise to thrombocytopenia, but full-scale disseminated intravascular coagulation is rare in the nonepidemic typhus fevers.

Clinical Features

Scrub and Tick Typhus

Case History 3
A 24-year-old female backpacker presented on her return from a 4 week visit to Thailand with a 'flu-like illness associated with macular rash. On examination, there was an eschar on her upper arm, with regional lymphadenopathy. She was treated with oral doxycycline and made a good recovery. The diagnosis of scrub typhus was subsequently confirmed serologically.

Headache, myalgia and feverishness—a nondescript 'flu-like illness—are the first, and often the only, symptoms of tick and scrub typhus and typically start quite abruptly between 5 and 7 days after the arthropod bite. Examination will reveal an eschar at the site of a tick bite in most cases. This typically has a black necrotic centre, resembling a black scab, up to 1 cm in diameter surrounded by an area of acute inflammation about 3 cm across. It is often dismissed as a secondarily infected insect bite. A dull maculopapular rash, usually involving palms and soles, appears about 5 days after the onset of illness. Cough with radiographic evidence of a patchy pneumonitis is common in scrub typhus. Untreated, symptoms usually settle spontaneously after about 10 days, but with appropriate treatment recovery is usually apparent after 2 days.

Rocky Mountain Spotted Fever

The illness ranges from a mild 'flu-like illness to the picture of overwhelming sepsis with multiorgan failure and a generalised maculopapular rash, which typically appears on the third day. Purpura are common and the picture then resembles meningococcaemia, except that in the latter condition the purpuric rash typically appears within hours of the onset of symptoms and a maculopapular element is absent. The incubation period ranges from 2 to 10 days but as the ticks responsible for transmission are tiny, and their bites are seldom noticed, this is usually of little help in establishing the diagnosis in endemic areas. Outside these, the fact of having walked or camped in rural North America, especially in the Carolinas, Virginia, Maryland, Georgia, Tennessee and Oklahoma between June and September, is enough to justify empirical treatment in an individual who is ill with compatible symptoms (reviewed in Silber, 1996).

Diagnosis

Empirical therapy of patients ill with suspected rickett-sioses is vital because there is no reliable early diagnostic test (reviewed in La Scola and Raoult, 1997). In practice, patients with 'flu-like symptoms, a normal white cell count and thrombocytopenia in some cases, are likely to receive antimalarials if they have travelled in a malarious area, but such patients should always be inspected care-fully for an eschar and, if a compatible lesion is seen, they should also be treated for possible typhus. The diagnosis can be confirmed later by a rise in antibody titre.

Treatment

Tetracyclines have been used most extensively in rickett-sial infection and remain the treatment of choice. Doxycycline 100 mg daily is effective in tick and scrub typhus, whereas double this dose is advised in Rocky Mountain spotted fever. As with most infections, there is no good evidence on optimal duration of treatment: con-tinuing for 2 days after defervescence is conventional.

Prevention

When walking in endemic areas, travellers should try to minimise pushing through dense vegetation and stay in relatively open areas as far as possible. Inspecting the body for ticks every few hours, and removing them by steady traction, will help to protect travellers but the best, ultimate protection is the preparedness of physicians to administer tetracyclines promptly on the first reasonable suspicion of rickettsial infection.

LEPTOSPIROSIS

Definition

A spirochaetal infection, the severity of which ranges from inapparent to a life-threatening illness with multi-system involvement. Infection is usually acquired as a result of exposure to fresh water contaminated with the urine of domestic or wild animals.

Epidemiology

A zoonosis with a worldwide distribution, the polar re-gions excepted. Infected reservoir animals excrete spirochaetes in their urine and humans are infected either by direct exposure (chiefly in farm workers, for example in milking parlours in the case of serovar Hardjo) or via contact with contaminated water during activities such as wading through streams or in paddy fields or while wash-ing, etc. The contact may not, however, have been obvi-ous to the subject (see case history 4). The incubation period is about 10 days, with a range of between 4 and 19 days.

Reservoir of Infection

Serovars pathogenic to humans are harboured by domes-tic animals, including dogs, and livestock including cattle, pigs and horses. A variety of wild animals may harbour pathogenic serovars but rats are the most important natural reservoir.

Pathology

In severe cases with multisystem involvement (Weil's dis-ease) there is extensive vasculitis with focal haemorrhage in many organs. The kidneys are swollen, with evidence of interstitial ephritis, and there may be necrosis of proximal tubular epithelium. Spirochaetes have been seen between the necrotic cells. Meningeal involvement suggests viral meningitis, in that lymphocytes usually predominate, but a polymorphonuclear leucocytosis is usual in the blood. Multisystem infection may be immunologically mediated.

Clinical Features

Most infections are subclinical but clinical illness usually consists of a 'flu-like illness with headache and muscle pain. This may progress seamlessly to a multisystem dis-ease (see case history 4) or the patient may recover before apparently relapsing with recurrence of fever, and in some cases aseptic meningitis, hepatitis, renal failure and a haemorrhagic rash.

> Case History 4
> A 46-year-old man was admitted with 'flu-like symptoms 4 days after returning from staying with relatives in Jamaica. On admission, he was pyrexial, jaundiced and had photophobia but no

neck stiffness. There was no rash. Immediate investigations revealed a neutrophil count of 17×10^9 per litre and evidence of a mild hepatitis. Despite immediate commencement of penicillin, he developed anuric renal failure and required dialysis for 3 weeks before complete recovery. Leptospirosis was diagnosed serologically during convalescence. He recalled seeing rats around the 'outside privy' and said he had worn sandals throughout his visit.

Diagnosis

A high index of suspicion is required as the disease presents in a nonspecific manner. The diagnosis can usually be made serologically, with positive results appearing from day 6 to 12 of illness; however, some patients may remain seronegative throughout if their infecting serotype is not detected by the currently available assays. Leptospires can be cultured from blood or cerebrospinal fluid in the first few days of illness, and subsequently in urine. Culture requires specialised media and takes 5–6 weeks.

Management and Treatment

Early treatment may be life-saving. Those patients with a biphasic illness who are not treated until there is evidence of multisystem disease may show no response to antibiotics and require supportive therapy. The spirochaetes are sensitive to penicillin, tetracyclines and macrolides (e.g. erythromycin).

Prevention

Immunisation is not justified by the low risk to travellers; advice to travellers who intend to walk in Africa or Southeast Asia should include a caution against wading barefoot through water likely to be contaminated by rat urine, especially still or slow-flowing water close to human habitation.

BRUCELLOSIS

Definition

A zoonosis transmitted to humans via contact with infected animals or by ingestion of their unpasteurised milk. Now virtually extinct as an endemic infection in Britain, it is still seen occasionally in returned travellers.

Nature of the Infectious Agent

The genus *Brucella* includes three species pathogenic to man: *B. melitensis* (enzootic in sheep and goats), *B. abortus* (cattle) and *B. suis* (pigs). Brucella organisms are slow growing, Gram-negative fastidious aerobes. Growth is encouraged by vigorous aeration and many strains require supplementary carbon dioxide.

Epidemiology

The reservoirs of infection are wild and domestic animals. Cattle, pigs, sheep and goats are the main sources of human infection but related wild species are also reservoirs of the organisms. Globally, most cases arise in farmers and others whose work or way of life brings them into regular contact with reservoir animals; the occasional cases now imported to Britain are usually the result of ingestion of unpasteurised milk products. An epizootic in Arabian Gulf countries in the last two decades led to thousands of human cases in Bedouin and other indigenous people, with occasional cases in western expatriates who had received their hospitality.

Clinical Features

There is a range of clinical presentations from an acute 'flu-like illness, with chills, myalgia and headache, to a more chronic disease with an insidious onset in which the fever may be low-grade or intermittent and focal symptoms may eventually emerge. Meningitis, with lymphocytes predominating in the cerebrospinal fluid, has been comparatively common in the recent Arabian Gulf epidemic but sacroilitis, vertebral discitis with later extension to adjacent vertebrae, and infection of the genitourinary tract are well documented, as is endocarditis. Depression is a common accompaniment to chronic infections.

Diagnosis

Positive blood or bone marrow cultures provide the only conclusive proof of infection and are present in a majority of those with acute febrile presentations, but in only a minority of those with chronic illness. Using traditional blood culture methods, growth of brucellae may not be apparent for 3 weeks or more, but new semiautomatic rapid isolation systems (e.g. Bactec) may allow detection in as little as 3 days (Gedikoglu *et al.*, 1996). Serological tests are reliable if IgM is detected, although when IgG antibody predominates it may be difficult to distinguish between active and past infection (Gad El-Rab and Kambal, 1998).

Treatment

Best results have been obtained with doxycycline 100 mg twice daily with rifampicin 15 mg kg^{-1}, both for 45 days. This length of treatment is necessary to prevent relapse because of the intracellular persistence and low growth rate of brucellae.

DIPHTHERIA

Definition

An acute infection of tonsils and pharynx, less often of larynx or nose, or of skin. In individuals immunised against the exotoxin produced by *Corynebacterium diphtheriae*, infection may still occur but gives rise to no more than moderate inflammation of the infected site. In the unimmunised, the production of toxin leads to the characteristic leathery pharyngeal exudate, swelling of the neck, cranial and peripheral demyelinating neuropathy and myocarditis. In toxaemic cases, early administration of antitoxin is vital.

Nature of the Infectious Agent

C. diphtheriae is a nonsporulating pleomorphic Gram-positive bacillus. The species is subdivided into three types, *gravis*, *intermedius* and *mitis*, based on *in vitro* culture characteristics. The ogranisms is generally not particularly invasive, remaining in the superficial layers of pharyngeal mucosa; the major virulence determinant is the production of a potent exotoxin which inhibits protein synthesis in mammalian cells. *Gravis* biotypes are most likely to be toxigenic. Nontoxigenic strains can cause local inflammation without systemic complications.

Epidemiology and Reservoir

Carriage of *C. diphtheriae* and diphtheria are confined to humans. Although immunisation does not prevent acquisition and carriage of *C. diphtheriae*, and even a minor inflammatory reaction at the site of infection, clinical infection of any kind is extremely rare in immunised communities. Furthermore, clinical infection is rare even in many unimmunised communities, including most of sub-Saharan Africa, but cases are comparatively common in the Indian subcontinent, the Middle East and in the Russian Federation, especially the southern republics and in emigrants from these areas to St Petersburg and Moscow. Travel to these areas poses a theoretical risk to older travellers in whom immunity might be waning, but the last case in Britain was in an unimmunised child who acquired the infection in Pakistan.

Clinical Features

Diphtheria typically starts with a sore throat and difficulty in swallowing. The patient appears 'toxic', is flushed with a rapid pulse, and examination of the throat typically reveals a grey membrane adherent to the tonsils. Within a few days there may be swelling of the neck and evidence of myocarditis or peripheral neuropathy.

Diagnosis

The diagnosis is usually a presumptive one, based on the clinical features. The organism can occasionally be identified on throat swab or smears of the membrane, but definitive identification is based on culture of *C. diphtheriae* from such samples. Selective media are required for optimal growth, and thus the laboratory must be alerted if there is clinical suspicion of diphtheria.

Treatment

C. diphtheriae is sensitive to penicillins but this has no effect on toxaemia, at the first sign of which antitoxin should be administered. Evidence of disordered conduction on ECG is enough to justify immediate administration of antitoxin, which is ineffective once the toxin has bound to target cells (reviewed in Bonnet and Begg, 1999).

Prevention

Travellers visiting areas where diphtheria is known to be prevalent should receive a booster of low-dose vaccine if more than 10 years have passed since a primary course. This is most important for longer-term travellers who will be living or working with the indigenous population.

RELAPSING FEVER

Definition

A systemic spirochaetal disease characterised by periods of fever lasting from 2 to 10 days, separated by fever-free intervals of 2–4 days. The epidemic louse-borne variety, caused by *Borrelia recurrentis*, is now confined to the Horn of Africa and poses a threat to visiting health-care and aid workers, whereas the endemic tick-borne variety, caused by at least 15 *Borrelia* species, occurs in pockets in Asia, Africa and South America.

Nature of the Infectious Agent

Borreliae are microaerophilic spirochaetes that give rise to relapsing fevers because mutation of their surface antigens allows them to 'escape' from antibody produced by the host. Relapses eventually cease, but as many as 10 or more have been observed in untreated cases.

Epidemiology

For distribution, see Definition. Louse-borne strains of *B. recurrentis* are spread by lice from person to person, but, as human carriage has not been documented, it is possible that in some cases epidemics may originate from endemic tick-borne disease in circumstances in which lice are prevalent, i.e. where populations are displaced and crowded as a result of war or national disaster. Endemic cases are zoonoses with a reservoir in small rodents and other mammals. The vectors are soft ticks of the genus *Ornithodoros*, which also act as a reservoir because *Borrelia* are passed transovarially to the next generation. These ticks abound in dwellings with mud walls and earth floors; they feed at night, engorging rapidly before dropping off so that the host is usually unaware of having been bitten.

Pathology

Disappearance of spirochaetes from the blood coincides with a rise in temperature and pulse rate, with neutropenia and thrombocytopenia. This is thought to represent a Jarisch–Herxheimer reaction triggered by the relapse of cellular pyrogens. Eventual recovery is usual in endemic disease but widespread haemorrhage in the skin and viscera is seen in fatal cases of the epidemic form.

Clinical Features

After a mean incubation period of 7 days, the onset of spirochetaemia coincides with fever, rigors, headache and muscle pains. The subsequent relapsing pattern of disease is very characteristic (see Definition). Neutropenia and thrombycotopenia are usual and there may be slight elevation of liver enzymes. The diagnosis is established by seeing extracellular spirochaetes in Giemsa- or Wright-stained blood smears taken during febrile relapses.

Management

A single dose of a tetracycline or erythromycin is usually curative. Antibiotic treatment typically triggers a Jarish–Herxheimer reaction, with pyrexia, hypotension and leucopenia. This is thought to represent an extreme form of the febrile response associated with clearance of organisms from the blood stream in the untreated host, and is not prevented by prior administration of steroids.

Prevention

Travellers to endemic areas should be warned of the danger of sleeping in mud huts. Those working with refugees should ensure that they remain louse-free by regular dusting of clothing with insecticides.

REFERENCES

Bonnet JM and Begg NT (1999) Control of diphtheria: guidance for consultants in communicable disease control. *Communicable Disease and Public Health*, **2**, 242–249.

Dedicoat M and Venkatesan P (1999) The treatment of Legionnaires' disease. *Journal of Antimicrobial Chemotherapy*, **43**, 747–752.

Gad El-Rab MO and Kambal AM (1998) Evaluation of a Brucella enzyme immunoassay (ELISA) in comparison with bacteriological culture and agglutination. *Journal of Infection*, **36**, 197–201.

Gedikoglu S, Helvaci S, Ozakin C *et al.* (1996) Detection of *Brucella melitensis* by BACTEC NR730 and BACTEC 9120 systems. *European Journal of Epidemiology*, **12**, 649–650.

Joseph CA, Harrison TG, Ilijic-Car D *et al.* (1999) Legionnaires' disease in residents of England and Wales: 1998. *Communicable Disease Public Health*, **2**, 280–284.

La Scola B and Raoult D (1997) Laboratory diagnosis of rickettsioses: current approaches to diagnosis of old and new rickettsial diseases. *Journal of Clinical Microbiology*, **35**, 2715–2727.

Plouffe JF, File TM, Breiman RF *et al.* (1995) Reevaluation of the definition of Legionnaires' disease: use of the urinary antigen assay. *Clinical Infectious Diseases*, **20**, 1286–1291.

Silber JL (1996) Rocky Mountain spotted fever. *Clinics in Dermatology*, **14**, 245–258.

8

Vector-borne Parasitic Diseases

Indran Balakrishnan and Stephen H. Gillespie

Royal Free and University College Medical School, London, UK

INTRODUCTION

Vector-borne parasites are an important consideration for all involved in travel medicine; these parasites include the causative agents of malaria, trypanosomiasis, leishmaniasis, and filariasis. Travellers are often unable to control the environment fully and therefore must take particular care to prevent insect bites and, consequently, vector-borne diseases. In this chapter, each of the main vector-borne parasitic diseases will be described, together with the means whereby they may be prevented.

MALARIA

Introduction

Malaria is one of the most important human diseases. About 40% of the world's population are at risk of acquiring this infection, and there are 300–500 million clinical cases of malaria each year (Croft, 2000). For travellers, malaria is both a common disease and more importantly, if not diagnosed and treated correctly, may result in death. At present, about 100 countries or territories are considered malarious, nearly half of which are in sub-Saharan Africa (Figure 8.1). Each year 25–30 million people from nontropical countries visit malaria-endemic areas, of whom between 10 000 and 30 000 contract malaria. This makes malaria the single most important travel-related infection.

Classification and Life Cycle

There are four plasmodium species that are responsible for human malaria: *Plasmodium falciparum, P. vivax, P. ovale* and *P. malariae*. The malaria parasites belong to the phylum Apicomplexa and are thus closely related to *Babesia, Toxoplasma, Cryptosporidium* and *Isospora*. All these organisms are characterised by the presence, at specific stages of their life-cycles, of an apical complex comprising several specialised organelles, such as micronemes, rhoptries, polar rings and a conoid. Human malaria parasites have adapted to a complex life cycle involving the female *Anopheles* mosquito, within which the sexual reproduction phase of the life cycle takes place. The asexual phase takes place in the human host. It should be noted, however, that there are many species of *Plasmodium* that infect other mammals and birds.

Infection is initiated when an infected feeding female *Anopheles* mosquito injects sporozoites that have migrated to its salivary glands (Figure 8.2). The sporozoites rapidly migrate to the liver, where they are taken up by hepatocytes within which multiplication (by binary fission) and differentiation occur to produce extraerythrocytic schizonts, each of which contains thousands of merozoites. Two sporozoite proteins, circumsporozoite (CS) and thrombospondin-related adhesive protein (TRAP), have been shown to play important roles in the invasion of both mosquito salivary gland cells and human hepatocytes. CS protein is a multifunctional protein involved in sporogony, invasion of salivary glands, the arrest of sporozoites in hepatic sinusoids, the gliding motility of sporozoites and hepatocyte recognition and entry. TRAP has been shown to be critical for sporozoite infection of mosquito salivary glands and hepatocytes, and is essential for sporozoite gliding motility (Sultan, 1999; Menard, 2000). After a period that varies between species, the infected hepatocytes rupture, releasing merozoites which attach to and invade circulating red cells. The duration of exoerythrocytic schizogony is shortest for *P. falciparum* and longest for *P. malariae* (Table 8.1).

In *P. vivax* and *P. ovale*, a subset of organisms undergo change in which they become dormant within the hepatocytes. These cells are known as hypnozoites and are responsible for the late relapses that are a characteristic of these species. One important consequence of this feature is that prophylaxis with some antimalarial agents must continue until 6 weeks after leaving a malarious area.

The merozoites attach to the red cells via a variety of receptors, the nature of which exhibits interspecific

Principles and Practice of Travel Medicine. Edited by Jane N. Zuckerman.
© 2001 John Wiley & Sons Ltd.

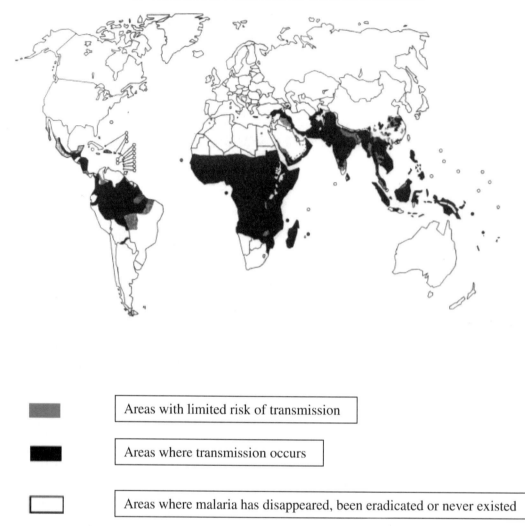

Figure 8.1 Global malaria status. (From WHO, 1998b, by permission of the World Health Organization)

variation, as each of the different malaria species infects a different subpopulation of red cells. *P. vivax* can only infect reticulocytes, as attachment to a reticulocyte-specific receptor and a specific interaction between a 135–140 kDa *P. vivax* protein and the Duffy (FyFy) blood group glycoprotein are also required for cell invasion to occur (Wertheimer and Barnwell, 1989). *P. ovale* also exhibits a reticulocyte preference. As this subpopulation only accounts for approximately 1% of the total red cell number, *P. vivax* and *P. ovale* parasitaemias are limited to approximately 1%. *P. malariae* is only capable of infecting senescent red cells and this also limits the maximum parasitaemia that can be achieved. *P. falciparum* is able to infect red cells of all ages using receptors that vary between merozoite isolates, and include sialic acid (Facer,

1983), glycophorins (Pasvol *et al.*, 1982) and band 3 (Okoye and Bennett, 1985), and is hence able to develop very high parasitaemias, with the inevitable serious pathological consequences.

The merozoite surface exhibits considerable antigenic variation, and contains several proteins that have a role in erythrocyte attachment and invasion. Five merozoite surface proteins (MSP-1–5) have been found on the surface of *P. falciparum*, all of which cooperate in erythrocyte invasion. MSP-1 varies in antigenicity among parasites; only the C-terminal 19 kDa fragment, which is carried with the merozoite during invasion, is relatively conserved. The rest of MSP-1, which is shed during invasion, exhibits antigenic variation. Erythrocyte membrane-binding protein (EBA-175), another merozoite surface

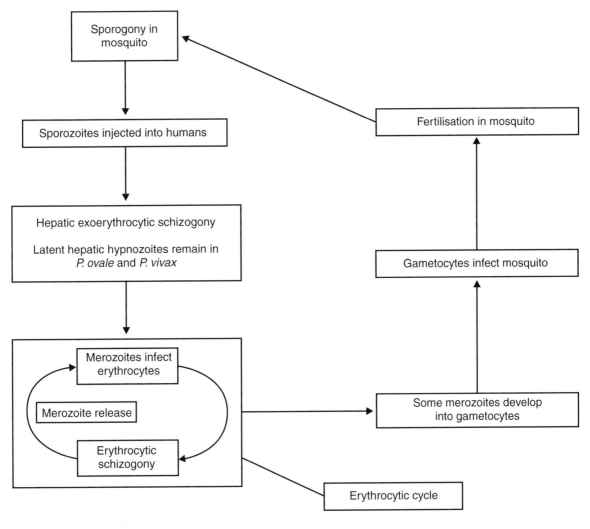

Figure 8.2 Life-cycle of the malarial parasite

polypeptide, also plays a role in merozoite attachment to glycophorin of human erythrocytes; it, too, varies among isolates (Sim *et al.*, 1994). Another group of antigens that are almost certainly involved in erythrocyte attachment/ invasion are the Pf60 antigens, which are located in the rhoptry in the merozoite apex and are deposited on the erythrocyte surface during invasion (Carcy *et al.*, 1994). This polypeptide is encoded by the Pf60 multigene family, each haploid genome having about 140 gene copies; there is evidence that genetic rearrangement or modification occurs in the parasite genome (Bonnefoy *et al.*, 1997). While the number of these genes that are expressed by a single merozoite remains unknown, the capacity for antigenic variation is obviously vast.

Within the red cells, the parasites differentiate, passing through the trophozoite stages, and multiply asexually to develop into an erythrocytic schizont (Figure 8.3). Eventually the schizont ruptures, releasing free merozoites into the bloodstream, completing the erythrocytic cycle. It is the release of merozoites that is associated with spikes of fever. The time that the erythrocytic cycle takes varies between species, being fastest for *P. falciparum*, *P. vivax* and *P. ovale* (48 h) and slowest for *P. malariae* (72 h). At first, the erythrocytic cycle is asynchronous but, with prolonged infections, the cycle becomes synchronised, resulting in sudden increases in the numbers of parasites present in the blood. Once synchronised schizont rupture is established, peaks of fever occur every 48 h in *P. fal-*

Table 8.1 Some characteristics of the four species of human *Plasmodium* (modified from Gilles, 1993)

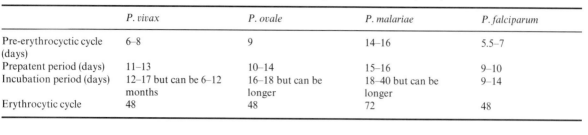

	P. vivax	*P. ovale*	*P. malariae*	*P. falciparum*
Pre-erythrocyctic cycle (days)	6–8	9	14–16	5.5–7
Prepatent period (days)	11–13	10–14	15–16	9–10
Incubation period (days)	12–17 but can be 6–12 months	16–18 but can be longer	18–40 but can be longer	9–14
Erythrocytic cycle	48	48	72	48

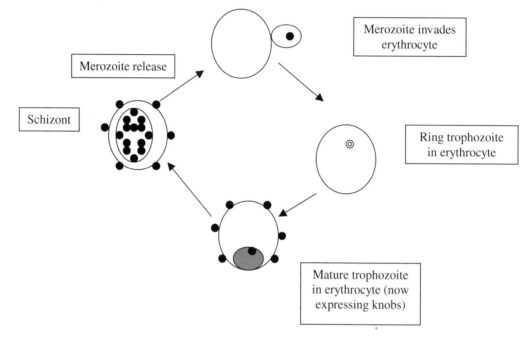

Figure 8.3 The erythrocytic cycle

ciparum, P. vivax and *P. ovale* malaria and every 72 h in *P. malariae* infection. However, it should be noted that in *P. falciparum* infection in immunologically naive subjects, very high parasitaemia will occur before synchronisation develops and thus this form of malaria rarely exhibits the classical periodic fever (see below).

Upon invasion of the erythrocyte, malaria parasites extensively remodel the cell, both externally and internally, making structural modifications necessary for their survival and proliferation. The most obvious ultrastructural alteration to the parasitised erythrocyte (pRBC) membrane is the appearance of electron-dense protrusions or 'knobs' (in *P. falciparum* and *P. malariae*) about 100 μm in diameter (Luse and Miller, 1971). These knobs are thought to consist of several parasite polypeptides, including *P. falciparum* erythrocyte membrane protein 1 (PfEMP1), and are the sites where pRBCs bind to other cells, particularly erythrocytes (producing the phenom-

enon termed 'rosetting') and vascular endothelium (cytoadherence). Several parasite-derived polypeptides, including PfEMP1, rosettins/rifins, sequestrins and modified band 3 are inserted into the erythrocyte membrane, resulting in considerable loss of deformability of the erythrocyte. PfEMP1 is a 200–400 kDa variable multidomain polypeptide which is encoded by the multiple *var* gene family (Smith *et al.*, 1995; Su *et al.*, 1995). It is likely that the different domains function independently; hence, PfEMP1 would appear to be a highly antigenically variable ligand with multiadhesive properties, allowing binding of pRBCs to a wide range of receptors, including intercellular adhesion molecule 1 (ICAM-1), chondroitin sulphate A (CSA) and CD36 on endothelia and heparan sulphate-like glycosaminoglycans (HS-like GAGs), complement receptor 1 (CR1, CD35) and CD36 on erythrocytes (Baruch *et al.*, 1996, Barragan *et al.*, 1999). There are several other receptors

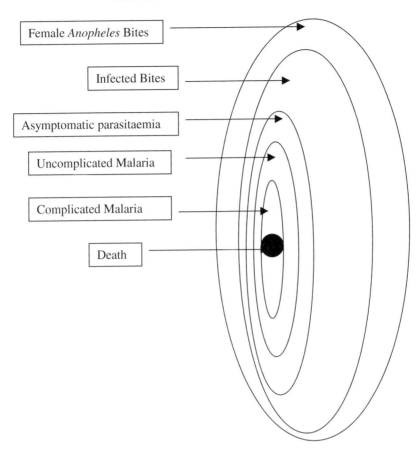

Female *Anopheles* Bites

Infected Bites

Asymptomatic parasitaemia

Uncomplicated Malaria

Complicated Malaria

Death

Figure 8.4   Conceptual diagram of epidemiology

for which the PfEMP1 is the likely (but not definite) parasite ligand, such as blood group antigens A and B on erythrocytes and thrombospondin and CD31 on endothelia. Rosettins or rifins are parasite-derived low molecular weight polypeptides encoded by the large *rif* multigene family (Fernandez *et al.*, 1999). Their abundance on the pRBC surface suggests that they contribute significantly to antigenic variation; other possible roles for these proteins are still being investigated. Special channels or pores are created by the parasite in the erythrocyte membrane to enable the acquisition of nutrients.

A proportion of the multiplying parasites develop into the sexual form, the gametocytes. The male and female gametocytes are taken up by mosquitoes, in which fertilisation occurs. The zygote develops into an oocyst, which ruptures to release about 1000 sporozoites into the mosquito body cavity. These sporozoites migrate to the salivary glands, and a further bite allows the life cycle to be completed (Figure 8.2).

Epidemiology

Malaria was once widespread in the world but the sponsored malaria eradication campaign of the 1960–1970s, sponsored by the World Health Organization (WHO), resulted in its eradication from most parts of central America. Europe was declared malaria-free in 1976. In many countries of Asia, malaria became an uncommon disease but in recent years has begun to return. The risk of malaria is highest in sub-Saharan Africa where there remain many areas of intense transmission.

The term 'endemic malaria' is used to describe an area where there has been a constant incidence both of cases and of transmission of malaria over a number of years. Endemicity is said to have ceased if there has been no evidence of transmission in the area over at least 3 years. If the vector is still present in the area, malaria remains potentially endemic. The malariogenic potential of the area then depends on its receptivity (i.e. number of new cases of malaria that could theoretically originate from one single imported case) and vulnerability (i.e. rate of entry of imported cases). Levels of endemicity may be classified as follows:

- *Holoendemicity.* Perennial transmission of high degree. Considerable immunity in all age groups, particularly adults.
- *Hyperendemicity.* Intense but seasonal transmission. Immunity insufficient to prevent clinical malaria.
- *Mesoendemicity.* Varying intensity of transmission depending on local circumstances.
- *Hypoendemicity.* Little transmission with minimal effects on population.

Not all female mosquitoes carry malaria parasites. The proportion of infected mosquitoes influences the endemicity of infection. Once sporozoites are injected into a human host, infection is not inevitable; indeed, only approximately half of infective bites will result in infection. Of these, only a proportion will result in clinical disease, and an even smaller amount will be serious and result in death if untreated (Figure 8.4). The risk of malaria is also influenced by other vector factors. Mosquitoes bite between dusk and dawn and thus travellers who protect themselves during this period are at much lower risk of acquiring infection. Mosquitoes are positively attracted to heat and smells emitted by the human body. Also, mosquitoes have a limited flight range of approximately 500 metres; hence, siting of housing estates away from breeding areas, the use of larvicides and environmental control where mosquito breeding habitats are destroyed can do much to reduce the risk of malaria. In endemic countries most serious disease is found in children under the age of 5 years. Since recurrent bouts of infection result in partial immunity, adults living in endemic areas are able to control the degree of parasitaemia and minimise the pathological consequences. Travellers who travel to endemic areas are immunologically naive and are thus at risk of severe disease.

Malaria appears some time after travel to an endemic area. The incubation period is shortest for *P. falciparum* (9–14 days) and longest for *P. malariae* (18–40 days or longer). Clinical disease is unlikely to occur in less than 9 days. The majority of cases occur within 3 months and almost all within 1 year of return from an endemic area. There are reports of malaria occurring many years after this time but this is very unusual.

Clinical Features

The incubation period of malaria varies from 9 days to more than 1 year. Clinical infection commences with a prodromal illness characterised by fever, myalgia and weakness. Patients then develop a 'flu-like illness with high temperature, weakness and prostration, often accompanied by a cough. Some patients may develop diarrhoea due to parasites in mesenteric vessels. Periodic fevers, with the classical cold and hot stage, may develop in patients with vivax or ovale malaria but is often absent

in falciparum disease—the diagnosis has been missed in many patients by doctors who have assumed this fever pattern is essential for the diagnosis of malaria. The cold stage lasts 15–60 min, and is characterised by an inappropriate feeling of cold and apprehension. The patient is usually shivering, has a rapid low-volume pulse and exhibits intense peripheral vasoconstriction despite a high core temperature. The hot stage lasts 2–6 h, during which the patient suffers unbearable heat, running temperatures of 40–41 °C. Other characteristics include confusion, delirium, severe headache, nausea, prostration and postural syncope. Vomiting and diarrhoea may also feature, adding confusion to the clinical picture. The patient has a rapid, bounding pulse and dry, flushed, burning skin. Febrile convulsions are particularly common in children. This is followed by defervescence over 2–4 h, accompanied by profuse sweating, whereupon the exhausted patient sleeps. *P. vivax*, *P. ovale* and *P. malariae* infection may progress but the severity of symptoms is limited by parasitaemia. In contrast, *P. falciparum* infection may progress rapidly, and patients may develop the serious complications set out below in a matter of hours.

Complications of *P. falciparum* Malaria

The most serious complication of *P. falciparum* infection is cerebral malaria, which is most common among children aged 3–4 years. This is caused by massive sequestration of pRBCs, often accompanied by uninfected red cells in the cerebral vasculature—a phenomenon unique to *P. falciparum*. This massive sequestration is the result of upregulation of endothelial cytoadherence receptor expression by a variety of cytokines, including tumour necrosis factor α (TNF α) and interferon γ (IFNγ) (Jakobsen et al., 1995). These cytokines also upregulate nitric oxide production, which causes local damage at sites of sequestration (Green et al., 1994). In cerebral malaria, overproduction of these cytokines and nitric oxide is stimulated by the glycophosphatidylinositol (GPI) anchor of several transmembrane toxins (Gowda and Davidson, 1999). Patients with cerebral malaria present with fever, a disordered level of consciousness, confusion or inappropriate behaviour, which progresses rapidly to generalised convulsions, coma and death. Retinal haemorrhages are seen in 15% and these are associated with a bad prognosis. The typical neurological pattern in adults is that of a symmetrical upper neuron lesion and absent abdominal reflexes; however, patients, particularly children, may be hypotonic. The cerebrospinal fluid (CSF) opening pressure is often raised in children, with cerebral herniation sometimes occurring (Newton et al., 1991). Cerebral malaria carries a mortality of 15–20% in areas where good standards of management are available, most deaths occurring within 24 h of admission. Patients who recover become rousable after being comatose for 30–40 h. Neurological sequelae, such as focal epilepsy, mononeuritis multiplex, cranial nerve palsies, mental deficit, behavioural disturbances and generalised spasticity, occur in more than 10% of children but are much less common in adults (Molyneux *et al.*, 1989).

Sequestration also occurs in several other organs, with parasitisation being greatest in the brain, heart, liver, lung and kidney.

The intense haemolysis that may occur in severe malaria may be associated with haemoglobinuria, resulting in the syndrome known as blackwater fever. This used to be a common manifestation of severe malaria, but haemoglobinuria is now usually the result of intravascular haemolysis brought on by oxidant antimalarial drugs in patients with glucose-6-phosphate dehydrogenase (G6PD) deficiency.

A rare but severe form of malaria, termed 'algid malaria', is characterised by cardiovascular collapse. In some patients with algid malaria, Gram-negative bacteraemia has been documented.

Other complications of malaria include anaemia, hepatic and renal dysfunction (failure is rare), hypoglycaemia (> 5% of children with severe malaria), metabolic (largely lactic) acidosis, haemostatic disturbances and adult respiratory distress syndrome (ARDS) which carries a mortality in excess of 50%.

Malaria should form part of the differential diagnosis of any patient presenting with fever following travel to a malaria-endemic country. Because the parasites may adhere to microvasculature throughout the body, it has the capacity to mimic almost any infectious disease. Patients frequently have a mild cough and this may be mistaken for pneumonia, especially when travel occurs during the winter months in temperate countries or during influenza epidemics, where the clinical symptoms and signs may resemble a lower respiratory tract infection. Intestinal symptoms, which are common, may result in a false diagnosis of enteric infection. Symptoms of cerebral malaria may be mistaken for CNS infection and behavioural abnormalities or confusion may be blamed on alcohol misuse. In surveys of fatal cases of malaria, in almost all instances fatal outcome is associated with delayed diagnosis.

Diagnosis

Diagnosis of malaria is made simply by taking samples of capillary blood for morphological diagnosis. Parasites are found in the blood when the patient is febrile and for more than 4 h afterwards. A malaria examination must be undertaken on any patient complaining of fever who has recently travelled to a malaria-endemic area. Further samples should be taken in the presence of fever and the diagnosis should not be excluded unless three satisfactorily taken negative blood films are obtained. In the laboratory, capillary blood is examined by a Romanowsky-stained thick and thin film. The thick film is a 1 μl blood spot which places many red cells together, the lysis of these cells that occurs during the staining process making the parasites apparent (Figure 8.5). This technique has the effect of concentrating the blood and hence increasing the

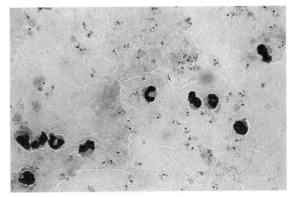

Figure 8.5 Giemsa-stained thick film showing malarial parasites. × 1000

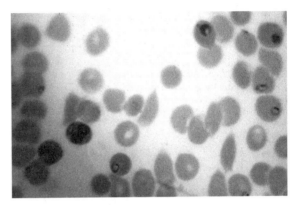

Figure 8.6 Giemsa-stained thin film showing several ring trophozoites. × 1000

sensitivity of the tests. A satisfactorily prepared thick film, examined by a competent microscopist, has a sensitivity of about 0.0004% (Bruce-Chwatt, 1984). It is most suitable for returning travellers in whom parasitaemias may be low. However, thick film examination is technically demanding, as parasites may be difficult to identify; only experienced technologists should perform the test. The thin film is useful in speciating the parasite and defining the degree of parasitaemia (Figure 8.6).

Conventional blood film examination has been modified in attempts to improve rapidity of diagnosis, particularly when parasitaemias are low. The refinements introduced have sought to concentrate pRBCs by centrifugation of heparinised blood, density gradient centrifugation and selective magnetic separation, and facilitate identification by the use of fluorochrome stains. One such commercially available centrifugation/fluorochrome technique is the quantified buffy coat (QBC) technique (Spielman *et al.*, 1988). This technique is easy to perform and rapid, but requires specialised equipment (a microcentifuge and fluorescence microscope) and a supply of costly QBC tubes. The sensitivity of the QBC technique is similar or slightly better than that of conventional microscopy.

Rapid immunological antigen detection methods for falciparum malaria are now available using dipstick technology. In the Parasight-F test, a monoclonal antibody captures the falciparum antigen *P. falciparum* histidine-rich protein II (*Pf*HRPII). A positive result is indicated by a visible line on the dipstick produced by a second, labelled, anti-HRPII antibody (Shiff *et al.*, 1993). One problem with tests based on HRPII detection is the persistence of HRPII antigenaemia after effective treatment; this makes the test unreliable for the identification of treatment failures. There are newer tests based on the detection of parasite-specific lactate dehydrogenase—these have the advantages of being able to diagnose infection with any of the malarial parasites, and of becoming negative with effective treatment (Makler *et al.*, 1998). Although commercially available, these tests have not been evaluated as thoroughly as the Parasight-F test in the field. These methods approach the sensitivity and specificity of conventional blood film examination but have the advantage that they are much less time-consuming (the Parasight-F test takes only 10 min) and do not require an experienced parasitologist or any additional equipment for their use. They may be of particular value in hospitals which have a low throughput of samples for malaria diagnosis.

Treatment

The treatment of malaria depends on the species of parasite identified, its drug susceptibility profile, the level of parasitaemia and severity, and any factors pertinent to the patient in question. Patients infected with *P. vivax*, *P. ovale*, *P. malariae* and chloroquine-susceptible *P. falciparum* should be treated with chloroquine, which may be administered either orally, in uncomplicated malaria, or parenterally (by intravenous, intramuscular or subcutaneous routes) in severe disease (Tables 8.2–8.5). Chloroquine is a 4-aminoquinoline which has marked, rapid blood schizontocidal and gametocytocidal activity. Against sensitive parasites, chloroquine is more potent than quinine, usually requiring fewer doses to clear parasitaemia (White *et al.*, 1989). Chloroquine is also better tolerated; however, rapid intravenous administration causes life-threatening arrythmias, hypotension, seizures and cerebral oedema. Hence, oral administration is preferred. Haemolysis occurs in patients with hereditary defects of the pentose phosphate shunt, most commonly G6PD-deficiency. Methaemoglobinaemia may also occur. The most common side-effect of chloroquine in dark-skinned people is pruritus, which can affect compliance. Other adverse effects include dizziness, rash and blurring of vision. In susceptible patients, severe attacks of acute intermittent porphyria and of psoriasis may be precipitated.

Since *P. vivax* and *P. ovale* have a latent hypnozoite stage in the liver (see above) against which chloroquine is inactive, radical cure can only be achieved by the addition

Table 8.2 Antimalarial chemotherapy for uncomplicated falciparum malaria (modified from Hommel and Gilles, 1998)

Chloroquine-sensitive areas	Chloroquine-resistant areas or sensitivity unknown
Chloroquine	Quinine[a]
Adults: 600 mg base on days 1 and 2	Adults: 600 mg of the salt t.d.s. for 7 days
300 mg base on day 3	Children: 10 mg kg^{-1} of the salt t.d.s. for 7 days
Children: 10 mg base kg^{-1} on days 1 and 2	OR
5 mg base kg^{-1} on day 3	*Sulfonamide-pyrimethamine*
	Sulfadoxine or sulfalene (500 mg) plus pyrimethamine (25 mg)
	Adults: 3 tablets as a single dose
	Children: 5–6 kg—0.25 tablet
	7–10 kg—0.5 tablet
	11–14 kg—0.75 tablet
	15–18 kg—1 tablet
	19–29 kg—1.5 tablets
	30–39 kg—2 tablets
	40–49 kg— 2.5 tablets
	> 50 kg—3 tablets
	OR
	Amodiaquine
	25–35 mg kg^{-1} over 3 days
	OR
	Mefloquine
	Adults: 15–25 mg base kg^{-1} given as two doses 6 h apart
	Children: 25 mg base kg^{-1} given as two doses 6 h apart
	OR
	Atovaquone-proguanil[b]
	Atovaquone (250 mg) plus proguanil (100 mg)
	Adults: 4 tablets o.d. for 3 days
	Children: 11–20 kg—1 tablet o.d. for 3 days
	21–30 kg—2 tablets o.d. for 3 days
	31–40 kg—3 tablets o.d. for 3 days
	> 40 kg—dose as for adults
	OR
	Qinghaosu derivatives
	Loading dose: Artesunate or artemether[c] 3.2 mg kg^{-1} orally (day 1)
	Maintenance dose: Artesunate or artemether[c] 1.5 mg kg^{-1} orally (days 2–7)
	OR
	Loading dose: Artesunate or artemether[c] 3.2 mg kg^{-1} orally (day 1)
	Maintenance dose: Artesunate or artemether[c] 2.0 mg kg^{-1} orally (days 2–5)
	plus
	Mefloquine 25 mg kg^{-1} in two divided doses

[a] In areas where a 7 day course of quinine is not curative (e.g. the Mekong region), therapy should be supplemented with an oral course of tetracycline 4 mg kg^{-1} q.d.s. or doxycycline 3 mg kg^{-1} o.d. for 3–7 days once the patient can swallow. This is contraindicated in children below the age of 8 years and pregnant and lactating women, who should receive clindamycin 10 mg kg^{-1} b.d. for 3–7 days instead.
[b] Safety in pregnancy unknown.
[c] Contraindicated in first trimester of pregnancy.

Table 8.3 Management of severe chloroquine-sensitive malaria (modified from WHO, 2000a)

Chloroquine
10 mg kg^{-1} base in isotonic fluid over 8 h by controlled i.v. infusion
followed by:
15 mg kg^{-1} given over the next 24 h
OR
25 mg kg^{-1} base in isotonic fluid over 30 h by controlled i.v. infusion
OR
3.5 mg kg^{-1} base every 6 h I.M. or S.C. up to a total dose of 25 mg kg^{-1}

Oral therapy should be substituted once the patient can swallow

Table 8.4 Management of *P. vivax* and *P. ovale* malaria (modified from Hommel and Gilles, 1998)

Chloroquine
10 mg base kg^{-1} on days 1 and 2
5 mg base kg^{-1} on day 3
plus (for radical cure)
Primaquine[a]
0.25–0.33[b] mg base kg^{-1} o.d. (days 4–17)

[a]Contraindicated in pregnant and lactating women. Daily doses also contraindicated in G6PD-deficient patients but radical cure may be obtained with an 8 week course of 0.75 mg kg^{-1} once weekly.
[b]For Oceania and Southeast Asia strains.

Table 8.5 Management of *P. malariae* malaria (modified from Hommel and Gilles, 1998)

Chloroquine
10 mg base kg^{-1} on days 1 and 2
5 mg base kg^{-1} on days 3 and 4

of primaquine, an 8-aminoquinoline derivative with potent hypnozoitocidal activity and gametocytocidal activity (Table 8.4). This is unnecessary for *P. malariae* and *P. falciparum* as they lack a hypnozoite stage. Primaquine is an oxidant drug, causing intravascular haemolysis in patients with hereditary defects of the pentose phosphate shunt, most commonly G6PD deficiency. It may be administered at a reduced dose (0.75 mg kg^{-1} per week for 6 weeks) to patients with mild variants but is contraindicated in patients with with severe variants of the disease. Methaemoglobinaemia is common, particularly in G6PD deficiency, and may be severe, resulting in cyanosis and shock.

For patients with potentially chloroquine-resistant malaria (defined as malaria acquired in an area in which chloroquine resistance exceeds 5%, as shown in Figure 8.7), the drug most commonly used is quinine. However, WHO guidelines suggest that antimalarial therapy should differ depending on disease severity and presence of complications (WHO, 2000b). For severe disease, quinine remains the drug of first choice. Quinine is an alkaloid, derived from the bark of the cinchona tree, with blood schizontocidal activity. It should be administered by slow, rate-controlled intravenous infusions (never injections). Where this is not possible, intramuscular administration is an effective alternative. Oral medication should be substituted as soon as the patient has improved sufficiently and can swallow: this can take the form of quinine tablets (to complete a 7 day course) or a single dose of sulphadoxine-pyrimethamine (details of treatment regimens are shown in Table 8.6 (WHO, 2000a)). Quinine is a relatively toxic drug with a poor therapeutic index. Its principal adverse effect is hypoglycaemia; both the disease itself and quinine may promote insulin secretion, hence reducing blood sugar (White *et al.*, 1983). This is particularly common in children and pregnant women, occurring in 50% of the latter, and blood glucose should therefore be monitored regularly. Quinine is a Vaughan-Williams class 1a antiarrhythmic agent, i.e. it has the effect of lengthening the duration of cardiac action potentials and refractory periods. Toxicity is manifest by prolongation of the QT interval and widening of the QRS complex. However, very high drug concentrations need to be achieved before cardiac function is seriously affected, and electrocardiographic monitoring is necessary only in patients with pre-existing heart disease. Seizures may also occur at high drug levels. A troublesome but considerably less serious side-effect of quinine is cinchonism (tinnitus, headache, blurred vision, altered hearing, nausea and diarrhoea), which is often seen in recovering patients after about 3 days of treatment. Hypersensitivity reactions, including haemolytic uraemic syndrome, bronchospasm and pancytopenia, occur rarely.

In some countries, notably the USA, quinine is not available. In these situations, quinidine, its dextrorotatory diastereomer, may be used instead. Quinidine is four times more cardiotoxic than quinine, making electrocardiographic monitoring mandatory in all patients.

In uncomplicated falciparum malaria acquired in areas where the parasite is resistant only to chloroquine, the treatment recommended by WHO is either sulfadoxine-pyrimethamine or amodiaquine (WHO, 2000b; Table 8.2). Sulfadoxine-pyrimethamine is a combination product that contains a dihydrofolate reductase inhibitor (pyrimethamine) and a dihydropteroate synthase inhibitor (sulfadoxine), which synergise to inhibit folate metabolism. The combination is an effective blood schizontocide against *P. falciparum* and *P. vivax*, a single dose being sufficient treatment. The major contraindication to its use is sulphonamide hypersensitivity, which is manifest by cutaneous reactions that may be life-threatening (e.g. Stevens–Johnson syndrome, toxic epidermal necrolysis), erythema multiforme and myelotoxicity. Haemolysis may occur in patients with G6PD deficiency. Amodiaquine is a 4-aminoquinoline that has been shown to be more effective than quinine and is more palatable than chloroquine (White, 1996). It is more effective than chloroquine

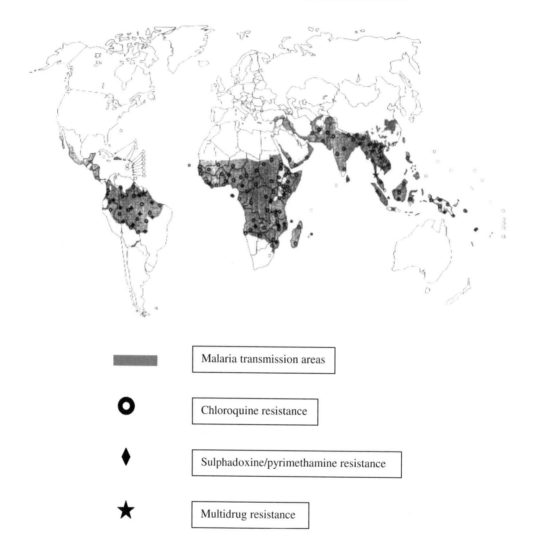

	Malaria transmission areas
O	Chloroquine resistance
◆	Sulphadoxine/pyrimethamine resistance
★	Multidrug resistance

Figure 8.7   Reported *P. falciparum* drug resistance. (From WHO, 1998, by permission of the World Health Organization)

in areas of low-grade chloroquine resistance (such as Africa). Following reports of agranulocytosis and serious hepatotoxicity, WHO recommended that it should cease to be used in 1990. However, a recent overview of 40 randomised trials concluded that the likelihood of toxicity associated with amodiaquine treatment is not significantly different from that with chloroquine or sulfadoxine-pyrimethamine, and the twentieth report of the WHO Expert Committee on Malaria recommends its use (Olliarro *et al.*, 1996; WHO, 2000b). Clinicians using amodiaquine should, however, be wary of its partial crossresistance with chloroquine.

In the face of resistance to chloroquine, sulfadoxine-pyrimethamine and amodiaquine, the WHO recommend mefloquine (WHO, 2000b). Mefloquine is a 4-aminoquinoline methanol with blood schizontocidal activity. Owing to its long elimination half-life, mefloquine is effective as single-dose treatment. The principal problem with mefloquine is that it can cause virtually immediate vomiting, which is a major concern in a single-dose regimen. Hence, patients need to be observed for 1 h post-treatment, and retreatment with either full-dose or half-dose administered if vomiting occurs within 30 and 60 min of the initial dose, respectively. Mefloquine also causes serious but reversible neuropsychiatric disturbances, and is therefore contraindicated in patients with a pre-existent

Table 8.6 Antimalarial chemotherapy of severe falciparum malaria that is chloroquine-resistant or of unknown sensitivity (modified from WHO, 2000a)

Quinine[a]

Loading dose[b]: 20 mg kg^{-1} salt in 10 ml kg^{-1} isotonic fluid by i.v. infusion over 4 h

Then, 8 h[d] after the loading dose began:

Maintenance regimen: 10 mg kg^{-1} salt[e] by i.v. infusion[c] over 4 h[f], given 8-hourly[d], calculated from the beginning of the previous infusion, until the patient can swallow

This is followed by:

Quinine tablets 10 mg kg^{-1} 8-hourly to complete a 7 day course of treatment

OR

Sulfadoxine 25 mg kg^{-1} and pyrimethamine 1.25 mg kg^{-1} as a single dose (max. 1500 mg sulfadoxine and 75 mg pyrimethamine)

[a]In areas where a 7 day course of quinine is not curative (e.g. the Mekong region), therapy should be supplemented with an oral course of tetracycline 4 mg kg^{-1} q.d.s. or doxycycline 3 mg kg^{-1} o.d. for 3–7 days once the patient can swallow. This is contraindicated in children below the age of 8 years and pregnant and lactating women, who should receive clindamycin 10 mg kg^{-1} b.d. for 3–7 days instead.
[b]Should not be given if patient has received quinine, quinidine or mefloquine in preceding 12 h.
[c]If intravenous infusion is not possible, quinine can be given at the same dose intramuscularly with half the dose being given into the anterior of each thigh, diluted in normal saline to a concentration of 60–100 mg ml^{-1}.
[d]12 h in children.
[e]If parenteral therapy exceeds 48 h, maintenance doses should be reduced by one-third to one-half.
[f]2 h in children.

OR

Artenusate

Loading dose: 2.4 mg kg^{-1} i.v.[g]

Maintenance regimen: 1.2 mg kg^{-1} at 12 and 24 h[g]

1.2 mg kg^{-1} o.d. for 6 days[h]

[g]Dissolved in 0.6 ml of 5% sodium bicarbonate diluted to 3–5 ml with 5% dextrose and given as an i.v. bolus.
[h]May be given orally if patient can swallow.

OR

Artemether[i]

Loading dose: 3.2 mg kg^{-1} i.m.

Maintenance regimen: 1.6 mg kg^{-1} o.d. for 6 days[j]

[i]Contraindicated in first trimester of pregnancy.
[j]May be given orally if patient can swallow.

If parenteral administration is not possible, artemisinin or artenesunate suppositories can be given

Artemisinin

Loading dose: 40 mg kg^{-1} P.R.

Maintenance regimen: 20 mg kg at 24, 48 and 72 h P.R.

This is followed by:

An oral antimalarial drug such as mefloquine 25 mg kg^{-1} in two divided doses (10 and 15 mg kg^{-1}–24 h apart

---

history. The alternative to mefloquine is quinine, possibly in combination with tetracycline or doxycycline to ensure cure (see below).

In some areas, particularly the greater Mekong region (i.e. the region including Thailand, Vietnam, Laos PDR, Cambodia and Myanmar, see Figure 8.7), multidrug resistance has begun to emerge: strains of *P. falciparum* with resistance to all the drugs mentioned have been documented. The treatment of choice in this situation is with qinghaosu and its analogues, given orally in combination with mefloquine in uncomplicated disease and either intravenously or intramuscularly in complicated disease. The artemisinin derivatives remain over 90% effective even in the face of multidrug resistance, and might also reduce transmission by their gametocytocidal action (Looareesuwan *et al.*, 1992; Price *et al.*, 1996). An alternative approach, in areas where the qinghaosu derivatives are unavailable, such as Europe, the USA and Australasia, is to supplement quinine therapy with a course of tetracycline or doxycycline, except in children below the age of 8 years and pregnant or lactating women, in whom clindamycin should be considered.

Malarone, a formulation combining 250 mg atovaquone and 100 mg proguanil, has recently been shown to be another safe and highly effective alternative (Looareesuwan *et al.*, 1999). Atovaquone is a hydroxynaphthoquinone which acts by inhibiting the cytochrome bc_1 complex, resulting in inhibition of dihydro-orotate dehydrogenase and disruption of pyrimidine biosynthesis. Whereas monotherapy with atovaquone has been shown to have an unacceptably high failure rate (30% recrudescence rate), combination therapy with proguanil, an arylbiguanide inhibitor of dihydrofolate reductase, produces synergistic blood schizontocidal activity against all species of malarial parasite. However, atovaquone-proguanil remains unevaluated in the management of complicated falciparum malaria, and the combination lacks activity against the hypnozoites of *P. vivax*. Atovaquone-proguanil has a favourable safety profile and is well tolerated. Although data from animal studies are encouraging, the safety of atovaquone-proguanil in human pregnancy is unproven, and mothers receiving the agent should not breast-feed.

Treating Malaria in Pregnancy

Pregnant women with malaria should always be managed as inpatients. Long-acting sulphonamides near term, the oral artemisinin derivatives in the first trimester, tetracyclines, primaquine and halofantrine are contraindicated. Chloroquine, pyrimethamine, proguanil and quinine are safe in pregnancy, but quinine-induced hypoglycaemia is a greater concern (see above). There is inadequate data on atovaquone-proguanil or mefloquine to recommend their use, but animal studies on the former are encouraging and mefloquine seems safe in the second and third trimesters. Tetracyclines, sulfonamide-pyrimethamine, atovaquone-proguanil and primaquine should be avoided in lactating women.

The management of severe malaria goes far beyond the administration of antimalarial chemotherapy. The patient may have any combination of the complications mentioned above. The following measures form an essential component of correct management:

- Admission to intensive therapy unit if available.
- Frequent monitoring of vital signs to facilitate early detection of complications.
- Careful attention to fluid balance and urine output. If indicated, rehydration should be done cautiously with 0.9% saline, as overhydration may precipitate fatal acute pulmonary oedema. Haemoglobinuria or oliguria may indicate incipient renal failure, and renal replacement therapy may need to be instituted.
- Frequent blood glucose monitoring. Hypoglycaemia is particularly problematic in patients with severe disease, especially children, patients treated with quinine or quinidine, and pregnant women. It should be corrected with an infusion of 50 ml of 50% dextrose ($1.0 \, \text{ml} \, \text{kg}^{-1}$ of body weight in children) followed with a continuous intravenous infusion of 5 or 10% dextrose.
- Other treatable causes of coma need to be excluded. Meningitis due to other causes should be excluded by lumbar puncture (if there is no evidence of papilloedema) or covered empirically.
- Temperature control by tepid sponging, fanning and antipyretic therapy.
- Empirical broad-spectrum antibacterial therapy (following blood cultures) if shock supervenes.
- Regular monitoring of clinical and parasitological response, together with haematological and biochemical parameters.
- Specific complications may require particular interventions, e.g. convulsions may require anticonvulsant therapy, anaemia (haemoglobin $< 7 \, \text{g} \, \text{dl}^{-1}$) may require packed cell transfusion and hyperparasitaemia ($> 10\%$) may require exchange transfusion.

Prevention

WHO has brought together a new initiative called 'Roll Back Malaria', which is intended to halve the suffering caused by this disease by 2010 (Nabarro, 1999). Roll Back Malaria consists of a worldwide partnership, in which all partners contribute their skills and resources to maximise impact. Hence, high-quality, consistent technical advice regarding the various aspects of malaria is made available to national authorities by networks of experts based in research, academic and disease control institutions. The initiative also supports research and development in the fight against malaria. The technical basis of this project is the 'Global Malaria Control Strategy'.

The Global Malaria Control Strategy emphasises the selective use of preventive measures wherever this will produce sustainable results. Selective vector control contributes significantly to reducing the morbidity associated with malaria. Nonselective coverage, as was performed using DDT and other insecticides previously, is no longer recommended because of its environmental risks. Indoor residual spraying should be reserved for well-defined, special risk situations; in some countries, where the *Anopheles* mosquito is still susceptible, DDT continues to be used for this purpose. The targeted application of insecticides to indoor walls serves to interrupt transmission, with little dispersion into the environment. Resistance of the malarial vector to insecticides is a growing concern. Resistance to dieldrin, which became widespread in the 1960s, is still prevalent amongst *Anopheles* populations despite the agent having been abandoned. Moreover, the resistance mechanism also confers cross-resistance to a new class of insecticides called the phenyl-pyrazoles. In contrast, DDT resistance developed more slowly and was never as widespread. Of greater concern is a novel resistance mechanism called *kdr* (knock-down resistance), which has emerged in West Africa. *Kdr* results from a mutation in sodium channels, and confers cross-resistance to DDT and a wide range of pyrethroids.

For the traveller, prevention of malaria is the most important aim and depends on risk awareness, bite avoidance and chemoprophylaxis. If these measures fail and the traveller is unfortunate enough to get malaria, early diagnosis and treatment are of paramount importance.

Bite Avoidance

Several means are available for avoiding mosquito bites. Besides malaria, these measures protect against a wide variety of mosquito-borne diseases such as dengue fever, yellow fever and arboviral encephalitis.

The risk of mosquito bites can be reduced significantly by avoiding outdoor areas between dusk and dawn, covering the skin as much as possible and using mosquito repellents on exposed areas. Eucalyptus oil has been used successfully on the skin, but its effect only lasts 15–20 min. Successful synthetic mosquito repellents include indalone, Rutgers 612, dimethyl phthalate (DMP) and dibutyl phthalate (DBP), which offer protection for 2–4 h. The best repellent currently available is *N,N*-diethyl-*m*-toluamide (DEET), a synthetic organic chemical which remains active for at least 10 h. Repellents should be applied to exposed areas of skin, avoiding the mouth, nose, eyes and broken skin. Cream-based preparations are generally preferred, and offer protection for longer periods than liquid formulations. Synthetic repellents are solvents of plastic materials, and direct contact with spectacles, pens, sleeping-bags, etc. must be avoided. However, repellents may be applied to clothing or mosquito nets for greater protection.

Houses should be screened with mosquito netting that prevents the ingress of mosquitoes. In order to be effective, not only the screen but also the building itself has to be in an adequate state of repair so that mosquitoes do not find an alternative means of entry. Once in place, it is then possible to use knock-down sprays containing permethrin to kill any mosquitoes already present. Additionally, mosquito coils containing pyrethrum, or, electrical devices which vaporise a pyrethroid compound, can reduce the risk of bites.

Mosquito nets, the final line of defence at night, should be in good repair and put in position before dusk. When travelling, travellers should carry a repair kit to enable unexpected holes in the net to be repaired. Nets that have been impregnated with pyrethrum are much more effective and should be used where possible (Alonso *et al.*, 1991).

Antimalarial prophylaxis

Antimalarial prophylaxis is a controversial subject, with varying opinions on the correct prophylactic agents for each area. The use of prophylaxis has also been complicated by the rising tide of resistance. WHO recommendations for malaria prophylaxis are shown in Figure 8.8 (WHO, 1998a; see Table 8.7 for dosage schedules). For areas with chloroquine-susceptible *P. falciparum* (such as North Africa, the Middle East and Central America north of the Panama Canal), *P. ovale* or *P. malariae*, chloroquine is recommended. Chloroquine is still the recommended prophylactic agent for areas with *P. vivax*, but this advice may need to be re-evaluated in the light of reports of chloroquine-resistant *P. vivax* in Papua New Guinea, Irian Jaya, Myanmar and Vanuatu (WHO, 1998a). Chloroquine-resistant *P. falciparum* is now so widespread, however, that most travellers require an additional or alternative agent. In countries where there is chloroquine resistance but where mefloquine resistance has not emerged, mefloquine is the drug of choice. Alternatively, chloroquine/proguanil may be used. In areas where multidrug-resistant *P. falciparum* is also mefloquine-resistant (on the eastern and western borders of Thailand, Cambodia and Burma), and for patients unable to take chloroquine or mefloquine, doxycycline is the drug of first choice. Prophylaxis should be commenced 1 week before travel (1 day for proguanil or doxycycline and 2 weeks for mefloquine) and continued for 4 weeks after leaving an endemic area.

The choice of antimalarial prophylaxis is always a balance between the risk of disease and the complications of prophylaxis. None of the agents used are without risk of adverse events and over the last many years several agents (e.g. sulfadoxine-pyrimethamine and amodiaquine) have had to be withdrawn as a result of unacceptable toxic events. Doxycycline may cause skin photosensitivity; people likely to be exposed to prolonged direct sunlight should use a highly protective sunscreen. The rate of (neuropsychiatric) adverse events attributable to mefloquine is controversial, and how it compares with that of chloroquine/proguanil remains unclear. A survey indicated serious side-effects in 1 : 10000 recipients but British data suggest a higher incidence (Bradley and Warhurst, 1995). As it would clearly be dangerous to discontinue antimalarial prophylaxis while in an endemic area, mefloquine should be started at least 2 weeks before travel so that these effects can be identified (70% of disturbances occur within the first three doses) and a suitable alternative given. Mefloquine is not recommen-

Table 8.7 Antimalarial prophylactic regimens (modified from Bradley and Warhurst, 1995; WHO, 1998b)

Drug	Dosage
Chloroquine (100 or 150 mg base tablets)	5 mg base kg^{-1} weekly
Proguanil[a] (100 mg tablets)	3 mg kg^{-1} daily
Mefloquine[b] (250 mg tablets)	5 mg kg^{-1} weekly
Doxycycline[c] (100 mg tablets)	1.5 mg salt kg^{-1} daily
Pyrimethamine (12.5 mg) and dapsone (100 mg) (Maloprim)[a]	10–19 kg: $\frac{1}{4}$ tablet weekly 20–39 kg: $\frac{1}{2}$ tablet weekly > 40 kg: 1 tablet weekly

[a]Folate supplementation required in pregnancy. Maloprim is not recommended in the first trimester of pregnancy and in children below 6 weeks of age.
[b]Contraindicated in the first trimester of pregnancy, during lactation and in children below 2 years of age. Pregnancy should be avoided for 3 months following cessation of prophylaxis.
[c]Contraindicated in pregnancy, lactation and children below 8 years of age. Pregnancy should be avoided for 1 week following cessation of prophylaxis.

ded in the first trimester of pregnancy and, as the drug is excreted slowly, pregnancy should be avoided for 3 months after stopping prophylactic mefloquine.

Combination therapy comprising chloroquine and proguanil provides substantial protection in areas with chloroquine-resistant malaria, but less so than mefloquine.

Pyrimethamine/dapsone has been largely superseded by mefloquine. However, used as a fixed dose combination of pyrimethamine 12.5 mg and dapsone 100 mg (Maloprim) together with chloroquine, it remains a second-line prophylactic agent for Oceania and elsewhere when the other drugs are not usable (Bradley and Warhurst, 1995). A maximum adult dose of 1 tablet weekly must be adhered to because of the risk of agranulocytosis.

Atovaquone-proguanil has been shown recently to have an excellent safety/efficacy profile for the chemoprophylaxis of falciparum malaria (Shanks *et al.*, 1998; van der Berg *et al.*, 1999). In addition to the blood schizontocidal activity of atovaquone and the erythrocytic schizogony-inhibiting action of proguanil, both agents inhibit development of the primary exoerythrocytic liver forms and hence have causal as well as suppressive prophylactic activity. They also inhibit development of the mosquito stages of the parasite, an activity which could have significant impact on transmission.

Vaccine

Although malaria vaccination still appears a distant hope, prospects for malaria vaccine look to be favourable in the long run. Several approaches have been identified. Antigens present in the sporozoite could be used to prevent infection of liver cells and thus provide sterile immunity. Irradiated sporozoites do provide good protec-

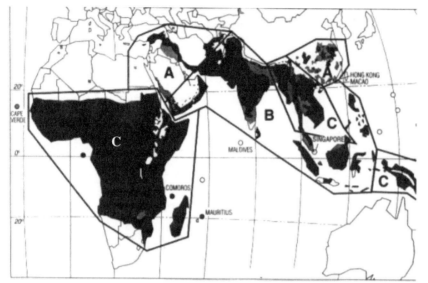

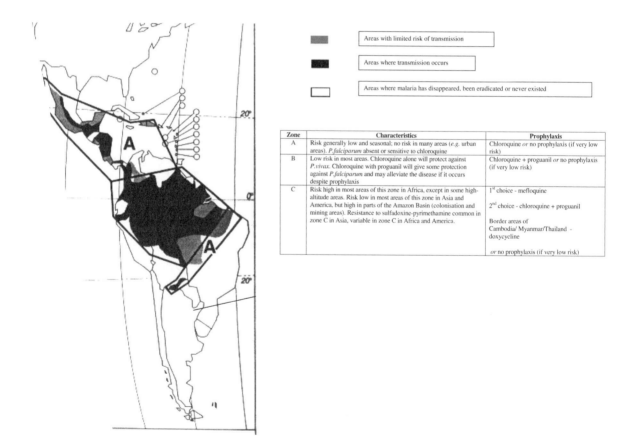

Zone	Characteristics	Prophylaxis
A	Risk generally low and seasonal; no risk in many areas (*e.g.* urban areas). *P.falciparum* absent or sensitive to chloroquine	Chloroquine *or* no prophylaxis (if very low risk)
B	Low risk in most areas. Chloroquine alone will protect against *P.vivax*. Chloroquine with proguanil will give some protection against *P.falciparum* and may alleviate the disease if it occurs despite prophylaxis	Chloroquine + proguanil *or* no prophylaxis (if very low risk)
C	Risk high in most areas of this zone in Africa, except in some high-altitude areas. Risk low in most areas of this zone in Asia and America, but high in parts of the Amazon Basin (colonisation and mining areas). Resistance to sulfadoxine-pyrimethamine common in zone C in Asia, variable in zone C in Africa and America.	1st choice - mefloquine 2nd choice - chloroquine + proguanil Border areas of Cambodia/ Myanmar/Thailand - doxycycline *or* no prophylaxis (if very low risk)

Figure 8.8 WHO recommendations for malaria drug prophylaxis. (From WHO, 1998b, by permission of the World Health Organization)

Table 8.8 Choice of stand-by treatment (modified from WHO, 1998b)

Prophylactic regimen	Stand-by treatment
None	Chloroquine (zone A in Figure 8.8) $25\,mg\,kg^{-1}$ over 3 days *Sulfadoxine or sulfalene (500 mg) and pyrimethamine* (25 mg) (zone B in Figure 8.8 and sub-Saharan Africa) Single-dose therapy Adults: 3 tablets Children: 5–6 kg—0.25 tablets 7–10 kg—0.5 tablets 11–14 kg—0.75 tablets 15–18 kg—1 tablet 19–29 kg—1.5 tablets 30–39 kg—2 tablets 40–49 kg—2.5 tablets > 50 kg—3 tablets *Mefloquine* $15\,mg\,kg^{-1}$ (single dose) *Quinine* $8\,mg\,base\,kg^{-1}$ t.d.s. for 7 days Supplement with doxycycline 100 mg salt o.d. or tetracycline 250 mg o.d. for 7 days in areas of high levels of quinine resistance, except in pregnancy, lactation and children below the age of 8 years
Chloroquine + / − Proguanil	*Sulfadoxine or sulfalene* (500 mg) *and pyrimethamine* (25 mg) *(see above)* (zone B in Figure 8.8 and sub-Saharan Africa) *Mefloquine* $15\,mg\,kg^{-1}$ *Quinine* (see above)
Mefloquine	*Sulfadoxine or sulfalene* (500 mg) *and pyrimethamine* (25 mg) *(see above)* (zone B in Figure 8.8 and sub-Saharan Africa) Quinine (see above)
Doxycycline	Mefloquine $25\,mg\,kg^{-1}$ in two doses (10 and $15\,mg\,kg^{-1}$ 6–24 h apart) *Quinine + tetracycline* (see above)

tion but this is not practical for a mass vaccine. Early studies with CS protein, the major surface antigen of this stage of the parasite, did not prove successful due to a failure to induce strong T-cell immunity (Nussenzweig and Nussenzweig, 1989). A new vaccine candidate, using CS protein linked to hepatitis B surface antigen to induce T-cell immunity, is currently under trial. Vaccines based on the merozoite surface proteins would not protect against infection but could provide protection against severe disease. Vaccines directed against adhesion molecules, similarly, would not prevent disease but could reduce the severity of the most dangerous complications. Another vaccine approach has been to target antigens on the gametocyte. This would neither protect against infection nor reduce the severity of disease but would reduce transmission in the community.

A recent attempt to produce a malaria vaccine using a combination of CS protein and synthesised peptides based on merozoite antigens (the Spf66 vaccine) was shown to produce a strong immunological response and significant protection in studies in South America (Valero *et al.*, 1996); however, studies in sub-Saharan Africa found protective efficacy to be inadequate (Metzger *et al.*, 1999). These apparently disappointing studies do, however, prove the principle that a malaria vaccine can be effective. New vaccine candidates are being identified, and DNA vaccines are being investigated.

Stand-by Emergency Treatment

For the minority of travellers unable to obtain prompt medical attention when malaria is suspected, WHO advise the issue of antimalarial drugs for self-administration. It must be emphasised that stand-by emergency treatment is a first-aid measure, and not a substitute for medical help, which should be sought urgently. The choice of stand-by treatment is influenced by the resistance pattern of the parasites in the area being visited, the prophylactic regimen taken and factors pertinent to the individual patient (Table 8.8).

The Pregnant Traveller

Pregnant women are advised not travel to malarious areas. Malaria poses serious hazards to both mother and fetus, increasing the risks of both maternal and neonatal death, miscarriage and stillbirth. Chloroquine and proguanil are considered safe, as is mefloquine after the first trimester. Doxycycline is contraindicated throughout pregnancy and lactation; hence, areas of mutidrug resistance should be avoided if at all possible. In the event of unplanned pregnancy, malaria chemoprophylaxis is not regarded as an indication for termination.

LEISHMANIASIS

Leishmania are trypanosomatid parasites that produce a chronic granulomatous disease. This may be limited to the skin (cutaneous leishmaniasis or oriental sore) or can be widespread (visceral leishmaniasis or kala-azar).

Leishmania are members of the trypanosomatid family, characterised by possession of a kinetoplast. Leishmaniasis can be classified in several ways, either clinically or taxonomically. It is conveniently divided into Old and New World leishmaniasis, or clinically into visceral and cutaneous disease (Tables 8.9, 8.10). Leishmaniasis occurs sporadically throughout tropical and temporal countries. It is endemic in parts of southern Ethiopia, Sudan, northern Kenya and central Asia, and large epidemics can occur (as reported amongst refugees in southern Sudan) (Zijlstra *et al.*, 1994). It can be acquired in various parts of the Mediterranean littoral as well as in Africa, Central and South America and India and other parts of Asia. It is transmitted to humans by the bite of the female sandfly. In the Old World these belong to the *Phlebotomus* genus and in the New World to the *Lutzomyia* genus.

Life cycle

Leishmaniasis is mainly a zoonotic disease with a varied animal reservoir including rodents, dogs and wild foxes; humans are accidentally infected and also serve as a reservoir, particularly during epidemics. The life cycle is dimorphic. The insect stage consists of promastigotes that are injected into humans (and other susceptible mammals) when the insect bites. The promastigotes are rapidly taken up by macrophages and transform into amastogotes, which are able to survive inside the macrophage phagolysosome. The amastigotes multiply, infecting new macrophages and setting up a chronic granulomatous infection, which can last from months to years. In cutaneous leishmaniasis the amastigotes remain confined to the skin. In visceral disease there may be an initial skin lesion, but infection is spread throughout the reticuloendothelial system. The life cycle is complete when the host is bitten and the female sandfly takes up a blood meal. For transmission of cutaneous disease to occur, the sandfly must bite a cutaneous lesion.

Clinical Features

Visceral Leishmaniasis or Kala-azar

Visceral leishmaniasis is the most serious form of this infection. It is typically caused by *Leishmania donovani*, *L. infantum* (which mainly affects young children) or *L. chagasi*. The disease has a typical incubation period of 2–6 months and is accompanied by a low-grade fever; however, onset may be delayed for many years. Cells of the reticuloendothelial system are invaded and the patient presents with weight loss, malaise, anorexia, left hypochondrial discomfort, shivering and chills. On clinical examination the patient is cachectic and anaemic; hepatosplenomegaly and lymphadenopathy may be present. The symptoms and signs are due to the effects of chronic cytokine release; TNFα is known to have anorectic and catabolic effects (Pearson *et al.*, 1992). Uncontrolled activation of the immune system results in inability to

respond to bacterial and viral infections, and death can result from pneumonia, dysentery, measles or tuberculosis. Once symptoms have developed, the patient declines progressively and dies within 2 years in the absence of effective treatment. The course of the disease can be quite variable, depending on the health and nutritional state of the patient; there may be acute onset of symptoms with rapid progression to life-threatening disease within a fortnight, or the disease may follow a far more insidious course (Badaró *et al.*, 1986).

Laboratory findings include leucopenia, normochromic normocytic anaemia and hypergammaglobulinaemia. Circulating immune complexes and rheumatoid factors are usually present (Pearson *et al.*, 1983).

Cutaneous Leishmaniasis

Cutaneous leishmaniasis is a chronic but self-limiting cutaneous infection, characterised by a circular granulomatous lesion that heals leaving a fine 'cigarette paper' scar and brings about solid immunity to that particular species of parasite. It is typically caused by *L. tropica*, *L. major*, *L. aethiopica*, certain strains of *L. infantum* and, rarely, *L. donovani* in the Old World (where the disease is also called 'oriental sore') and 12 of the 14 neotropical species of *Leishmania* in Latin America (where it has been assigned various names, depending on its presentation and location, such as bush yaws, uta or Chiclero ulcer). Infection is complicated by secondary bacterial infection or by cosmetic consequences at the site of the lesion.

Mucocutaneous Leishmaniasis (Espundia)

South American leishmaniasis may be complicated by chronic destructive disease at the mucocutaneous junctions. This may occur many years after the original infection, causing severe destruction of the nose and face. Blockage of the nasal passages by developing lesions usually results in respiratory distress, mouth breathing and pneumonia that may be fatal. The vast majority of infections are caused by *L. (Viannia) braziliensis*.

Disseminated Cutaneous Leishmaniasis

This may occur in primary *L. aethiopica* infection or when other cutaneous leishmaniasis infection (*L. (L.) pifanoi*, *L. (L.) mexicana*, *L. (L.) amazonensis*) occurs in individuals with little cell-mediated immunity. Uncontrolled multiplication occurs over much of the surface of the skin, producing large, swollen plaques and nodules that do no ulcerate. There is immunological anergy, neither arm of the immune system being activated. This is a protracted illness which can cause serious morbidity for the patient's lifetime.

Table 8.9 Leishmaniasis in the Old World (modified from Ashford and Bates, 1998)

Species	Disease in humans	Geographical distribution	Important mammalian hosts
L. major	Rural, zoonotic, cutaneous leishmaniasis	North Africa, Sahel of Africa, Central and West Asia	Great gerbil, fat sand rat
L. tropica	Urban, anthroponotic cutaneous leishmaniasis	Central and West Asia	Humans
L. aethiopica	Cutaneous and diffuse cutaneous leishmaniasis	Ethiopia, Kenya	Rock hyraxes
L. donovani	Visceral leishmaniasis, PKDL	India, East Africa	Humans
L. infantum	Infantile visceral leishmaniasis	Mediterranean basin, Central and West Asia	Domestic dog

Table 8.10 Leishmaniasis in the New World (modified from Pearson *et al.*, 2000)

Clinical syndromes	Species	Location
Visceral leishmaniasis	*L. (L.) chagasi*	Latin America
	L. (L.) amazonensis	Brazil
Cutaneous leishmaniasis	*L. (L.) mexicana*[a]	Central and South America, Texas
	L. (L.) amazonensis	Amazon Basin, Brazil
	L. (L.) pifanoi	Venezuela
	L. (L.) garnhami	Venezuela
	L. (L.) venezuelensis	Venezuela
	L. (V.) braziliensis[a]	Central and South America
	L. (V.) guyanensis[a] (forest yaws)	Guyana, Surinam, northern Amazon basin
	L. (V.) peruviana (uta)[b]	Peru, Argentinian Highlands
	L. (V.) panamensis[a]	Panama, Costa Rica, Columbia
	L. (V.) columbiensis[a]	Panama, Columbia
	L. (L.) chagasi	Central and South America
Diffuse cutaneous leishmaniasis	*L. (L.) amazonensis*	Amazon Basin, Brazil
	L. (L.) pifanoi	Venezuela
	L. (L.) mexicana[a]	Central and South America, Texas
Mucosal leishmaniasis	*L. (V.) braziliensis*[a] (espundia)	Central and South America

[a]Reservoirs are small sylvatic rodents.
[b]Reservoir is the dog.

Leishmaniasis Recidivans

This relapsing, tuberculoid form of cutaneous leishmaniasis is caused by *L. tropica*. It is seen in central Asia and Iran, and is characterised by lesions, usually facial, which heal centrally and spread outwards. It is a chronic illness that can last 20–30 years.

Diagnosis

Relative unfamiliarity with leishmaniasis amongst clinicians in nonendemic areas may lead to misdiagnosis.

Clinical diagnosis of cutaneous leishmaniasis is made on the basis of the characteristic cutaneous lesions. Typical lesions are easily diagnosed by their painlessness, raised edges, exudative, necrotic centre with granulomatous base and persistence. Not all lesions have these features, and less typical lesions can be confused with leprosy, tuberculosis, basal cell carcinoma and fungal infection.

The clinical diagnosis of visceral leishmaniasis depends largely on awareness, as none of the signs or symptoms are diagnostic.

In the laboratory, leishmaniasis can be diagnosed by demonstration of amastigotes in tissue or isolation of promastigotes in culture. Serodiagnosis is also possible in visceral leishmaniasis.

Parasitological Diagnosis

Suitable specimens for parasitological diagnosis include slit-skin smear taken from the rim of a cutaneous lesion, splenic aspirate, bone marrow biopsy, lymph gland puncture or blood buffy coat. In visceral leishmaniasis, splenic aspiration is the most sensitive technique (Chulay and Bryceson, 1983). Smears should be stained with Wright or

Giemsa stain, preferably at pH 7.2. Parasites may be scanty and are mostly extracellular in slide preparations, so careful examination is necessary. Amastigotes are recognised by their possession of a nucleus and kinetoplast. In addition to microscopic examination, specimens can also be cultured in Novy, McNeal and Nicolle medium, or one of several liquid media with fetal calf serum, and maintained at 22–26 °C. Prolonged incubation is required as promastigotes may not be detectable for several weeks. Speciation can then be carried out using isoenzyme profiles, gene probes and monoclonal antibodies.

Serology

Antibodies to leishmania may be detected using a number of techniques including immunofluorescent antibody testing (IFAT), direct agglutination testing (DAT), or enzyme-linked immunosorbent assay (ELISA) (Kar, 1995). The main advantages of IFAT are that the antibody response is detectable very early in infection and is short-lived, becoming negative 6–9 months after cure; hence, IFAT is useful for the detection of relapses. The use of amastigote antigens overcomes the problem of crossreaction with trypanosomiasis. The advantages of DAT are its simplicity, robustness, use of inexpensive reagents and exquisite sensitivity. Interpretation of the results of any of these tests must be done cautiously. Positive results are often obtained in patients without clinical evidence of leishmaniasis, either as a result of 'natural' crossreacting antibodies or other infections such as Chagas disease, malaria and schistosomiasis. Negative results are often obtained in HIV patients with concurrent infection, in whom antibodies are frequently absent or of low titre.

Molecular Diagnosis

Although not yet commercially available, techniques using monoclonal antibodies and DNA probes (with or without polymerase chain reaction (PCR) amplification) for the identification of parasites have been developed.

Treatment

Uncomplicated single lesions in cutaneous leishmaniasis due to *L. major* and *L. tropica* will heal naturally over several months. They need only to be kept clean, disinfected and dressed. Chemotherapy is, however, indicated for lesions that are multiple or disfiguring.

Amphotericin B

This lipophilic polyene antibiotic is the drug of choice for the treatment of visceral leishmaniasis. It is also used for mucocutaneous leishmaniasis unresponsive to the pentavalent antimonials. It can only be administered by slow intravenous infusion, preferably via a central venous catheter. The recommended dose is $0.5–1 \, mg \, kg^{-1}$ on alternate days, a cumulative dose of 1–3 g usually being required.

Amphotericin B is a toxic drug. Chills, fever and vomiting are frequent during infusion: the severity of these reactions may be reduced by administration of 5 mg of hydrocortisone 1 h before infusion. Deterioration of renal function is to be expected, and may not be fully reversible. This may necessitate dosage reduction. Other adverse effects include hypokalaemia (requiring potassium supplementation) and bone marrow depression. Safe use in pregnancy has not been established.

More recently, liposomal amphotericin B has proved to be safe and effective, resulting in a very high rate of cure (Seaman *et al.*, 1995). This is the only drug currently approved by the US Food and Drug Administration for the treatment of visceral leishmaniasis. A dosage regimen of $3.0 \, mg \, kg^{-1}$ is given on days 1 to 5, 14 and 21 in immunocompetent people. For immunocompromised people, $4.0 \, mg \, kg^{-1}$ is given on days 1 to 5, 10, 17, 24, 31 and 38.

Pentavalent Antimonials

The drug of choice for cutaneous leishmaniasis is pentavalent antimony, in the form of either meglumine antimoniate or sodium stilbogluconate. Uncomplicated single lesions may be treated by intralesional infiltration of 1–3 ml, repeated once or twice at intervals of 1–2 days. The agent may also be administered intramuscularly or intravenously, the recommended dosage being $10–20 \, mg \, Sb^{5+} \, kg^{-1}$ o.d. until a few days after clinical cure (WHO, 1995a). If infection is caused by *L. (V.) braziliensis*, a regimen of $20 \, mg \, Sb^{5+} \, kg^{-1}$ o.d. until clinical cure and for at least 4 weeks is recommended. Treatment should be continued for several months after clinical improvement in diffuse cutaneous leishmaniasis due to *L. (L.) amazonensis*, as relapses are frequent. Visceral leishmaniasis is treated with intramuscular injection of $20 \, mg \, Sb^{5+} \, kg^{-1}$ o.d. (to a maximum of 850 mg) for at least 20 days. Treatment should continue until parasitological cure is achieved (no parasites are seen in splenic or bone marrow aspirates taken 14 days apart). Follow-up is essential owing to the high relapse rate: biopsies should be repeated at 3 and 12 months after apparent cure.

L. aethiopica and *L. guyanensis* infections are unresponsive to treatment with antimonials.

These drugs are remarkably free of adverse effects if administered correctly. However, hepatic and renal function may deteriorate, and dose-dependent, reversible electrocardiographic changes may occur, preceding dangerous arrythmias; hence, monitoring of hepatic and renal function and ECG is recommended, with dose reduction should changes occur. Safe use in pregnancy has not been established.

Aromatic Diamidines

For cutaneous disease unresponsive to antimony, pentamidine is the drug of choice (WHO, 1995a). Deep intramuscular injection is the preferred route of administration. Intravenous infusions must be delivered over at least 1 h to reduce the risk of acute hypotension and syncope. It is given at a dose of $4\,mg\,kg^{-1}$ thrice weekly in visceral and mucocutaneous leishmaniasis for 5–25 weeks or longer until parasitological and clinical cure, respectively. For diffuse cutaneous leishmaniasis, a regimen of 3–$4\,mg\,kg^{-1}$ once weekly is recommended; this should continue for at least 4 months after parasitological cure (i.e. parasites are no longer detectable in slit-skin smears). A regimen of 3–$4\,mg\,kg^{-1}$ once or twice a week until clinical cure is recommended in cutaneous leishmaniasis.

Pentamidine is considerably more toxic than the pentavalent antimonials. Besides the cardiovascular risks (see above), pentamidine also causes pancreatic damage, resulting initially in hypoglycaemia and subsequently in permanent insulin-dependent diabetes mellitus. Other adverse effects include confusion, hallucinations, bone marrow toxicity and nephrotoxicity. Pentamidine can induce abortion in pregnancy.

Post-Kala-azar Dermal Leishmaniasis (PKDL)

PKDL is a relatively common consequence of therapeutic cure from visceral leishmaniasis. It is only associated with *L. donovani* infection. It can antedate cure, but can be delayed as long as 2 years. Manifestations of the disease vary from a widespread punctate, progressive cutaneous depigmentation to an extensive surface of coalescing papules. Recent evidence suggests that patients with PKDL may serve as reservoirs for *L. donovani* infection (Addy and Nandy, 1992).

Prevention

Prevention of leishmaniasis depends on avoiding, where possible, sandfly bites. Travellers should avoid the more remote areas, where most bites occur, particularly at night when the sandfly is most active. Permethrin applied to clothing, DEET-containing insecticides to skin and impregnated bed nets provide partial protection (Schreck et al., 1982; Maroli and Majori, 1991).

Individuals with HIV are at particular risk of leishmaniasis. About 40% of cases of visceral leishmaniasis in France were found to be HIV-positive (Pratlong et al., 1995). The diversity of strains found is much greater, and strains usually associated with cutaneous infection may disseminate and cause visceral disease in both HIV-positive patients and transplant recipients (Agostoni et al., 1998; Golino et al., 1992). Leishmaniasis in these patients is also more difficult to treat successfully. Careful consideration should therefore be given to the need to be exposed to the risk of leishmaniasis.

On a larger scale, environmental management, such as the destruction of desert rodent colonies in inhabited areas, has been successful in central Asia. In areas of peridomestic transmission, the use of residual insecticides has greatly reduced sandfly numbers, and the elimination of animal hosts has also been shown to have a significant impact on numbers of cases (Guan, 1991). During epidemics, person–sandfly–person transmission occurs, and case identification and treatment become an important component of disease control.

Unfortunately, in many areas leishmaniasis is a zoonosis involving sylvatic mammals. The disease is very much more difficult to control in areas of sylvatic transmission, as reservoir control is neither practical nor desirable, and residual insecticides are of no benefit.

Efforts to develop a vaccine are ongoing, and, based on experience with human and animal models, it is likely that an effective form of immunoprophylaxis will eventually be developed; however, although the work thus far is promising, an effective human vaccine remains some years away.

HUMAN TRYPANOSOMIASIS

Human trypanosomes are divided into three species: *Trypanosoma brucei* var. *gambiense*, *T. b.* var. *rhodesiense* and *T. cruzi*. The former two are the causative agents of African sleeping sickness, and the latter of Chagas disease.

AFRICAN TRYPANOSOMIASIS

Life Cycle

The life cycle of *T. brucei* is depicted in Figure 8.9. Development in the tsetse fly commences when an uninfected fly bites an infected vertebrate, ingesting trypomastigote forms of *T. brucei*. The trypanosomes in the vertebrate's blood migrate into the vector's midgut, where the short stumpy (SS) forms differentiate into the long slender (LS) procyclic stages. The procyclic forms develop further, undergoing more morphological changes, and, after numerous cycles of multiplication, migrate into the vector's salivary glands and differentiate into epimastigotes, which attach to the cells of the gland and continue multiplying. Eventually, some epimastigotes undergo a final transformation stage into nondividing metacyclic trypomastigotes, which are short, stumpy and highly motile. Mature metacyclic trypomastigotes detach from the salivary gland cells and are able to infect a vertebrate bitten by the vector.

After metacyclic trypomastigotes have been transmitted from the tsetse fly to the vertebrate host, they transform into LS forms (20–$40 \times 0.1\,\mu m$). These forms multiply by binary fission until a threshold population is

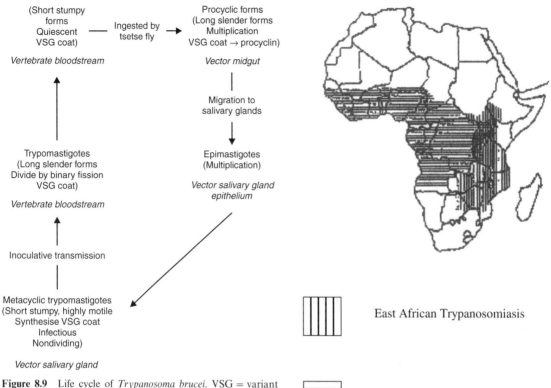

Figure 8.9 Life cycle of *Trypanosoma brucei*. VSG = variant surface glycoprotein

East African Trypanosomiasis

West African Trypanosomiasis

Figure 8.10 Distribution of East and West African trypanosomiasis. (Redrawn from Kirchhoff, 1990)

reached, whereupon a switch occurs, resulting in LS forms transforming first into intermediate forms and then into SS forms (15–25 × 3.5 µm). It is likely that the SS form is the form infective for the tsetse, and the switch from a predominance of LS forms to SS forms is therefore essential for the cycle to continue (Seed, 1998).

Epidemiology

Trypanosomiasis is found exclusively in sub-Saharan Africa between latitudes 14°N and 29°S. The geographical distributions of East and West African trypanosomiasis are shown in Figure 8.10. The at-risk population is about 60 million, and it is estimated that about 300 000 new cases occur annually. Regrettably, less than 10% of this number reach medical attention.

West African Trypanosomiasis

Although the tsetse fly is adapted to feeding on a wide variety of mammals, the slow rate of progression of this disease makes the human reservoir of prime importance. The main vectors are *Glossinia palpalis palpalis*, *G. p. gambiensis*, *G. fuscipes fuscipes* and *G. tachinoides*. These vectors inhabit forests and wooded areas along rivers, where favourable conditions of temperature, moisture

and darkness are combined with the availability of mammalian blood. This distribution of the vectors restricts the occurrence of human infection to the tropical rain forests of central and west Africa. Transmission is related to the site, intensity and frequency of contact between humans and the tsetse fly and occurs mainly in the following situations.

- Savannah and forest galleries—places which humans visit during their daily domestic schedule (e.g. for washing, fetching water), work (e.g. fishing) or while walking by or across rivers.
- Forest habitats—areas of human activity attract tsetse fly.
- Mangrove swamps—transmission mainly occurs in areas of human activity (e.g. encampments).

Other transmission sites include mango plantations and patches of forest around villages. Peridomestic transmission is relatively rare, occurring mainly when there are few zoonotic hosts or when the ecological environment around human habitations is unfavourable for the tsetse fly. Epidemic peaks can result from minor alterations in the environment, such as changes in temperature, humidity and vegetation, that alter the ecological balance.

East African Trypanosomiasis

The epidemiology of endemic disease is zoonotic in nature, human infection being acquired from species of tsetse fly which inhabit the savannah and usually feed on a wide variety of domestic and wild animals. The bushbuck is probably the most important animal reservoir as it can live close to human habitation; important domestic reservoirs include cattle, dogs, sheep and goats. Human infection usually follows entry into woodland areas infested by the tsetse fly, the principal species involved being *G. morsitans morsitans*, *G. m. centralis*, *G. swynnertoni*, *G. pallidipes* and *G. f. fuscipes*. Hence, the infection tends to have a patchy distribution, affecting predominantly adult men.

Epidemic disease is associated with changes in the distribution of *G. morsitans* populations resulting in increased feeding on humans by tsetse flies, possibly caused by an alteration in the distribution of wild animals. It has a different transmission cycle, the human and domestic animal reservoirs predominating. In consequence, men, women and children are equally affected.

Pathogenesis and Clinical Features

The signs and symptoms of East and West African trypanosomiasis are very similar; however, the former is a more acute illness, with overt clinical manifestations appearing within days to weeks of infection, and death supervening in weeks to months. The latter runs a more indolent course, with an incubation period of months to years.

The haemolymphatic stage of trypanosomiasis is characterised by a chancre which develops 2–3 days after the bite of an infecting tsetse fly as a tender, erythematous swelling. It is more common in *T.b.* var. *rhodesiense* infection, and subsides within 3 weeks. Posterior cervical lymphadenopathy (the Winterbottom sign) often occurs with West African trypanosomiasis, lymphadenopathy being more generalised in East African disease. Fever, arthralgia, headache and myalgia are the commonest symptoms; unfortunately these symptoms occur in numerous febrile illnesses and are of little diagnostic value. The fever takes the form of recurrent febrile episodes coinciding with each wave of parasitaemia, each bout lasting 1–3 days; trypanosomes are notoriously successful at evading the host immune response by periodically changing the variant surface glycoprotein in their surface coat by the phenomenon of antigenic variation. The haemolymphatic stage of trypanosomiasis is also marked by anaemia, hepatosplenomegaly and characteristic cutaneous ring-like patches with polycyclic contours, called trypanids. Other manifestations that can develop in the haemolym-

phatic stage and progress in the meningoencephalitic stage include oedema, ascites, albuminuria, endocrine and cardiac dysfunction (including pericardial effusion) and intercurrent infection.

Although the clinical features of the haemolymphatic stage may persist, the meningoencephalitic stage is characterised by the onset of neurological phenomena. These can manifest in a myriad of ways, the loss of the circadian sleep–wake rhythm being commonest. Daytime somnolence develops, sometimes alternating with nightime insomnia. The progressive severity of the somnolence has resulted in the use of the term 'sleeping sickness'. Other manifestations include hyperreflexia, presence of primitive reflexes, coordination disorders, sensory disorders, tremor and choreoathetosis, hyper- or hypotonia, convulsions, impairment of conscious level and alteration of the mental state, including confusion, disorientation, alteration of mood (e.g. depression or euphoria) and behavioural changes marked by progressive indifference.

Diagnosis

Parasite Detection

Diagnosis is made most accurately by demonstration of the parasite in body fluids. In early *T.b.* var. *rhodesiense* infection, trypanosomes can be detected in serous fluid aspirates from the trypanosomal chancre, when present. In acute illness, trypanosomes can be detected in blood films. Wet blood films can be used for the visualisation of motile trypanosomes, and have a detection limit of 25 parasites ml^{-1} of sample; thin (Figure 8.11) and thick blood smears fixed in methanol and stained with Fields or Giemsa stain should also be made and have detection limits of 33 and 17 parasites ml^{-1}, respectively. The number of parasites in the blood is often very low, and multiple sampling and a variety of concentration techniques may be employed to facilitate detection:

- Capillary tube centrifugation (microhaematocrit centrifugation) technique—microscopic examination of the buffy coat of blood spun in microhaematocrit tubes. Detection limit is about 16 parasites ml^{-1} (WHO, 1998a)
- Quantitative buffy coat technique—a glass haematocrit tube precoated with acridine orange and anticoagulant is centrifuged, with a float forcing the sedimentation of erythrocytes. Motile fluorescent trypanosomes are concentrated in the buffy coat around the float. Detection limit is about 16 parasites ml^{-1}.
- Miniature anion-exchange centrifugation technique—the difference in electrical charge on the surface of trypanosomes from that in blood is used to effect a separation on an anion exchange (diethylaminoethyl cellulose) chromatography column. Trypanosomes are detected in the eluate after the passage of infected blood through the column followed by centrifugation. This is

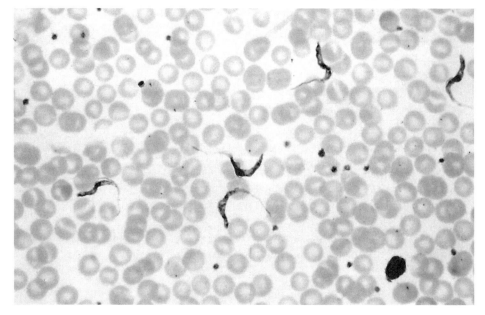

Figure 8.11 Giemsa-stained peripheral blood smear demonstrating African trypanosomes. × 1000

the most sensitive of the blood concentration techniques, with a detection limit of 3–4 parasites ml^{-1} (WHO, 1998a).

- Density gradients and differential haemolytic agents can be employed to enable separation of trypanosomes from erythrocytes by centrifugation.

In early illness, lymph node aspiration is carried out easily and microscopic examination of a wet preparation of aspirates often enables visualisation of trypanosomes. Examination of CSF is of particular use in demonstrating cerebral involvement. The double centrifugation technique substantially enhances sensitivity to a detection limit of 1 parasite ml^{-1}. In the absence of trypanosomes in CSF, a raised leucocyte count (> 5000 ml^{-1}), the presence of morula cells and raised protein are all indicators of possible cerebral trypanosomiasis. In late disease, elevated IgM titres are also of diagnostic value, and can now be determined through a latex agglutination test (latex/IgM) which is sensitive, simple and stable (Lejon et al., 1998). CSF examination should not be undertaken until haemolymphatic system infection is treated, to avoid accidental inoculation of trypanosomes.

In vivo and *in vitro* culture systems may be used for the isolation of trypanosomes, but neither technique is currently practical for routine diagnosis.

Indirect Diagnosis

As the density of trypanosomes in body fluids is often beyond the limits of even the most sensitive detection systems, indirect diagnostic techniques employing detection of antibodies, antigens or nucleic acids often need to be employed.

Antibody tests. Various antibody detection tests have been developed, including ELISA, immunofluorescence, immune trypanolysis, direct agglutination, indirect haemagglutination, latex agglutination, Western blot and dot blot. The card agglutination test for trypanosomiasis (CATT) uses a reagent made of fixed, stained intact trypanosomes of variable antigen type LiTat 1.3 (Büscher et al., 1999). This test has the advantages of high sensitivity and specificity, low cost, simplicity and speed, results being obtained within 5 min in the field; however, the LiTat 1.3 gene is not present in a small proportion of isolates, and nonexpression of this gene could also produce a false-negative result. CATT is not equally effective in all geographical areas and is only currently available for *T.b.* var. *gambiense* infection. Preliminary studies show that the trypanosomiasis agglutination card test (TACT) could be a promising development in the serological diagnosis of *T.b.* var. *rhodesiense* infection (Akol et al., 1999).

Antigen tests. Several direct, indirect and sandwich ELISA antigen detection systems are being developed. The card indirect agglutination test for trypanosomiasis (*Tryp*Tect CIATT) uses specific antibodies coupled to latex beads to detect circulating trypanosomal antigens in patients' blood (Asonganyi et al., 1998). The antigens are invariant antigens expressed on the surface of procyclic forms of *T. brucei*, and are common to all *T.b.* var. *gambiense* and *T.b.* var. *rhodesiense* stocks. *Tryp*Tect CIATT has been shown to have high sensitivity and specificity (both > 99%), and is simple and quick to perform. It is applicable for both *T.b.* var. *gambiense* and *T.b.* var. *rhodesiense* infection.

PCR techniques have been developed for trypanosome detection both in CSF and in blood, and sensitivity thresholds of 1 parasite ml^{-1} have been reported; however, further evaluation is required before they are used for routine diagnosis.

Treatment

The clinical course of trypanosomiasis divides into two stages, an earlier haemolymphatic stage and a later meningoencephalitic stage. Management of the two stages is different, and determination of the stage by examination of CSF must therefore always be performed once parasites have been detected in other body fluids. The criteria for diagnosing the meningoencephalitic stage are an elevated CSF leucocyte count (> 5 mm^{-3}) or protein concentration (> 37 mg 100 ml^{-1}). Detection of trypanosomes in the CSF is not essential.

Haemolymphatic Stage

Suramin, a polysulphonated naphthylamine derivative of trypan red, is usually successful in treating patients with trypanosomiasis not involving the central nervous system. It is effective against both *T.b.* var. *gambiense* and *T.b.* var. *rhodesiense*, but cannot be used in the meningoencephalitic stage as it does not cross the blood–brain barrier. Suramin is a relatively toxic drug. Immediate side-effects include nausea, vomiting, shock, loss of consciousness, fever, urticaria and occasionally death. Later side-effects that may occur include optic atrophy, nephrotoxicity, adrenal insufficiency, chronic diarrhoea and prostration. Agranulocytosis and haemolytic anaemia occur rarely. Pre-existing renal or hepatic disease are relative contraindications to suramin administration. Suramin is suitable only for intravenous administration. All doses are given by slow intravenous infusion of a 10% aqueous infusion; a test dose of 5 mg kg^{-1} is given on the first day, followed by doses of 20 mg kg^{-1} (maximum dose 1 g) on days 3, 10, 17, 24 and 31.

Pentamidine isethionate was identified as a trypanocidal agent in the 1930s. Like suramin, it is highly protein bound, and therefore does not cross the blood brain–barrier and is not effective in meningoencephalitic disease. Pentamidine has a lower cure rate than suramin in *T.b.* var. *gambiense* infection, and some cases of *T.b.* var. *rhodesiense* infection do not respond to this agent. Toxicity is a serious concern with pentamidine (see section on leishmaniasis for details on administration and adverse effects). The recommended dosage regimen is 4 mg kg^{-1} daily or on alternate days to a total of 7–10 injections; however, recent pharmacokinetic data and *in vitro* experiments suggest that cure may be achieved with lower dosages and shorter durations of therapy. The cure rate achieved with the current treatment regimen is 98%; relapse rates of 7–16% have been reported.

Meningoencephalitic Stage

Eflornithine (DL-α-difluoromethylornithine) is now the treatment of choice for *T.b.* var. *gambiense* meningoencephalitis. *T.b.* var. *rhodesiense* is not susceptible to the drug (Bacchi *et al.*, 1990). It acts by irreversibly inhibiting the enzyme ornithine decarboxylase, which is involved in trypanosomal polyamine synthesis (Haegele *et al.*, 1981). Eflornithine readily crosses the blood–brain barrier. Adverse effects include myelosuppression, diarrhoea, convulsions, vomiting and fever. The current recommended dosage regimen is 400 mg kg^{-1} intravenously in four divided doses for 14 days; however, comparative studies with a view to reducing the duration of treatment are underway. Treatment regimens based on oral administration of the drug have resulted in a failure rate, and are hence not recommended. Eflornithine is a much less toxic drug than suramin, pentamidine or melarsoprol and is likely eventually to replace them as the treatment of choice for *T.b.* var. *gambiense* infection. It is not currently used as a first-line agent in West Africa for economic and logistic reasons (Pécoul and Gastellu, 1999).

Melarsoprol, an arsenical compound, used to be the most effective drug for trypanosomal meningoencephalitis before the introduction of eflornithine, and remains so for *T.b.* var. *rhodesiense* meningoencephalitis. Melarsoprol is a highly toxic drug, its most serious complication being a reactive encephalopathy which affects 5–10% of patients in the first four days of therapy and carries a 6% mortality (Arroz, 1987). Other adverse effects include a Guillain–Barré-like syndrome, hepatotoxicity, agranulocytosis, exfoliative dermatitis, myocardial damage, gastrointestinal disturbances, polyneuropathy and allergic reactions. Patients with G6PD deficiency can develop severe haemolysis on treatment with melarsoprol. Various treatment regimens are used in different areas. In general, three series of three or four daily injections are given for 3–4 days, separated by a week's rest period; the dosage is increased from 1.2 to 3.6 mg kg^{-1} within each series, to a total dose of 26–27 mg kg^{-1}; however, a recent trial suggests that a shorter treatment schedule comprising 10 daily injections of 2.2 mg kg^{-1} is equally efficacious (Burri *et al.*, 2000). Melarsoprol treatment is usually preceded by one or two injections of either pentamidine or suramin to eliminate parasites from the blood and lymph.

There is evidence that the incidence and severity of adverse reactions to melarsoprol may be reduced by simultaneous administration of corticosteroids. The recommended regimen is prednisolone 1 mg kg^{-1} day^{-1} up to a maximum of 40 mg day^{-1}. Corticosteroid treatment should be commenced 1 day before the first dose of melarsoprol and continued throughout therapy.

Patients should be followed up at 3-month intervals for the first 6 months and at 6-month intervals for the next 18 months. At each session, blood and CSF examination should be carried out in addition to clinical assessment. CSF cell counts and protein levels usually take several months to return to normal; preliminary work shows that PCR may a useful technique for staging African trypanosomiasis.

Prevention

Travellers should be cautious in known endemic areas and try to avoid being bitten by the tsetse fly.

On a national scale, strategies for the prevention and control of trypanosomiasis are based on reducing infection by vector control and suppression of disease in infected people by early treatment.

Vector Control

The goal of programmes aimed at controlling the tsetse fly population is to reduce their numbers to a level where transmission is greatly diminished or interrupted. Total eradication is no longer regarded as achievable. Numerous techniques have been developed and tried with varying degrees of success. Techniques that cause significant environmental damage, such as eradication of animal reservoirs and bush clearance, are no longer permitted. Biological control techniques have been found to be ineffective and the mainstay of tsetse fly control is now based on the use of insecticides and traps and screens. Older insecticides such as diphenyltrichloroethane (DDT), dieldrin and endosulfan are effective but difficult to use in large-scale programmes, owing to cost, environmental pollution and the time required. Fortunately, the recently developed synthetic pyrethroid compounds (e.g. cypermethrin and deltamethrin) overcome these problems to a large extent. The development of ultralow-volume aerial spraying techniques has also contributed significantly by reducing both the time and quantity of insecticide required; however, the feasibility of aerial spraying is limited by the terrain, and is not possible in forests.

The main advantage of using traps and screens to reduce the tsetse fly population is that these techniques are virtually harmless to the environment. Traps are enclosures which may be hung from posts, into which tsetse flies enter and then die either by contact with insecticide or sun exposure. Screens are flat pieces of blue and black cloth suspended by wooden posts. They are impregnated with insecticide and trap flies in flight.

Disease Suppression

Suppression of disease in infected individuals requires an efficient system of case detection to be in place. This is hampered by a failure of patients to present in the early stages of illness and the inability of medical staff to diagnose trypanosomiasis correctly, owing to the nonspecificity of signs and symptoms in the early stages and the relative insensitivity of parasitological techniques. The development of simple, cheap serodiagnostic techniques has greatly facilitated case detection, and the approach that has been adopted is that of initial serological screening and subsequent parasitological confirmation of positive cases. The main problems with serological screening are that the sensitivity of these techniques varies between areas and a significant proportion of cases are seropositive but parasite-negative; this proportion also exhibits considerable interregional variation. Whereas these cases could represent serological false positives, it is possible that some of them are infected patients with parasitaemias too low to be detected; hence, these patients require 3–6-monthly follow-up for 1–2 years unless they become seronegative. Treatment is not usually commenced unless trypanosomiasis is confirmed parasitologically.

SOUTH AMERICAN TRYPANOSOMIASIS

Life Cycle and Epidemiology

Trypanosoma cruzi is transmitted to humans via the bite of reduviid bugs. These large insects bite at night and, on biting, defaecate. The victim then inoculates the faeces (containing metacyclic trypomastigotes) into the itchy bite, initiating the infective cycle. The trypomastigotes penetrate cells, forming the lesions described below, and transform into amastigotes, which multiply by binary fission, forming a pseudocyst. The amastigotes then transform back into trypomastigotes, which are released into surrounding tissue, either to continue the intracellular cycle or circulate in the bloodstream. The latter may be taken up by feeding reduviid bugs, in which they multiply and develop through several stages, into infective metacyclic trypomastigotes.

The natural life cycle of *T. cruzi* is between the reduviid bugs and sylvatic animals (e.g. rodents, birds, reptiles) but development in South America has resulted in periurban dwelling places with poor quality housing providing a habitat for the bugs and initiation of an urban cycle of infection. Important domestic hosts, apart from humans, are dogs, guinea-pigs, cats, rats, mice and any mammals closely associated with humans. Infected mammals and reduviid bugs have been found from the southern USA to central Argentina (Kirchhoff, 2000).

For most travellers who will stay in hotels, this infection is not a significant risk; however, exposure may occur to travellers in more remote environments and those living in poor quality housing, especially during trips to rain-forest areas. Moreover, contamination with infected bug faeces is not the only route of transmission, and transfusion-associated transmission of Chagas disease is a major hazard, both for the indigenous population and for the traveller. This applies both in endemic areas as well as in other parts of the world, such as the USA, that have a large immigrant population from endemic areas.

The prevalence of *T. cruzi* infection in the donor populations of Bolivia and Los Angeles is about 63% and 1 in 8800 respectively (WHO, 1991; Leiby *et al.*, 1997). It is likely that thousands of infections each year occur by this route in South America, and at least six cases of transfusion-associated Chagas disease have occurred in the USA and Canada (Kirchhoff, 2000).

Congenital transmission of Chagas disease is well recognised. Other more minor routes whereby transmission of Chagas disease could occur include consumption either of reduviid bugs or of food contaminated with bug faeces, organ transplantation and accidental laboratory infection (WHO, 1991).

Clinical Features and Pathogenesis

Acute Chagas disease is diagnosed as such in only 1–2%, passing unnoticed in the remaining cases. Those particularly afflicted are children and those who have acquired infection congenitally. Trypomastigote entry through the skin sometimes gives rise to a cutaneous lesion called a chagoma. If the parasites cross the conjunctiva, painless periophthalmic oedema and conjunctivitis results, and is termed Romãna's sign. Systemic features may occur at the acute stage, including fever, hepatosplenomegaly, generalised lymphadenopathy and oedema. Early ECG changes may also occur, and 2–3% of patients develop fatal myocarditis (Ochs *et al.*, 1996). Meningoencephalitis may also develop, and carries a poor prognosis with a mortality as high as 50% (Villanueva, 1993).

Patients who survive the acute phase enter the indeterminate stage 8–10 weeks later. In this stage, there is no clinical evidence of infection; however, the patient remains seropositive and parasitaemia may be detected by xenodiagnosis in 20–60% (WHO, 1991). This stage may last many years or even decades, and may persist indefinitely, forming a large asymptomatic human reservoir of *T. cruzi*.

The final, chronic phase of the disease is associated with destruction caused by the presence of the organism in cardiac and neurological tissue. The heart is the organ most commonly affected, the most common cardiac manifestations being cardiomyopathy, arrythmias and thromboembolism (Hagar and Rahimtoola, 1995). Autonomic disturbances are a particular problem in the gastrointestinal tract, resulting in megaoesophagus or megacolon. These disorders may be complicated by recurrent aspiration pneumonia, weight loss and intestinal perforation (Kobayasi *et al.*, 1992). Involvement of the central and peripheral nervous system can also occur. The manifestations of chronic Chagas disease are rare in travellers.

The pathogenesis of Chagas disease remains poorly understood. It is tempting to hypothesise that neuronal damage in the acute phase is caused by a direct destructive effect mediated by *T. cruzi* antigens. A cell-mediated autoimmune reaction, triggered by persistent exposure of the immune system to these antigens, then further damages cardiac and neuronal tissue, with crossreacting epitopes in chronic disease (Kalil and Cunha-Neto, 1996).

Diagnosis

In acute infection, trypanosomes can be visualised in Giemsa-stained thick blood films or by microscopy of blood after application of a concentration technique, such as haematocrit concentration followed by buffy coat examination, allowing blood to coagulate, followed by examination of centrifuged serum and red cell lysis (with 0.85% ammonium chloride), followed by centrifugation.

Techniques also exist to demonstrate the parasites in peripheral blood by culture in liquid media and xenodiagnosis (Marsden *et al.*, 1979; Chiari *et al.*, 1989). The major problem with these techniques is that they take about 1 month to complete, which makes them far too slow to have any influence on acute management. While PCR-based molecular techniques have been developed, none are commercially available as yet.

The mainstay of diagnosis in travellers is by serology. A variety of tests exist, including a complement fixation test (CFT), an IFAT, an ELISA and an indirect haemagglutination test (IHAT) (Carvalho *et al.*, 1993). The main drawback with all these tests is that crossreactions may occur with other infections, notably leishmaniasis, malaria and syphilis. Tests for anti-*T. cruzi* IgM are neither widely available nor standardised, and hence serodiagnosis of acute Chagas disease is unreliable.

Treatment

Treatment is difficult and drugs are most effective during the acute stages of the disease. The question as to whether patients in the indeterminate or chronic stages of Chagas disease should be treated has been debated for some time. However, several long-term follow-up studies have now shown that treatment reduced significantly the appearance or progression of cardiac pathology, and an international panel of experts has recommended recently that patients with any stage of infection should be treated (Kirchhoff, 2000). Two drugs are currently available: nifurtimox and benznidazole.

Nifurtimox is a synthetic nitrofuran derivative which markedly reduces the duration and severity of both acute and congenital Chagas disease; however, the rates of parasitological cure achieved are variable, being as high as 80–90% in some areas but lower in others. Compliance is often a problem as prolonged treatment is required: the recommended dosage schedule is $8–10 \, mg \, kg^{-1} \, day^{-1}$ orally in three divided doses for 90 days in adults and $15–20 \, mg \, kg^{-1} \, day^{-1}$ orally in four divided doses for 90 days in children (WHO, 1995a). Adverse events are frequent, and include gastric pain, insomnia, vertigo, myalgia and convulsions. Nifurtimox should not be used in the first trimester of pregnancy.

Benznidazole is a nitroimidazole derivative with similar efficacy to nifurtimox. The recommended dosage is $5-7 \, mg \, kg^{-1} \, day^{-1}$ orally in two divided doses for 60 days in adults and $10 \, mg \, kg^{-1} \, day^{-1}$ orally in two divided doses for 60 days in children (WHO, 1995a). Adverse effects are frequent, and may necessitate cessation of treatment. They include severe rashes, peripheral neuropathy and agranulocytosis. Treatment in pregnancy should be deferred until the second trimester.

Additional treatment is an important part of management in both acute and chronic Chagas disease. Severe acute infections may require treatment for fever, cardiac failure, convulsions, diarrhoea and vomiting. In the chronic stages, treatment of cardiac failure, antiarrythmics, anticonvulsants, pacemaker implantation and cardiac and gastrointestinal surgery may be required.

Prevention

The disease may be prevented by ensuring that houses are maintained to an adequate standard and are regularly fumigated to prevent reduviid bugs living in close proximity to humans. The most appropriate insecticides are the synthetic pyrethroids, which have a long residual activity and low toxicity. Insecticide resistance has not been a significant problem so far. The combination of insecticide spraying, health education/community participation and housing improvement has been the basis of successful national control programmes (Wanderley, 1993).

The traveller should take particular care in forest areas; the use of insect repellents and mosquito nets will prevent bites.

Transfusion-associated transmission in several South American countries has been drastically reduced by the mandatory serological screening of donors. Where seropositive rates are very high, trypomastigotes in donated blood can be eliminated by treating seropositive units with 125 mg of crystal violet per 500 ml and storing the unit at 4 °C for 24 h. There is no evidence that this treatment has any adverse effects, except transient blue staining of skin and mucosa. In nonendemic areas, prospective donors at high risk of *T. cruzi* infection should be identified (by means of a questionnaire) and deferred from donation.

Pregnant women and organ donors who may have been exposed to risk should be subjected to serological screening. Seropositivity should be a contraindication to organ donation. However, if no compatible alternative donor can be found, risk of transmission can be considerably reduced by treatment of the donor for 2 weeks prior to transplantation, and of the recipient for 2 weeks after it. Infants of seropositive mothers should be followed up for 12 months after birth and treated if they remain seropositive.

SCHISTOSOMIASIS

There are five species of schistosomes that are mainly responsible for human infection: *Schistosoma mansoni, S. haematobium, S. japonicum, S. intercalatum* and *S. mekongi*. The areas in which these occur are illustrated in Figure 8.12.

Life Cycle and Epidemiology

The life cycle of the schistosome is complex. Eggs of the parasite are excreted in the faeces or urine of the human host and hatch in fresh water. Emerging miracidia go on to infect species of fresh-water snails (the intermediate host), these species differing for each of the main human schistosomes. After a complex life cycle within the snails, a cercaria emerges after several weeks; it is adapted to invade the human host. It is negatively geotropic and positively photo- and thermotropic; thus it homes in on individuals in the water. Proteolytic enzymes in the cercaria enable it to attack and burrow through skin, allowing the organism to develop within the human host. Over 6 weeks the cercaria develops into an adult. Male and female adult schistosomes mate and migrate to the mesenteric (*S. mansoni, S. japonicum, S. intercalatum* and *S. mekongi*) and vesical plexus (*S. haematobium*), where they live *in copulo*, the female producing large numbers of eggs. The eggs emerge through the bladder wall or the intestinal wall to enter the urine and faeces, respectively, completing the life cycle. Transmission depends on snails and the snails prefer to live in slow-moving, dark water. Development projects involving irrigation and damming have resulted in a global upsurge in the number of cases of human schistosomiasis.

Pathogenesis and Clinical Features

Three major disease syndromes occur in schistosomiasis: dermatitis, Katayama fever and the chronic fibro-obstructive sequelae. These syndromes are associated with the three different stages of development of the schistosome within the host: cercaria, adult worm and egg.

The penetration of cercariae through the skin may result in an itchy, papular rash, known as swimmer's itch. This is a sensitisation phenomenon because it rarely occurs on primary exposure. This reaction is most severe when the skin is penetrated by avian schistosomes, which die in the dermis. Migration and development of the cercariae into adult worms then occurs. Between four and eight weeks after acute infection, oviposition results in an acute immune response, which may result in fever, eosinophilia, skin rashes, hepatosplenomegaly and abdominal pain. This syndrome is most severe with the *S. japonicum* form of the disease but also occurs in immunologically naive travellers; it is known as Katayama fever (Doherty, 1996). Although symptoms and signs usually subside within a few weeks, Katayama fever may be fatal. The next symptoms that develop are associated with the emergence of eggs into the faeces (*S. japonicum, S. mekongi, S. intercalatum* and *S. mansoni*) or urine (*S. hae-*

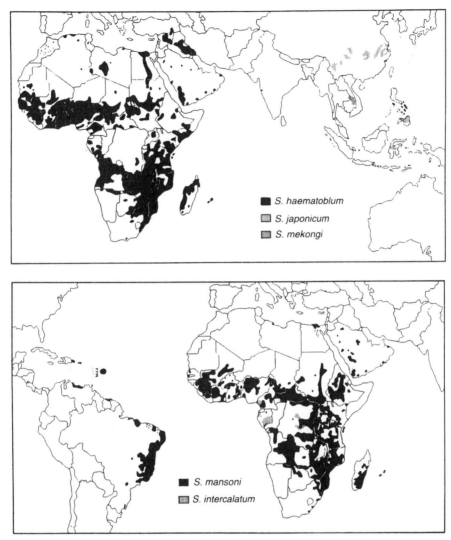

Figure 8.12   Distribution of schistosomiasis (from WHO, 1985, by permission of the World Health Organization)

matobium) and are characterised by bloody diarrhoea or haematuria, respectively. The serious and long-term complications of schistosomiasis are associated with the retention or ectopic deposition of eggs in viscera and the granulomatous reaction they induce. Eggs retained in the bladder can lead to bladder wall thickening and eventually to obstructive uropathy, and those in the gut wall cause dysentery, colicky pain and polyps (Siongok *et al.*, 1976). Some eggs are swept backwards in the portal circulation to lodge in the liver, where they produce hepatic fibrosis, or are swept onwards to the lungs, where they produce lung fibrosis (and eventually portal and pulmonary hypertension, respectively) (von Lichtenberg *et al.*, 1971). Rarely ectopic eggs may be found in the brain, causing epilepsy (*S. japonicum*), or in the spinal cord, producing a transverse myelitis (*S. mansoni* and *S. haematobium*) (Ariizumi, 1963).

The severity of disease depends on the infecting dose. Thus, travellers rarely suffer from the long-term complications of schistosomiasis unless they are resident and exposed to the infection extensively over a period of years. More commonly travellers present with undiagnosed fevers 6 weeks to 3 months after exposure. Because the burden of infection is low, the symptoms and signs may be subtle and difficult to diagnose; the patient might even be asymptomatic.

Diagnosis

The classical means of making a diagnosis of schistosomiasis is to detect the presence of eggs in urine (*S. haematobium*) or stool (other species). Since travellers are not heavily infected, egg counts are often very low and beyond the limit of detection. Sensitivity (for all species) can be enhanced by taking rectal biopsies (Harries *et al.*, 1986).

For *S. haematobium* infection, urine should be concentrated using a filter. The maximum concentration of eggs occurs in urine passed between 10.00 and 14.00, and such a specimen should ideally be obtained (Marshall, 1995). The total volume passed, as opposed to the terminal few drops, should be collected. Examination of a single specimen is not adequate to exclude the diagnosis, and up to four specimens passed on different days may be necessary. It is important to distinguish opaque, black, empty eggs, which are dead and do not by themselves merit treatment, from translucent, pale yellow/colourless, miracidium-containing, live eggs, which do.

In intestinal schistosomiasis, 3–5 stool specimens passed on different days should be examined before the diagnosis is excluded.

For many travellers, these techniques fail to make a diagnosis. A variety of serodiagnostic techniques are available and all travellers should have serum tested for the presence of schistosoma antibodies at least 3 months after a potential exposure. ELISA is widely used in diagnosis. ELISAs for the detection of circulating anodic antigen (CAA) and circulating cathodic antigen (CCA) in serum and urine have been developed, and have been shown to have substantially higher sensitivities than single egg counts (Polman *et al.*, 1995).

Treatment

Treatment of schistosomiasis is with a single dose of praziquantel 40–60 mg kg^{-1} (WHO, 1995a). This agent is exceptionally well tolerated but may cause abdominal discomfort, nausea, drowsiness and dizziness in patients with high worm loads. Praziquantel has not been shown to be teratogenic.

Recently, the existence of an *S. mansoni* isolate insusceptible to praziquantel has been reported from Senegal (Fallon *et al.*, 1995). This insusceptibility has been termed 'tolerance' rather than 'resistance', indicating an innate insusceptibility of the parasite to a drug to which it has never been exposed. Resistant isolates have also emerged in Egypt, where praziquantel has been extensively used: 1–2.4% of villagers harbour schistosomes that remain viable even after repeated high-dose treatment (Ismail *et al.*, 1996). These reports could have serious implications for schistosomiasis control programmes.

An alternative agent for the treatment of *S. mansoni* intestinal schistosomiasis is a tetrahydroquinoline derivative called oxamniquine. The effective dose varies with geographical location (Table 8.11). Oxamniquine produces cure rates of between 60 and 90%. Resistant strains have been reported particularly in South America, but subsequent treatment with praziquantel has been

Table 8.11 Oxamniquine dosage schedule

Region	Dosage
West Africa, South America, Carribean	Adults: 15 mg kg^{-1} single dose Children: 20 mg kg^{-1} in two divided doses
East and Central Africa, Arabian Peninsula	Adults/children: 30 mg kg^{-1} in two divided doses
Egypt, southern Africa	Adults/children: 60 mg kg^{-1} over 2–3 days^a

^{a}Maximum single dose must not exceed 20 mg kg^{-1}.

successful. This agent is not as well tolerated as praziquantel: dizziness and drowsiness occur in about one-third of patients, levels of serum transaminases may be transiently raised, and many patients in the eastern Mediterranean region develop the Loeffler syndrome after treatment. Hallucinations and convulsions have also been reported rarely. Patients should be warned that their urine may be discoloured orange-red. Oxamniquine has not been shown to be teratogenic.

Whereas oxamniquine has no activity against *S. haematobium*, metrifonate, an organophosphorous cholinesterase inhibitor, has been used extensively in large-scale control programmes. This agent is administered at a dose of 7.5–10 mg kg^{-1} at fortnightly intervals, and cures 40–80% of cases (WHO, 1995a). Metrifonate is well tolerated and is not teratogenic.

Animal studies suggest that artemether is effective in the treatment of schistosomiasis; the results of field trials are awaited (Xiao *et al.*, 1995).

Prevention

Schistosomiasis is transmitted to humans by contact with slow-moving, shady water areas near to human habitations. Bathing in rivers and lakes in these environments may be risky and other sports, such as canoeing and windsurfing, may bring the traveller into contact with the parasite. Although there have been many research studies, a vaccine for schistosomiasis is not available.

On a national scale, snail control by molluscicides (such as sodium pentachlorophenate and B-2 (sodium 2,5-dichloro-4-bromophenol) has been shown to drastically reduce transmission (WHO, 1985). Unfortunately, these agents are not suitable for application into water sources that are in daily use. A safe supply of water and good sanitation are therefore crucial components of any control programme.

Engineers in water resource projects need to be aware of possible design and management practices that will minimise adverse effects on public health. Periodic removal of vegetation from irrigation canals, lining of canals and modification to improve flow will all reduce the size of the snail population. The use of night storage tanks

Table 8.12 Main types of human filariasis (modified from Muller and Wakelin, 1998)

Species	Vector	Primary pathology	Distribution
Wuchereria bancrofti	Mosquito (*Culex*, *Anopheles* and *Aedes*)	Lymphatic and lung	Africa, Asia, Australia, Pacific, Latin America
Brugia malayi	Mosquito	Lymphatic and lung	Southeast Asia
B. timori	Mosquito	Lymphatic and lung	Indonesia
Loa loa	Tabanid fly (*Chrysops*)	Allergic (calabar) cutaneous swellings	Africa
Onchocerca volvulus	Black fly (*Simulium* spp)	Skin and eyes	Sub-Saharan Africa, Yemen, Central and South America

in irrigation schemes should be avoided, human settlements should be sited well away from canals and proper drainage is essential so that new snail habitats are not created.

Water bodies around villages can act as transmission sites, and should be filled, drained or made less accessible. Aquatic vegetation should be cleared.

FILARIASIS

There is a wide range of filarial parasites that infect humans. They are rarely of a significant health threat to travellers.

Classification and Epidemiology

The filaria of major importance to humans, together with their vectors and distribution, are outlined in Table 8.12.

Clinical Features and Pathogenesis

Lymphatic Filariasis

The primary features are the consequence of the host's immune response to adult filaria in the lymphatic channels. Acute disease is characterised by recurrent intermittent fever and eosinophilia, accompanied by systemic symptoms, such as headache, malaise and acute lymphadenitis and lymphangitis of the groin and axillae. Each attack lasts 3–15 days, and there may be several attacks each year. Eventually, after 10–15 years, the lymphatic channels are permanently damaged, and chronic disease supervenes. The incompetent lymphatics become fibrosed, and the nodes calcify. Lymph accumulates in tissues, producing lymphoedema and eventually elephantiasis. Secondary bacterial and fungal infection is common. Hydrocele, orchitis and epididymitis occur in men. Rarely an abnormal connection between ureter and thoracic duct results in chyluria.

The presence of microfilaria in the tissues, especially the lungs, produces the disease syndrome termed tropical pulmonary eosinophilia. This disorder reflects immunological hyperresponsiveness to filarial antigens, and is characterised by dry cough, wheezing and dyspnoea. Patients may be systemically unwell, with scattered lymphadenopathy, weight loss, malaise and anorexia. Auscultation reveals crackles and wheeze, and chest radiography shows scattered reticulonodular shadowing. Eosinophilia is invariably present. Microfilaraemia is absent, often confounding diagnosis; however, filarial serology is positive, and the diagnosis is ultimately confirmed by an appropriate response to treatment.

Loiasis

This disease is characterised by the presence of transient, painless, oedematous, cutaneous swellings called Calabar swellings. These reflect hypersensitivity reactions to the adult worm antigens as it migrates through connective tissue. The patient also often develops a fever and generalised pruritus. Sometimes adult worms may be seen migrating across the conjunctiva.

Onchocerciasis

The adult onchocerca are found within subcutaneous nodules: these are usually of cosmetic significance only, although pressure symptoms can occur. Most of the damage that occurs in onchocerciasis is due to the host's immune response to dead/dying microfilaria, released from these nodules, that invade the skin and eyes. Both granulomatous and nongranulomatous inflammation occur.

The commonest symptom is pruritus, which may be very severe. A variety of other acute reactive skin manifestations may occur, including papular eruptions (reflecting intraepithelial abscesses) and transient oedema. Subsequent cutaneous changes resemble those of ageing (wrinkling, atrophy and hyper/hypopigmentation). Lymphadenopathy may also occur.

Ocular damage is the most devastating consequence of onchocerciasis. It only occurs in patients with moderate/high worm loads. Both anterior uveitis and chorioretinitis may occur.

Diagnosis

Lymphatic Filariasis

Lymphatic filariasis is diagnosed by identifying microfilaria in smears of peripheral blood. The microfilaria synchronise their appearance in blood with the time the insects feed, and thus blood should be taken as close to midnight as possible in most areas. To facilitate diagnosis in scanty microfilaraemia, a larger volume of blood can be passed through a filter (e.g. Nuclepore or Millipore), which is then stained and examined microscopically (Dennis and Kean, 1971; Desowitz et al., 1973). A sensitive dot ELISA technique that detects circulating filarial antigen has been developed and has the advantage of remaining positive during the day. Results should be interpreted cautiously, however, because false-positive results have been obtained in patients with other filarial infections (Zheng et al., 1990).

Loiasis

Loa loa exhibits diurnal periodicity, so microfilaraemia is best detected at midday. Occasionally, the adult worm can be extracted from the eye.

Onchocerciasis

In onchocerciasis, 'pinch biopsies' should be taken from any affected area, together with samples from usual infected sites, i.e. the shoulder blade, the buttocks and thighs. The biopsies should be placed in normal saline or distilled water and, on microscopic examination, microfilaria can be seen to emerge between 30 min (60%) and 24 h (> 75%) later. Further identification can be performed by staining with Giemsa or Mayer's haemalum. If negative, the Mazzotti test may be performed. This is a provocative test in which a 50 mg dose of diethylcarbamazine is given to the patient, and the diagnosis is suggested by the appearance of pruritus, rash and lymphadenitis (as a result of microfilarial death) 1–24 h after the dose. Pinch biopsies taken at this time are more likely to be positive. Heavily infected patients may have severe reactions, and the test should therefore only be done in patients with negative punch biopsies.

Rarely, ocular microfilaria may be detected in the anterior chamber by slit-lamp examination.

Reliable serological and molecular tests are not yet in general use.

Treatment

Lymphatic Filariasis

The management of lymphatic filariasis remains unsatisfactory. Diethylcarbamazine administered at a dosage of

Table 8.13 Dosage schedule for diethylcarbamazine

Day	Dose
1	50 mg
2	50 mg t.d.s.
3	100 mg t.d.s.
4–21	3 mg kg^{-1} t.d.s.

6 mg kg^{-1} daily in divided doses for 12 days is the treatment of choice. This agent is a piperazine derivative that kills microfilaria, as well as some adult worms. Severe immunological reactions similar to the Mazzotti reaction may be precipitated. The dying worms can also stimulate an acute inflammatory reaction which develops into a granulomatous process and ultimately progressive fibrosis. Diethylcarbamazine should not be used in pregnancy. Single-dose therapy with ivermectin (200–400 μg kg^{-1}), preferably in combination with albendazole (400 mg), has been shown to be effective and may replace diethylcarbamazine as first-line treatment (Addiss et al., 1997).

Loiasis

Diethylcarbamazine has been used for many years in the treatment of loiasis. In the presence of heavy worm loads, encephalitis may be precipitated. The dose should hence be built up gradually. (Table 8.13).

Treatment with ivermectin at a single dose of 200 μg kg^{-1} has also been shown to be effective in reducing microfilaraemia (Gardon et al., 1997).

Onchocerciasis

The first-line treatment of onchocerciasis is ivermectin, a semisynthetic compound that has been shown to be a suppressive microfilaricide in onchocerciasis (WHO, 1995a). It has little effect on adult worms, and hence does not produce radical cure. This agent is administered as a single dose of 150 μg kg^{-1} once or twice a year. It is contraindicated in children below the age of 5 years, pregnant women and mothers nursing babies below the age of 1 week. Ivermectin is well tolerated, although mild Mazzotti reactions may occur. It has been shown to be safer and more effective than diethylcarbamazine, which used to be the treatment of choice for onchocerciasis (Van Laetham and Lopes, 1996).

Suramin does have macrofilaricidal action and has been used for curative treatment of onchocerciasis. Owing to its extreme toxicity (see section on African trypanosomiasis for details) its use should be considered only for the curative treatment of selected individuals in areas without disease transmission, of individuals leaving an endemic area and for severe hyperreactive onchodermatitis with persistent symptomology despite repeated

Table 8.14 Dosage schedule for suramin in onchocerciasis

Week	Dose (mg kg^{-1})
1	3.3
2	6.7
3	10.0
4	13.3
5	16.7
6	16.7

treatment with ivermectin (WHO, 1995b). A total dose of 4.0 g is administered intravenously, as shown in Table 8.14.

Prevention and Control

Lymphatic filariasis is prevented by avoiding mosquito bites and mosquito control measures. It has recently been identified as a potentially eradicable disease and WHO is coordinating efforts towards this end. These efforts entail both environmental vector control (e.g. adequate maintenance of open drains and septic tanks, spraying a film of oil over water surfaces, the addition of larvivorous fish to ponds and the use of larval insecticides) and mass chemotherapy. It has recently been shown that single annual doses of diethylcarbamazine and/or ivermectin have potent, sustained activity in reducing microfilaraemia and that additional treatment with albendazole has macrofilaricidal activity (WHO, 1992; Ottesen and Ramachandran, 1995). These findings lay the foundations for a successful international eradication campaign.

The prevention of loiasis is based on the avoidance of tabanid fly bites. This involves the avoidance of places where flies are numerous and the use of insect repellents and protective clothing. Prophylactic diethylcarbamazine administered to travellers at a dose of 300 mg once weekly is effective in preventing loiasis (Nutman *et al.*, 1988). Transmission has been successfully interrupted by the mass treatment of villages with diethylcarbamazine 5 mg kg^{-1} day^{-1} for 3 consecutive days each month or quarterly doses of ivermectin (Ranque *et al.*, 1996).

For the traveller, onchocerciasis is best prevented by the avoidance of endemic areas and the use of protective clothing and insect repellents. Onchocerciasis is an important public health problem in West Africa and, as such, several intensive efforts to control this devastating disease using different approaches are ongoing. Successful vector control was first achieved in 1951 by removal of all the riverside shade trees from a small area in Kenya. Subsequent efforts at vector control have focused on the larval stage. The Onchocerciasis Control Programme (OCP) began in 1974, and has successfully reduced transmission over approximately 1.3 million km^2 in 11 countries. The basis of the OCP is the aerial spraying of five insecticides (temephos, phoxim, pyraclofos, permethrin and carbosulphan) used in rotation, guided by entomological and hydrological data that is updated weekly. This programme is estimated to have prevented 250 000 cases of blindness and currently protects some 20 million people at a cost of less than $US1 per person per year. A mass chemotherapy programme is also underway: whole populations (about 7 million people in total) are being treated using ivermectin donated free to WHO by the manufacturers.

REFERENCES

Addiss DG, Beach MJ, Streit TG *et al.* (1997) Randomised placebo-controlled comparison of ivermectin and albendazole alone and in combination for *Wuchereria bancrofti* microfilaraemia in Haitian children *Lancet*, **350**, 480–484.

Addy M and Nandy A (1992) Ten years of kala-azar in West Bengal Part 1. Did post kala-azar dermal leishmaniasis initiate the outbreak in 24 Parganas? *Bulletin of the World Health Organization*, **70**, 341–346.

Agostoni C, Dorigoni N, Malfitano A *et al.* (1998) Mediterranean leishmaniasis in HIV-infected patients: epidemiology, clinical and diagnostic features of 22 cases. *Infection*, **26**, 93–99.

Akol MN, Olaho-Mukani W, Odiit, M *et al.* (1999) Trypanosomiasis agglutination card test for *Trypanosoma brucei rhodesiense* sleeping sickness. *East African Medical Journal*, **76**, 38–41.

Alonso PL, Lindsay SW, Armstrong JR *et al.* (1991) The effect of insecticide-treated bed nets on mortality of Gambian children. *Lancet*, **337**, 1499–1502.

Ariizumi M (1963) Cerebral schistosomiasis japonica. Report of one operated case and fifty clinical cases. *American Journal of Tropical Medicine and Hygiene*, **12**, 40–55.

Arroz JO (1987) Melarsoprol and reactive encephalopathy in *Trypanosoma brucei rhodesiense*. *Transactions of the Royal Society of Tropical Medicine and Hygiene*, **81**, 192.

Ashford RW and Bates PA (1998) Leishmanasis in the Old World. In *Topley and Wilson's Microbiology and Microbial Infections* (eds FEG Cox, JP Kreier and D Wakelin), 9th edn, vol. 5, pp 215–240. Arnold, London.

Asonganyi T, Doua F, Kibona SN *et al.* (1998) A multi-centre evaluation of the card indirect agglutination test for trypanosomiasis (*Tryp*Tect CIATT). *Annals of Tropical Medicine and Parasitology*, **92**, 837–844.

Bacchi CJ, Nathan HC and Livingston T (1990) Differential susceptibility to DL-alpha-difluoromethylornithine in clinical isolates of *Trypanosoma brucei rhodesiense*. *Antimicrobial Agents and Chemotherapy*, **34**, 1183–1188.

Badaró R, Jones TC, Lorenco R *et al.* (1986) New perspectives on a subclinical form of visceral leishmaniasis. *Journal of Infectious Diseases*, **154**, 639–649.

Barragan A, Spillmann D, Carlson J *et al.* (1999) The role of glycans in *Plasmodium falciparum* infection. *Biochemical Society Transactions*, **27**, 487–493.

Baruch DI, Gormley JA, Ma C *et al.* (1996) *Plasmodium falciparum* membrane protein 1 is a parasitized erythrocyte receptor for adherence to CD36, thrombospondin and intercellular adhesion molecule 1. *Proceedings of the National Academy of Sciences of the USA*, **93**, 3497–3502.

Bonnefoy S, Bischoff E, Guillotte, M *et al.* (1997) Evidence for distinct prototype sequences with the *Plasmodium falciparum* Pf60 multigene family. *Molecular Biochemical Parasitology*, **87**, 1–11.

Bradley DJ and Warhurst DC (1995) Malaria prophylaxis: guidelines for travellers from Britain. Malaria Reference Laboratory of the Public Health Laboratory Service, London. *BMJ*, **310**, 709–714.

Bruce-Chwatt LJ (1984) DNA probes for malaria diagnosis. *Lancet*, **i**, 795.

Burri C, Nkunku S, Merolle A *et al.* (2000) Efficacy of new, concise schedule for melarsoprol in treatment of sleeping sickness caused by *Trypanosoma brucei gambiense*: a randomised trial. *Lancet*, **355**, 1419–1425.

Büscher P, Lejon V, Magnus E *et al.* (1999) Improved latex agglutination test for detection of antibodies in serum and cerbrospinal fluid of *Trypanosoma brucei gambiense* infected patients. *Acta Tropica*, **73**, 11–20.

Carcy B, Bonnefog S, Guillotte M *et al.* (1994) A large multigene family expressed during the erythrocytic schizogony of *Plasmodium falciparum*. *Molecular Biochemical Parasitology*, **68**, 221–233.

Carvalho MR, Krieger MA, Almeida E *et al.* (1993) Chagas' disease diagnosis: evaluation of several tests in blood bank screening. *Transfusion*, **33**, 830–834.

Chiari E, Dias JCP, Lana M *et al.* (1989) Hemocultures for the parasitological diagnosis of human chronic Chagas' disease. *Revista Da Sociedade Brasileira de Medicina Tropical*, **22**, 19–23.

Chulay JD and Bryceson AD (1983) Quantitation of amastigotes of *Leishmania donovani* in smears of splenic aspirates from patients with visceral leishmaniasis. *American Journal of Tropical Medicine and Hygiene*, **32**, 475–479.

Croft A (2000) Extracts from 'Clinical Evidence'. Malaria: prevention in travellers. *BMJ*, **321**, 154–160.

Dennis DT and Kean BH (1971) Isolation of microfilariae: report of a new method. *Journal of Parasitology*, **57**, 1146–1147.

Desowitz RS, Southgate BA and Mataika JU (1973) Studies on filariasis in the Pacific. 3. Comparative efficacy of the stained blood-film, counting-chamber and membrane-filtration techniques for the diagnosis of *Wuchereria bancrofti* microfilaraemia in untreated patients in areas of low endemicity. *Southeast Asian Journal of Tropical Medicine and Public Health*, **4**, 329–335.

Doherty JF, Moody AH and Wright SG (1996) Katayama fever: an acute manifestation of schistosomiasis. *BMJ*, **313**, 1071–1072.

Facer CA (1983) Erythrocyte Sialoglycoproteins and *Plasmodium falciparum* invasion. *Transactions of the Royal Society of Tropical Medicine and Hygiene*, **77**, 524–530.

Fallon PG, Sturrock RF, Niang, AC *et al.* (1995) Short report: diminished susceptibility to praziquantel in a Senegal isolate of *Schistosoma mansoni*. *American Journal of Tropical Medicine and Hygiene*, **53**, 61–62.

Fernandez V, Hommel M, Chen Q *et al.* (1999) Small clonally variant antigens on the surface of the *Plasmodium falciparum*-infected erythrocyte are encoded by the *rif* gene family and are the target of human immune responses. *Journal of Experimental Medicine*, **190**, 1393–1403.

Gardon J, Kamgno J, Folefack G *et al.* (1997) Marked decrease in *Loa loa* microfilaraemia six and twelve months after a single dose of ivermectin. *Transactions of the Royal Society of Tropical Medicine and Hygiene*, **91**, 593–594.

Gilles HM (1993) The malaria parasites. In *Bruce-Chwatt's Essential Malariology* (eds HM Gilles and DA Warrell), 3rd edn, pp 12–34. Arnold, London.

Golino A, Duncan JM, Zeluff B *et al.* (1992) Leishmaniasis in a heart transplant patient. *Journal of Heart and Lung Transplantation*, **11**, 820–823.

Gowda DC and Davidson EA (1999) Protein glycosylation in the malaria parasite. *Parasitology Today*, **15**, 147–152.

Green SJ, Scheller LF, Marletta MA *et al.* (1994) Nitric oxide: cytokine-regulation of nitric oxide in host resistance to intracellular pathogens. *Immunology Letters*, **43**, 87–94.

Guan L-R (1991) Current status of kala-azar and vector control in China. *Bulletin of the World Health Organization*, **69**, 595–601.

Haegele KD, Alken RG, Grove J *et al.* (1981) Kinetics of alpha-difluoromethylornithine: an irreversible inhibitor of ornithine decarboxylase. *Clinical Pharmacology and Therapeutics*, **30**, 210–217.

Hagar JM and Rahimtoola SH (1995) Chagas' heart disease. *Current Problems in Cardiology*, **20**, 825–924.

Harries AD, Fryatt R, Walker J *et al.* (1986) Schistosomiasis in expatriates returning to Britain from the tropics: a controlled study. *Lancet*, **i**, 86–88.

Hommel M and Gilles HM (1998) Malaria. In *Topley and Wilson's Microbiology and Microbial Infections* (eds FEG Cox, JP Kreier and D Wakelin), 9th edn, vol. 5, pp 361–409. Arnold, London.

Ismail M, Metwally A, Farghaly A *et al.* (1996) Characterisation of isolates of *Schistosoma mansoni* from Egyptian villagers that tolerate high doses of praziquantel. *American Journal of Tropical Medicine and Hygiene*, **55**, 214–218.

Jakobsen PH, Bate CA, Taverne J *et al.* (1995) Malaria: toxins, cytokines and disease. *Parasite Immunology*, **17**, 223–231.

Kalil J and Kunha-Neto E (1996) Autoimmunity in Chagas disease cardiomyopathy: fulfilling the criteria at last. *Parasitology Today*, **12**, 396–399.

Kar K (1995) Serodiagnosis of leishmaniasis. *Critical Reviews in Microbiology*, **21**, 123–152.

Kirchhoff LV (1990) *Trypanosoma* species (American trypanosomiasis, Chagas' disease): biology of trypanosomes. In *Principles and Practice of Infectious Diseases* (eds GL Mandell, RG Douglas and JE Bennett), 4th edn, pp 2077–2084. Churchill Livingstone, New York.

Kirchhoff LV (2000) *Trypanosoma* species (American trypanosomiasis, Chagas' disease): biology of trypanosomes. In *Mandell, Douglas and Bennett's Principles and Practice of Infectious Diseases* (eds GL Mandell, JE Bennett and R Dolin), 5th edn, vol. 2, pp 2845–2853. Churchill Livingstone, Philadelphia.

Kobayasi S, Mendes EF, Rodrigues MAM *et al.* (1992) Toxic dilatation of the colon in Chagas' disease. *British Journal of Surgery*, **79**, 1202–1203.

Leiby DA, Read EJ, Lenes BA *et al.* (1997) Seroepidemiology of *T. cruzi*, etiologic agent of Chagas' disease, in US blood donors. *Journal of Infectious Diseases*, **176**, 1047–1052.

Lejon V, Büscher P, Sema NH *et al.* (1998) Human African trypanosomiasis: a latex agglutination field test for quantifying IgM in cerebrospinal fluid. *Bulletin of the World Health Organization*, **76**, 553–558.

Looareesuwan S, Viravan C, Vanijanonta S *et al.* (1992) Randomised trial of artesunate and mefloquine alone and in sequence for acute uncomplicated falciparum malaria. *Lancet*, **339**, 821–824.

Looareesuwan S, Chulay JD, Canfield CJ *et al.* (1999) Malarone (atovaquone and proguanil hydrochloride): a review of its clinical development for treatment of malaria Malarone Clinical Trials Study Group. *American Journal of Tropical Medicine and Hygiene*, **60**, 533–541.

Luse SA and Miller LH (1971) *Plasmodium falciparum* malaria: ultrastructure of parasitised erythrocytes in cardiac vessels. *American Journal of Tropical Medicine and Hygiene*, **20**,

655–660.

Makler MT, Palmer CJ and Ager AL (1998) A review of practical techniques for the diagnosis of malaria. *Annals of Tropical Medicine and Parasitology*, **92**, 419–433.

Maroli M and Majori G (1991) Permethrin impregnated curtains against phlebotomine sandflies: laboratory studies. *Parassitologia*, **33**(suppl.), 399–404.

Marsden PD, Barreto AC, Cuba CC et al. (1979) Improvements in routine xenodiagnosis with first instar *Dipetalogaster maximus* (Uhler 1894) (Triatominae). *American Journal of Tropical Medicine and Hygiene*, **28**, 649–652.

Marshall I (1995) Schistosomiasis. In *Medical Parasitology: A Practical Approach* (eds SH Gillespie and PM Hawkey), pp 191–208. Oxford University Press, Oxford.

Menard R (2000) The journey of the malaria sporozoite through its hosts: two parasite proteins lead the way. *Microbes and Infection*, **2**, 633–642.

Metzger WG, Haywood M, D'Alessandro U et al. (1999) Serological responses of Gambian children to immunization with the malaria vaccine SPf66. *Parasite Immunology*, **21**, 335–340.

Molyneux ME, Taylor TE, Wirima JJ et al. (1989) Clinical features and prognostic indicators in paediatric cerebral malaria: a study of 131 comatose Malawian children. *Quarterly Journal of Medicine*, **71**, 441–459.

Muller R, Wakelin D (1998) Lymphatic filariasis. In Topley and Wilson's Microbiology and Microbial Infections, 9th edn, vol. 5, pp 609–619. Arnold, London.

Nabarro D (1999) Roll back malaria. *Parassitologia*, **41**, 501–504.

Newton CR, Kirkham FJ, Winstanley PA et al (1991) Intracranial pressure in African children with cerebral malaria. *Lancet*, **338**, 573–576.

Nussenzweig RS and Nussenzweig V (1989) Antisporozoite vaccine for malaria: experimental basis and current status. *Reviews of Infectious Diseases*, **11**(suppl. 3), S579–585.

Nutman TB, Miller KB, Mulligan M et al. (1988) Diethylcarbamazine prophylaxis for human loiasis Results of a double-blind study. *New England Journal of Medicine*, **319**, 752–756.

Ochs DE, Hnilica V, Moser DR et al. (1996) Postmortem diagnosis of autochthonous acute chagasic myocarditis by polymerase chain reaction amplification of a species-specific DNA sequence of *Trypanosoma cruzi*. *American Journal of Tropical Medicine and Hygiene*, **34**, 526–259.

Okoye VC, Bennett V (1985) *Plasmodium falciparum* malaria: band 3 as a possible receptor during invasion of human erythrocytes. *Science*, **227**, 169–171.

Olliaro P, Nevill C, LeBras J et al. (1996) Systematic review of amodiaquine treatment in uncomplicated malaria. *Lancet*, **348**, 1196–1201.

Ottesen EA and Ramachandran CP (1995) Lymphatic filariasis and disease: control strategies. *Parasitology Today*, **11**, 129–131.

Pasvol G, Jungery M, Weatherall DJ et al. (1982) Glycophorin as a possible receptor for *Plasmodium falciparum*. Lancet, **2**, 947–950.

Pearson RD, de Alencar JE, Romito R et al. (1983) Circulating immune complexes and rheumatoid factors in visceral leishmaniasis. *Journal of Infectious Diseases*, **147**, 1102.

Pearson RD, Cox G, Jeronimo SM et al. (1992) Visceral leishmaniasis: a model for infection-induced cachexia. *American Journal of Tropical Medicine and Hygiene*, **47**, 8–15.

Pearson RD, De Queiroz Sousa A and Jeronima SMB (2000) *Leishmania* species: visceral (kala-azar), cutaneous and mucosal leishmaniasis. In *Mandell, Douglas and Bennett's Principles and Practice of Infectious Diseases* (eds GL Mandell, JE Bennett and R Dolin), 5th edn, vol. 2, pp 2831–2845. Churchill Livingstone, Philadelphia.

Pécoul B and Gastellu M (1999) Production of sleeping-sickness treatment. *Lancet*, **354**, 955–956.

Polman K, Stelma FF, Gryseels B et al. (1995) Epidemiologic application of circulating antigen detection in a recent *Schistosoma mansoni* focus in northern Senegal. *American Journal of Tropical Medicine and Hygiene*, **53**, 152–157.

Pratlong F, Dedet JP and Marty P (1995) *Leishmania*-human immunodeficiency virus co-infection in the Mediterranean basin: iso-enzymatic characterisation of 100 isolates of the *Leishmania infantum* complex. *Journal of Infectious Diseases*, **172**, 323–327.

Price RN, Nosten F, Luxemburger C et al. (1996) Effects of artemisinin derivatives on malaria transmissability. *Lancet*, **347**, 1654–1658.

Ranque S, Garcia A, Boussinesq M et al. (1996) Decreased prevalence and intensity of *Loa loa* infection in a community treated with ivermectin every three months for two years. *Transactions of the Royal Society of Tropical Medicine and Hygiene*, **90**, 429–430.

Schreck CE, Kline DL, Chaniotis BN et al. (1982) Evaluation of personal protection methods against phlebotomine sand flies including vectors of leishmaniasis in Panama. *American Journal of Tropical Medicine and Hygiene*, **31**, 1046–1053.

Seaman J, Boer C, Wilkinson R et al. (1995) Liposomal amphotericin B (AmBisome) in the treatment of complicated kala-azar under field conditions. *Clinical Infectious Diseases*, **21**, 188–193.

Seed JR (1998) African trypanosomiasis. In *Topley and Wilson's Microbiology and Microbial Infection* (eds F Cox, J Kreier and D Wakelin), 9th edn, vol. 5, pp 267–282. Arnold, London.

Shanks GD, Gordon DM, Klotz FW et al. (1998) Efficacy and safety of atovaquone-proguanil as suppressive prophylaxis for *Plasmodium falciparum* malaria. *Clinical Infectious Diseases*, **27**, 494–499.

Shiff CJ, Premij Z and Minjas JN (1993) The rapid ParaSight™-F. A new diagnostic tool for *Plasmodium falciparum* infection. *Transactions of the Royal Society of Tropical Medicine and Hygiene*, **87**, 29–31.

Sim BKL, Chinis CE, Wasniowska K et al. (1994) Receptor and ligand domains for invasion of erythrocytes by *Plasmodium falciparum*. *Science*, **264**, 1941–1944.

Siongkok TKA, Mahmoud AAF, Ouma JH et al. (1976) Morbidity in schistosomiasis mansoni in relation to intensity of infection: study of a community in Machakos, Kenya. *American Journal of Tropical Medicine and Hygiene*, **25**, 273.

Smith JD, Chitnis CE, Craig AG et al. (1995) Switches in expression of *Plasmodium falciparum var* genes correlate with changes in antigenic and cytoadherent phenotypes of infected erythrocytes. *Cell*, **82**, 101–110.

Spielman A, Perrone JB, Teklehaimanot A et al. (1988) Malaria diagnosis by direct observation of centrifuged samples of blood. *American Journal of Tropical Medicine and Hygiene*, **39**, 337.

Su X-Z, Heatwole VM, Wertheimer F et al. (1995) The large diverse gene family *var* encodes proteins involved in cytoadherence and antigenic variation of *Plasmodium falciparum*-infected erythrocytes. *Cell*, **82**, 89–99.

Sultan AA (1999) Molecular mechanisms of malaria sporozoite motility and invasion of host cells. *International Microbiology*, **2**, 155–160.

Valero MV, Amador R, Aponte JJ et al. (1996) Evaluation of SPf66 malaria vaccine during a 22-month follow-up field trial in the Pacific coast of Colombia. *Vaccine*, **14**, 1466–1470.

van der Berg JD, Duvenage CS, Roskell NS *et al.* (1999) Safety and efficacy of atovaquone and proguanil hydrochloride for the prophylaxis of *Plasmodium falciparum* malaria in South Africa. *Clinical Therapeutics*, **21**, 714–749.

Van Laetham Y and Lopes C (1996) Treatment of onchocerciasis. *Drugs*, **52**, 861–869.

Villanueva MS (1993) Trypanosomiasis of the central nervous system. *Seminars in Neurology*, **13**, 209–218.

von Lichtenberg F, Sadun EH, Cheever AW *et al.* (1971) Experimental infection with *Schistosoma japonicum* in chimpanzees. Parasitologic, clinical, serologic, and pathological observations. *American Journal of Tropical Medicine and Hygiene*, **20**, 850–893.

Wanderley DM (1993) Control of *Triatoma infestans* in the State of Sao Paulo. *Revista Da Sociedade Brasileira de Medicina Tropical*, **26**(Suppl. 3), 17–25.

Wertheimer SP and Barnwell JW (1989) *Plasmodium vivax* interaction with the human Duffy blood group glycoprotein: identification of a parasite receptor-like protein. *Experimental Parasitology*, **69**, 340–350.

White NJ (1996) Can amodiaquine be resurrected? (letter: comment). *Lancet*, **348**, 1184–1185.

White NJ, Warrell DA, Chanthavanich P *et al.* (1983) Severe hypoglycemia and hyperinsulinemia in falciparum malaria. *New England Journal of Medicine*, **309**, 61–66.

White NJ, Krishna S, Waller D *et al.* (1989) Open comparison of intramuscular chloroquine and quinine in children with severe chloroquine-sensitive falciparum malaria. *Lancet*, **ii**, 1313–1316.

WHO (1985) The control of schistosomiasis: report of a WHO expert committee. *World Health Organization Technical Report Series*, **728**, 1–113.

WHO (1991) Control of Chagas disease. *World Health Organization Technical Report Series*, **811**, i–vi, 1–95.

WHO (1992) Lymphatic filariasis: The Disease and Its Control. Fifth Report of a WHO Expert Committee on Lymphatic Filariasis. *World Health Organization Technical Report Series*, **821**, i–vi, 1–71.

WHO (1995a) *WHO Model Prescribing Information. Drugs used in Parasitic Diseases*, 2nd edn. World Health Organization, Geneva.

WHO (1995b) Onchocerciasis and its control: report of a WHO expert committee on onchocerciasis control. *World Health Organization Technical Report Series*, **852**, i–viii, 1–103.

WHO (1998a) Control and surveillance of African trypanosomiasis: report of a WHO expert committee. *World Health Organisation Technical Report Series*, **881**, I–VI, 1–114.

WHO (1998b) *International Travel and Health. Vaccination Requirements and Health Advice: Situation as on 1 January 1998*. World Health Organization, Geneva.

WHO (2000a) *Management of Severe Malaria: A Practical Handbook*, 2nd edn. World Health Organization, Geneva.

WHO (2000b) WHO expert committee on malaria (20th report). *World Health Organization Technical Report Series*, **892**, i–v, 1–74.

Xiao SH, You JQ, Yang YQ *et al.* (1995) Experimental studies on early treatment of schistosomal infection with artemether. *Southeast Asian Journal of Tropical Medicine and Public Health*, **26**, 306–318.

Zheng HJ, Tao ZH, Cheng WF *et al.* (1990) Comparison of Dot-ELISA with Sandwich-ELISA for the detection of circulating antigens in patients with bancroftian filariasis. *American Journal of Tropical Medicine and Hygiene*, **42**, 546–549.

Zijlstra EE, Hassan AM, Ismael A *et al.* (1994) Emdemic kalaazar in eastern Sudan: a longitudinal study on the incidence of clinical and subclinical infection and post kala-azar dermal leishmaniasis. *American Journal of Tropical Medicine and Hygiene*, **51**, 826–836.

Section III

Prevention and Management of Travel-Related Disease

9

Tropical Skin Infections

Francisco Vega-López and Verity Blackwell

University College London Hospitals NHS Trust, London, UK

INTRODUCTION

Skin infections and tropical diseases may represent a primary condition or a secondary manifestation of illness elsewhere in the body. Cutaneous larva migrans, Madura foot and localized cutaneous simple leishmaniasis are examples of the former, whereas the latter can be exemplified by systemic conditions such as leprosy, disseminated leishmaniasis secondary to kala-azar, and paracoccidioidomycosis.

The clinical approach to a patient with tropical disease of the skin involves a thorough exercise in history-taking. This must include detailed information on previous skin disease, travel history, activities while travelling, occupation, duration of signs and symptoms, evolution of clinical signs, symptoms in relatives or travel companions, and a fast practical assessment of the patient's immune status. The identification of extracutaneous signs, such as fever, enlarged lymph nodes, hepatosplenomegaly, and general malaise, indicates systemic illness and these findings should prompt immediate action for further investigations or an appropriate referral. Particular epidemiological settings in the tropics determine exposure and attack rates of specific diseases and, hence, an understanding of the global geographical pathology and living conditions of the overseas population is required in the practice of travel medicine.

The prevalence of skin diseases in the tropics is similar to that found in developed countries and Table 9.1 summarises the main dermatological problems diagnosed in the outpatients in a Latin American hospital. The main differences found in tropical dermatology when compared with the practice of this specialty in northern European hospitals are a higher incidence of endemic infectious diseases, a lower frequency of skin malignancy, and the lack or decreased availability of dermatological services and travel medicine specialists. Moreover, poor living conditions, overcrowding, and malnutrition account for a variety of cutaneous signs and symptoms related to poverty.

Our specialised clinic in 'Tropical Dermatology and Skin Infections' was established in 1997 at the Hospital for Tropical Diseases in London and provides clinical service for travellers as well as for individuals with HIV/AIDS-related skin conditions. Our experience from this tertiary centre indicates that 75% of the total of referrals present with a skin condition related to a travelling event. Seventy per cent of this population is represented by holiday-makers returning from the Caribbean, Latin America, India, and northern, central, and eastern Africa, but cases returning from other tropical regions are also well represented. The remaining 30% of our patients travel for professional or family reasons. Only a minority of individuals included in the last group travel to the tropics, to carry out aid missions, army exercises in the jungle, or else correspond to immigrants that have been displaced from tropical regions of the world. The relative frequencies and most common diagnoses in travellers who have been referred to our clinic are presented in Table 9.2.

This chapter presents a description of the most relevant conditions grouped by aetiological agents and the main emphasis has been placed on clinical findings and diagnosis as a practical guide to everyday work in clinical medicine. Pathogenesis of disease and management of conditions have also been included, and the chapter concludes with a brief description of noninfectious skin conditions that are relevant in travel medicine.

DISEASES CAUSED BY PARASITES, ECTOPARASITES, AND BITES

Cutaneous Larva Migrans

Aetiology and Pathogenesis

This dermatosis results from the accidental penetration of the human skin by parasitic larvae from domestic canine and feline hosts. Cats and dogs pass ova of these helminths with the stools, and larval stages develop in the

Principles and Practice of Travel Medicine. Edited by Jane N. Zuckerman.
© 2001 John Wiley & Sons Ltd.

Table 9.1 Common dermatological conditions in the outpatients department at the National Medical Centre, IMSS, Mexico City, 1993–1998

Eczema (acute, contact, chronic, stasis)
Psoriasis
Pyogenic infections
Pemphigus
Dermatophyte infections
Benign tumours
Lupus erythematosus
Viral infections
Leprosy
Leg ulcers
Drug reactions
Malignant tumours

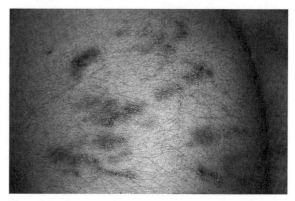

Figure 9.1 Cutaneous larva migrans acquired on a Caribbean beach. Erythematous papular lesions and serpiginous tracks in a multiple infection on the buttocks

Table 9.2 Travel-related skin conditions in 875 patients referred to the Hospital for Tropical Diseases in London

Condition	%
Pyogenic infections	23
Eczema and eczematisation	18
Urticaria	11
Insect bites and insect bite reactions	9
Dermatophyte and other fungal infections	9
Cutaneous larva migrans	7
Leishmaniasis, onchocerciasis, schistosomiasis	6
Pruritus, scabies, prurigo, and other	17

soil or beach sand. A close contact with human skin allows the infective larvae to burrow into the epidermis and cause clinical disease. The main aetiological agents are *Ancylostoma brasiliensae, A. caninum, A. ceylanicum,* and *A. stenocephalae* but other species affecting ruminants and pigs can also cause human disease. Following penetration into the skin, the larvae are incapable of crossing the human epidermodermal barrier and stay in the epidermis, creeping across spongiotic vesicles, until they die a few days or weeks later. Multiple infections can, however, last for several months.

Clinical Findings and Diagnosis

The plantar regions of one or both feet represent the main anatomical site affected by cutaneous larva migrans, but any part of the body in contact with infested soil or sand can be involved. Individuals of all age groups and both sexes can be affected and the disease is a common problem for tourists on beach holidays where they walk on bare feet or lie on the infested sand. A report of 44 cases presenting in returning travellers attending our specialised clinic in London revealed that 70% of the lesions were located on one foot, but the buttocks were also commonly affected, as shown in Figure 9.1 (Blackwell and Vega-López, 2000). The initial lesion is a prurigi-

nous papule at the site of penetration that appears within a day following the infestation. An erythematous, raised, larval track measuring 1–3 mm in width and height starts progressing in a curved or looped fashion. New segments of larval track reveal that the organism can advance at a speed of 2–5 cm daily. Commonly, the larval track measures between a few millimetres up to several centimetres in the region adjacent to the penetration site, but uncommon cases may present long larval tracks surrounding large areas of the foot, with a well-defined perimalleolar distribution. Localized clinical pictures on the toes may present with only papular lesions but other presentations include blisters and urticarial wheals. Secondary complications to the presence of the parasite in the epidermis include an inflammatory reaction, eczematisation, impetiginised tracks or papules, and even deeper pyogenic infections. Variable in severity, but most commonly intense, pruritus and a burning sensation are the main symptoms.

The diagnosis is based on the clinical history and physical findings on the affected skin. The histopathological investigation has little, if any, value in the diagnosis of cutaneous larva migrans. The study of 332 cases in central Mexico throughout 10 years in the 1980s (L. R. Orozco, personal communication, 1993) revealed that H&E preparations of affected skin show a spongiotic acute or subacute dermatitis with a variable presence of larval structures. A mild perivascular lymphocytic infiltrate was frequently observed in the dermis and a low proportion of cases may develop peripheral eosinophilia, but this is not a constant finding.

Management and Treatment

The treatment of choice is the systemic administration of albendazole for 3 days. Topical options include a 10% tiabendazole cream applied several times daily for 10 days, and one or more sessions of cryotherapy with liquid nitrogen. Resistant cases may respond to a single dose of systemic ivermectin (Caumes *et al.*, 1992).

Leishmaniasis

Aetiology and Pathogenesis

Leishmania spp parasites are protozoan organisms transmitted to humans and other vertebrates by the bite of female sandflies of the genera *Phlebotomus* or *Lutzomya*. Most *Leishmania* species can cause skin or mucocutaneous disease, but a few of them affect internal organs as well. It is estimated that 15 million individuals are infected by *Leishmania* in 88 countries. The main endemic foci are found in Asia, the Middle East, Africa, southern Europe, and Latin America. Hot and humid environment, such as that found in rain-forest jungles, provides adequate habitat for the vectors in Latin America. In contrast, desert conditions favour breeding sites for the vectors in the Middle Eastern and North African endemic regions (WHO, 1990).

Following the bite from a *Leishmania*-infected sandfly, humans can heal spontaneously or else develop localised or disseminated skin disease. Sandfly and *Leishmania* species causing skin disease in humans have been classified in geographical terms as Old World and New World cutaneous leishmaniasis. Both can affect one area of exposed thin skin but multiple infective bites or disseminated forms may present with lesions on several anatomical regions. Common inoculation sites include facial bone prominent regions, external aspects of wrists, and malleolar regions. The bite of the sandfly commonly targets exposed areas, such as the external ankles during walking or medial regions of the foot when the host is at rest. Depending on the area left uncovered by light footwear, the foot dorsum, heel, toes, lateral aspect, and plantar region can also be affected by bites.

Leishmania parasites can resist phagocytosis and damage by complement proteins from the host by the action of lipophosphoglycan and glycoprotein antigens. Following phagocytosis, the intracellular forms of *Leishmania* parasites induce a delayed-type hypersensitive granulomatous reaction, which adds to the tissue damage (Meñdoza-Léon *et al.*, 1996).

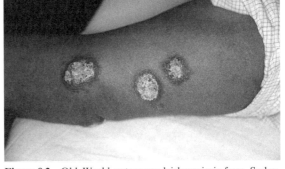

Figure 9.2 Old World cutaneous leishmaniasis from Sudan. Disseminated violaceous nodular and ulcerated lesions covered by crusts

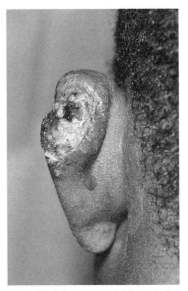

Figure 9.3 New World cutaneous leishmaniasis from Belize's jungle. Typical 'chiclero ulcer' with destructive inflammatory granuloma on the helix

Clinical Findings and Diagnosis

The clinical picture of cutaneous leishmaniasis has recently been reviewed by Chopra and Vega-López (1999). The bite of a sandfly may induce an inflammatory papular or nodular lesion of prurigo but it may go unnoticed for several weeks. The incubation period can be as short as 15 days but commonly it is estimated at around 4–6 weeks. Certain forms may take longer to develop clinically. A nonhealing papule with surrounding erythema and pain may also indicate superimposed bacterial infection, which subsequently develops ulceration. On average, 6–8 weeks after the sandfly bite a violaceous nodule with or without nodular borders starts enlargement and ulceration. The ulcer is partially or completely covered by a thick crust that, after curettage, reveals a haemorrhagic

and vegetating bed. Cutaneous leishmaniasis on the upper limbs can manifest clinically as nodules covered with crust, ulceration with a raised inflamed solid border, tissue necrosis, and lymphangitic forms (Figure 9.2). Advanced late forms present with scarring, skin atrophy, and pigmentary changes. A particular localised form caused by *L. braziliensis* is called 'chiclero ulcer' and affects the helix of one ear (Figure 9.3) but this species commonly manifests as a single violatious ulceration of the skin (Figure 9.4). Other regions of the body surface may be affected by pigmented and hyperkeratotic lesions in a clinical form named post-kala-azar dermal leishmaniasis. This clinical form presents after an episode of visceral leishmaniasis caused by *L. donovani* in cases originating from India and Africa.

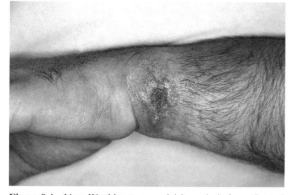

Figure 9.4 New World cutaneous leishmaniasis from Central America. Ulcerated lesion with nodular violaceous border on the external aspect of the wrist

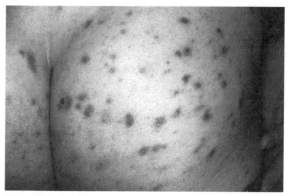

Figure 9.5 Onchocerciasis from Central Africa. Erythematous and pruriginous papules and nodules on the buttocks

The clinical picture of cutaneous leishmaniasis and the history of exposure in an endemic region of the world strongly suggest the diagnosis. Complementary tests include histology of lesional skin, slit-skin smears stained with Giemsa for direct microscopy, and tissue samples for culture in NNN medium, and for genetic analysis by polymerase chain reaction (PCR) techniques.

Management and Treatment

The general public and health personnel easily establish the diagnosis of cutaneous leishmaniasis in endemic areas of the world and, following referral to a physician, one or more treatment options are available. However, in nonendemic regions, and particularly in nontropical countries, the returning traveller requires attention by an experienced doctor in tropical medicine, infectious diseases, or dermatology. Several drugs are effective against *Leishmania* parasites and these include pentavalent antimonials, amphotericin B, triazole and alylamine antifungal compounds; however, the only treatment of choice for a number of species is the intravenous administration of antimonials carefully monitored in hospital and administered only by experienced personnel. In our experience, a dose of $20\,\text{mg}\,\text{kg}^{-1}$ body weight daily for 3 weeks has been effective in curing most of our patients with New World cutaneous leishmaniasis caused by *L. braziliensis*. Patients require long-term follow up as leishmaniasis may relapse in some cases.

Onchocerciasis

Aetiology and Pathogenesis

This filarial disease is acquired through the inoculation into the skin of *Onchocerca volvulus* by blackflies of the genus *Simulium*. This infection, also named 'river blindness' and 'Robles disease', is highly prevalent in Africa within latitudes 15°N and 15°S, and affects tropical coun-

tries in Central and South America. Fast flowing brooks and small rivers provide breeding sites for the blackfly vectors and only the female individuals are haematophagous. They can bite potential hosts throughout the day, principally those pursuing outdoors activities. Holiday-makers as well as those travelling for professional reasons risk acquiring this parasitic disease, but it is the local population that suffers the highest toll from both clinical disease and subsequent disability.

Following an approximate incubation period of 1 year, the adult worms live freely in the skin or within fibrotic nodules or cysts named onchocercomas. The female adult worm releases microfilaria into the dermis, and they are disseminated by the lymphatic system. Adult worms may live and reproduce for up to 15 years in the human host.

Clinical Findings and Diagnosis

The main clinical manifestations include pruritus and skin lesions, consisting of lichenified plaques, papular or prurigo eruptions, nodules, atrophic changes, and pigmentary abnormalities. Early symptoms include fever, arthralgia, and transient urticaria affecting face and trunk. Pruritus and scratching lead to eczematization, revealed as patches of lichenified and excoriated skin on the trunk and lower limbs. The buttocks are commonly involved (Figure 9.5) and oedematous plaques are characteristic in Latin American cases, named locally 'mal morado'. Late skin lesions show atrophy and hyper- and hypopigmented patches, giving the appearance of leopard skin described in African cases. The presence of filaria in the ocular anterior chamber causes acute symptoms and late ocular lesions lead to blindness.

The parasitological diagnosis includes the identification of microfilaria in samples taken from skin snips from the back, hips, and thighs, specimens for histopathological investigation and serology. Most patients develop peripheral hypereosinophilia.

Management and Treatment

The treatment of choice for onchocerciasis is a single dose of systemic ivermectin every 6 months. The surgical excision of nodules is indicated and all patients require specialised attention in tertiary medical centres, including a comprehensive ophthalmological assessment. An active programme of mass therapy for individuals living in endemic regions of the world has been in place for more than a decade.

Gnathostomiasis

Aetiology and Pathogenesis

A number of *Gnathostoma* species live as adult worms in the intestine of domestic cats. Travellers can acquire the disease by eating contaminated fish that have ingested small crustaceans, acting as intermediary hosts in this condition. The larval stages do not reach maturation in the human body and can cause disease in several internal organs as well as in the skin. The disease is prevalent in Southeast Asia, China, Japan, Indonesia, and Mexico.

Clinical Findings and Diagnosis

Episodes of migrating intermittent subcutaneous oedema with pruritus constitute the main clinical picture and cases can adopt a chronic protracted course for years. The episodes of oedema can be quite inflammatory and painful and the larvae can erupt out from the affected skin. The feet are not affected commonly.

Management and Treatment

The surgical extraction of the larva from the skin represents the curative therapeutic approach (Taniguchi *et al.*, 1992).

Tungiasis

Aetiology and Pathogenesis

Tungiasis is a localised skin disease commonly affecting one foot and caused by the burrowing flea *Tunga penetrans*. This is also known as chigoe infestation, jigger, sandflea, chigoe, and puce chique (Fr.). It has been reported that this flea originated in Central and South America (Ibanez-Bernal and Velasco-Castrejón, 1996) and was subsequently distributed in Africa, Madagascar, India, and Pakistan. It is a very small organism, ~ 1 mm in length, and lives in the soil near pigsties and cattle sheds. Fecundated females require blood and their head and mouthparts penetrate the epidermis to reach the blood and other nutrients from the superficial dermis.

After taking nourishment for several days, eggs are laid to the exterior and the flea dies.

Clinical Findings and Diagnosis

These fleas commonly affect one foot, penetrating the soft skin on the toe web spaces, but other areas of toes and plantar aspects on the foot can be affected (Douglas-Jones *et al.*, 1995). The initial burrow and the flea body can be evident in early lesions but within 3–4 weeks a crateriform single nodule develops, with a central haemorhagic point. Superimposed bacterial infections may be responsible for impetigo, ecthyma, cellulitis, and gangrenous lesions.

The diagnosis is clinical but skin specimens for direct microscopy and histopathology with H&E stain reveal the structures of the flea and eggs.

Management and Treatment

Curettage, cryotherapy, surgical excision, or else careful removal of the flea and eggs are the curative therapeutic choices. Early treatment and avoidance of secondary infection are of the utmost importance in all infested travellers, and particularly in individuals with diabetes mellitus, leprosy, or other debilitating conditions of the feet. A haemorrhagic nodule caused by *T. penetrans* may pose differential diagnostic difficulty with an inflamed common wart or a malignant melanoma but the short duration of the lesion and the history of exposure indicate the acute nature of this parasitic disease.

Myasis

Aetiology and Pathogenesis

A number of diptera species in larval stages (maggots) may colonize the human skin. The infestation mechanisms include direct deposition of eggs, contamination by soil or dirty clothes, other insects acting as vectors, or else by actual penetration into the skin by larvae. Species of *Dermatobia* and *Cordylobia* are the commonest found in the tropics, respectively in the Americas and Africa, whereas European cases originate from *Hypoderma* spp. (Lui and Buck, 1992). A local inflammatory reaction to the larvae, with secondary infection, is responsible for the signs and symptoms of disease.

Clinical Findings and Diagnosis

Elderly and debilitated individuals of both sexes with exposed chronic wounds or ulcers are at a higher risk of suffering from this infestation. Furunculoid and subcutaneous forms may affect any part of the body, but in children the scalp is a commonly affected site. Chronic ulcers of the lower legs and feet represent a predisposing factor and myasis often complicates severe infections by bacteria or fungi. Larvae feed on tissue debris and may not cause discomfort or symptoms at all. Cases are observed throughout the year in tropical regions where the standards of hygiene, nutrition, and general health are poor. The diagnosis is based on clinical suspicion and physical findings. This problem is rarely seen in the returning traveller.

Management and Treatment

The treatment of choice is the mechanical removal or surgical excision of the larvae (Lui and Buck, 1992). Single furunculoid lesions can be covered by thick petroleum jelly or paste to suffocate the larvae, which can then be extracted. Superficial infestations respond to repeated topical soaks or baths in potassium permanganate, at a 1:10 000 dilution in water, carried out for a few days. Cases with secondary pyogenic infection require a full course of β-lactam or macrolide antibiotics.

Scabies

Aetiology and Pathogenesis

Scabies is a cosmopolitan problem but individuals in poor tropical countries with low standards of hygiene, and particularly overcrowding, suffer from cyclical outbreaks of severe and chronic forms. Travellers often acquire this infestation by personal contact. The human scabies mite *Sarcoptes scabiei* commonly affects the skin of both feet of infants and children. Adults rarely manifest scabies on the lower limbs below the knees (Hebra lines), but exceptional cases of crusted or Norwegian scabies may present with lesions on both feet. The scabies mite burrows a tunnel of up to 4 mm into the superficial layer of the epidermis, where eggs are laid. The eggs hatch and reach the stage of nymph and subsequently become an adult male or female mite. Female individuals live up to 6 weeks and lay up to 50 eggs. A new generation of fecundated females penetrates the skin in regions adjacent to the nesting burrow, but the mite infestation can also be perpetuated by clothes, or by reinfestation from another host in the family.

Clinical Findings and Diagnosis

Papules, with or without excoriation, and S-shaped burrows are the elementary classical lesions of scabies. Infants and young children present with papular, vesicular, and/or nodular lesions on both plantar regions but other parts of the feet can be affected. In contrast, adult travellers present with bilateral lesions on hands, upper limbs, anterior axillary lines, periumbilical region, external genitalia, and buttocks. Travellers of all age groups suffering from chronic crusted scabies may present with eczematisation, impetiginised plaques, and hyperkeratosis, masking the typical clinical signs of this infestation. Large crusts covering inflammatory papular lesions contain a large number of parasites and a careful examination is required to prevent health personnel from acquiring the infestation.

The clinical findings and intense pruritus support the diagnosis. Confirmation is obtained by direct microscopy of skin scrapings from a burrow, revealing the structures or faecal pellets of the mite. This test is carried out on a glass slide in 10–15% KOH solution under low power; it has a low sensitivity if carried out by inexperienced hands.

Management and Treatment

Topical treatment overnight with benzyl benzoate, malathion, lindane, or permethrine, lotion or cream, is usually effective. A second course is recommended 10–14 days after the original application, and all the affected members of a household or travelling party require treatment at the same time to prevent cyclical reinfestations. Severe cases or individuals in particular community settings, such as those living in homes for the elderly, orphanages, prisons, or psychiatry wards, require oral treatment with a single dose of ivermectin, as originally described by E. Macotela in 1991 (personal communication). Severe outbreaks often require a second dose of ivermectin after a 2 week interval (150–200 μg kg^{-1} of body weight). This drug can only be prescribed by a qualified physician. Other therapeutic measures are directed to controlling the symptoms, inflammation, and infection. Clothes and bedlinen require washing at high temperature to kill all young fecundated females but a number of authors have demonstrated that this is not necessary. In the right epidemiological context, scabies may represent a venereal disease. Pruritus may last for several weeks after cure.

Ticks

Aetiology and Pathogenesis

Ticks are cosmopolitan ectoparasites capable of transmitting severe viral, rickettsial, bacterial, and parasitic diseases. The transmission of infectious agents takes place at the time of taking a blood meal from a human host, who becomes infested accidentally. Soft ticks of the family Argasidae are more prevalent in the tropics and subtropical regions of the world and transmit agents of tick-borne relapsing fever. The main genera of hard ticks are *Ixodes*, *Dermacentor*, *Haemaphysalis*, and *Amblyomma* and these can transmit arboviral, bacterial, and rickettsial diseases.

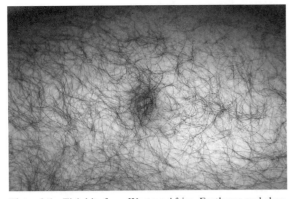

Figure 9.6 Tick bite from Western Africa. Erythema and characteristic eschar in a patient who subsequently developed typhus

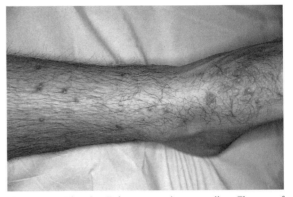

Figure 9.7 Bites by *Pulex irritans* in a traveller. Clusters of erythematous and pruriginous papules on the lower limbs

Clinical Findings and Diagnosis

The bite of a tick is painful and the patient is aware of this episode. The bite produces a local inflammatory reaction suggesting initially an ordinary papular insect bite that subsequently causes localized superficial vascular damage with necrosis. The characteristic clinical picture manifested as an eschar can be easily recognised on careful physical examination (Figure 9.6). An area of circular scaling of the skin surrounding the original haemorrhagic bite can be seen after a week or 10 days. Residual chronic lesions may leave hyperpigmentated patches with a central induration.

Management and Treatment

Removal of the tick can be carried out by applying a tight dressing or cloth impregnated with chloroform, petrol, or ether to the tick body. The organism is carefully removed a few minutes later, avoiding the rupture of head and mouth-parts, which can be left behind, into the skin. A careful follow-up and self-surveillance is indicated as systemic illness may start a few days or weeks following the tick bite. Symptoms such as a fever, skin rash, lymph node enlargement, fatigue, and night sweats indicate systemic disease and the patient requires referral to a hospital physician or to a specialist in tropical or travel medicine.

Fleas

Aetiology and Pathogenesis

The common human flea *Pulex irritans* is cosmopolitan but a number of other species show preference for tropical climates. Such is the case of the tropical rat flea *Xenopsylla cheopis*. Fleas bite humans in order to get a blood meal and in doing so produce a localised inflammatory reaction. History of exposure can reveal an individual host or family members recently moving house or acquir-

ing a second-hand piece of wooden furniture, in which fleas can live for months without taking blood meals.

Clinical Findings and Diagnosis

A clinical picture of prurigo with papules, vesicles, or small nodules on both feet and lower legs is characteristic and the lesions are often found in clusters (Figure 9.7). The papular discrete lesions may reveal a central haemorrhagic punctum and the lesions in clusters often show a remarkable asymmetry. Modification of the initial pruriginous lesions may result from intense scratching and superimposed secondary bacterial infection.

Management and Treatment

Fumigation can be successfully achieved by using common insecticide products approved for domestic use. Severe reactions of prurigo require a topical steroid cream, and impetiginised cases topical or systemic antibiotics. Antihistamine lotions or tablets may provide symptomatic relief. Severe cases are treated with a single dose or short course of systemic corticosteroids.

BACTERIAL INFECTIONS

Pyogenic Infections

Aetiology and Pathogenesis

Common bacterial infections in the skin of the traveller are caused by *Staphylococcus* and *Streptococcus* species. These infectious agents are ubiquitous in both urban and rural environments and are capable of causing disease in travellers of all age groups. Healthy and immunocompromised hosts develop pyogenic infections of the skin following direct inoculation of bacteria. Less often, haematogenous dissemination and even a septicaemic state may develop as a result of a minor skin injury. The port of entry for these pathogenic organisms is often unnoticed

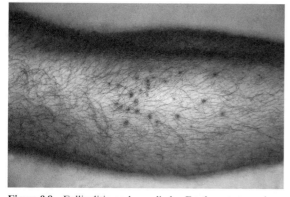

Figure 9.8 Folliculitis on lower limbs. Erythematous and excoriated follicular papules

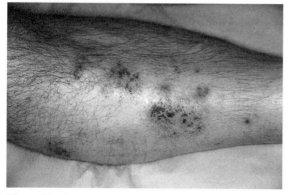

Figure 9.9 Impetigo in a returning traveller. Plaques with erythema and yellowish thin crust showing superficial excoriation

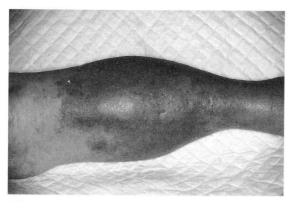

Figure 9.10 Cellulitis on the leg of an elderly traveller. Localised plaque of shiny erythematous skin with dermal thickening

by both the patient and doctor, but minor injuries, insect bites, friction blisters, or superficial fungal infection are the commonest found in clinical practice. Other clinical circumstances such as burns, use of indwelling catheters in children, and surgical procedures also play a role as risk factors for these infections.

Pyogenic bacteria cause damage in the infected tissue

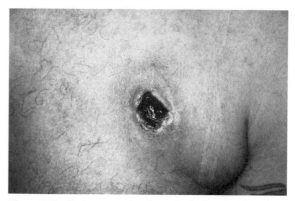

Figure 9.11 Ecthyma on the chest of a backpacker. Pyogenic ulcer following a friction blister caused by the strap of a rucksack

by the pathogenic action of proteases, haemolysins, lipoteichoic acid, and coagulases. Erythrogenic toxins are responsible for the erythema commonly observed in infections by *Streptococcus* spp (Bisno and Stevens, 1996).

Clinical Findings and Diagnosis

The clinical spectrum of skin pyogenic infections includes folliculitis (Figure 9.8) and furuncle and carbuncle formation on areas with hair follicles. Plaques of impetigo and infiltrated thickened dermis commonly affect the lower limbs (Figure 9.9) and are respectively caused by *Staphylococcus* and *Streptococcus* species. Abscess formation, cellulitis (Figure 9.10), and necrotic ulceration represent the more severe end of the spectrum. The perimalleolar regions are by far the most commonly affected areas of the foot as they are exposed to mechanical trauma while travelling. The dorsum, toes, and heels follow in frequency.

Common clinical signs of pyogenic infections include a variety of manifestations, such as erythema, inflammation, pus discharge, abscess formation, ulceration, blistering, necrotising lesions, and gangrene. Severe scarring may result from pyogenic ulcers caused by friction injury (Figure 9.11). Most pyogenic skin infections in the traveller are painful and the diagnosis is based on the clinical history and findings.

Bacteriological investigations and sensitivity profile to antibiotics must be carried out if available. Disseminated, chronic, or severe infections require an immediate referral to a dermatologist or to an infectious disease specialist. Uncommon cases of streptococcal infection of the throat may express clinically with a sudden eruption of guttate psoriasis as a result of bacterial superantigen stimulation (Figure 9.12).

Management and Treatment

Mild infections are successfully treated with bathing or soaking of the affected skin in potassium permanganate

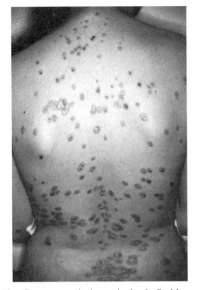

Figure 9.12 Guttate psoriasis on the back. Sudden eruption in a young traveller, characterised by erythemato-scaling 'drops' and small plaques

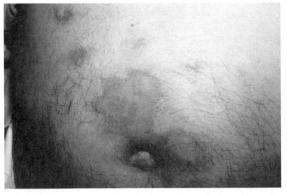

Figure 9.13 Fatal septicaemia by *Vibrio vulnificus* from the Gulf of Mexico. Violaceous and purpuric patches affecting abdominal skin

solution (1:10 000 dilution in water) for 15 min daily. Other mild superficial infections, like isolated plaques of impetigo or impetiginised eczema, respond well to antiseptic or antimicrobial creams and ointments containing cetrimide, chlorhexidine, fucidic acid, or mupirocin. Acute or chronic eczema requires treatment with potent topical steroids in order to eliminate risk factors for infection. Infections with multiple lesions, or those involving larger areas of the skin, require a complete course of systemic β-lactam or macrolide antibiotics in addition to the above topical treatments. Recurrent episodes of cellulitis require longer courses of these antibiotics, and hospitalisation followed by surgical debridement is mandatory in necrotic lesions, gangrenous plaques, and deeper infections with severe fasciitis. Superficial infections of the foot skin complicated by deeper involvement with necrosis of soft tissues carry a high mortality rate of up to 25% (Elliot *et al.*, 1996).

Treponemal Infections

Cosmopolitan treponemal diseases such as secondary *syphilis* present with an asymptomatic, symmetrical papular eruption and scaling of plantar regions. Other clinical features, such as concurrent palmar involvement, as well as the history of a primary chancre and the characteristic trunkal rash, while travelling, confirm the clinical suspicion. A definitive diagnosis can be established by specific tests such as positive dark-field microscopy from early skin lesions, as well as from highly sensitive treponemal serology (Young, 1992). Despite the fact that syphilis is not strictly a tropical disease, it represents a significant problem for the returning traveller involved in high-risk sexual activities while in the tropics (WHO, 1986). The treatment of choice is penicillin but allergic individuals respond to erythromycin or tetracyclines.

Yaws is a treponemal tropical disease manifesting on the feet and periorificial skin on the face. This condition affects mainly the male rural population in South America, sub-Saharan Africa, and Southeast Asia. It is associated with poverty in the humid tropics (Sehgal *et al.*, 1994) and one of the characteristic clinical presentations is that of plantar hyperkeratosis. Late tertiary infection results in asymptomatic palmoplantar keratoderma that develops nodular hyperkeratotic lesions, leading to painful disability; hence, the characteristic walk known as 'crab yaws'. The clinical picture can be difficult to differentiate from other types of infectious and noninfectious plantar keratodermas. Tests for diagnosis include darkfield microscopy of early lesions and treponemal serology. The treatment of choice is penicillin but *Treponema pallidum pertenue* also responds to tetracyclines and macrolides.

Other Bacterial Infections in the Traveller

Tropical *seaborne infections* by halophilic *Vibrio vulnificus* can produce localised or systemic disease manifested by acute and painful erythema, purpura, oedema, and necrosis, particularly affecting the lower limbs. Cases of returning travellers presenting in inland metropolitan areas can be very difficult to diagnose and these patients carry a high mortality risk. Fatal septicaemia manifests with coalescing purpuric patches on one or both lower limbs that subsequently spread to the periumbilical region (Figure 9.13). The infection is acquired by direct traumatic inoculation in estuaries and seawaters, or by ingestion of raw seafood, particularly oysters. Male individuals with a history of liver disease and iron overload states are the group at highest risk for this infection (Serrano-Jaen and Vega-López, 2000). Severe cases require immediate referral to a specialist hospital physician as intravenous antibiotics and early surgical debridement represent the treatment of choice.

Exfoliation of the plantar skin is part of the complex and severe picture in cosmopolitan cases with *staphylococcal scalded-skin syndrome* (SSSS) (Cribier *et al.*, 1994), whereas necrotic ulceration of the foot can result from tropical *cutaneous diphtheria* caused by *Corynebacterium diphtheriae* (Belsey and Leblanc, 1975). Cutaneous diphtheria commonly manifests as a nonhealing, single ulcerated lesion on the toe or toe cleft, lasting between 4 and 12 weeks.

Mycobacterial Infections

Aetiology and Pathogenesis

Several mycobacterial species can cause primary or secondary infection in the traveller. The 'swimming' or 'fish-tank granuloma' is an infection caused by *Mycobacterium marinum*. Other common chronic mycobacterial tropical infections include leprosy, tuberculosis, and Buruli ulcer, but these conditions are not relevant for travellers. They are caused by *M. leprae*, *M. tuberculosis*, and *M. ulcerans*, respectively. Mycobacterial skin diseases can be acquired by direct skin contact with a patient, by direct accidental or occupational inoculation, and by inhalation of the infective organisms. Particular clinical forms of cutaneous tuberculosis result following haematogenous dissemination from a primary infection elsewhere. The respiratory route is particularly important for leprosy and diverse forms of pulmonary tuberculosis. In the case of Buruli ulcer it has been suggested recently that contact with infected water in rural areas of Africa may represent the main source of infection. A toxin called mycolactone seems to be responsible for the severe tissue destruction and ulceration seen in patients with Buruli ulcer (Thangaraj *et al.*, 1999). In general, however, it is accepted that agents causing mycobacterial skin diseases have a low pathogenic potential, as most infected individuals in endemic regions do not develop clinical mycobacterial diseases.

Mycobacteria are very complex organisms, most of them ubiquitous in nature as saprophytes, but a number of species cause disease in other animals. A very thick wall surrounds the cytoplasmic membrane of mycobacteria and contains virulence factors, such as proteins and glycolipids. Mycobacteria can inhibit an efficient phagocytosis and intracellular killing by macrophages and also interact with the host's immune cells. This interaction results in chronic inflammation, tissue damage, and immunopathology, all of which account for the signs and symptoms observed in the wide range of mycobacterial diseases.

Clinical Findings and Diagnosis

The *fish-tank granuloma* affects more commonly the fin-

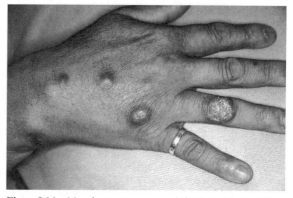

Figure 9.14 *Mycobacterium marinum* infection of the hand in a patient from Hong Kong. Fish-tank granuloma with violaceous nodules showing proximal lymphangitic dissemination

gers or dorsum of the hand but it has also been described on the foot and other anatomical sites. *M. marinum* frequently infects freshwater fish and, hence, individuals handling fish tanks represent the main population at risk (Gray *et al.*, 1990). Direct inoculation into the foot presents with similar clinical findings to those found in infections of the upper limb. The disease manifests as a localised, progressing swelling with variable pain, and the appearance, within a few weeks, of nodular or verrucous skin lesions on the affected area. These lesions can show ulceration and bleeding from the disease process itself but also from mechanical trauma. The nodular lesions, measuring a few millimetres up to 2–3 cm, may resolve spontaneously after a few months, but they can also disseminate proximally by haematogenous or lymphatic spread (Figure 9.14). The dorsal aspects of the hand, foot, and the malleolar regions are exposed to trauma and therefore direct inoculation commonly takes place on these regions. Once the condition is suspected, microbiological and histopathological investigations are the most sensitive tests to confirm the clinical diagnosis.

Leprosy is a chronic disease that affects not only the skin but particularly the peripheral nerves bilaterally. The hands and feet are the anatomical sites where inflammation, characteristic skin lesions, and nerve damage occur in the course of leprosy. The commonest skin lesions are nodules, erythematous plaques, or hypopigmented patches. Symptoms like hypo- or dysaesthesia, together with motor/sensory nerve abnormalities and obvious thickening of peripheral nerve branches, suggest the characteristic demyelinating neuropathy of leprosy. Advanced disease manifests with skin atrophy, pigmentary changes, and in severe cases chronic ulceration leading to mutilation and disability (Figure 9.15). Mutilating lesions of the hands and feet result from bone resorption, mechanical trauma, and secondary bacterial infection.

The clinical diagnosis of leprosy can be easily established in most cases that occur in endemic regions of the world (Bryceson and Pfaltzgraff, 1990). Epidemiological, clinical, histopathological, bacteriological, and immunological criteria have been used for many years to

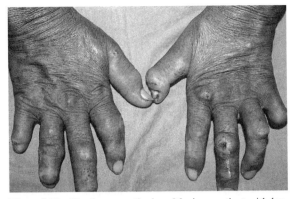

Figure 9.15 Hand neuropathy in a Mexican patient with leprosy. Atrophic and dysautonomic skin with ulceration and distal mutilation in a patient with bilateral ulnar, radial, and median nerve damage

diagnose and classify the cases of leprosy within a disease spectrum. This spectrum considers two polar groups or forms, called tuberculoid and lepromatous, as well as intermediate forms of the disease defined as borderline. Early disease may not present characteristics of any of the above groups and such cases are called indeterminate. The evolution of leprosy is a dynamic process and a significant number of cases cannot be classified easily at the time of diagnosis. All patients require long-term follow-up as their place within the spectrum involves not only therapeutic, but most importantly, prognostic implications. Patients with early disease, and particularly those presenting to the travel specialist in countries nonendemic for leprosy, often pose diagnostic difficulties. The delay in establishing an accurate diagnosis and treatment inevitably results in irreversible nerve damage and chronic complications with variable degrees of disability.

Skin tuberculosis affects individuals of all ages and both sexes, presenting with a wide variety of clinical pictures that frequently affect the lower limbs and particularly one or both feet (Chopra and Vega-López, 1999); however, lupus vulgaris and papulonecrotic tuberculide are more common in females, whereas tuberculosis verrucosa cutis is rare in children. By far the main clinical presentation of cutaneous tuberculosis affecting the adult foot is called tuberculosis verrucosa cutis, whereas cases of lupus vulgaris are commonly observed on the face. The tuberculous bacilli cause disease following direct inoculation into the skin but clinical disease can also result from haematogenous dissemination. Unilateral and asymmetrical involvement is the rule in almost all cases of skin tuberculosis. Commonly observed asymptomatic lesions include dry patches of atrophic skin, pigmentary changes, nodules, and plaques of verrucous lesions. The typical plaque of tuberculosis can measure between 2 and 12 cm in diameter, but chronic and larger lesions can involve most of the foot dorsum and lateral aspects. The course of cutaneous tuberculosis is indolent and chronic, but determines skin atrophy and variable degrees of scarring with

a consequent degree of local skin insufficiency. The clinical diagnosis can be confirmed by histopathology, bacteriology, and PCR investigations.

Buruli ulcer affects mainly young individuals in rural Africa, and particularly in West Africa, where an increase in incidence has been reported (Thangaraj *et al.*, 1999). More than two-thirds of the total of cases present in children below age 15. The initial lesions present as papules or small nodules that slowly increase in size to the point of causing an area of inflammation and subsequently ulceration of the skin. The ulcer characteristically presents with undermined edges and manifests active indolent phagedenism, often involving large areas of the affected limb. A single ulcer or smaller, coalescing ulcers present more frequently on the lower leg above the ankles but other regions of the foot can be involved as well. Oedematous forms may progress rapidly and cause a panniculitis, with destruction of underlying tissues such as fascia and bone. In cases where a large ulceration is followed by healing, contractures of the affected limb result from scarring. Severe scarring and contractures have been identified as a high morbidity factor for disability and up to 10% of these cases require amputation of the deformed limb (Josse *et al.*, 1994).

Management and Treatment of Mycobacterial Infections

All mycobacterial diseases require highly specialised diagnostic investigations that in many cases can only be carried out in a tertiary hospital setting. Most mycobacterial diseases affecting the skin represent public health priorities, not only for the endemic countries where they occur but also at an international level, as established by the World Health Organization (WHO). Following the diagnosis of individual cases, a long-term multidrug therapeutic regimen can be prescribed only by specialised physicians. Mycobacteria are known to develop resistance to antibiotics and it is imperative that all cases are treated with combinations of at least two drugs. The main drugs with antimycobacterial activity are rifampicin, ethambutol, pyrazinamide, clofazimine, sulfone, isoniazid, macrolide antibiotics, tetracyclines, and quinolones. The management of all mycobacterial diseases must include not only the medical treatment but also a full range of educational initiatives aimed at the patient, the community, and health personnel. Early lesions of fish-tank granuloma, skin tuberculosis, and particularly those caused by Buruli ulcer require surgical excision.

Bacterial Mycetoma

Aetiology and Pathogenesis

Nocardia, *Actinomadura*, and *Streptomyces* species are the common aetiological agents of 'Madura foot' or

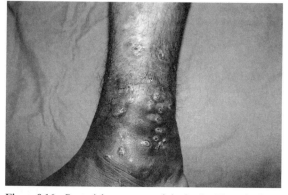

Figure 9.16 Bacterial mycetoma of the leg by *Nocardia braziliensis*. Deformity of the region with hiperpigmented skin, sinus tract formation, and scarring

actinomycetoma. This form of bacterial mycetoma occurs in tropical countries and the main case series have been reported from Sudan, Senegal, Nigeria, Saudi Arabia, India, and Mexico. The infection is acquired by direct inoculation of bacteria into the skin and does not seem to represent a risk for travellers. Young male individuals living in endemic regions and dedicated to agricultural activities have been reported with the highest incidence of actinomycetoma (López-Martínez *et al.*, 1992). Bacteria causing actinomycetoma have a thick wall surrounding the cytoplasmic membrane, which is rich in lipid and carbohydrate compounds. Some of these compounds, such as lipoarabinomannan and mycolic acids, have been identified as virulence factors. These bacteria are capable of blocking the adequate killing mechanisms of the cells of the infected host; however, it is considered that they have a low pathogenic potential and most of them live as saprophytes in the soil.

Clinical Findings and Diagnosis

The clinical disease is characterised by a chronic course, with inflammation, formation of sinus tracts discharging 'grains', and progressive deformity of the affected foot. Healing of discharging sinus tracts over years determines scarring, with atrophic skin plaques and secondary pigmentary changes (Figure 9.16). Asymptomatic nodular or verrucous lesions can also be found, and in a few cases a variable range of symptoms is present. These include pain that often results from superimposed pyogenic infection, acute inflammation, and bone involvement. The chronic infection with deformity of the foot determines periosteal involvement and subsequently osteomyelitis. Variable but often severe degrees of disability complete the chronic course of actinomycetoma.

The clinical picture manifested on one foot is highly suggestive of the diagnosis. The main differential diagnosis includes mycetoma caused by fungi (see Eumycetoma below) but other forms of 'cold' abscess formation, histoplasmosis, chromoblastomycosis, cutaneous

tuberculosis, and sarcoidosis are the main conditions to consider. Direct microscopy to disclose the 'grains' discharged from sinus tracts confirms the diagnosis and the culture of this material also provides a definite diagnosis of actinomycetoma.

Management and Treatment

Effective drugs against the agents of bacterial mycetoma include streptomycin, dapsone, and trimethoprim–sulfamethoxazole (Welsh, 1991). Recently, a report revealed efficacy with a combination of trimethoprim-sulfamethoxazole, amikacin, and immunomodulators (L.G. Serrano-Jaén, personal communication, 1999). The treatment has to be administered for several months and the therapeutic response is variable. Early cases of mycetoma presenting with small lesions can be cured by surgical excision. In contrast, advanced cases with periosteal involvement and those with osteomyelitis do not respond to medical treatment and radical surgery of the foot represents the only therapeutic option.

DISEASES CAUSED BY RICKETTSIAE

Rickettsiae are Gram-negative bacterial obligate intracellular parasites transmitted by blood-sucking arthropods. The rickettsiae are released from the salivary glands of the tick or mite directly into the dermis or, in the case of flea or louse vectors, infected faeces are deposited on to the skin and rubbed into puncture wounds made by the organism. The rickettsiae may infect endothelial cells or macrophages, causing intravascular thrombosis and infarcts; increased capillary permeability results in extravascular fluid loss; and sometimes frank vasculitis occurs in the skin, brain and heart. In the typhus group they spread from cell to cell by lysis of the infected cell. In the spotted fever group the infecting organisms spread rapidly using actin-based motility.

Diagnosis can be made by indirect immunofluorescence or enzyme-linked immunosorbent assay (ELISA)-based detection of IgG and IgM antibodies against type specific rickettsial proteins. Treatment with antibiotics may rarely delay the rise in antibody titre. In addition, the organisms may be demonstrated in tissue samples by immunohistochemistry or direct immunofluorescence utilising monoclonal antibodies (Mab) against rickettsial proteins. The organisms may be cultured but are fastidious in their growth requirements. PCR performed on tissue, blood or urine may allow early diagnosis but currently lacks sensitivity.

Spotted Fever group

These include Rocky Mountain spotted fever, tick typhus and rickettsialpox.

Table 9.3 Tick-borne typhus diseases

	Organism	Vector	Reservoir	Distribution
African tick typhus (boutonneuse fever/Mediterranean spotted fever)	*Rickettsia conorii*	Ixodid tick	Rodents, dogs	Africa, Mediterranean
Siberian tick typhus	*R. sibirica*	Ixodid tick	Rodents	Russia, Central Asia
Queensland tick typhus	*R. australis*	Ixodid tick	Marsupials, rodents	Australia

Rocky Mountain Spotted Fever

Organism: *Rickettsia rickettsii*.
Vector: dog tick *Dermacentor varaiblis*; wood tick *D. andersoni*.
Reservoir: dogs.
Distribution: western hemipshere: Rocky mountains of North America, Maryland, Virginia, North Carolina, Mexico, Colombia, Brazil.

Clinical features. The incubation period is between 3 and 12 days after the tick-bite but a good 40% of patients are unaware of the tick bite episode. Young adult males are more commonly affected, with a seasonal peak in April to September in the USA. Prodromal symptoms of headache, malaise and high fever (39–40 °C) are followed 3–4 days later by a maculopapular rash on wrists and ankles. This spreads centrally to affect the trunk and face. Palms and soles are usually involved. The rash becomes haemorrhagic and may become confluent. Acral gangrene may occur but 13% of patients may have no rash and in 20% it develops later in the illness. General examination may reveal hepatosplenomegaly, shock, altered consciousness and renal failure. Recovery usually occurs over 3 weeks, with fatality rates of 1.5–6%. Mortality is higher in the elderly, those with coexisting disease and those with no known tick bite or rash.

Tick typhus

Clinical features. The clinical features of the tick-borne typhus diseases (Table 9.3) are very similar and usually milder than those of Rocky Mountain spotted fever. Fatal cases are rare. The initial lesion develops at the site of the tick bite with an erythematous papule, which vesiculates and develops an overlying eschar, also called 'tache noir' (Figure 9.6) and local lymphadenopathy. Fever and headache develop and after about 5 days a widespread exanthem evolves, which usually involves the palms and soles. This is an erythematous maculopapular eruption but may become haemorrhagic.

Rickettsialpox

Organism: *R. akari*.
Vector: mites.

Reservoir: house mice, rodents.
Distribution: USA, Russia, Africa.

Clinical features. Rickettsialpox is a mild self-limiting disease. The initial skin lesion, which develops at the site of the mite bite after 7–10 days, is a 1–1.5 cm painless erythematous papule. Central vesiculation subsequently develops and becomes covered with a black eschar. This lesion heals slowly to leave a scar. Regional lymph nodes may be enlarged. Fever develops 3–7 days after the initial lesions and a widespread exanthem evolves. The rash has a widespread distribution and is maculopapular and vesicular in nature. Palms and soles are usually spared. The eruption heals without scarring.

Typhus group

Epidemic Typhus

Organism: *R. prowazeki*
Vector: louse.
Reservoir: humans, flying squirrels.
Distribution: worldwide.
Epidemics are usually associated with displaced populations and refugees.

Clinical features. The incubation time is 7–14 days. Prodromal symptoms consist of headache, fever, and malaise and after 4–7 days a rash develops in the majority of patients. Crops of erythematous macules appear on the trunk and spread centrifugally but spare the palms and soles. Conjunctival haemorrhage may be a feature. The skin lesions progress to purpuric lesions and gangrene of extremities may occur.

Sporadic Typhus (Brill–Zinsser disease)

This is the recrudescence of epidemic typhus in individuals who have had an attack of the disease previously. It is usually milder and the skin features are not prominent.

Murine Typhus

Organism: *R. mooseri*.
Vector: rat flea.

Reservoir: rodents.
Distribution: worldwide but increased in Central and South America.

Clinical features. Similar to epidemic typhus, but milder with less-marked cutaneous features. Recovery occurs within 2 weeks.

Management of Rickettsial Infections

This includes general supportive treatment and specific antirickettsial therapy. The drugs of choice are doxycycline (100 mg b.d. p.o./i.v.) and tetracycline (25–50 mg kg^{-1} day^{-1} qds). Alternative treatments include chloramphenicol (50–75 mg kg^{-1} day^{-1}) and ciprofloxacin (1.5 g day^{-1}).

DISEASES CAUSED BY FUNGI

Dermatophyte Infections and Malasseziosis

Aetiology and Pathogenesis

Superficial fungal infections by dermatophytes are cosmopolitan and affect any anatomical site, including scalp and nails; however, one of the commonest presentations in the traveller affects one or both feet. These fungi are transmitted to humans by direct skin contact from their habitat in the soil, vegetation, or other individuals. Local conditions on the skin, such as a moist and hot environment while travelling, are predisposing factors. Dermatophyte infections are highly prevalent in tropical climates as this represents an ideal environment for these organisms: numerous case series and epidemiological studies from Latin America have been reported to the Spanish and Portuguese literature. The main genera involved in human infections are *Trychophyton*, *Epidermophyton*, and *Microsporum*, but infections of the foot including the toenails, are particularly caused by *T. rubrum*, *T. mentagrophytes*, and *E. floccosum*. Dermatophytes are keratinophylic organisms and exert their pathogenesis through attachment to the skin, nail, or hair surfaces.

Clinical Findings and Diagnosis

Individuals of both sexes and all age groups are affected by dermatophytes; however, children under the age of 10 rarely present with tinea pedis. The main clinical pictures are those of localised tinea pedis, interdigital, plantar hyperkeratotic, and onychomycosis. Common names for these conditions include ringworm and athlete's foot. Dermatophyte infections can manifest as localised single or multiple circinate plaques with erythema and variable degrees of scaling on the body in cases of tinea corporis (Figure 9.17). Athlete's foot involves the dorsum or per-

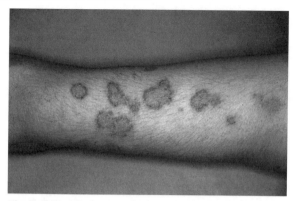

Figure 9.17 Tinea corporis from Southeast Asia. Discrete erythematous plaques with a circinate polycyclic border and pruritus

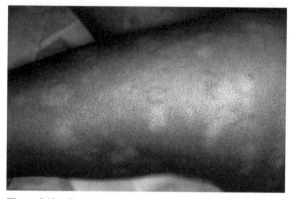

Figure 9.18 Tinea corporis in a traveller with atopic eczema. Erythematous polycyclic plaques from fungal infection and hypopigmented patches on eczematous skin

imalleolar regions. Toe-web involvement is commonly bilateral, presenting with erythema, a burning sensation, pruritus and scaling, particularly of the fourth interdigital toe web space. Severe acute forms present with painful erythema and blistering in a similar pattern to that found in cases of acute eczema or pompholix. Patients with a history of atopy are predisposed to superficial infections by dermatophytes, and in these cases erythematous inflammatory fungal lesions coexist with patches of eczematous skin (Figure 9.18). Chronic plantar lesions develop asymptomatic large hyperkeratotic plaques and a particular form of toenail infection by *T.rubrum* manifests clinically as a subungual white onychomycosis. Varying degrees of temporary disability may result from severe infections. Children manifest scalp infections under the kerion clinical form with patches of nonscarring alopecia and boggy inflammation of the skin (Figure 9.19). Less commonly, adult travellers manifest granulomatous inflammation with varying degrees of scarring in infections caused by other species of *Trychophyton* (Figure 9.20).

Discrete plaques of granuloma annulare have to be considered in the differential diagnosis of localised ringworm, whereas thickenned plaques of plantar psoriasis

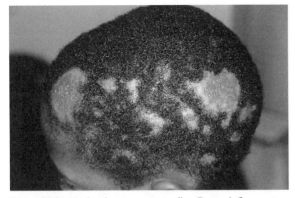

Figure 9.19 Kerion in a young traveller. Boggy inflammatory plaques on nonscarring alopecic patches of the scalp

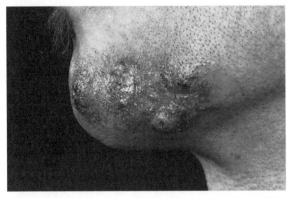

Figure 9.20 *Trychophyton mentagrophytes* granuloma of the chin from South America. Erythema and nodular lesions with areas of scarring

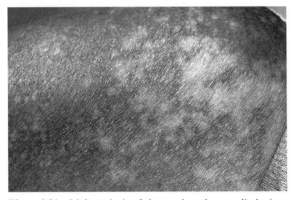

Figure 9.21 Malasseziosis of the trunk and upper limbs in a returning traveller. Small and coalescing hypopigmented asymptomatic patches

may pose diagnostic difficulties with chronic hyperkeratotic infections by dermatophytes. Other superficial skin and nail infections of the foot, such as those caused by *Candida* and *Scytalidium* species, may also present a diagnostic difficulty. The returning traveller from the tropics is often referred to our specialised clinic with

severe or recurrent superficial yeast infections by *Malassezia furfur* (Figure 9.21).

The diagnosis of dermatophyte infection on the skin is made on clinical grounds. Additional diagnostic measures include direct microscopy of skin scrapings in 10–12% KOH solution, and the identification of the causative organism by culture in Sabouraud medium. A similar strategy is recommended for the laboratory diagnosis of pityriasis versicolor (malasseziosis), which requires special oily additives for successful isolation in culture.

Management and Treatment

The therapy of choice includes the use of topical and/or systemic azole or alylamine antifungal compounds. Localised infections require topical therapy for 3–4 weeks but cases with interdigital athlethe's foot may require up to 6–8 weeks. Topical steroids are often required to control the inflammatory picture, but are administered only when effective antifungal treatment is already in place. Systemic therapy with antifungals is indicated in severe skin infections and onychomycosis of the toenails. *M. furfur* infection responds to selenium sulphide preparations, ketoconazole shampoo, and other imidazolic or alylamine topical compounds applied for 6 weeks. Cases also respond to systemic triazoles. Other therapeutic measures address the control of symptoms, secondary eczematisation, and superimposed bacterial infection. Measures of general hygiene and appropriate shoewear are useful to prevent reinfection, which is a common problem in the traveller.

Sporotrichosis

Aetiology and Pathogenesis

This infection is acquired by direct inoculation into the skin or subcutaneous tissue of mycelia or conidia from *Sporothrix schenckii*. Inhalation of infective organisms can also produce clinical disease; accidental exposure takes place outdoors as a result of an accidental or professional contact involving splinters, thorns, straw, wood shavings, or other sharp objects. This dimorphic fungus is ubiquitous in nature and lives in the soil, bark of trees, shrubs, and plant detritus. This is a disease of temperate humid and tropical areas and represents a risk for travellers. *S. schenckii* has a low pathogenic potential and causes disease by virulence factors that include extracellular enzymes and polysaccharides, as well as showing thermotolerance. The infective structures display a strong acid phosphatase activity and mannan compounds are capable of inhibiting phagocytosis by macrophages.

Clinical Findings and Diagnosis

Sporotrichosis may manifest as a systemic illness in pulmonary forms but in most cases the disease is limited to

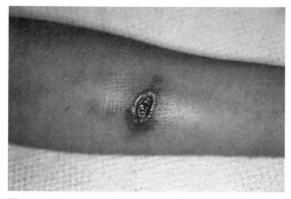

Figure 9.22 Sporotrichosis from Brazil. Forearm with erythematous nodular ulcer and lymphangitic track proximally. (Courtesy of Professor A.Bryceson)

the skin and subcutaneous and lymphatic tissues. The upper and lower limbs are the usual sites of inoculation. Following the traumatic episode the disease manifests with a localised skin nodule involving only the affected limb. This inoculation chancre develops a suppurative and granulomatous infection that remains fixed, or else disseminates proximally via the lymphatic system (Figure 9.22). Superimposed bacterial infection may occur and verrucous lesions show a tendency to ulceration. The gold standard of laboratory diagnosis is the identification of the fungus in culture, but direct microscopy and histopathological investigations also have a diagnostic value. Outbreaks in parties of travellers require full epidemiological investigation.

Management and Treatment

Potassium iodide in increasing daily doses is the treatment of choice in the tropics but systemic itraconazole and amphotericin B have also resulted in cure in a hospital context. As the disease is acquired by direct inoculation into the skin, preventive measures are of the outmost importance. Protective footwear, clothing, and avoidance of skin contact with splinters, rough bark, plant detritus, and soil are the most efficient methods of preventing the disease.

Eumycetoma

Aetiology and Pathogenesis

Madurella mycetomatis, *Pseudoallescheria boydii*, and *Leptosphaeria senegalensis* are the main aetiological agents of true fungal mycetoma, also known as eumycetoma. A generic term 'Madura foot' is currently used to describe all forms of bacterial and fungal mycetoma (see Bacterial Mycetoma above). Eumycetoma occurs in Sudan, Senegal, and Saudi Arabia, particularly in arid or semiarid regions (Abbott, 1956). Cases also occur in India and Central and South America. Infective organisms pen-

etrate the skin of the foot or other exposed regions by direct traumatic inoculation, and in the host's tissue the agents multiply and infect adjacent structures. Changes in the fungal cell wall and melanin production are the main virulent factors involved in local pathogenesis.

Clinical Findings and Diagnosis

Eumycetoma affects predominantly young male individuals between 20 and 50 years of age. It has been estimated that more than 70% of cases with eumycetoma manifest on one foot. Other anatomical regions identified as port of entry for the accidental, professional, or traumatic inoculation include the trunk, face, and scalp. The perimalleolar region and the foot dorsum are the most commonly affected sites but any region of the foot can suffer the direct inoculation of infective organisms. The characteristic clinical signs include a nodule or irregular swelling followed by sinus tract formation and discharge of purulent material containing the characteristic grains. Pigmentary changes of the skin and scarring result from the persistent and chronic inflammatory process over months or years. Periosteal involvement is the starting point of bone resorption, osteolysis, and irreversible osteomyelitis.

The epidemiological context and characteristic clinical picture are diagnostic. This is confirmed by direct microscopy of pale or black grains that measure 0.5–1 mm and contain fungal structures measuring 2–4 μm. This material grows in agar containing glucose and peptone, and the histological sections of deep skin specimens reveal the characteristic, and in many cases pathognomonic, grains of particular fungal species. Radiological investigation of the affected region discloses periosteal involvement, cortical resorption, and osteolysis.

Management and Treatment

Early nodular lesions or small papular forms, called micromycetoma, can be treated by complete surgical excision; however, delay in diagnosis results in advanced cases that respond poorly to medical treatment. Systemic antibiotics in combination, such as streptomycin, cotrimoxazole, amikacin, dapsone, and rifampicin, are the drugs of choice and require long-term administration. Nearly two-thirds of cases caused by *M. mycetomatis* respond to ketoconazole (Mahgoub and Gumaa, 1984). Severe cases with bone involvement can only be cured by radical surgery.

Chromoblastomycosis

Aetiology and Pathogenesis

This is a chronic infection caused by fungi of *Fonsecaea*, *Cladosporium*, and *Phialophora* species. The disease is widely distributed in the tropics and affects predominant-ly agricultural workers who acquire the infection through direct inoculation into the skin. Numerous cases have been reported, mainly from Costa Rica, Cuba, Brazil, Mexico, Indonesia, and Madagascar.

Clinical Findings and Diagnosis

The initial lesion starts as a papular or nodular inflamma-tory reaction that subsequently develops a warty appear-ance. In time this lesion enlarges at a slow rate and becomes characteristically a large verrucous asympto-matic plaque. The commonest site affected in sporadic infections is the foot, and the chronic verrucous plaque appears on the dorsum or the perimalleolar region. The plaque may become very thick over several years and cause gross deformity of the affected foot. Varying de-grees of disability and recurrent secondary infections and/ or infestations are a common problem for the foot with chromoblastomycosis.

The diagnosis is made on clinical grounds and con-firmed by direct microscopy and mycological culture in glucose–peptone agar. The histopathology of skin speci-mens is characteristic, showing acanthosis with a granuloma formation and the presence of typical fungal structures known as 'fumagoid' cells.

Management and Treatment

Flucytosine and tiabendazole have been used in combi-nation without consistent efficacy. Triazole compounds, such as itraconazole, have resulted in cure but in general it is accepted that chromoblastomycosis is not easy to treat medically, and patients require long-term treatment. Localized and early cases respond successfully to com-plete surgical excision of the lesion, and thermosurgery has also been reported to be of benefit. All patients af-fected by chromoblastomycosis require attention and fol-low-up by specialists in mycology, infectious diseases, and/or dermatology.

Systemic Mycosis Manifesting on the Skin

Infections by *Coccidioides immitis*, *Histoplasma cap-sulatum*, and *Paracoccidioides brasiliensis* commonly manifest with disease of the lungs but haematogenous dissemination results in the appearance of skin lesions.

Coccidioidomycosis is acquired through inhalation of infective spores in tropical but also subtropical desert regions of the world, particularly in the American conti-nent. Southern and western States in USA and north-western regions of Mexico are well-recognised endemic regions, and the disease is acquired most commonly in urban areas. Travellers acquire the infection in urban areas where a high proportion of the resident population manifest a positive intradermal reaction on skin testing

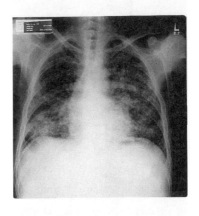

Figure 9.23   Paracoccidioidomycosis from Venezuela. Chest X-rays with bilateral nodular infiltrate of the lungs

using coccidioidin. This systemic mycosis presents a risk particularly for the immunocompromised traveller. The skin becomes involved in a small proportion of cases and lesions manifest as erythematous, verrucous, or scaling nodules on the face, upper limbs, or on the plantar surface or any other part of the foot. A history of exposure in endemic regions followed by an episode of erythema nodosum supports the diagnostic possibility. Other in-vestigations such as serology, chest X-rays, and culture for the isolation of the organism confirm the diagnosis. Culture of agents causing systemic mycoses should only be carried out in specialized laboratories, as they repre-sent a serious biological hazard. Systemic therapeutic options for coccidioidomycosis include amphotericin B and triazole compounds.

Paracoccidioidomycosis occurs in Mexico, Central, and South America, predominantly affecting male individuals who live and acquire the infection in rural areas. Actual evidence of the mode of transmission is incomplete but the respiratory route seems to be common in acquisition of the infection. Following a chronic picture of lung in-volvement (Figure 9.23), weight loss, and fatigue, the skin of one or both feet can be affected. Painful nodular, haemorrhagic, ulcerated, and verrucous lesions can be observed, covered by a thick crust (Figure 9.24), and severe disability results in advanced forms of the disease. The diagnosis is based on the history of exposure in an endemic region and the clinical picture, supported by investigations to reveal the presence of the typical large, budding yeast cells. These can be observed by direct microscopy and in H&E preparations for histology and are easily identified in culture. Effective systemic treat-ment has been reported with triazole compounds and amphotericin B.

Patients with foot involvement from systemic fungal

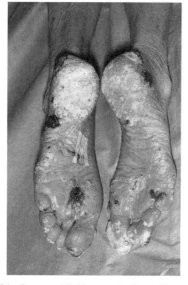

Figure 9.24 Paracoccidioidomycosis from Venezuela. Disseminated verrucous, hyperkeratotic and haemorrhagic ulcerated lesions on lower limbs

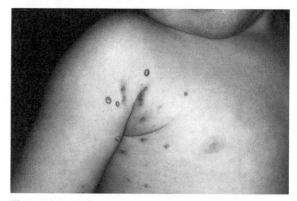

Figure 9.25 Molluscum contagiosum in a child. Umbilicated and erythematous/whitish millimetric papules on the trunk and upper limb

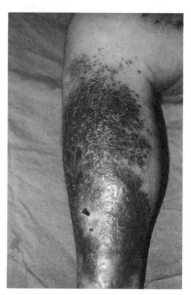

Figure 9.26 Kaposi sarcoma of the leg. Lymphangiomatous form in a traveller with AIDS

disease require immediate referral to an experienced hospital physician or specialists in mycology, infectious diseases, or dermatology.

DISEASES CAUSED BY VIRUSES

Most common viral skin diseases are cosmopolitan but the onset may coincide with a trip to the tropics and pose problems in the differential diagnosis of the returning traveller. Viral infections that are prevalent in the tropics include *molluscum contagiosum* in children (Figure 9.25), *plantar warts* in adults, *Kaposi sarcoma* in patients with AIDS (Figure 9.26), and severe blistering forms of *varicella*. Severe cases require a full diagnostic protocol with specimens for culture, electron microscopy, serology, and histopathology, followed by specialised treatment in tertiary referral centres.

SUN-RELATED SKIN DISEASES AND CANCER

Many dermatoses may be provoked by exposure to ultraviolet (UV) radiation and they may be acute or chronic. In addition, a number of other dermatoses may be exacerbated by exposure to sunlight; these include acne, atopic eczema, dermatomyositis, erythema multiforme, herpes simplex, Darier disease, lichen planus, autoimmune blistering disorders, psoriasis, rosacea, and seborrhoeic dermatitis. Some of the more common problems included in this section are presented in Table 9.4.

It is important to take a specific history of sun exposure and the following points are helpful in delineating some of the photodermatoses:

1. *Length of time taken in sun to provoke reaction?*
   Solar urticaria lesions appear within minutes.
2. *Can the reaction be provoked through glass, i.e. UVA exposure?*
   Solar urticaria may be provoked by UVA.
3. *Is there a past history of photosensitivity?*
   Polymorphic light reaction is often recurrent.
4. *Is there a family history of photosensitivity?*
   Porphyrias may affect several family members.
5. *Does the eruption itch or burn?*
   Phototoxic reactions tend to produce burning sensa-

Table 9.4 Disorders caused by exposure to ultraviolet irradiation

Chronic photosensitivity	Acute photosensitivity
Photoageing	Sunburn
Skin cancer	Phototoxicity
	Drug-induced
	Plant-induced
	Photoallergy
	Drug-induced
	Solar urticaria
	Idiopathic
	Polymorphic light eruption
	Systemic lupus erythematosus

tions.

6. *What medications are you taking?*
   Many drugs may cause photosensitive reactions.
7. *What creams, perfumes, etc. do you apply to your skin?*
   Photoallergic contact dermatitis may occur.
8. *Do you have any other symptoms?*
   Systemic lupus erythematosus (SLE) may be associated with systemic symptoms.

Some patients may not specifically relate their skin problem to light exposure and thus distribution of skin lesions may provide a clue to the aetiology, i.e. face, V of neck, hands and forearms with sparing of eyelids, submental areas and areas under clothing, watch straps, or those partially covered by footwear.

Sunburn

This is an acute delayed transient response to UV radiation and the clinical features are easily identified by travellers. These include erythema and tenderness, but severe cases manifest with blistering, oedema and pain. Systemic symptoms of headache and malaise are common. Prevention with adequate sunscreens is most important. The acute treatment consists of topical corticosteroids, cool wet dressings, systemic aspirin, and bed rest away from direct, reflected, or refracted sunlight.

Polymorphic Light Eruption

This acquired idiopathic condition is the commonest of the photodermatoses. The average age of onset is the second decade and women are more commonly affected. All races and skin types may be affected, although Caucasians are affected more frequently. The condition often occurs in people from northern latitudes travelling to the tropics in winter. It occurs in spring/early summer and may improve by the end of the summer. The eruption occurs 18–24 hours after UV exposure of several hours and lasts 7–10 days. The condition may be provoked by UVA and therefore can be precipitated by exposure

through window glass.

Clinical Findings and Diagnosis

Pruritus occurs and then erythematous papules and papulovesicles develop, less commonly urticated plaques. The rash affects arms, trunk and anterior chest but areas habitually exposed, such as the face and hands, are often spared. The disease tends to follow a recurrent and chronic course and the clinical features tend to follow the same pattern in recurrences within a single patient. The diagnosis is usually made on history and clinical features, although phototesting may be helpful in some cases. SLE is an important differential diagnosis and serology for autoimmune screening must be checked. Histopathological investigation of lesional skin is necessary in complex clinical cases, particularly if the clinical picture manifests with urticated plaques.

Management and Treatment

Prevention is important, with the use of adequate high factor sunblock creams. Systemic treatment with β-carotene and antimalarials (hydroxychloroquine 200 mg b.d.) is recommended 1 week prior to and during travel. Psoralen–UVA (PUVA) phototherapy may help by inducing tolerance if given in a course (i.e. three times a week for 4 weeks) before exposure.

Solar Urticaria

This is a rare disorder in which UVA, UVB and visible light may produce itchy wheals after a few minutes exposure. Tingling sensation and erythema precede the development of whitish wheals which fade within a few hours. It is more common in female individuals, who become affected between 10 and 50 years of age. It may rarely be associated with lupus erythematosus and the treatment includes avoidance of exposure, use of adequate sunscreens, and antihistamines.

Cutaneous Lupus Erythematosus

All forms of cutaneous lupus may manifest photosensitivity. Cases with *acute SLE* may present with the characteristic butterfly facial rash in addition to constitutional symptoms, whereas *subacute cutaneous lupus* occurs in about 10% of patients with lupus erythematosus. Common skin presentations include an annular scaly erythematous, psoriasiform rash involving light-exposed areas, which may present abruptly, extensor surfaces of arms, dorsa of hands, V of chest and upper back and face. Patients may also manifest a diffuse nonscarring alopecia. The treatment of choice is topical steroids in mild cases but systemic therapy with antimalarials, corticosteroids,

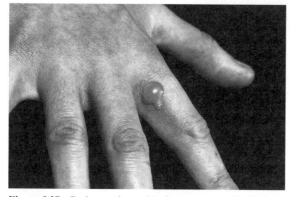

Figure 9.27 Berloque dermatitis from a gardening holiday. Phytophotodermatitis with erythema and severe blistering

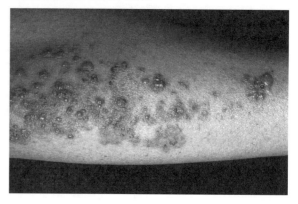

Figure 9.28 Erythema multiforme and photosensitivity during a beach holiday. Erytematous, urticated and blistering lesions with a photorreactive pattern on the forearms

and immunosupressants is usually required. Chronic forms of *discoid LE* present with weeks-to-months history of erythematous papules and plaques with follicular plugging and atrophy, with subsequent scar formation. The rash tends to occur on habitually exposed areas of the face, scalp, external ears, and hands. Scalp involvement results in scarring alopecia and approximately 5% of these patients develop systemic disease. DLE can be controlled with supervised use of potent topical steroids and adequate sunscreens. When systemic therapy is required, antimalarials are effective.

Porphyria Cutanea Tarda

Porphyria cutanea tarda is the most common of the porphyrias, with significant cutaneous involvement. This form may be hereditary but far more frequently is due to an exogenous agent, such as alcohol, oestrogens, iron, antimalarials (high doses), hexachlorobenzene, and chlorinated phenols. Other predisposing factors include diabetes mellitus and hepatitis C. While patients do have photosensitivity, there is some delay between sun exposure and the development of the lesions and they actually complain of skin fragility and, conversely, may appear sun-tanned.

Other main clinical features include bullae and erosions on a background of normal skin with atrophic scars from healed previous lesions. Small milia may also be present. Patients may develop hypertrichosis and sclerodermatous changes on the face. The diagnosis is made by history, clinical features and elevated urinary porphyrins and the treatment includes the discontinuation of exacerbating factors, phlebotomy or low-dose chloroquine, 125 mg twice a week.

Phytophotodermatitis (Berloque)

Phytophotodermatitis is inflammation of the skin caused by contact with certain plants during or subsequent to exposure to UV light. The inflammation is a consequence of photosensitising chemicals present in several plant families, e.g. lime, lemon, wild parsley, celery, giant hogweed, parsnip, carrot and fig, plus plant oils such as bergamot used in perfumes or aromatherapy. Gardening holidays represent a risk for travellers (Figure 9.27). Complex clinical presentations of erythema multiforme reveal a photosensitive pattern on exposed areas of the skin (Figure 9.28). Phytophotodermatitis manifests as an acute eruption of erythema, vesicles and bullae. These are often in a bizarre distribution, indicating an exogenous cause for the rash. Taking a careful history makes the diagnosis and the acute picture responds to treatment with local antiseptics and wet dressing for the vesicular lesions plus topical steroids. The eruption will fade spontaneously over a few days.

Skin Cancer and Photoageing

Chronic effects of sun exposure include skin wrinkles, pigmentation, premalignant skin lesions (actinic keratoses), basal cell carcinoma, squamous cell carcinoma and malignant melanoma. Several aetiological studies support the role of UV radiation in the development of skin cancers.

Actinic Keratoses

Actinic keratoses (solar keratoses) are sun-induced premalignant lesions, common in Caucasian patients who have had significant sun exposure over several years. Clinically they present as erythematous scaly lesions which gradually enlarge. They may occasionally develop extensive scale and form cutaneous horns. They are most frequently seen on exposed areas of the scalp (Figure 9.29), face, and hands. The diagnosis is made clinically and is confirmed by biopsy, which demonstrates dysplastic cells within the epidermis and solar damage. Thera-

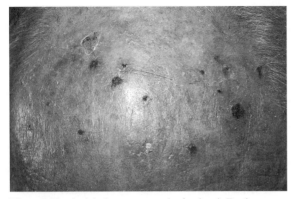

Figure 9.29 Actinic keratoses on the forehead. Erythematous lesions with superficial ulceration in a patient with severe sun damage

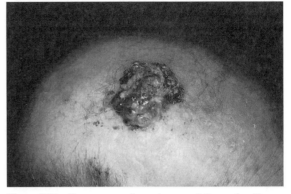

Figure 9.31 Squamous cell carcinoma of the scalp. Hyperkeratotic and verrucous ulcer with tissue destruction and fast growth

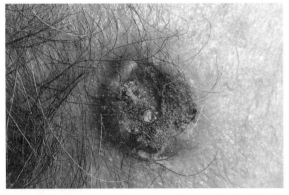

Figure 9.30 Basal cell carcinoma on the temple. Nodular-ulcerative form in a patient with white skin and history of intense sun exposure in the tropics

peutic options include cryotherapy, excision, or topical cytotoxic cream with 5-fluorouracil.

Basal Cell Carcinoma

This is the most common cutaneous malignancy in Caucasians, being four times as common as squamous cell carcinoma. They present most commonly on the head and neck, are locally invasive and rarely metastasise (Figure 9.30). The most common clinical forms include nodular, cystic, superficial spreading, and morpheic. The lesions can be pigmented and manifest slow growth, affecting predominantly exposed areas of the skin. The diagnosis is made clinically and confirmed by biopsy; the treatment of choice is surgical excision but this depends upon anatomical location. Other therapeutic approaches include radiotherapy and cryotherapy. Micrographic surgery is indicated in centrofacial lesions.

Squamous Cell Carcinoma

Squamous cell carcinoma also occurs more commonly in

fair-skinned individuals with excessive sun exposure. Other aetiological agents may be relevant, such as arsenic ingestion, human papilloma virus infection, polycyclic aromatic hydrocarbons, industrial carcinogens (tar, pitch, crude paraffin oil), previous radiotherapy and chronic ulceration. Lesions arising in sun-exposed sites have a low risk of metastasis but this is increased in tumours arising on the lower lip, in scars or ulcers, anogenital mucosa or in immunocompromised patients. These carcinomas usually present as slowly evolving plaques or nodules, which may become eroded or ulcerate, usually on the head (Figure 9.31) and neck. They can also occur in the genital area and oral mucosa. Surgical excision is the treatment of choice but adjuvant radiotherapy or node dissection are required in metastatic lesions.

Malignant Melanoma

The incidence of melanoma is increasing and represents a common malignancy among young people. The cause of melanoma is multifactorial and includes UV light exposure and genetic factors such as mutations in, or loss of, tumour suppressor genes. The risk is increased in individuals with fair skin, numerous atypical moles or a family history of melanoma. These tumours classically present as a new or changing pigmented lesion. The ABCD features of pigmented lesions can be helpful in the clinical assessment of suspicious-looking moles:

A Asymmetry—asymmetry of shape is a suspicious feature.
B Border—the border of a mole should be clearly defined and smooth.
Bleeding—any mole which bleeds should be assessed.
C Colour—moles should show even pigmentation of a single colour hue.
D Diameter—most melanomas are > 6 mm in diameter, although smaller irregular lesions may still be malignant.

Malignant melanoma most commonly presents on the

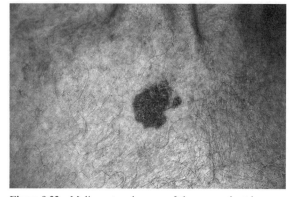

Figure 9.32 Malignant melanoma of the upper chest in a patient with a history of sun exposure in the tropics

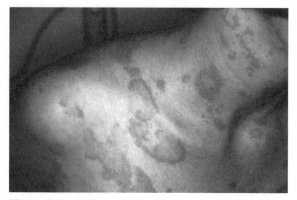

Figure 9.33 Acute urticaria from drugs, showing large erythematous wheals lasting for a few hours in a recurring pattern

trunk in males (Figure 9.32) and lower leg in females. The main clinical variants are:

- *Superficial spreading*: most common form; irregularly pigmented macule.
- *Nodular*: less common, presents as pigmented nodule and may ulcerate.
- *Acral lentiginous*: most common form in black-skinned and Asian individuals; presents as pigmented macule on palms or soles or nail bed.
- *Lentigo maligna melanoma*: presents as irregular pigmented macule or chronically photodamaged skin, often on the face of elderly patients.
- *Amelanotic melanoma*: nonpigmented friable nodule; clinically may be confused with other benign skin lesions such as pyogenic granuloma.

The treatment of melanoma must be managed by experienced physicians and includes excision with adequate margins, evaluation for metastases, chemotherapy and immunotherapy, as appropriate.

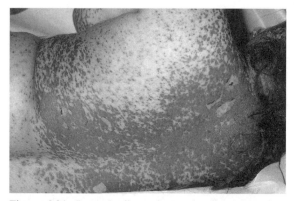

Figure 9.34 Brocq–Lyell syndrome in a patient from Bangladesh. Severe toxic epidermal necrolysis from carbamazepine

DRUG-RELATED SKIN DISEASES

Drug reactions occur worldwide but may coincide with a trip to the tropics, and in some cases result from sun exposure. A variety of medicines induce moderate-to-severe reactions and the patient's history often identifies the use of antibiotics, carbamazepine, sulphonamides, diuretics, or β-blockers. More than three-quarters of all patients with drug reactions present with erythema (rash) and/or urticaria (Figure 9.33). Other severe forms of drug reaction include erythema multiforme and toxicodermias. Specialised management in hospital is required for all severe cases, as mortality can be high for toxic epidermal necrolysis (Brocq–Lyell syndrome) (Figure 9.34) and Stevens–Johnson syndrome. The finding of vasculitis presenting with purpura (Figure 9.35) or severe exfoliation with hyperpigmented lesions and epidermal detachment indicate systemic illness due to a drug reaction.

A number of skin eruptions may suggest the aetiologi-

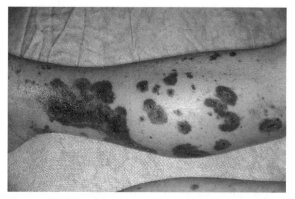

Figure 9.35 Vasculitis of lower limbs with leucocytoclasia in a traveller

cal factor involved; for instance, the *oral contraceptive pill* combines an oestrogen with a progestogen and can have a number of cutaneous complications, listed below.

Chloasma

Common; 90% of patients are female. Pregnancy and the oral contraceptive pill are important aetiological factors. There is facial hyperpigmentation, exacerbated by sun exposure. On examination, there is macular symmetrical hyperpigmentation on cheeks, forehead, nose, upper lip, and chin; less frequently on the dorsae of arms. Pathogenesis is unknown and treatment includes preventive measures by use of sunscreens, cessation of contraceptive pill use, and topical depigmenting compounds.

Alopecia

Androgenic or telogen effluvium related to stopping the oral contraceptive pill.

Erythema Nodosum

This is a rare but well-recognised complication.

Provocation of Porphyria Cutanea Tarda (see above)

Photosensitivity

Antimalarials such as chloroquine and hydroxychlorquine may be associated with:

- *Pigmentary changes.* Occur in 25% of patients receiving antimalarials for more than 4 months: blackish-purple patches on shins and brown-grey hyperpigmentation on sun-exposed sites. Nails may also be affected.
- *Photosensitivity.* Phototoxic drug reactions may occur and chloroquine may precipitate porphyria.
- *Psoriasis.* The deterioration of psoriasis in association with antimalarial treatment is well recognised but probably uncommon in those treated with standard doses.
- *Lichenoid reactions.* These are well documented but uncommon, i.e. itchy violaceous flat-topped papules with or without oral lesions.

Mepacrine

There is yellow staining of the skin and conjunctivae. Lichenoid eruptions occur. Pigmentation similar to that associated with chloroquine may occur after prolonged administration.

Quinine

Purpura may occur, in association with thrombocytopenia. Bullous and fixed drug eruptions have been recorded. Lichenoid eruptions are rare.

Drug-induced Photosensitivity

Phototoxic

This is an exaggerated sunburn response. It may occur in all individuals, regardless of skin type and age. Many drugs may be responsible: thiazides, tetracyclines, oral hypoglycaemics, chlorpromazine, nonsteroidal anti-inflammatory drugs, oral contraceptive pills, amiodarone, and phenothiazines. The patients present with symptoms of sunburn in sun-exposed sites only, and the reactions clear on cessation of the causative drug.

Photoallergic

These reactions are less common and can also affect all skin types but occur in sensitised individuals only. The main clinical feature is an eczematous reaction with erythema, scaling and lichenification, primarily on sun-exposed sites but may extend locally to nonexposed skin. Topically applied photosensitisers are the most common cause, e.g. benzocaine, musk in aftershave, 6-methyl-coumarin in sunscreens. Systemic drugs may also cause a photoallergic reaction, e.g. phenothiazines, halogenated salicylamides, and sulphonamides.

MISCELLANEOUS CONDITIONS

Ainhum

This uncommon condition affecting the fifth toe of adults in tropical Africa is also called spontaneous dactylolysis. A painful constricting band of fibrotic tissue results in spontaneous amputation of the toe. A number of contributing factors have been identified, including familial occurrence, decreased blood supply locally, mechanical trauma from walking on bare feet, and chronic diseases with neuropathy, such as leprosy and diabetes mellitus. General hygiene measures, avoidance of infection, and surgical amputation, if required in advanced cases, are the therapeutic interventions of choice (Browne, 1976).

Pellagra

Pellagra is caused by a nutritional deficiency of niacin and classically manifests with the triad dermatitis, diarrhoea, and dementia (3Ds). Clinically, it manifests with a remarkable photosensitive rash that may show an eczematoid pattern with hyperpigmentation. Most lesions affect the face and neck, and both lower limbs present with signs similar to those found in stasis dermatitis. Eczematoid changes, xerosis, and hyperpigmented patches are present symmetrically on both feet (Stratigos and Katsambas, 1977). Oral treatment with niacin amide is indicated and podiatry care includes general hygiene, moisturizing, and avoidance of infections or mechanical trauma.

Finally, a number of chronic skin conditions, eczematous in nature, result in bilateral and remarkably symmetrical hyperpigmented skin patches. A symmetrical rash suggests contact dermatitis, but complex cases involve a vascular deficit secondary to venous hypertension. Psoriasis may also present with a chronic recurrent eczematous picture affecting the heel and medial plantar aspects on both feet.

Seaborne, Waterborne Conditions

Holiday-makers in tropical seawaters present to local doctors following contact with or traumatic skin injury from jelly fish, coral reefs, anemones, sea-urchins, and venomous fish. A variety of acute clinical pictures manifest as contact eczema, stings, burns, as well as penetrating injuries, whereas vasoactive phenomena represent the common pathogenic mechanism in direct skin poisoning. The returning traveller commonly has postinflammatory lesions characterised by hyperpigmentation and scarring. Chronic eczematous reactions and secondary bacterial infections require specific treatment.

Cercarial Dermatitis

This name describes a group of skin disorders with a common cause, namely penetration of the skin by free-living cercarial stages of schistosomes. These conditions have a number of local names, e.g. swimmer's itch or clam digger's itch. The clinical features are very similar for the different classes of cercaria, with differing intermediate and definitive hosts: freshwater avian cercarial dermatitis, seawater avian cercarial dermatitis and freshwater mammalian cercarial dermatitis.

The initial clinical feature is that of tingling on contact with the water, followed up to an hour later with a fine diffuse macular erythema of exposed areas. After 10–15 h a more florid itchy papular eruption develops, which may evolve into vesicles. More severe reactions occur in previously sensitised individuals. The reaction settles spontaneously after about a week, with no long-term sequelae. Symptomatic treatment can be achieved by antihistamines.

Sea-bather's Eruption

This eruption is due to exposure to the larvae of the sea anemone *Edwardsiella lineata*. It presents with monomorphic erythematous inflammatory papules or vesicles hours or days after exposure at sites covered by the patient's swimming costume. Some patients may recall feeling a stinging sensation while in the seawater. The rash may persist for up to 2 weeks. Topical steroids provide symptomatic relief.

REFERENCES

Abbott PH (1956) Mycetoma in the Sudan. *Transactions of the Royal Society of Tropical Medicine and Hygiene*, **50**, 11–24.

Belsey MA and LeBlanc DR (1975) Skin infections and the epidemiology of diphtheria: acquisition and persistence of *C. diphtheria* infections. *American Journal of Epidemiology*, **102**, 179–184.

Bisno AL and Stevens DL (1996). Streptococcal infections of skin and soft tissues. *New England Journal of Medicine*, **334**, 240.

Blackwell V and Vega-López F (2000) Two years of cutaneous larva migrans in London. *British Journal of Dermatology*, **143** (Suppl. 57), 53–54.

Browne SG (1976) Ainhum. *International Journal of Dermatology*, **15**, 348–350.

Bryceson A and Pfaltzgraff RE (1990) Symptoms and signs. In *Leprosy*, 3rd edn, pp 25–55. Churchill Livingstone, Edinburgh.

Caumes E, Datry A and Paris L (1992) Efficacy of ivermectin in the therapy of cutaneous larva migrans. *Archives of Dermatology*, **128**, 995–996.

Chopra S and Vega-López F (1999) Skin granulomas in clinical practice. In *The Granulomatous Disorders* (eds G. James and A. Zumla), pp 507–510, 513–517. Cambridge University Press, Cambridge.

Cribier B, Piemont Y and Grosshans E (1994) Staphylococcal scalded skin syndrome in adults. *Journal of the American Academy of Dermatology*, **30**, 319–324.

Douglas-Jones AG, Llewelyn MB and Mills CM (1995) Cutaneous infection with *Tunga penetrans*. *British Journal of Dermatology*, **133**, 125–127.

Elliot DC, Kufera JA and Myers RA (1996) Necrotizing soft tissue infections. Risk factors for mortality and strategies for management. *Annals of Surgery*, **224**, 672–683.

Gray SF, Smith RS and Reynolds NJ (1990) Fish tank granuloma. *BMJ*, **300**, 1069–1070.

Ibanez-Bernal S and Velasco-Castrejón O (1996) New records of human tungiasis in Mexico (Siphonaptera: Tungidae). *Journal of Medical Entomology*, **33**, 988–999.

Josse R, Guedenon A, Aguiar J *et al.* (1994) Buruli's ulcer, a pathology little known in Benin. Apropos of 227 cases. *Bulletin de la Société de Pathologie Exotique*, **87**, 170–175.

López-Martínez R, Méndez-Tovar LJ, Lavalle P *et al.* (1992) Epidemiología del micetoma en México: estudio de 2105 casos. *Gaceta Médica de México*, **128**, 477–481.

Lui H and Buck W (1992) Cutaneous myasis: a simple and effective technique for extraction of *Dermatobia hominis* larvae. *International Journal of Dermatology*, **31**, 657–659.

Mahgoub ES and Gumaa SA (1984) Ketoconazole in the treatment of eumycetoma due to *Madurella mycetomi*. *Transactions of the Royal Society of Tropical Medicine and Hygiene*, **78**, 376–379.

Meñdoza-León, Shaw JJ and Tapia F (1996) In *Molecular and Immune Mechanisms in the Pathogenesis of Cutaneous Leishmaniasis* (eds F Tapia, G Cáceres and M Sánchez), pp 1–21, 25–47. Springer, Heidelberg.

Sehgal VN, Jain S, Bhattacharya SN *et al.* (1994) Yaws control and eradication. International Journal of Dermatology, **33**, 16–20.

Serrano-Jaén L and Vega-López F (2000) Fulminating septicaemia caused by *Vibrio vulnificus*. *British Journal of Dermatology*, **142**, 386–387.

Stratigos JD and Katsambas A (1977) Pellagra: a still existing disease. *British Journal of Dermatology*, **96**, 99–106.

Taniguchi Y, Ando K and Isoda K (1992) Human gnathostomiasis: successful removal of *Gnathostoma hispidum*. *International Journal of Dermatology*, **31**, 175–177.

Thangaraj HS, Evans MRW and Wansbrough-Jones MH (1999) *Mycobacterium ulcerans* disease; Buruli ulcer. *Transactions of the Royal Society of Tropical Medicine and Hygiene*, **93**, 337–340.

Welsh O (1991) Mycetoma. Current concepts in treatment. *International Journal of Dermatology*, **30**, 387–398.

WHO (1986) Expert committee on venereal diseases and treponematoses: sixth report. *World Health Organization Technical Report Series*, **736**.

WHO (1990) Control of leishmaniasis: report of a WHO expert committee. *World Health Organization Technical Report Series*, **793**.

Young H (1992) Syphilis: new diagnostic directions. *International Journal of Sexually Transmitted Diseases and AIDS*, **3**, 391–413.

10

Travelers' Diarrhea

Luis Ostrosky-Zeichner

University of Texas Houston Medical School, Houston, Texas, USA

Charles D. Ericsson

University of Texas Houston Medical School, Houston, Texas, USA

INTRODUCTION

Travelers' diarrhea is arguably the most common and important health problem affecting travelers. It has a high frequency and economic impact on both the business and vacationing traveler. The syndrome occurs in 20–50% of travelers, resulting in considerable morbidity of untreated disease (DuPont and Ericsson, 1993). Fortunately, mortality due to typical travelers' diarrhea is extremely uncommon (Petola and Gorbach, 1997). Nearly 40% of persons with travelers' diarrhea change their itinerary, about 20% are confined to bed for a day, and approximately 1% of suffers are admitted to hospital (Ericsson and DuPont, 1993; Petola and Gorbach, 1997). A whole trip may be ruined by a particularly severe case. Travelers' diarrhea is preventable and should be extensively addressed when giving medical travel advice. New approaches to prevention, self-treatment and the prospect of new vaccines have modified the course and impact of this disease substantially (Ericsson and Rey, 1997; Petrucelli *et al.*, 1997).

GENERAL CONSIDERATIONS

Travelers' diarrhea, also known as Montezuma's revenge, Aztec two-step, Delhi belly, Gyppy tummy, Turkey trots and turista, is usually defined as the passage of 3–4 unformed stools in a 24 h period plus at least one symptom of enteric disease, such as abdominal pain, cramps, nausea, vomiting, fever, or tenesmus (DuPont and Ericsson, 1993; Ericsson and DuPont, 1993). Less severe forms of the syndrome (e.g. 1–2 loose stools per day) are frequently caused by the same enteropathogens but probably do not need to be treated symptomatically or specifically because they are mild and short-lived (Ericsson *et al.*, 1994). Some definitions of diarrhea consider the volume of unformed stool passed over a period of time. Such a definition might fail to account for classic dysentery in which many small volume bloody stools are passed. The total volume of dysenteric stools might not meet the volume definition of diarrhea. Travelers' diarrhea lasting longer than 2 weeks, by definition, becomes chronic diarrhea.

Travelers might decide to treat illness even though it does not meet the standard definition of diarrhea. For instance, a traveler might treat one large volume watery stool associated with a severe cramp. Advice about how to begin self-therapy must be practical and should not be driven simply by study criteria.

Due to changes in habits (e.g. increased fruit/vegetable consumption, fat intake, irritating spices) and stress, travelers commonly experience benign changes in bowel movement consistency or frequency. Watery stools can be passed following ingestion of alcohol or associated with menstruation. Although troublesome, most patients and experts do not address these episodes as 'travelers' diarrhea'.

ETIOLOGY

The frequency with which specific microorganisms cause disease varies somewhat around the world (Table 10.1), but the majority of the identified causal organisms are bacterial (Petola and Gorbach, 1997). The most common cause of travelers' diarrhea is enterotoxigenic *Escherichia coli* (ETEC). In some regions of the world *Campylobacter jejuni* is a relatively common cause of travelers' diarrhea, especially during the winter season. *Aeromonas* species are a frequent cause of diarrhea in parts of Southeast Asia. Invasive bacterial pathogens (*Shigella*, *Salmonella* and *Campylobacter*) on average cause more severe, longer-lasting disease than that caused by ETEC. *Salmonella*

Principles and Practice of Travel Medicine. Edited by Jane N. Zuckerman.
© 2001 John Wiley & Sons Ltd.

Table 10.1   Regional distribution of pathogens causing travelers' diarrhea (%)

Pathogen	Latin America	Africa	Asia
No pathogen identified	24–62	15–53	10–56
Bacterial			
Escherichia coli			
Enterotoxigenic	17–70	8–42	6–37
Others[a]	7–22	2–9	3–4
Campylobacter jejuni	1–5	1–28	9–39
Salmonella spp	1–16	4–25	1–33
Shigella spp	2–30	0–9	0–17
Plesiomonas shigelloides	0–6	3–5	3–13
Aeromonas spp	1–5	0–9	1–57
Viral			
Rotavirus	0–6	0–36	1–8
Parasitic			
Giardia lamblia	1–2	0–1	1–12
Entamoeba histolytica	<1	2–9	5–11
Cryptosporidium	<1	2	1–5
Cyclospora cayetanensis	?<1	?<1	?1–5

[a]Including enteroaggregative, enteroinvasive and enterohemorrhagic.

typhi and *Vibrio cholerae*, both potentially deadly causes of diarrhea, are uncommon causes of travelers' diarrhea.

Viruses (e.g. rotaviruses, Norwalk agent, adenoviruses, caliciviruses and other small round viruses) are uncommon causes of travelers' diarrhea compared with bacteria. Specific antimicrobial therapy for viral diarrhea is not available, but bismuth subsalicylate preparations have been effective in treating it. Using nonantimicrobial symptomatic medications such as loperamide likely affords some relief when the cause of diarrhea is viral. This is one reason why combination therapy with loperamide plus an antimicrobial agent was studied as empiric treatment of the travelers' diarrhea syndrome.

Parasites are an uncommon cause of travelers' diarrhea in the developing world (Petola and Gorbach, 1997); therefore, their treatment need not be included in the self-therapy regimen for most travelers. When trekkers in eastern Europe and Russia might be far removed from medical care, arming them with medication (e.g. metronidazole or tinidazole) to treat possible *Entamoeba histolytica* or *Giardia lamblia* disease seems reasonable. In Nepal, *Cyclospora* can cause disease with some regularity. This organism responds only to trimethoprim-sulfamethoxazole. No adequate therapy exists for *Cryptosporidium* disease; fortunately, it is not a common cause of travelers' diarrhea. Amebiasis should always be considered in a traveler to an endemic area who has bloody diarrhea that fails to respond to antibiotics.

Many cases of travelers' diarrhea occur without an obvious known etiology (Petola and Gorbach, 1997). Also, new causes of travelers' diarrhea have been discovered (e.g. enteroinvasive and enteroaggregative *E. coli*)

and the role of other enteric organisms is being investigated (e.g. toxin-producing *Bacteroides fragilis* or *Klebsiella*). As a general rule, clinical disease associated with no identified pathogen has responded to antimicrobial agents, implying that a substantial proportion of this subset of travelers' diarrhea will eventually be found to be caused by bacterial enteropathogens.

EPIDEMIOLOGY

The incidence of travelers' diarrhea is highest among persons moving from developed to developing countries, with some variation in risk among developing countries (Petola and Gorbach, 1997). The risk of travelers' diarrhea averages about 7% in developed areas such as the United States, Canada, Europe, Australia, New Zealand, and other industrialized nations. The risk increases to about 20% in southern Europe, Israel, Japan, South Africa, and certain Caribbean Islands. The risk is highest (20–50%) in the rest of Africa, Latin America, the Middle East and most of Asia (Petola and Gorbach, 1997). The risk of diarrhea for a person moving from one developed country to another is about the same as it is for a traveler moving from a developing country to a developed country.

Prior experience as a short-term traveler to high-risk areas does not appear to confer much, if any, protection. Expatriates residing in Nepal for a prolonged period of time appear to remain substantially at risk for travelers' diarrhea. Conversely, the rate of diarrhea dropped among US adult medical students as they became long-term residents in Mexico, implying that a degree of protection (whether by immunity or risk avoidance) might develop in some expatriate populations (Ericsson and DuPont, 1993). Such protection was measurably lost when medical students returned to Mexico after a 6–8 week vacation in the USA. The implication is that continued exposure to enteropathogens in a developing country might be necessary for protection against disease to persist. Also, persons who reside in a developing country and move to another developing country appear to have a degree of protection against the development of diarrhea, because their rates of diarrhea are lower compared with those of travelers coming from industrialized countries.

Studies of Swiss and Austrian travelers have indicated that 90% of travelers' diarrhea occurs during the first 2 weeks of stay in a developing country. On the other hand, studies of diarrhea prevention and prospective 1 month studies of diarrhea incidence among adults newly arrived in Mexico (Ericsson *et al.*, 1994) have indicated that the first-month rate of diarrhea among US college-age students living in Mexico was 54%. Fifty-seven percent of the cases occurred in the first 2 weeks of stay in Mexico and 43% of the cases occurred in the second two weeks of stay. Such studies help to explain the wide variation in the reported incidence of travelers' diarrhea (Petola and Gorbach, 1997). By definition, incidence numbers must include the time of stay in the developing country to be valid.

Perhaps because they mouth their environment indiscriminately, the very young are at increased risk for travelers' diarrhea. Young adults in the 20–29 year age group have the next highest risk. This group is probably fairly adventuresome and willing to sample foods and beverages indiscriminately. They often travel on a shoestring budget and might not have received advice about risk factors and their avoidance. Residing in high- or low-budget hotels has no apparent bearing on the risk of travelers' diarrhea, perhaps attesting to the ubiquity of the risk. Failure to adhere to dietary advice appears to be universal behavior that is not limited to the younger age groups.

Some enteropathogens are more likely to cause disease during certain seasons. Among Finnish tourists, *Campylobacter* and *Salmonella* caused disease in Morocco more often in the winter than the fall, and ETEC causes disease more often in the fall than the winter. Similarly, *Campylobacter* causes diarrhea among US adults in Guadalajara, Mexico predominantly in the winter, dry season, and ETEC causes diarrhea in the summer, rainy season (Ericsson and DuPont, 1993). When an effective vaccine becomes available, these observations might be helpful in deciding which short-term traveler to vaccinate against ETEC.

Seasonality of pathogen occurrence does not guide adequately the choice of an antibiotic for the treatment of travelers' diarrhea. *Campylobacter* disease, for instance, can occur in the 'off' season, and its inherent resistance to an antibiotic like trimethoprim-sulfamethoxazole is more important than seasonality when choosing an antibiotic for empiric treatment. Increasing antimicrobial resistance worldwide among many enteropathogens, including common *E. coli*, is pivotally important when choosing an antimicrobial agent for empiric use.

RISK FACTORS

Food and, to a lesser extent, water consumption are well-documented risk factors for travelers' diarrhea. The problem is ingestion of fecally contaminated food or water. Sometimes dirty hands or insects are the vectors for fecal contamination of food. Other important risk factors are host-related (e.g. immune status, gastrointestinal disease and behavior) and should be taken into consideration when counseling patients.

Water

Travelers should take care to drink safe beverages, even though contaminated water usually accounts only for a minority of travelers' diarrhea. Tap water in developing countries can be chlorinated, but crosscontamination can occur after water leaves the chlorinating plant. Tap water was the probable vehicle of transmission of predominately nonbacterial diarrhea in Mexico during the winter

(Ericsson *et al.*, 1994). Infection with *Salmonella typhi* has been related to ingestion of contaminated food and water or other noncarbonated beverages. Fortunately, typhoid fever is rare among travelers. Cryptosporidiosis is probably acquired via ingestion of contaminated water. It is an infrequent cause of travelers' diarrhea except in regions like Russia and Nepal. The number of cysts necessary to cause cryptosporidiosis is small, but the level of contamination of chlorinated water is also usually low.

Travelers should avoid swimming in freshwater rivers and lakes, which might be a sewer for the local population. Also, salt water can be contaminated by a river emptying into it or by emptying recreational boat bilge near swimming areas. Adequate chlorination and acidification of pool water is not always found in countries without high standards of public health practices.

The risk of diarrhea is probably not high when ice is made in a machine with clean water. Slab ice is more likely to be or become contaminated. Unwashed hands can contaminate ice in the process of chipping off portions for beverages. Alcohol in a drink cannot be assumed to have sterilized contaminated ice. The concentration of alcohol used in mixed drinks takes more time to kill microorganisms than the time taken to consume the drink. The tiny amount of water involved with brushing teeth or taking a shower is probably a safe exposure, especially if the water is hot.

Food

The use of human excreta as fertilizer, inadequate public health practices, and poor personal hygiene of food handlers jeopardize the food hygiene chain in developing countries. Fresh salads have been incriminated consistently as a risk for travelers' diarrhea. Ideally, produce should be rinsed thoroughly, soaked in a halide solution and rinsed in clean water. Kitchen personnel must wash their hands properly after defecation. The riskiest foods are generally raw and moist. Dry foods are generally safe because microorganisms do not grow well on a dry surface. An especially risky setting appears to be the buffet. Food is usually kept at room temperature for long periods of time, leading to bacterial overgrowth and exposure to contaminated hands and surfaces.

Cooked food is usually safe to eat once the temperature at its interior has reached 70°C (160°F). Enterohemorrhagic *E. coli* can contaminate ground meat at the processing plant. The cook can introduce microorganisms into the middle of a hamburger patty during its preparation. Thorough cooking is critical. Ice cream and other frozen or unfrozen dairy products can also be contaminated and cause disease.

Host-related Factors

Differences in host susceptibility to travelers' diarrhea are difficult to demonstrate, because exposure to enteropathogens is frequent in a developing country. Persons with blood group O appear to be more susceptible to cholera but not to ETEC, even though the heat-labile enterotoxin of *E. coli* is similar immunologically to cholera toxin.

Achlorhydria is a risk factor for travelers' diarrhea. Stomach acid decreases the inoculum of ingested pathogens to a number that is incapable of causing disease in most instances. An exception is *Shigella*, which is still pathogenic when less than 100 organisms survive stomach acid. H-2 blockers and proton pump inhibitors are thought to be risks for diarrhea, because they inhibit acid strongly for prolonged periods, including meal times. The role of antacids as a risk factor for travelers' diarrhea is less certain, particularly if they are used only well after ingestion of food.

Patients with AIDS and low CD4+ counts are known to be susceptible to enteric pathogens. After institution of highly active antiretroviral therapy, patients feel better and are more likely to travel. Rises in CD4+ cells should be sustained over at least a 3 month period before the patient can assume they are protected from opportunistic infections consistent with the new number of CD4+ cells. While data are lacking, AIDS patients who travel might be considered for antimicrobial prophylaxis if their CD4+ count is less than 200, and bismuth subsalicylate prophylaxis if the count is less than 500. Other immune-deficient hosts, such as patients receiving cancer chemotherapy or corticosteroids, as well as those with common IgA deficiency, should also be considered to be at special risk for the development of travelers' diarrhea.

Some hosts are not necessarily more at risk of developing diarrhea, but when they do develop diarrhea the consequences are worse compared with the average host. Such persons include those with underlying gastrointestinal diseases, such as Crohn's disease and ulcerative colitis, and persons with an ileostomy. Dehydration in such patients is an important concern. Elderly patients with diarrhea might become confused and forget to rehydrate themselves or they might continue diuretic therapy in the face of developing dehydration. Small children and infants are at special risk of becoming dehydrated when they develop diarrhea. On the other hand, travelers' diarrhea in the healthy adult is usually not dehydrating (Ericsson and DuPont, 1993).

Adventurous travelers are difficult to advise. They may plan to eat indiscriminately and might ask for chemoprophylaxis against diarrhea. Such patients serve to remind us that we should not be overly judgmental about quality-of-life decisions as long as such persons are fully informed about the risks and benefits of medications and behavioral change (Ericsson and Rey, 1997).

SALIENT CLINICAL FEATURES

Travelers' diarrhea is a clinical syndrome. The clinical manifestations of the various microbiological causes of travelers' diarrhea overlap considerably (Mattila, 1994). It usually begins within 2–3 days of arrival to the destination. The average frequency of associated symptoms are: cramps, 40–60%; nausea, 10–70%; vomiting, 5–10%; and fever 10–30% (Petola and Gorbach, 1997). Because of considerable overlap in the clinical syndromes categories of diarrhea like 'secretory' or 'invasive' do not adequately differentiate the specific etiology of diarrhea in an individual. Patients infected with a classic invasive pathogen like *Shigella* often present early with watery diarrhea and not the frequent, small-volume, bloody, and mucus-laden stools that characterize dysentery. Alternatively, patients infected with a classic secretory pathogen like ETEC can sometimes present with low-grade fever and a small amount of occult blood in the stool. The more severe the diarrhea is, the more likely that an invasive pathogen will be found, but the relationship is not strong enough for clinical decision-making in the individual patient (Mattila, 1994). Cholera usually presents as a very high output 'rice water' diarrhea with low-grade temperature and quickly leads to life-threatening dehydration. Patients should be advised to seek prompt medical help when such characteristics are present.

MANAGEMENT, TREATMENT AND CONTROL

General Principles

Some authorities feel that symptomatic or specific therapy of travelers' diarrhea is frequently not necessary because travelers' diarrhea is a self-limiting disease (Petrucelli *et al.*, 1997). It is considered that fluid and electrolyte replacement is the preferred approach to diarrhea management. Electrolyte replacement solutions are increasingly readily available in pharmacies or grocery stores in developing countries. An antimicrobial agent might be used when results of a stool culture show the cause of diarrhea is an invasive pathogen. However, a well-trained physician, who also speaks the traveler's language, can be difficult to locate in a developing country. Delay in treatment while waiting for stool culture results can increase time lost from planned activities.

Another approach to therapy is to reserve empirical antibiotic treatment for occasions when clinical parameters suggest disease caused by an invasive pathogen. The problem is that neither patients nor physicians can reliably predict when an invasive pathogen is causing disease based solely on clinical symptoms and signs. While the positive predictive power of symptoms of dysentery is very high, the negative predictive power is low. If only patients with dysentery were treated with an antibiotic, many patients with disease caused by an invasive pathogen would be denied the benefits of antibiotics.

Empiric self-therapy, regardless of the cause of diarrhea, has emerged as a valid approach to the treatment of travelers' diarrhea (DuPont and Ericsson, 1993; Ericsson

Table 10.2 Antimicrobial agents recommended for the treatment of travelers' diarrhea

Agent	Dose	Comments
Trimethoprim-sulfamethoxazole	Two DS[a] tablets as a single dose One DS tablet b.i.d. for 3 days Two DS tablets (loading dose), then one DS b.i.d. for 3 days	The loading dose regimen led to a statistical benefit that is not clinically relevant. Rising resistance worldwide has limited its usefulness
Fluoroquinolones		
Norfloxacin	400 mg b.i.d. for 3 days	Double doses can be used for single-dose
Ciprofloxacin	500 mg b.i.d. for 3 days	therapy. Other fluoroquinolones like
Ofloxacin	200 mg b.i.d. for 3 days	fleroxacin and pefloxacin should be effective
Levofloxacin	500 mg q.d. for 3 days	
Azithromycin	500 mg (loading dose) then 250 mg q.d. for 4 days 1000 mg as a single dose	Optimal dosing is under investigation. Highly effective agent in recent studies
Rifaximin	200–400 mg t.i.d. for 3 days	Not absorbed
Aztreonam	—	Not absorbed. Effective in studies but not available

[a]Trimethoprim-sulfamethoxazole DS = 160 mg TMP plus 800 mg SMX.

and DuPont, 1993). Choice of a specific antimicrobial agent has been determined, in part, by a growing understanding of the many causes of travelers' diarrhea and increasing antimicrobial resistance among some of the enteropathogens (Petola and Gorbach, 1997).

Oral Rehydration Therapy and Feeding

Oral rehydration solution is a cost-effective, elegantly simple treatment for dehydrating diarrhea. The addition of glucose to electrolyte-containing solutions facilitates absorption of electrolytes. The output of fluid is increased by as much as 50% by aggressive fluid replacement with traditional oral rehydration solutions. Furthermore, travelers' diarrhea is not usually a dehydrating disease. The addition of oral rehydration solution to therapy with loperamide makes no difference to the recovery of the patient with the usual travelers' diarrhea. The use of oral rehydration solutions that contain complex sugars derived from rice or cereal can lower the output of diarrhea, and such solutions should be studied in the treatment of travelers' diarrhea.

Early refeeding is recommended in children with diarrhea. In adults, dietary adjustment is often not necessary because diarrhea abates so quickly with modern therapy. When symptoms linger despite treatment, common sense suggests that milk, fruits, vegetables, red meat, caffeine and alcohol should be added to the diet only when diarrhea has abated. Persisting or recurring symptoms should prompt consideration of parasitic disease.

Antimicrobial Therapy

Kean first demonstrated the successful prevention of travelers' diarrhea with antimicrobial agents in 1963.

Many studies have verified the efficacy of antimicrobial agents in both the prevention and the treatment of the syndrome. Antibiotics can limit the course of diarrhea to approximately 1 day. Untreated diarrhea lasts over 3 days. The benefits of antibiotic therapy include significant reductions in the total duration of diarrhea, earlier relief of accompanying symptoms like cramps, and a decrease in the amounts of time spent in bed and missing or altering planned activities. Some experts still consider that antibiotics have little role in the empiric treatment of travelers' diarrhea (Petrucelli et al., 1997). While it is true that travelers' diarrhea is a self-limited disease, in the authors' opinion the considerable relief afforded by antibiotic treatment argues against therapeutic nihilism.

A number of antibiotics have been shown to be useful in the treatment of travelers' diarrhea. For years trimethoprim-sulfamethoxazole (TMP-SMX) was an excellent choice for treatment of travelers' diarrhea, and trimethoprim alone could be substituted for patients who were allergic to sulfa preparations. TMP-SMX resistance around the world has increased so much that it is no longer a preferred empiric treatment choice.

Currently, the most readily available of the active antibiotics for treatment are fluoroquinolones such as norfloxacin, ciprofloxacin, ofloxacin, enoxacin, fleroxacin and others (Table 10.2). All appear to be highly effective, so the choice of one should probably be based solely on the price.

Nonabsorbed antibiotics (e.g. bicozamycin, aztreonam, and rifaximin) were predicted to be less effective for the treatment of diarrhea because antibiotic absorption and high mucosal levels were thought to be necessary. However, these agents have been proven to be efficacious in treating diarrhea due to the full range of causal bacterial agents, including those like *Salmonella* that cause intracellular infection. The theoretic reason for preferring nonabsorbed agents is that they should engender fewer side-effects and should be safer to use in children and pregnant women, in whom the currently preferred quinolones are contraindicated. With the exception of rifaximin, which is available in some countries but not worldwide, companies have been slow to develop such agents further, presumably because the market is not large enough to satisfy their economic motivations.

Erythromycin is effective in *Campylobacter* disease and has been shown to be effective in the prevention of travelers' diarrhea, probably owing to its activity against Gram-negative enteric organisms in the alkaline milieu of the gut. Erythromycin, however, has not been studied for the treatment of travelers' diarrhea. The azalide, azithromycin, has been studied in *Campylobacter* disease, and it is also efficacious (Kuschner *et al.*, 1995). *In vitro* studies predict that azithromycin should be active in treating travelers' diarrhea.

Certain antibiotics are available over the counter in many developing countries and local physicians might recommend them. These include ampicillin, which is simply not active enough around the world to be an effective choice. Furazolidone is active not only against bacterial causes of travelers' diarrhea but also against *Giardia*. This feature can be a benefit in some regions of the world like Russia, where the risk of acquisition of *Giardia* appears to be exceptionally high. The problem is that furazolidone is only about one-half as effective as the preferred quinolones in the treatment of the common bacterial causes of travelers' diarrhea.

Increasing resistance around the world has limited the usefulness of doxycycline. Chloramphenicol is cheap and readily available over the counter in many countries, but its rare but devastating bone marrow toxicity limits its widespread recommendation. Clioquinol was studied many years ago with variable results. It was taken off the market in many countries because of serious ophthalmologic adverse effects. Doxycycline, chloramphenicol and clioquinol cannot be recommended.

The duration of treatment with antibiotics has steadily decreased with ongoing study. Now a single dose of antibiotic can be recommended for most patients (DuPont and Ericsson, 1993; Ericsson and Rey, 1997). The invasive pathogens and severe disease are the causes and clinical state that might require lengthier therapy than a single dose. As a rule *Shigella* responds to single dose therapy, but disease caused by *S. dysenteriae* appears best treated with a 3-day course of antibiotic. Fortunately, *S. dysenteriae* is an uncommon cause of travelers' diarrhea. More study is needed before single-dose therapy can be recommended confidently for *Campylobacter* disease. In areas of the world where *C. jejuni* is especially prevalent (e.g. Southeast Asia), at least a 3 day course of antibiotic is recommended. Probably 3 day therapy should be preferred over single-dose therapy to treat winter-time diarrhea, because *Campylobacter* is a relatively more common cause of winter-time diarrhea in regions where it is otherwise not a common cause of travelers' diarrhea during peak summer-time travel (e.g. Morocco and Mexico).

Antibiotic resistance has developed during treatment of *Campylobacter* disease with the quinolones. Symptoms have relapsed despite having responded initially. When quinolones are used as agents of choice for self-therapy in areas where *Campylobacter* are common causes of travelers' diarrhea, the patient might need to be armed with a course of azithromycin to take in the event that quinolone-treated disease relapses. Alternatively, rifaximin could be prescribed in place of a fluoroquinolone if it is available. Azithromycin needs more study before it can be advocated as front-line therapy.

We provide clients with 3 day courses of a quinolone for self-therapy. We ask them to re-evaluate themselves when the next dose of antibiotic would be due. If they are still passing unformed stools, or fever or passage of bloody stools was a feature of their disease, we recommend that they finish the full 3 days of antibiotic. Otherwise, we feel that single-dose antibiotic therapy usually suffices.

Symptom Management

Less severe disease can be treated with a variety of nonantibiotic agents (Table 10.3). Bismuth subsalicylate (BSS)-containing compounds decrease the number of unformed stools passed after beginning treatment by almost 50%. The antisecretory and antimotility agent, loperamide, is more efficacious than BSS. Neither is as effective as an antibiotic.

Some studies with antimotility agents such as diphenoxylate suggested that the agents might prolong the course of disease caused by invasive enteropathogens. In a small number of prisoners, shigellosis was treated with an antibiotic and diphenoxylate. Shedding of *Shigella* and fever where prolonged. Patients with bloody diarrhea treated with diphenoxylate alone had a longer course of disease than did placebo-treated subjects. The use of antimotility agents should be avoided in the treatment of *Clostridium difficile* disease. Conversely, current research indicates disease is not prolonged when patients are able to take an antibiotic when they feel they are not getting enough relief from loperamide. Also, ciprofloxacin plus loperamide treats *Shigella* dysentery more effectively than ciprofloxacin alone (Murphy *et al.*, 1993).

Loperamide is absorbed rapidly and acts more quickly than BSS preparations, which take nearly 4 h to begin having their effect. Loperamide is a safe drug that is available over the counter. It is approved for use in children as young as 3 years old.

The prescription product diphenoxylate plus atropine (Lomotil) is popular, but the drug is not as efficacious as loperamide in the treatment of diarrhea and has a relatively unfavorable side-effect profile. Elderly men can suffer urinary retention due to the atropine. Lomotil is habit forming and central nervous system side-effects are possible.

Other symptomatic drugs that have been advocated in

Table 10.3 Symptomatic treatment of travelers' diarrhea

Therapeutic agent	Dose	Comments
Attapulgite	3 g initially and after each loose stool for a total of 9 g per day	Safe in pregnancy but only marginally effective
Bismuth subsalicylate preparations	30 ml (1 ounce) every half hour for a total of 240 ml (8 ounces)	Rinse mouth carefully. Brush teeth and tongue after evening dose
Loperamide	4 mg loading dose, then 2 mg after each loose stool, not to exceed 16 mg per day	Over-the-counter directions limit total daily dose to 8 mg. Oral hydration does not add to symptomatic relief afforded by loperamide
Zaldaride maleate	—	Not yet marketed. Calmodulin antagonist
SP 303	—	Mechanism of action not known. Not yet approved but alternatively available as a natural preparation

the past include the anticholinergic agents, activated charcoal, *Lactobacillus* preparations, polycarbophil, methylcellulose, psyllium, and kaolin/pectin preparations (Petrucelli *et al.*, 1997). All of these are not effective for the treatment of travelers' diarrhea with the exception of attapulgite (a hydrated aluminum silicate clay preparation), which performed well enough in trials to recommend it for mild diarrhea. Attapulgite is a safe product that can be recommended for use in pregnant women. It causes a more formed stool; however, net losses of water and electrolytes persist unabated.

Recent studies have shown that a new and novel calmodulin inhibitor, zaldaride, is useful in decreasing the duration of diarrhea from an average of 42 h in untreated subjects to an average of 20 h (DuPont *et al.*, 1993; Okhuysen *et al.*, 1995). The drug worked both in ETEC disease as well as in other bacterial diseases, suggesting a common role for calmodulin for the pathogenesis of diarrhea. A loading dose will likely be necessary for optimal use. Zaldaride is not yet marketed worldwide. Still another agent, the antisecretory drug SP303, shows promise in the symptomatic relief of travelers' diarrhea.

The combination of an antibiotic and loperamide has been studied with the usual dose of each agent. In one study more than half of the patients passed no further unformed stools once combination therapy was begun. The average duration of diarrhea was only a few hours, even when patients had blood in stools at enrollment. This result was superior to treatment with either agent alone and was confirmed in subsequent studies (Ericsson *et al.*, 1997). Some studies have not verified such remarkable results, either when *Campylobacter* was a common cause of disease or when disease among placebo controls was relatively mild.

Algorithmic Approach to Treatment

Among all travelers developing diarrhea, approximately 40% will have mild self-limiting disease that ceases within a day or two, with passage of no more than two unformed stools per day (Ericsson and DuPont, 1993). Once a third loose stool is passed within a 24 h period, diarrhea can be predicted to become more severe or last many days. We advise longer-term travelers such as expatriates to withhold antibiotic treatment for travelers' diarrhea unless more than two loose stools are passed. Some disease begins so explosively that therapy should logically be begun before passage of a third loose stool. Figure 10.1 outlines our approach to the treatment of travelers' diarrhea.

HEALTH ADVICE AND PROTECTIVE MEASURES

As shown in Figure 10.2, options for the prevention of travelers' diarrhea include education, vaccination and chemoprophylaxis with either BSS-containing compounds or antibiotics (Ericsson and Rey, 1997). Although vaccination is a promising option, vaccines against all enteropathogens that cause travelers' diarrhea will probably never be possible or cost-effective owing to the large number of strains that cause disease. Promising vaccines against ETEC and *Shigella* are not available for routine use (Ericsson and Rey, 1997).

Education

The problem with education as an approach to prevention is achieving and maintaining behavior modification among tourists. The tourist too often has a carefree attitude, wants intentionally to sample new culture and food and has consumed alcohol, which disinhibits all travelers. Catchy phrases like 'boil it, cook it, peel it—or forget it' are simply not practiced. Business travelers appear to have fewer episodes of diarrhea than do most tourist travelers. The business traveler faces occasionally meals of exotic and risky foods that cannot be refused easily. While not studied, a single dose of an effective antimicrobial should be effective in preventing most causes of diarrhea after such a risky meal.

Many travel experts have given up trying to educate travelers about safe culinary practices. The problem is

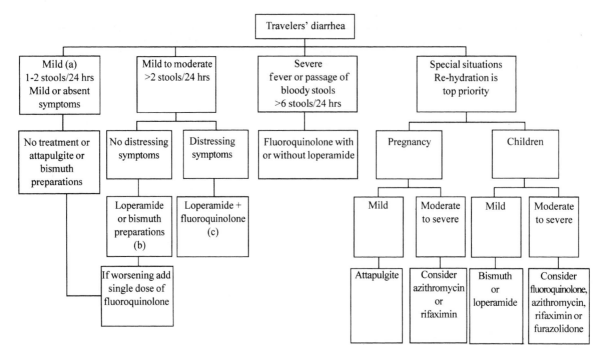

Figure 10.1 Algorithmic approach to the treatment of travelers' diarrhea. (a) Long-term travelers are encouraged to endure mild diarrhea to develop some immunity. (b) Business travelers on short, critical trips might consider earlier addition of a single dose of antibiotic. (c) Reassess symptoms when second dose of fluoroquinolone is due. Discontinue therapy if diarrhea has abated. A single dose of antibiotic usually suffices

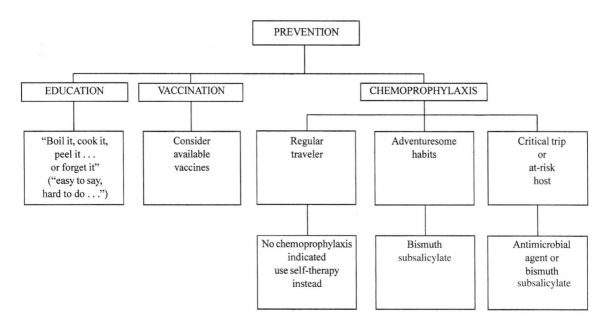

Figure 10.2 Approach to prevention of travelers' diarrhea

Table 10.4 Dietary advice for avoiding travelers' diarrhea

	Safe	Probably safe	Unsafe
Culinary practices	Careful Considers heat of food	Recognized restaurants Judicious alcohol	Adventurous Vendors Buffet food at room temperature Excessive alcohol
Beverages	Carbonated soft drinks Boiled water Iodized water Irradiated milk	Fresh citrus juices Packaged, machine-made ice Bottled water	Tap water Uncarbonated, bottled fruit juices Chipped ice Unpasteurized milk or butter
Food	Piping hot Peeled fruit Processed/packaged Cooked vegetables	Dry Jelly/syrup Washed vegetables	Cold salads Uncooked, cold sauces Undercooked hamburgers Unpeeled fruit Some cold desserts Fresh soft cheese Raspberries/strawberries

Table 10.5 Comparison of bismuth subsalicylate and antibiotics for the prevention of travelers' diarrhea

	Major side-effects (%)	Minor side-effects (%)	Protection against diarrhea (%)
Antimicrobial agent	0.01	3	90[a]
Bismuth subsalicylate	0	1	65

[a]Percent protection for fluoroquinolones; trimethoprim-sulfamethoxazole efficacy is lower.

that creative efforts at education have not been employed either because of ignorance of behavioral modification techniques or too much pressure on the practitioner's time. If travelers visit a specialized travel medicine clinic, it is considered that time should be devoted to their education, particularly when the traveler is paying personally for the visit. Table 10.4 shows the main specific recommendations to be given regarding food and beverage consumption, as well as eating attitudes.

Chemoprophylaxis

As shown in Table 10.5, BSS-containing compounds can be as much as 65% effective for the prevention of travelers' diarrhea (Ericsson and Rey, 1997). Protection rises substantially if travelers are also careful in what and where they eat. BSS is an antimicrobial and also has antisecretory and antiinflammatory properties. When the daily dose of BSS is taken as two divided doses, it is less effective than when the same total dose is taken as four smaller doses. Chewed tablets are as effective as liquid preparations. Bismuth toxicity is rare with ingestion of BSS. Serum bismuth concentrations are well below the level associated with encephalopathy, even after 2 weeks of use. Salicylate, however, is nearly completely absorbed. Chewing two tablets four times a day approximates taking 3–4 adult aspirins in terms of the salicylate absorbed. Taking aspirin should be avoided when BSS compounds are taken. Patients taking oral anticoagulants should cautioned against the use of BSS, even though the influence on the prothrombin time is not as high with salicylate as it is with acetylsalicylic acid. At standard doses of BSS, tinnitus was no more common in subjects who took active drug than in those who took placebo. Black insoluble bismuth salts in stools can be confused with melena. After a bedtime dose of BSS, tongues should be gently brushed and mouths carefully rinsed to avoid awakening with a black tongue.

Antibiotics are up to 90% effective in preventing travelers' diarrhea as long as they are active against the causal enteropathogens (Table 10.5) (Ericsson and Rey, 1997). Concentrations of antibiotic in stool are probably the best predictive of activity of antibiotics in preventing or treating enteropathogens. 'High-level' resistance, usually defined in terms of inadequate serum concentrations, predicts clinical ineffectiveness in the treatment and prevention of diarrhea only if adequate concentrations are also not achieved in stool. Antibiotics that can be recommended at present for the prevention of travelers' diarrhea are outlined in Table 10.6. The nonabsorbed antibiotics are theoretically appealing for the prevention of travelers' diarrhea because of predictable high efficacy and low potential for adverse reactions. One nonabsorbed antibiotic, bicozamycin, was regrettably never developed further despite an excellent record in the safe and efficacious treatment and prevention of travelers' diarrhea. Other nonabsorbed antibiotics, aztreonam and rifaximin, have been studied in the successful treatment of travelers' diarrhea but not in its prevention.

Table 10.6   Agents for the prevention of travelers' diarrhea

Agent	Dosing regimen	Comments
Activated charcoal	Variable	May adsorb important medications; not efficacious, not currently recommended
Lactobacillus preparations	Variable	Safe; efficacy not proven, not recommended; new genetically engineered strains hold promise
Bismuth subsalicylate preparations	Two 262 mg tablets chewed 4 times a day	Rinse mouth to avoid black tongue; 65% protective; may cause constipation and black stools
Trimethoprim-sulfamethoxazole	One double-strength tablet q.d.	Resistance rising worldwide; 70–80% protective
Fluoroquinolones		Over 90% protective; currently most effective
Norfloxacin	400 mg q.d.	antimicrobial antidiarrheal agent; generally reserve
Ciprofloxacin	500 mg q.d.	for self-therapy; other fluoroquinolones should work
Levofloxacin	500 mg q.d.	as well
Ofloxacin	300 mg q.d.	

A 1985 Consensus Development Conference in Washington concluded that travelers' diarrhea was self-limiting and did not cause mortality; therefore, antibiotic prophylaxis should not be used owing to rare but severe side-effects. Further, the consensus was that BSS should not be used because patients might abuse an over-the-counter preparation.

In our clinic we do not offer prophylaxis routinely, but are willing to discuss the issue with any traveler who expresses an interest in using prophylaxis. We discourage prophylaxis of travelers' diarrhea with antibiotics except in certain high-risk hosts. We recommend BSS to most travelers who desire prophylaxis. We educate the traveler wanting prophylaxis about the pros and cons of chemoprophylactic agents and let the traveler make the final decision.

Chemoprophylaxis, however, is not so straightforward. In addition to possible adverse reactions, the cost of chemoprophylactic agents must be considered. Prophylaxis was found to be more cost-effective than treatment for many travelers, when treatment with an antibiotic took, on average, longer than a day to cure the patient. Expensive vacation time was often lost. Treatment with an antibiotic plus loperamide has so shortened the course of disease that vacation time is not often lost when diarrhea is treated empirically and quickly. Treatment is more cost-effective than prevention, with the exception of trips that last only a few days. Chemoprophylaxis may lead to complacency in food and beverage selection, thus adding additional behavioral risks for acquiring parasitic or viral disease against which an antibiotic has no or little activity.

The use of antibiotics can cause overgrowth of *Candida*, resulting in vaginitis. Overgrowth of *Clostridium difficile* can cause diarrhea. Some antibiotics seem to promote infection with certain organisms such as *Salmonella* and *Campylobacter*.

Early, effective antibiotic treatment can obviate the immune response to an enteropathogen. Expatriates probably should not take chemoprophylaxis to prevent diarrhea and should not treat mild disease with an antibiotic (Ericsson *et al.*, 1994). This approach might encour-age immunity to develop against some enteropathogens.

Might tourists using preventative antibiotics in a developing country promote the emergence of antibiotic resistance? Subtherapeutic doses of antibiotic used by indigenous persons in a developing country are probably much more important to the development of resistance than antibiotic use by a relatively small number of tourists.

The bivalent cation in BSS interferes with the absorption of doxycycline. This interaction might jeopardize malaria prevention by lowering serum doxycycline concentrations below effective levels. Since the interaction occurs when the two drugs are taken concomitantly, and since prophylactic BSS is taken four times a day, plenty of opportunity exists for drug–drug interaction. The combination of BSS and doxycycline should be avoided.

Finally, parasites, viruses and *Clostridium difficile* become relatively more likely causes of diarrhea when a short-term traveler takes a prophylactic antibiotic and still develops diarrhea. These causes are ideally evaluated in conjunction with a visit to a physician, who can order stool studies in order to prescribe logical treatment. However, empiric treatment with metronidazole (followed by trimethoprim-sulfamethoxazole to treat *Cyclospora* if diarrhea persists) is an option for the trekker or others when they are far removed from reliable medical care.

Immunization

Vaccination to prevent travelers' diarrhea is limited by the number of available vaccines against the etiologic agents and their efficacy.

An oral vaccine for prevention of cholera (cholera whole cell/recombinant B subunit) is available in some parts of the world, and it appears to crossprotect somewhat against ETEC disease. Cholera vaccination is not necessary for most tourists, because they are simply not at risk unless they insist on eating raw seafood or are forced to live under deplorable conditions (e.g. some Peace Corps volunteers and refugee workers). Vaccination against typhoid with the preferred oral Ty21a (or parenteral Vi) vaccine is easy and devoid of bothersome side-effects. However, risk of typhoid is very low among tourists, and vaccination is generally limited to travelers who plan to stay longer than 3 weeks in a developing country or who avowedly are adventurous eaters. Vaccination against *Shigella* and other enteric agents is currently under investigation. New so-called DNA vaccine technology and novel vaccine delivery systems (e.g. fruit and vegetables) promise to revolutionize the field of vaccines and might have an important impact on risks for travelers' diarrhea in the future.

Milk immunoglobulins against ETEC have provided passive protection for a particular strain. Perhaps due to high development costs, further development of this approach has faltered.

REFERENCES

DuPont HL and Ericsson CD (1993) Prevention and treatment of travelers' diarrhea. *New England Journal of Medicine*, **328**, 1821–1827.

DuPont HL, Ericsson CD, Mathewson JJ *et al.* (1993) Zaldaride maleate, an intestinal calmodulin inhibitor, in the therapy of travelers' diarrhea. *Gastroenterology*, **104**, 709–715.

Ericsson CD and DuPont HL (1993) Travelers' diarrhea: approaches to prevention and treatment. *Clinical Infection Diseases*, **16**, 616–624.

Ericsson CD and Rey M (1997) Prevention of travelers' diarrhea: risk avoidance and chemoprophylaxis. In *Textbook of Travel Medicine and Health* (eds HL DuPont and R Steffen), pp 86–91. Decker, Hamilton, Ontario.

Ericsson CD, DuPont HL and Mathewson JJ (1994) Epidemiologic observations on diarrhea developing in US and Mexican students living in Guadalajara, Mexico. *Journal of Travel Medicine*, **2**, 6–10.

Ericsson CD, DuPont HL and Mathewson JJ (1997) Single dose ofloxacin plus loperamide compared with single dose or three days of ofloxacin in the treatment of travelers' diarrhea. *Journal of Travel Medicine*, **4**, 3–7.

Kuschner R, Trofa AF, Thomas RJ *et al.* (1995) Use of azithromycin for the treatment of *Campylobacter* enteritis in travelers to Thailand, an area where ciprofloxacin resistance is prevalent. *Clinical Infectious Diseases*, **21**, 536–541.

Mattila L (1994) Clinical features and duration of travelers' diarrhea in relation to its etiology. *Clinical Infectious Diseases*, **19**, 728–734.

Murphy GS, Bodhidatta L, Echeverria P *et al.* (1993) Ciprofloxacin and loperamide in the treatment of bacillary dysentery. *Annals of Internal Medicine*, **118**, 582–586.

Okhuysen PC, DuPont HL, Ericsson CD *et al.* (1995) Zaldaride malaete (a new calmodulin antagonist) versus loperamide in the treatment of travelers' diarrhea: randomized, placebo-controlled trial. *Clinical Infectious Diseases*, **21**, 341–344.

Petola H and Gorbach SL (1997) Travelers' diarrhea: epidemiology and clinical aspects. In *Textbook of Travel Medicine and Health* (eds HL DuPont and R Steffen), pp 78–86. Decker, Hamilton, Ontario.

Petrucelli BP, Kollaritsch H and Taylor DN (1997) Treatment of travelers' diarrhea. In *Textbook of Travel Medicine and Health* (eds HL DuPont and R Steffen), pp 92–100. Decker, Hamilton, Ontario.

11

Vaccine-preventable Disease

Jane N. Zuckerman

Royal Free and University College Medical School, London, UK

PRINCIPLES OF IMMUNITY BY VACCINATION

The provision of safe water and sanitation and the prevention of infectious diseases by immunisation have been the triumph of the twentieth century. This chapter is concerned with specific acquired passive and active immunity in relation to travel and routine vaccines, noting the International Health Regulations adopted by the World Health Organization (WHO). The purpose of these Regulations is to help prevent the international transmission of diseases and, in the context of international travel, to achieve this with the minimum inconvenience to the traveller. The vaccination requirements for international travel are listed conveniently in WHO's International Travel and Health publication, and are considered in greater detail in this and the chapters relating to particular infections.

Immunological Mechanisms of Immunisation

Active Immunisation

Currently, immunoprophylaxis is based on adaptive mechanisms which involve B and T lymphocytes. B cells produce humoral antibodies (immunoglobulins), which can be produced naturally, induced actively by antigenic stimulation or acquired passively by transfer, for example, from the mother to the fetus via the placenta or to the infant by breast milk or by immunisation. Such circulating antibodies react with the antigenic components of microorganisms and neutralise or destroy them. T cells induce specific cell-mediated immunity including cytotoxic T cells which destroy antigens bearing macromolecular structures, e.g. bacteria and viruses. This is achieved either directly or by means of T-helper and T-suppressor cells. These cells regulate the ability to make antibodies and cytokines and activate various different effector cells destroying foreign antigens on or in host cells. Advantage is taken of the specificity of anti-gen–antibody and antigen–T cell interactions, which recognise both surface and internal foreign antigens, and of the induced immunological memory by active immunisation with attenuated live vaccines and killed (inactivated) vaccines.

Live vaccines induce a cell-mediated response associated with a vigorous amnestic response, whereas inactivated vaccines initially raise a humoral response that is less efficient in terms of immune protection and often requires the administration of several doses of vaccine as part of the primary course. Consequently, for inactivated vaccines, long-lasting immunity is achieved by stimulation of both the cell-mediated and humoral response by the administration of regular boosters. Immunological or biological memory is dependent on prior selection or priming of lymphocyte clones with specific receptors, so that persistence of the microbial antigen or re-exposure to it maintains, activates and indeed expands the relevant immune functions.

Passive Immunisation

Passive immunisation consists of the administration of preformed polyclonal antibodies (immunoglobulins). The protection afforded is very rapid (within a few hours) but lasts for only a few weeks, measured according to the half-life of immunoglobulins. Immunological memory is not induced by passive immunisation.

Three principal types of immunoglobulin are used for passive immunsiation:

- Normal human immunoglobulin fractionated by the Cohn method from pooled plasma obtained from healthy individuals. This preparation is used as prophylaxis in immunodeficient patients and also for pre-exposure and post-exposure prophylaxis of some infections e.g. hepatitis A.
- Hyperimmune globulin which is fractionated from plasma of healthy individuals known to have a high titre of particular antibodies, e.g. hepatitis B,

Table 11.1   Type of vaccines

Live vaccines	Inactivated vaccines	Toxoid vaccines
BCG	Anthrax	Diphtheria
Measles, mumps,	Cholera (oral,	Tetanus
Rubella	parenteral)	
Oral cholera	Haemophilus (Hib)	
Oral poliomyelitis	Hepatitis A	
Oral typhoid	Hepatitis B	
Varicella	Influenza	
Yellow fever	Japanese	
	encephalitis	
	Pertussis	
	Plague	
	Pneumococcus	
	Inactivated	
	poliomyelitis	
	Rabies	
	Tick-borne	
	encephalitis	
	Inactivated	
	typhoid	

varicella zoster, rabies (induced by immunisation), tetanus, (induced by active immunisation with tetanus toxoid).

• Animal antisera produced specifically by toxoid immunisation, e.g. diphtheria, tetanus.

Vaccines: General Principles

The number of vaccines available currently and the introduction of multiple antigenic components (combined vaccines) have made immunisation schedules demanding and increasingly complex. Novel vaccines, such as mucosal, vector-based vaccines, DNA vaccines and edible vaccines produced by recombinant DNA technology in plants, stress the need to understand the immunobiology of these powerful tools of preventive medicine and their importance in the practice of travel medicine.

Types of Vaccine

There are two principal types of vaccine in current practice: live attenuated and killed (inactivated) vaccines (Table 11.1).

Live attenuated Virus Vaccines

These include oral poliomyelitis (Sabin type) vaccine, measles, rubella, mumps and yellow fever vaccine, which have been produced by essentially the random selection

of mutants, principally by serial passage in cells cultured *in vitro* and by adaptation to growth at low temperatures. With the development of recombinant DNA technology, genetic changes can be induced deliberately and precisely in a microorganism, and a virus, bacterium or yeast can also be used as a vector or carrier of genetic material from another source. Genetically-engineered 'site-directed' mutation is another technique to delete virulence. Attenuation of bacteria can also be attained: for example, bacillus Calmette–Guérin (BCG), an attenuated strain of *Mycobacterium bovis*, by culture on a glycerol–bile–potato medium; the production of an attenuated strain of *Salmonella typhi* by exposure to chemical mutagens; and the deletion of toxin from *Vibrio cholerae*.

Concurrent administration of live vaccines, with the exception of yellow fever, and immunoglobulins should be avoided due to the theoretical possibility of competitive inhibition of the immune response. It is recommended that a 3 month interval should be observed between their administration, although an exception may be made when travel is undertaken at short notice; for example, oral polio vaccine may be administered at the same time as human normal immunoglobulin when the risk of exposure to poliomyelitis is considered to be high. With the introduction of more immunogenic active vaccine preparations that have become available, the use of immunoglobulin preparations is expected to decrease significantly in the future.

It is still advised that, in circumstances where the administration of more than one live vaccine is recommended, live vaccines should either be given simultaneously in different anatomical sites, or be given separately, observing an interval of 3 weeks. Although this is based on a historical risk of immunological inhibition, it does apply in practice to the administration of live viral vaccines, e.g. measles vaccine, and tuberculin skin testing, which may result in a false-negative tuberculin skin test in individuals with tuberculosis. Otherwise it is probably of little relevance to the administration and subsequent immune response to live vaccines and consideration should be given to it in clinical practice and the immunisation of travellers.

Killed or Inactivated Vaccines

These are used when live attenuated vaccines are not available or where reversion of an attenuated strain to wild type occurs with relative ease. While killed vaccines are noninfective, they are generally less immunogenic (except toxoids) and several doses and boosters are required. Procedures used for inactivation include formaldehyde, β-propriolactone and, more recently, a variety of ethylenimines and psoralens for viruses. Bacteria are killed or inactivated with formaldehyde, phenol acetone or by heating.

Both inactivated and live vaccines may be given safely concurrently, although different anatomical sites of vaccination are recommended.

Toxoids

Toxoids are bacterial toxins that have been inactivated, usually by formaldehyde, such as tetanus toxoid and diphtheria toxoids. Such toxoids induce protective antibodies in high titre. Toxoids can also be used as carrier proteins for other antigens, but more usefully in the form of conjugate or combined vaccines where they also act as adjuvants, e.g. *Haemophilus influenzae* type b (Hib) vaccine.

Subcellular factors can also be used as immunogens: for example, the outer protein coat of hepatitis B virus—hepatitis B surface antigen; the polysaccharide capsule of pneumococci, *Haemophilus* and meningococci; and the experimental use of protein bacterial filaments (pili) of *Escherichia coli* and *Neisseria gonorrhoea*. A further extension of the use of subcellular fractions is the development of immunogenic peptides synthetically or by cloning.

Live attenuated vaccines are preferred when available, as such vaccines are more likely to be effective, inducing long-term immunity, because they mimic many of the features of the infection itself without causing an illness. Other advantages when compared with killed (inactivated) vaccines include replication of the attenuated virus strain, often localising to a particular site, e.g. poliomyelitis oral vaccine replicates in the gut inducing local as well as systemic immunity; the induction of IgA, IgG and cell-mediated immunity; a single dose may be sufficient (but see under individual vaccines); an adjuvant is not required; low cost and persistent immunity for many years. The disadvantages of live attenuated vaccines include the potential tendency to reversion to virulence, e.g. oral live attenuated polio vaccine-associated poliomyelitis in recipients of the vaccine and in contacts; such vaccines should not be used during pregnancy and in the immunocompromised; and live attenuated vaccines are heat labile and require cold storage or lyophilisation.

Combination Vaccines

In recent years, there has been considerable development in the availability of combination vaccines for both paediatric and adult immunisation. Examples include combination vaccines including inactivated antigenic components such as hepatitis A and hepatitis B, and hepatitis A and Vi antigen (*S. typhi*). Evaluation of the safety and immunogenicity of combination live and inactivated vaccines, e.g. yellow fever, hepatitis A and Vi antigen, are currently being undertaken on a clinical trial basis.

Combination vaccines are a useful addition to the portfolio of travel vaccines now available. The benefits include dual protection against disease with a single injection, so aiding compliance and completion of vaccination courses, as well as added convenience for the individual, particularly for those with needle phobia. Combination vaccines also provide an alternative site for administration of other monovalent vaccines that may need to be administered concurrently, which is of particular value to the traveller person at short notice and requiring several vaccinations.

Adjuvants

These are substances that enhance the immunological response when administered as a component with the antigen. At present only aluminium hydroxide, aluminium phosphate and calcium phosphate are licensed as adjuvants because of their safety and efficacy. Other formulations are under development.

The immunogenicity of an antigen can also be enhanced by using delivery systems in which the antigen is presented to the immune system on the surface of small particulate structures such as liposomes, which have a single or multiple phospholipid vesicles; micelles and immune-stimulating complexes of micelles (ISCOMS).

Other forms of adjuvant substances include bacteria, e.g. *Bordetella pertussis* in the triple DTP (diphtheria, tetanus, pertussis) vaccine; yet others are under investigation, such as BCG and, in particular, a small water-soluble molecule derived from mycobacterium, muramyl dipeptide (MDP), which is claimed to be less toxic.

Cytokines IL-1 and IL-2 and interferon γ have been used as adjuvants, e.g. in nonresponders to hepatitis B vaccine, but their value is controversial and cytokines are not in use.

Other Vaccine Components

Components other than antigen in vaccines include suspending fluids, such as sterile water, saline, culture media, adjuvants, stabilisers, preservatives and antibiotics to prevent bacterial contamination.

Thiomersal is a preservative that contains mercury and has been used as an additive in vaccines and biological substances for some 70 years because it prevents bacterial and fungal contamination, particularly in multidose containers. In 1999, the American Academy of Paediatrics and the US Public Health Service recommended, as part of the effort to reduce exposure to mercury, that the thiomersal content of vaccines should be reduced or replaced with formulations which do not contain thiomersal as a preservative as soon as possible, without unnecessary disruption of the vaccine system. It should be noted that the risk, if any, to infants from exposure to thiomersal is believed to be slight. The demonstrated risks for not vaccinating children far outweigh the theoretical risk for exposure to vaccines containing thiomersal during the first 6 months of life. Single and multiple antigen vaccine preparations, e.g. Hib and hepatitis B/Hib vaccines, are available and others are in preparation.

Storage of Vaccines

The recommendations of manufacturers for storage and

use of vaccines must be observed. Refrigerators must contain a maximum–minimum thermometer and refrigerators designed for vaccine storage should be used. Vaccines should not be stored with food and a secure supply of electricity should be used. Vaccines must not be kept at temperatures below 0 °C and the maximum–minimum temperatures must be recorded daily.

Reconstituted vaccine must be used within the recommended period, usually within 1–4 h, according to the instructions of the manufacturer. Spent or partly used vials and unused vaccine must be disposed of safely, preferably by heat sterilisation or by incineration. The disposal of unused attenuated live vaccines requires special care. The safe disposal of syringes, needles and other sharps without hazard to others and to children is imperative.

Route of Administration of Vaccines

The route of administration of vaccines varies according to the type of vaccine. Most vaccines are given by intramuscular injection.

1. By mouth. Oral polio vaccine (OPV) and oral typhoid vaccine are given by mouth.

2. Intramuscular and subcutaneous injection. With the exception of oral vaccines and BCG, all vaccines available currently should be given by intramuscular injection or by deep subcutaneous injection. The site of injection is important: the upper arm (the deltoid region) or the anterolateral aspect of the thigh are strongly recommended, and *not* the buttock. The injection of vaccine into deep fat in the buttocks is likely, particularly with needles shorter than 5 mm, and there is a lack of phagocytic or antigen-presenting cells in layers of fat. Another factor may involve the rapidity with which antigen becomes available to antigen-processing cells from deposition in fat, leading to delay in presentation to T and B cells. An additional factor may be denaturation of antigen by enzymes as a result of deposition in fat for many hours or days. This is well illustrated in the case of hepatitis B vaccines. There are over 100 reports of low antibody seroconversion rates after hepatitis B immunisation into the buttocks. One comprehensive study in the USA showed that participants who received the vaccine in the deltoid had antibody titres that were up to 17 times higher than those who received the inoculations into the buttock. Furthermore, those who were injected in the buttock were 2–4 times more likely to fail to reach a minimum antibody level of $10 \, \text{mIU} \, l^{-1}$ after vaccination. There are also reports which have implicated injection into the buttock as a possible factor in failure of rabies postexposure prophylaxis using a human diploid cell rabies vaccine. Finally, injection into the buttock, particularly at a site other than the upper outer quadrant, carries the risk of damage to the sciatic nerve.

Injection by the deep subcutaneous route and not intramuscularly is recommended for those with blood coagulation defects, e.g. patients with haemophilia.

3. The intradermal route. BCG vaccine is always given intradermally. A number of other vaccines, such as rabies vaccine, may also be given intradermally. However, apart from BCG vaccine, the use of the intradermal route for immunisation is controversial, particularly in the case of hepatitis B vaccine. One of the reasons for using the intradermal route, apart from BCG, is the possibility of reducing the antigen required for immunisation and thereby the cost of the vaccine. Another reason is more rapid presentation of the antigen to the immune system, resulting in a macrophage-dependent T-lymophcyte response via specific epidermal cells. In the case of hepatitis B vaccines, the immunogenicity of the vaccine given in doses of 0.1 ml (2 µg of antigen protein) has been clearly demonstrated. However, the booster injection at 6 months resulted in antibody titres which were 10 times higher after intramuscular injection than after intradermal inoculation. And there are data indicating that the decline in anti-HBs titre is inversely related to the antibody level attained after completion of primary immunisation. Indeed, trials of intradermal hepatitis B vaccine in children in Gambia have shown a high proportion (59%) of low protective antibody response of less than $10 \, \text{mIU} \, l^{-1}$ (i.e. failure to respond to the vaccine) in one study, and relatively poor antibody responses, as measured by geometric mean antibody titres after intradermal inoculation, in another study. In addition, intradermal inoculation in another requires skill and inadvertent subcutaneous injection into fat will result in a poor immune response.

Adverse reactions after intradermal injection are not marked, although painful local reactions at the site of injection can be severe. It should also be noted that international and national requirements for vaccine manufacture and licensure require assurance on safety, immunogenicity, and protective efficacy of the recommended dosage by an approved route of administration. It seems imprudent to ignore these requirements and recommendations.

Finally, the use of jet injectors for immunisation is not recommended. Current advice is that until studies clarify the risk of infection (such as with hepatitis B and the human immunodeficiency viruses) by different types of injectors, their use should be restricted to special circumstances where it is essential to immunise a large number of persons within a short time.

Adverse Events and Safety of Vaccines

Immunisation is one of the most effective and safest of all health interventions, and all vaccines are tested extensively and evaluated by the manufacturer before licensing, on the basis of quality, purity, safety and efficacy, and then assessed independently before release into general use. Surveillance and monitoring for adverse effects and safety continue after licensing, though organisations such as the World Health Organization and the Immunisation Safety Priority Project, the Global Advisory Committee on Vaccine Safety and the International Partnership Coalition, in addition to national regulatory and safety agencies.

Vaccination is obviously expected to be a safe medical procedure that will lead to no harm because vaccines are given to healthy children (often repeatedly) and to healthy adults. Paradoxically, the very success of immunisation and immunisation programmes in reducing markedly the incidence of infectious diseases, such as smallpox (now eradicated), wild-type poliomyelitis (virtually eradicated in many industrialised countries), measles, rubella, diphtheria and others, has led to increased concern about vaccine safety and adverse reactions. In addition, there have been a number of unwarranted reports alleging an association between vaccines and often diseases of unknown aetiology, e.g. mumps, measles, rubella (MMR) vaccine and Crohn's disease and autism, hepatitis B vaccine and multiple sclerosis and chronic fatigue syndrome (benign myalgic encephalomyelitis; ME). Such associations have not been confirmed by subsequent research, and subsequent studies which fail to confirm the original claim never receive the same publicity so a balanced view is very difficult to achieve.

Nevertheless, adverse events may occur after vaccination and may be either local, i.e. at the site of injection, or less commonly systemic, and may be mild or severe. Serious reactions to vaccines where there is evidence of a causal relationship include the following examples: anaphylaxis and acute encephalopathy with DTP; poliomyelitis in a vaccine recipient or contact of oral polio vaccine; anaphylaxis after MMR vaccine, hepatitis B and others; MMR and idiopathic thrombocytopenic purpura; acute arthropathy and acute arthritis after rubella vaccination, especially in adult women; and an association between some vaccines and Guillain–Barré syndrome and brachial neuritis. In addition, there are reports of postvaccination coincidental events, most of which are not related to vaccination.

The suspected adverse reactions reported on vaccines under the Yellow Card scheme in the UK from November 1990 to October 1995 serve as an example. Approximately 80 million doses of vaccines were distributed in the UK as part of the childhood immunisation programme (some of these vaccines were also given to adults), and there were 5433 reports of suspected adverse reactions to all vaccines. Most of the reports were of mild, self-limited reactions, such as local reactions at the site of injection, transient fever and rashes.

Contraindications to Vaccination

A number of general principles must be considered and several factors must be assessed before vaccination, and it is important to distinguish between true contraindi-

cations and other circumstances. These include the following:

- A careful medical history, and obviously consent for immunisation, must be obtained.
- Pregnancy and breast-feeding mothers.
- Allergy to protein (e.g. eggs) and to other components of the vaccine (e.g. antibiotics such as streptomycin and neomycin).
- Altered immunity.
- A definite history of a severe local or a general reaction to a preceding dose of the vaccine.
- Acute illness; immunisation should be deferred until recovery from the illness.

Pregnancy

Live vaccines should not be given to pregnant women or to women likely to become pregnant within the first 3 months after immunisation because of a theoretical possibility of teratogenic effects or other adverse effects on the fetus. However, where there is a significant risk of unavoidable exposure to infection such as yellow fever, the indication for immunisation outweighs any possible risk to the fetus. Immunoglobulin should be considered where there is a risk of exposure to measles (MMR is contraindicated during pregnancy).

Hepatitis B immunisation is not contraindicated because this is a recombinant purified (killed) surface antigen product. There is insufficient data on the safety of killed hepatitis A vaccine during pregnancy, but this is an inactivated vaccine and as such carries no risk to the fetus. If there is a significant risk of infection with poliomyelitis, oral (live) polio vaccine should not be used but the Salk-type of killed (inactivated) polio vaccine can be administered.

Allergies and Hypersensitivity Reactions

Anaphylactic reactions to a vaccine or to a vaccine constituent are an absolute contraindication to the use of that vaccine or to vaccines containing that constituent. A problem which is encountered frequently is allergy to eggs. Hypersensitivity to egg is a contraindication to influenza vaccine, and an anaphylactic reaction to egg contraindicates influenza and yellow fever vaccines. There is increasing evidence that MMR vaccine can be given safely to children even if they had previously had an anaphylactic reaction after eating food containing egg, but strict caution is advised and day admission to a hospital for the procedure is recommended.

It should be noted that asthma, hay fever or eczema are not contraindications to immunisation.

Altered Immunity

Great care is required in assessing the immunisation of

the immunocompromised. The administration of live attenuated vaccines to persons with altered immunity can result in disseminated infection and other serious effects and, whereas the administration of killed (inactivated) vaccines is not dangerous, the vaccines may be ineffective.

Immunocompromised Infants, Children and Adults

BCG, OPV, MMR or its single components—measles, mumps, rubella—are contraindicated and must not be given to the patient, their household or close contacts (see below for HIV infection and AIDS). Live attenuated vaccines must not be given to patients under treatment for malignant disease with chemotherapy or generalised radiotherapy, or within 6 months of terminating such treatments. Patients receiving corticosteroids orally or rectally (but not topical corticosteroids or by aerosol) at doses of 40 mg per day for 7 days should not be immunised with live vaccines, or an interval of least 3 months should be observed after cessation of the steroids. (Note that in the United States the following applies: live vaccines are contraindicated following the use of oral or rectal steroids at a dose of 20 mg per day for 14 days unless an interval of 1 month has been observed after the cessation of steroids.)

Tissue or organ transplant recipients, including bone marrow transplant recipients, who have received transplants within the previous 6 months must not be immunised with live attenuated vaccines. Antibody levels to diphtheria, tetanus, poliovirus, measles, mumps, rubella and Hib should be checked 6 months after transplant and then appropriate immunisation may be implemented.

Patients with impaired cell-mediated immunity including AIDS (see below), severe combined immunodeficiency syndrome, DiGeorge syndrome and other combined immunodeficiency syndromes must not be given live attenuated vaccines.

Minor antibody deficiency is not a contraindication but the advice of an immunologist should be sought. Patients with major antibody deficiencies receive immunoglobulin therapy and should not be given live vaccines.

Infection with HIV, With or Without Symptoms

Individuals with human immunodeficiency virus (HIV) infection must not receive BCG or yellow fever vaccine. MMR and live attenuated OPV have been given without harmful effects to asymptomatic individuals infected with HIV, who are at an increased risk of infection with these viruses. Note that prolonged excretion of polio virus may occur, and killed (inactivated) Salk-type of polio vaccine may be preferred. In cases of symptomatic HIV infection, the killed polio vaccine should be used and the administration of MMR vaccine must be given with caution and consideration of the risks of vaccination against those of contracting infection. Note that vaccine efficacy may be reduced in individuals with HIV infection and there is often rapid antibody decay and subsequent loss of protection. Other recommended vaccines for this group of individuals include pneumococcal and influenza vaccine, as the risk of infection with either of these respiratory diseases is considerable in terms of morbidity and mortality.

Although yellow fever vaccine is also contraindicated in this group, the vaccine has been administered safely to asymptomatic individuals infected with HIV who have a CD4 count of > 400 cells mm^{-3}, who are considered to be at high risk of infection, and are unable to avoid travelling to endemic areas.

TRAVEL AND ROUTINE VACCINES

All travellers should be advised to undergo a pretravel health risk assessment to determine the potential risks of exposure to infectious disease and other environmental hazards, according to their destination(s), the season in which they are travelling, the circumstances of their stay, i.e. rural or urban, camping or resident in a hotel, mode of transport, and planned activities. Travellers comprise a heterogeneous group whose travel health needs may vary according to their individual requirements, e.g. those of a business traveller may differ considerably from those of a backpacker. The appropriate use of vaccines is to be encouraged, including the use of those that may be optional and those from which travellers may benefit in the future. Achieving immunity against infectious diseases by vaccination often requires that a complete course of immunisation be administered at least 1 month before departure. It is therefore essential that travellers seek travel health advice well in advance of their proposed trip, particularly those who will be travelling for several months at a time; for those who are unable to do so, travel health professionals should consider the use of rapid schedules of administration of vaccines that may be given simultaneously, so as to afford some degree of protection within a short period of time.

The importance of travel health advice, particularly about vaccine-preventable diseases, cannot be overemphasised, as importation of infectious diseases, including the potential for public health concerns, has been realised in recent years. This is facilitated by the ease and rapidity of travel now occurring across the hemispheres of the world, often within the incubation period of many infectious diseases. The following section describes both the routine and the travel-related vaccines currently available (Tables 11.2 and 11.3). Consideration must be given to the fact that different licensing regulations, schedules of administration of vaccines and childhood immunisation programmes apply throughout the world and not all the listed vaccines are available in all countries. This section is based upon the vaccine requirements within the United Kingdom; where possible, the differences in other countries have been highlighted.

Table 11.2 Routine immunisations[a]

Vaccine	Route	Schedule	Booster	Potential interactions
Diphtheria (infants)	0.5 ml i.m. (as DTP)	3 doses at 4-weekly intervals	School entry and leaving	
Diphtheria (adults)	0.5 ml i.m.		10 years	
Tetanus (infants)	0.5 ml i.m. (as DTP)	3 doses at 4-weekly intervals	School entry and leaving	
Tetanus (adults)	0.5 ml i.m. (or as Td)		10 years	
Poliomyelitis (infants)	Oral/i.m.	3 doses at 4-weekly intervals	School entry and leaving	Human normal immunoglobulin, live viral vaccines, tuberculin skin test
Poliomyelitis (adults)		Single dose	10 years	
Haemophilus influenzae	0.5 ml i.m.	3 doses at 4-weekly intervals	NA	
Measles, mumps, rubella	0.5 ml i.m.	Single dose	School entry	Human normal immunoglobulin, live viral vaccines, tuberculin skin test
BCG (at birth for high risk or between 10 and 14 years)	0.1 ml i.d.	Single dose	NA	Live viral vaccines
Hepatitis B (universal)	0.5–1.0 ml i.m.	3 doses; 0,1 and 6 months	NA	
Influenza	0.5 ml i.m.	Single dose; 2 doses at 0, 4–6 weeks for < 13 years old	Annually	
Pneumococcal	0.5 ml i.m.	Single dose	5–10 years	

[a]Based upon schedules of immunisation applicable to the United Kingdom. Individual countries may follow different schedules.
i.d. = intradermal; i.m. = intramuscular; NA = not applicable.

Anthrax

Travellers' risk of infection with anthrax is extremely small and is only of relevance to those handling infected animals or to military personnel who may be exposed in terms of biological warfare. The inactivated vaccine is administered intramuscularly as four doses given at day 0, 3 weeks, 6 weeks and 6 months. Annual boosters may be given. This vaccine is used very rarely in any circumstances.

Cholera

Currently, cholera vaccine is unavailable in the United Kingdom as the inactivated vaccine previously licensed was proven to be of little efficacy in terms of protection against disease, with levels of seroprotection of < 50%. An inactivated, parenteral cholera vaccine is licensed for use in the United States and is administered intramuscularly as a two-dose primary course with 0.2 ml of vaccine given 1 week apart and a booster every 6 months. It is given either simultaneously with or 3 weeks apart from yellow fever vaccine, in order to avoid competitive immunological inhibition. However, an effective inactivated oral cholera vaccine, WC/rCTB, is available and licensed

in several European countries. Administered as two doses at day 0 and 2 weeks, the vaccine, containing inactivated components of *Vibrio cholerae*, provides 85% protection against infection for up to 3 years. It also simultaneously provides 65% crossprotection against *Eschericia coli*, a common cause of travellers' diarrhoea. A live attenuated oral cholera vaccine containing the CVD-103HgR strain has also been licensed in some European countries. The vaccine is given as a single dose and provides protection within 8 days, with duration of 6 months.

There is virtually no risk of cholera infection to travellers; the risk has been estimated at 1 per 1 million travellers. Consequently, travellers are advised to follow strict food and water hygiene precautions to avoid exposure when travelling to countries within the Indian and African subcontinents. Cholera vaccination is only recommended for use in very specific circumstances, e.g. aid workers deployed in an area where there is a confirmed outbreak. As validated by the WHO, no country in the world should expect proof of cholera vaccination before permitting entry; however, a few countries do occasionally request a certificate at remote borders, and in such circumstances a traveller would be well advised to carry a stamped letter of authority stating that cholera vaccine is not indicated.

In the United States, one dose of the inactivated

Table 11.3 Travel immunisations[a]

Vaccine	Route	Schedule	Booster	Potential interactions
Anthrax	i.m.	4 doses at 0, 3, 6 weeks and 6 months	Annually	
Cholera	i.m.	2 doses at 0, 7 days	6 months	(Yellow fever vaccine in USA)
	Oral (inactivated)	2 doses at 0, 14 days	3 years	
	Oral (live)	Single dose	6 months	Live vaccines
Hepatitis A	i.m.	2 doses at 0, 6–12 months	10 years	
Combined hepatitis A and typhoid	i.m.	Single dose	6–12 months for hepatitis A initially and then every 10 years and every 3 years for typhoid	
Hepatitis B	i.m.	3 doses at 0, 1, 6 months; 0, 1, 2, 12 months 0, 7, 21 days and 12 months	3–5 years	
Combined hepatitis A and hepatitis B	i.m.	3 doses at 0, 1, 6 months	10 years for hepatitis A and 5 years for hepatitis B	
Japanese encephalitis	s.c.	3 doses at 0, 7–14, 28 days or 2 doses 0, 7–14 days	2–4 years 3 months	
Lyme disease	i.m.	3 doses at 0, 1, 12 months	? Annually	
Meningococcal meningitis (AC and ACW135Y)	i.m.	Single dose	3–5 years for AC vaccine: at 1 year for children < 18 months old	Less immunogenic in children < 18 months
Plague	i.m.	3 doses at day 0, 1–3 months and 6–9 months	NA	
Rabies (pre-exposure)	i.m./i.d.	3 doses at 0, 7, 21–28 days 2 doses at 0, 28 days	2–3 years 6–12 months	Chloroquine and i.d. route
Typhoid	i.m. Oral	Single dose 3 doses alternate days (4 doses every 2 days in USA)	3 years (2 years in USA) Annually (5 years in USA	Mefloquine, antibiotics, live viral vaccines, oral polio with oral typhoid
Tick-borne encephalitis	i.m.	3 doses at 0, 4–12 weeks, 9–12 months or 2 doses at 0 and 4–12 weeks	3 years 1 year	
Varicella	s.c.	Single dose for 12 months—12 years old; 2 doses at 0, 4–8 weeks for > 13 years old and adults	NA	
Yellow fever	s.c.	Single dose	10 years	Live viral vaccines, tuberculin skin test (cholera vaccine in USA)

[a]Based upon schedules of immunisation applicable to the United Kingdom. Individual countries may follow different schedules.
i.d. = intradermal; i.m. = intramuscular; NA = not applicable; s.c. = subcutaneous.

parenteral vaccine is administered in order to satisfy the entry requirements of some countries. This is accompanied by a valid International Certificate of Vaccination against cholera, which is valid for a period of 6 months. Such procedures avoid travellers being subjected to quarantine rules or vaccination at a border, with its inherent risks.

Diphtheria

Routine childhood immunisation against diphtheria has been instigated for many years throughout the industrialised countries of the world. In the United Kingdom, diphtheria vaccine has been administered routinely as part of the national childhood immunisation programme since 1940, with a schedule of administration of 0.1 ml vaccine at 2, 3 and 4 months of age by the intramuscular route, now combined with tetanus and pertusis, (DTP). Booster doses of diphtheria and tetanus (DT) are given at school entry, followed by a dose of tetanus and low-dose diphtheria (Td) when leaving school. Consequently, travellers born before 1940 should be considered as either naturally immune or they might not have received a primary course of immunisation.

Although diphtheria has been eliminated in industrialised countries, travellers may continue to be exposed to a risk of diphtheria throughout the world, with disease being imported from Africa and the Indian subcontinent, as well as from the Russian Republic and Independent Federations, where there has been an epidemic for several years, since 1991. Therefore, adult travellers to endemic areas and expatriates and aid/health care workers deployed to such countries, who have previously received a primary course of diphtheria vaccine, should receive a low-dose booster, 0.5 ml at 10-yearly intervals. For children over the age of 10 years and adults who may not have been previously immunised against diphtheria, a primary course of three doses of low-dose monovalent diphtheria vaccine should be administered at monthly intervals in order to minimise any local or systemic side-effects or the possibility of a reaction, if naturally immune. A low-dose booster of diphtheria (d) alone or in combination with tetanus (Td), where appropriate, may then be given at 10-yearly intervals. It is strongly advised that infants receive a complete course of immunisation before travelling to developing countries.

An alternative for those who require protection against both diphtheria and tetanus is a combination vaccine using a full dose of diphtheria and tetanus toxoid vaccine (TD) intramuscularly, which is available as a paediatric preparation. It is also licensed for use in children over 10 years old and for adults, with this formulation containing low-dose diphtheria and a full dose of tetanus (Td). This is of value to those travellers who may require either a primary or a booster dose of both vaccines at the time of travel (see below, Tetanus). Neither the monovalent nor the combination vaccines are associated with serious side-effects, the most common of which are pain and swelling at the site of injection.

Haemophilus Influenza

Immunisation with Hib vaccine has now become a component of the routine childhood immunisation programme in industrialised countries, where it is administered simultaneously with the combination vaccine DTP. As a conjugate polysaccharide vaccine, it provides enhanced immunogenicity which is of particular importance in providing protection for infants under the age of 4 years, the highest risk group. It is also recommended for use in asplenic or immunosuppressed children and adults, in whom a single dose of vaccine will protect against serious respiratory disease. This may well be relevant for such individuals travelling where the risk of exposure may be high in developing countries. Booster doses are not recommended.

Hepatitis A

Vaccination against hepatitis A is recommended for all travellers visiting areas outside northwestern Europe, North America, Australia and New Zealand, where the risks of infection from contaminated food and water and close contact with the local population may be high. Those at risk include a wide group of travellers, e.g. short- and long-term travellers, expatriates, aid/health care workers, missionaries and military personnel, and those travellers with underlying medical conditions such as chronic liver disease, where infection with another hepatic virus may result in an increased burden on the liver, leading to morbidity and mortality in this group. The risks of infection with hepatitis A have been estimated as three cases per 1000 travellers per month of travel in a tourist resort, which rises to 20 cases per 1000 travellers per month of travel outside tourist resorts. As the prevalence of infection with hepatitis A has been estimated as 1.4 million cases per annum worldwide, this supports the fact that hepatitis A is the most frequent vaccine-preventable disease in travellers.

The available vaccines are both highly immunogenic and protective when administered intramuscularly at day 0 with a booster at 6–12 months, which confers long-term protection of between 10 and 20 years. Protective levels of hepatitis A antibody are reached within 7–10 days of the primary dose, and immunisation with a single dose of hepatitis vaccine only confers protection for up to 1 year. It is well known that compliance with the first booster at 6–12 months is often poor and so, in terms of practicalities, this first booster dose may be administered safely and effectively at any time after the first dose, which represents the primary course for this vaccine. At present, further booster doses are recommended at 10-yearly intervals but, as this is a highly immunogenic vaccine, further experience is likely to indicate that this may be unnecessary. Recent research has demonstrated the presence of protective antibody levels for up to 20 years by using a model of statistical extrapolation determining the kinetics of antibody decay.

As a result of the paradoxical shift in seroprevalence, adults over the age of 40 years, including those who may have a history of jaundice or have lived in an endemic area for several years, may be naturally immune to hepatitis A. In such circumstances, vaccination may not be necessary and natural immunity may be determined by serological testing of the presence of hepatitis A antibodies (IgG).

Both adult (0.1 ml) and paediatric (0.5 ml licensed for those over the age of 1 year) vaccine formulations are now available. Minor side-effects, such as swelling and pain at the site of injection, may be experienced, with systemic effects, such as nausea and fever, occurring infrequently. The availability of this immunogenic vaccine should dispense with the use of the hepatitis A immunoglobulin preparation whose immunological properties are much inferior to those of the active vaccine (see below, Immunoglobulins). Hepatitis A vaccine induces an adequate level of seroprotection within 7–10 days of vaccination and will provide some degree of protection to an individual travelling at short notice, depending upon their risk of exposure. Some travellers may not reach the high-risk destination for several days after immunisation. However, for those travellers who may be exposed more quickly, the human normal immunoglobulin preparation may be used simultaneously, but at a different anatomical site, with the vaccine in order to provide more immediate protection. Recent studies have demonstrated that hepatitis A vaccine is able successfully to prevent outbreaks of disease when used without the immunoglobulin preparation, by providing either protection or attenuation of infection with hepatitis A, which is afforded by use of the vaccine following exposure. This may therefore have implications for the use of hepatitis A vaccine for those travelling at short notice.

A recent communication from the Public Health Laboratory Service in the United Kingdom has recommended that, due to the lack of availability of human normal immunoglobulin, active vaccination using the licensed hepatitis A vaccines is the preferred option for the protection of travellers. Human normal immunoglobulin will only be made available for the protection of household contacts of confirmed cases of hepatitis A and to control outbreaks.

Combined Hepatitis A and B Vaccine

Recent advances in combination vaccines have resulted in the availability of two different multivalent vaccines, one containing hepatitis A and hepatitis B antigen (see below, Hepatitis B) and the other being hepatitis A and typhoid antigen (see below and Typhoid). These vaccines may be suitable for those travellers at dual risk of exposure to these diseases. The combined hepatitis A and B vaccine is licensed for both paediatric (0.1 ml; 1–15 years) and adult

(1.0 ml; over 16 years) use by the intramuscular route, with the primary course being administered at day 0, 1 month and 6 months. The corresponding levels of antibody protection achieved at each of these time points are 94%, 99% and 100% for hepatitis A, and 34%, 97% and 99% for hepatitis B. Booster doses of the monovalent hepatitis A vaccine should be administered at 10-yearly intervals, with that of the monovalent hepatitis B recommended at 5-yearly intervals at present for those travellers at continued high risk. No serious side-effects have been reported using this combination vaccine. Recent clinical trial data have demonstrated that the hepatitis A and B vaccine may be administered at an accelerated schedule on days 0, 7 and 21, with a booster at month 12, with effective levels of protection at 1 month of 99%, 96% at 12 months and 100% at 13 months for hepatitis A, and 82%, 94% and 100%, respectively, for hepatitis B. Travellers, especially those travelling at short notice, will certainly benefit from the availability of this schedule once licensure has been obtained.

Combined Hepatitis A and Typhoid Vaccine

Another combination vaccine recently licensed in the United Kingdom is that of hepatitis A and typhoid. Licensed currently for those aged 15 years and over, 1.0 ml of vaccine administered intramuscularly will confer protection against hepatitis A and typhoid within 14 days. Booster doses of the monovalent typhoid vaccine must be administered at 3-yearly intervals, while that of the monovalent hepatitis A vaccine must be given at 6–12 months initially, followed by 10-yearly intervals. Again, no serious side-effects have been reported with the use of this vaccine.

The future development of routine universal immunisation programmes against hepatitis A, such as those being introduced in the United States and several southern Mediterranean countries, will be of benefit to future generations of travellers, who will be protected well in advance of their travels. It could also be surmised that future universal immunisation programmes will include the use of the combination hepatitis A and B vaccine, therefore providing concurrent dual long-term protection against both types of viral hepatitis.

Hepatitis B

Protection against hepatitis B has gained greater importance for all types of travellers who may be exposed to hepatitis B by virtue of many risk activities as well as destination. It has been estimated that there are 2 billion people infected with hepatitis B and more than 350 million carriers of disease throughout the world. The risks of infection to travellers has been estimated to be 80–240 cases per 100 000 travellers per month of stay for long-term travellers and 2–10 times lower among short-term travellers. Therefore, hepatitis B is the second most common vaccine-preventable disease in travellers. The risk factors which may lead to subsequent infection with hepatitis B include sexual behaviour, medical or dental intervention, which may follow an accident or an adventure sports activity, acupuncture, tattooing, body piercing, haircuts, sharing razors and toothbrushes; all of these may result in transmission of bloodborne viruses. Travel health care professionals should consider vaccination against hepatitis B for those travelling outside northwestern Europe, North America, Australia and New Zealand, including long- and short-term travellers, those at occupational risk, e.g. aid/health care workers including expatriates, missionaries and the military, those with preexisting medical conditions who may require medical attention while abroad, and young children who may be in contact with other young children in an endemic area.

Hepatitis B vaccine is licensed for administration by the intramuscular route by several different schedules and is also available following the use of the combination hepatitis A and B vaccine (see above, Hepatitis A). Monovalent hepatitis B vaccine may be administered by the following schedules:

- 0, 1 and 6 months with a booster at 5-yearly intervals for those at continued high risk.
- 0, 1 and 2 months with a booster at 12 months.
- 0, 12 and 24 months (licensed schedule in the United States).
- Days 0, 7 and 21, with a booster at 12 months only for those over 18 years of age. The levels of seroprotection achieved are 65% within 1 week of the course and 98% 1 month after the booster dose. This schedule of immunisation is ideal for those travelling at short notice. It is currently only licensed for use in Europe.

The combined hepatitis A and B vaccine may be administered as follows:

- 0, 1 and 6 months.

Nonresponse to hepatitis B vaccine occurs in approximately 10–15% of adult vaccinees and is associated with several factors, including incorrect administration, male sex, increasing age (> 40 years), body mass index and haplotype. Hepatitis B vaccine must be administered intramuscularly in the deltoid muscle or anterolateral aspect of the thigh (see above, Route of Administration). Consequently, it is advisable to check the hepatitis B antibody response following vaccination with the primary course as well as boosters in the older traveller to ensure that adequate levels of protection have been achieved. The use of booster doses remains controversial, but for those at continued high risk, e.g. aid/health care professionals and expatriates deployed to areas of high endemicity, the administration of booster doses of hepatitis B vaccine is recommended at 5-yearly intervals. Travellers who have been exposed to a risk of infection with hepatitis B and are nonresponders or poor responders to hepatitis B vaccine should receive hepatitis B specific hyperimmune globulin as well as a booster dose of hepatitis B vaccine under specific medical guidance (see below, Immunoglobulins).

Universal immunisation against hepatitis B has been successfully implemented in more than 100 countries throughout the world, with the objective of eliminating this disease. Introduction of such programmes will ensure protection against infection for all high-risk groups, including those of travellers, both present and future. Dual and concurrent protection against both hepatitis A and B by use of the combination vaccine may be recognised in future universal immunisation programmes.

Immunoglobulins

The administration of immunoglobulins has been mostly superseded by the advent of improved methods of immunisation with new and improved active vaccines.

Human normal immunoglobulin provides immediate protection against infection with hepatitis A, measles, mumps, rubella and varicella in particular, as high titres of these circulating antibodies are found in the population from whom pooled plasma donations are sought. This preparation may, in theory, cause interference with the immune response to live virus vaccines by competitive inhibition. It is therefore recommended that live vaccines are administered a minimum of 3 weeks before or 3 months after human normal immunoglobulin in order to reduce this possibility. In practice, this may be difficult to achieve when a traveller is travelling at short notice. For those travellers who may be exposed to an immediate risk of disease, both an active live vaccine and human normal immunoglobulin may be administered simultaneously at different sites in order to confer immediate protection. This does not apply to the use of yellow fever vaccine as antibodies to yellow fever are not present in a significant quantity, in the human normal immunoglobulin preparations available from European countries, to cause any inhibition. Also, the potential of interference with the immune response to OPV and simultaneous administration of human normal immunoglobulin is negligible, particularly when OPV is given as a booster dose.

Inactivated and toxoid vaccines may be given simultaneously or at any time with human normal immunoglobulin but at different anatomical sites. Concurrent administration of human normal immunoglobulin and the first dose of hepatitis A vaccine may result in the production of lower hepatitis A antibody levels initially, which has little clinical significance owing to the subsequent synergistic effect, which provides a high hepatitis A antibody level overall.

Other immunoglobulin preparations include those which are specific for hepatitis B, tetanus, rabies and varicella-zoster. All these preparations are highly specific with greater antibody titres than those present in human normal immunoglobulin, as they are prepared from the pooled plasma of individuals who have recovered from infection or have been immunised (see under relevant headings).

Influenza

Infection with influenza virus has been considered in the context of travel-related diseases more recently, with travellers contracting infection and international travel also encouraging the spread of the virus. In general, vaccination is recommended for those aged 65 years and over, including those at high risk with chronic medical conditions, e.g. diabetes mellitus, chronic respiratory disease or cardiovascular disease. In temperate climates during the winter, the same population may be at risk of exposure to influenza after travel to tropical climates, where influenza can occur throughout the year, or to temperate climates of the southern hemisphere when influenza activity is at its peak between April to October. Apart from the environmental considerations, such as season and destination of travel, such individuals may be exposed to a greater than expected risk of infection by virtue of travelling with a group of people and contact with air conditioning, mechanisms by which respiratory-borne disease may be easily transmitted.

Identical or very similar strains of the influenza virus circulate in the different hemispheres, and travellers at high risk should be vaccinated with the current strain specific vaccine for that year. Although different strains of the influenza virus may circulate in tropical countries, the same advice applies to travellers as mentioned previously. Influenza vaccines are administered intramuscularly and are licensed for use for paediatrics and adults. Children under the age of 13 years should receive two doses of vaccine administered 4–6 weeks apart for the primary course. Adults require a single dose as the primary course and, as with children, a booster dose is administered annually. Influenza vaccine is a well-tolerated vaccine, occasionally associated with fever and general malaise which resolves within 48 h. Use of the vaccine is contraindicated in those with a severe egg allergy. It may also be advisable for travellers at high risk of the complications of influenza infection to take antiviral agents for use as either prophylaxis or treatment of infection, as appropriate.

Japanese Encephalitis

Vaccination against Japanese encephalitis is recommended for travellers to Southeast Asia and the Indian Subcontinent who will be visiting an endemic rural area, particularly for longer than 1 month during the appropriate season, which varies between countries within the Asian subcontinent. The risk of infection is extremely low and is estimated at approximately ≤ 1 per million travellers, which increases to 1 per 5000 for travellers visiting a rural endemic area. This risk depends upon the season, location and duration of travel as well as the actual activities of the traveller.

The vaccine is administered by deep subcutaneous injection at days 0, 7–14 and 28 and is licensed for paediatric (0.5 ml for those < 3 years) and adult (1.0 ml) use. A more rapid schedule may be considered for use, with two doses given at 1–2 weeks apart, and the last dose must be administered at least 10 days prior to travel to enable adequate levels of protection to develop. This schedule will confer immunity in 80% of vaccine recipients for between 3 and 12 months. In the United States the vaccine is also licensed for use in a schedule of days 0, 7 and 14. Booster doses are recommended at 2-yearly intervals and an additional 1 ml dose of vaccine is recommended a month after completion of the primary course for travellers over the age of 60 years. All travellers should also observe other methods of protection against mosquito bites.

Japanese encephalitis is a reactogenic vaccine with an incidence rate of severe reactions occurring following administration of 5–10 per 10 000 doses and within 2 weeks of the vaccination. Adverse reactions include urticaria and angiooedema; vaccination is therefore recommended at least 2 weeks prior to travel. The vaccine is unlicensed in the United Kingdom, where it must be given on a named-patient basis.

Lyme Disease

Lyme disease is a tick-borne disease endemic in the forested areas of northeast and north-central regions of the United States and Canada, as well as in parts of Asia and northern European countries, e.g. Scandinavia, where different strains of *Borrelia burgdorferi*, the causal organism, exist. Travellers hiking, trekking or camping in these areas may be exposed to a risk of infection, particularly in the spring and autumn.

Until recently, the only methods of prevention of exposure included the avoidance of walking through infested areas, the use of long-sleeved clothing and the use of insect repellent, i.e. *N,N*-dimethyl-*m*-toluamide (DEET), on clothes and exposed skin to reduce the risk of the tick attaching itself. These presently remain the mainstay of reducing exposure, except for people living in the United States where, recently, an effective recombinant inactivated vaccine against Lyme disease has been licensed: it provides protection against the specific strains of the disease prevalent in the USA.

The vaccine is administered intramuscularly, with three 0.5 ml doses at day 0, 1 month and 12 months with a level of seroprotection of 76% after three doses, which falls to 49% after two doses, clearly indicating that the use of the vaccine should be supplemented by the other methods of personal protection previously mentioned.

The vaccine is licensed for use in those aged between 15 and 70 years of age and is well tolerated with local side-effects being most commonly reported. Alternative schedules of administration are currently being evaluated and it is uncertain whether this vaccine will provide protection against infection with other strains of *B. burgdorferi*. Available data indicate that a booster dose of vaccine will probably be necessary a year after completion of the primary course. For detailed recommendations for the use of Lyme disease vaccine, see Further Reading.

Meningococcal Meningitis

Travellers are at risk of exposure to a specific strain of *Neisseria meningitides*, serogroup A, which is found predominately in sub-Saharan Africa (the meningitis belt), particularly during the dry season. Other countries where outbreaks of meningococcal meningitis group A occur include those within the Indian subcontinent. Travellers at particular risk of infection include aid/health care workers and expatriates visiting and living for extended periods within the indigenous population, backpackers, asplenic children and adults, who are at particular risk when visiting endemic areas. In recent years, following outbreaks of meningococcal disease in those attending the Hajj, a certificate of immunisation against meningococcal meningitis has become mandatory for those travelling to Mecca at the time of the Hajj; the certificate must have been issued less than 3 years, and not less than 10 days, before arrival in the country.

Protection is afforded by the administration of a single 0.5 ml dose of polysaccharide serogroup A and C vaccine administered intramuscularly, with booster doses recommended between 3 and 5 years. The polysaccharide A and C vaccine is a T-cell independent vaccine with poor immunogenicity in children under the age of 18 months, so a booster 1 year later is recommended for this age group. In 2000, a specific strain of *Neisseria meningitides*, serogroup W135, was identified as the cause of an outbreak of disease during the Hajj. Consequently, a quadrivalent polysaccharide, ACW135Y meningococcal meningitis vaccine has been developed and is now the required meningococcal meningitis vaccine for travellers specifically visiting Saudi Arabia for the Hajj.

Recently, a new conjugate serogroup C meningococcal meningitis vaccine has been licensed in the United Kingdom for use in all high-risk groups, including infants, children and adolescents. The introduction of this conjugate vaccine has been very effective, resulting in a 75% decrease in the incidence of disease in a period of 1 year. Infants receive three doses of 0.5 ml vaccine at 2, 3 and 4 months, with children receiving two doses and adolescents and adults receiving a single dose of vaccine. This vaccine does not provide crossprotection against the other serogroups; therefore, those individuals who have received the new conjugate C vaccine must be immunised with the polysaccharide A and C vaccine if travelling to an endemic area.

Current available data indicate that an interval of 6 months should be observed between the administration of the polysaccharide A and C and the subsequent administration of conjugate C vaccine in young children in order to provide enhanced protection. It is advisable for those children who may be exposed to a high risk of exposure to serogroup C to receive immunisation with the C conjugate vaccine within 2 weeks of the polysaccharide vaccine. If the C conjugate vaccine has been administered first and protection is required against serogroup A, a 2 week interval should be observed before the administration of the polysaccharide A and C vaccine. All other vaccines may be administered simultaneously with the C conjugate vaccine, although those vaccines containing diphtheria or tetanus should be administered at a 1 month interval in order to avoid enhanced reactogenicity, as the carrier protein used in the conjugation process includes the use of diphtheria toxin or tetanus toxoid.

Mumps, Measles and Rubella

The risk of travellers' exposure to measles, mumps and rubella is greatest from visits to tropical countries where these diseases remain endemic and routine vaccination programmes are not established, unlike those in industrialised countries. Infants and young children born in industrialised countries, who are going to live for prolonged periods in such areas, should receive their routine childhood immunisations, including MMR, before travel, which may necessitate immunisation at an earlier age than recommended for the national immunisation programme. For those that have defaulted or have not received a complete course of immunisation, the risks of infection should be clearly explained and immunisation strongly recommended and administered before departure. Susceptible adolescents, adults and women of childbearing age should also be vaccinated with MMR before travel or living abroad. Individuals born before 1957 are generally considered to have natural immunity and are therefore not susceptible to infection.

MMR vaccine is administered as a single 0.5 ml dose at 12–15 months of age, with a booster given at 3–5 years of age in the United Kingdom and during infancy and pre-school in other industrialised countries. The safety of these vaccines should not be questioned, as the causal relationship between MMR and autism and Crohn disease remains unproven.

Pertussis

As with other infectious diseases of childhood, pertussis immunisation is a well-established component of routine childhood immunisation programmes throughout the industrialised world. Administered as part of the triple combination vaccines against diphtheria and tetanus as three doses at monthly intervals, the whole cell pertussis vaccine has now been mostly superseded by the availability of the acellular formulation, the use of which is associated with less adverse events. It is strongly advisable that infants receive a complete course of immunisation before travelling to developing countries.

Plague

Regions of the world where the potential for a plague

epidemic to occur include the Indian Subcontinent, South America and Africa, but the risk to travellers is generally very low. If an epidemic were to occur, clearly travellers would be advised to avoid travel to such areas. Aid or health care workers deployed to an epidemic area may be vaccinated with an inactivated vaccine, which is not widely available. Three doses are administered intramuscularly at day 0, 1–3 months and 6–9 months and must be supplemented by methods of personal protection including the use of insect repellent, i.e. DEET, and appropriate clothing, as well as prophylactic antibiotics, e.g. tetracycline if there is a high risk of exposure. If vaccine is unavailable, it may be prudent to administer prophylactic antibiotics and advice regarding methods of personal protection if travel is absolutely unavoidable.

Pneumococcal Infection

Pneumoccocal infection may occur anywhere in the world but is of particular concern to those at high risk of infection in whom invasive disease may be a serious cause of morbidity and mortality. This group includes those who are over the age of 65 years, are immunocompromised, have an underlying chronic medical condition, e.g. diabetes mellitus or chronic respiratory or cardiovascular disease or have asplenia or have undergone a splenectomy. Asplenic individuals, travelling or otherwise, are advised to receive influenza, meningococcal and Hib vaccine as well as pneumococcal vaccine.

Immunisation consists of a single 0.5 ml dose of an inactivated polysaccharide vaccine administered intramuscularly with a booster dose at 5–10 years, which is only recommended for those at significant risk of serious illness. It should be noted that there is an association with rapid decay of antibody levels with polysaccharide vaccines as they are not T-cell dependent, resulting in a poor amnestic response.

Poliomyelitis

Although the objective of WHO and the Expanded Immunisation Programme is to achieve the eradication of polio throughout the world, the disease remains endemic in many countries in Africa and the Indian subcontinent. Although industrialised countries worldwide introduced national childhood immunisation programmes against polio between 1956 and 1962, polio remains endemic in some developing countries. Consequently, travellers, including aid/health care workers, are advised to receive booster doses to ensure maximum protection, particularly when visiting endemic countries. It should also be remembered that individuals born before 1958 may never have been immunised against poliomyelitis and so remain susceptible to infection and its consequences.

Immunisation against polio may be administered either orally or by injection, the latter being given when the oral formulation is contraindicated, e.g. if im-

munosupression is present. A primary course of the live trivalent OPV consists of 0.5 ml of vaccine given at 1-, 2- and 3-monthly intervals, and a booster dose is administered initially at 5 years and thereafter at 10-yearly intervals throughout adulthood. Unimmunised adults should receive the same schedule of immunisation. The oral preparation provides protection against wild virus poliomyelitis and contributes to the provision of herd immunity. However, faecal excretion of the vaccine strain of poliomyelitis virus occurs up to 6 weeks following immunisation. Consequently, oral administration of vaccine may be rarely associated with vaccine-associated poliomyelitis in individuals who are susceptible to infection, the incidence of which ranges from 1 : 520 000 after the first dose to 1 : 12 300 000 after subsequent doses. As this is a disease of faecal–oral transmission, individuals immunised with OPV must observe good methods of hygiene and sanitation in order to avoid transmission of the vaccine strain. In the United Kingdom, the incidence of transmission of the vaccine strain has been estimated as two contact or recipient cases per > 2 million doses of OPV administered. Therefore close and susceptible contacts of those who receive OPV should also be immunised or, if appropriate, receive a booster dose. Asymptomatic HIV individuals may be given live OPV but consideration must be given to the fact that there is likely to be increased faecal excretion of the vaccine virus strain. It may be also be administered to HIV symptomatic individuals, but only at the discretion of a medical practitioner.

Oral polio vaccine may be given simultaneously with other live vaccines. If this is not feasible, then a period of 3 weeks should elapse before administration of another live vaccine in order to avoid inhibition of the immune response to other live vaccines. Concurrent administration of oral polio and oral typhoid vaccines should be avoided because of the shared site of absorption and subsequent immune response. OPV should also be administered 3 weeks before or 3 months after human normal immunoglobulin to allow for a full immune response to develop. It also contains penicillin, neomycin and streptomycin and so its administration is contraindicated if there is extreme hypersensitivity to these constituents.

Inactivated polio vaccine, including the enhanced potency formulation, is administered intramuscularly for those in whom OPV is contraindicated, including the immunosuppressed, the pregnant and adults who have not previously been immunised, including siblings and other household contacts of immunosupressed individuals. Several countries recommend the use of the inactivated preparation in order to avoid any cases of vaccine-associated poliomyelitis. The schedule of administration is identical to that of the oral preparation.

In the United States, enhanced inactivated polio vaccine (eIPV) is administered routinely as part of the childhood immunisation programme at 2, 4 and 6–18 months, with a booster at 4–6 years. Unvaccinated adult travellers should receive eIPV at day 0, 4–8 weeks and 6–12 months. If rapid protection is required, three doses of vaccine may be given at 4-weekly intervals. If an unimmunised adult is travelling and there may be insufficient time to administer a course of eIPV, it would be advisable to provide immunisation using the oral preparation, as the risk of infection with wild virus poliomyelitis may be greater than that of the vaccine strain. A single adult booster at 10-yearly intervals is recommended. The oral and inactivated preparations may be used interchangeably; the latter does not contain penicillin.

Rabies

Although rabies is present throughout the world, the risk to travellers is minimal as this depends upon their chosen destination and activities, i.e. potential contact with animals where rabies is enzootic. Those specific groups of travellers at particular risk include those travelling to an endemic country where they will be more than 24 h away from medical assistance and the availability of rabies vaccine and immunoglobulin is poor, those staying for long periods in remote areas, and those at occupational risk while travelling, e.g. veterinarians, health and laboratory workers.

Pre-exposure immunisation includes the intramuscular administration of 1 ml doses of inactivated human diploid cell rabies vaccine at days 0, 7 and 21 or 28. Boosters are recommended at 2–3-yearly intervals for those at continued risk and may be associated with pain at the site of injection. An alternative schedule of intramuscular administration of rabies vaccine includes two doses of 1.0 ml of vaccine given 4 weeks apart, which confers 98% protection but is recommended for use as long as postexposure treatment is available. A further dose should be administered 6–12 months later for those at continued risk. Intradermal administration of rabies vaccine is licensed in the United States according to the 0, 7 and 21 or 28 day schedule and, if administered correctly, seroprotection may be achieved within 1 month of completion of the course. However, the antibody response following intradermal administration is less vigorous than that of intramuscular injection, which is the preferred method of immunisation. The intramuscular route is also preferred if antimalarial chemoprophylaxis is given concurrently because of the inhibitory effects of chloroquine or mefloquine on the rabies vaccine antibody response. The intradermal route may be used if it is completed in advance of antimalarial chemoprophylaxis, i.e. at least 1 month before travel; the intramuscular route should be used if this is not feasible. A rapid schedule of administration of rabies vaccine, presently unlicensed, may be used for both rapid pre-exposure immunisation and postexposure prophylaxis, with four single doses being administered into each limb.

If bites or scratches are sustained, pre-exposure vaccination does not circumvent the need for postexposure treatment nor the application of first-aid treatment; however, it does both eliminate the need for administration of rabies-specific immunoglobulin and reduce the number of doses of vaccine. In practical terms, preexposure prophylaxis provides a significant level of protection in situations where postexposure treatment may be delayed.

Postexposure immunisation with five doses of human diploid cell vaccine, at days 0, 3, 7, 14 and 30, is recommended within 24 h for those who are susceptible to infection, i.e. unimmunised or incompletely immunised individuals, and includes the administration of rabies-specific immunoglobulin. This must be given immediately and within 7 days, with at least half being injected directly into the site of the wound and the remainder given intramuscularly at a different anatomical site to that of the vaccine. Rabies-specific immunoglobulin is obtained from the plasma of immunised human donors and is administered for rapid postexposure protection simultaneously with active vaccine. For those previously immunised, two booster doses are recommended as soon as exposure has occurred and within 5 days to ensure maximum protection, e.g. day 0 and 3–5 days. There is no indication for the use of the immunoglobulin preparation in this situation.

Travellers who are immunosuppressed should be strongly advised to avoid travel to situations where they may be placing themselves at risk of exposure to rabies infection, as immunisation with rabies vaccine may not confer significant levels of protection.

Rubella

Rubella immunisation is administered as the MMR vaccine (see previously). It is strongly advisable for infants to receive a complete course of immunisation prior to travelling to developing countries. Susceptible adolescents, adults and women of childbearing age should also be vaccinated against rubella prior to travel or living abroad.

Immigrants may be susceptible to rubella infection as a result of the different epidemiological profile of disease in tropical climates. Individuals who immigrate after the age of completion of school immunisation programmes should therefore receive rubella vaccine as a single 0.5 ml injection to avoid infection and the possibility of subsequent transmission.

Tetanus

Vaccination against tetanus is recommended for all travellers visiting any destination throughout the world where the risk of infection remains high. Routine immunisation against tetanus as part of the childhood immunisation programme was introduced throughout the United Kingdom in 1961. Consequently, people born before this may not have received a primary course of vaccination and may be at risk of infection.

A primary course of inactivated tetanus vaccine is administered intramuscularly as three doses of 0.5 ml of vaccine at monthly intervals. Infants receive a combination DTP vaccine as part of their routine immunisations, with booster doses of tetanus when entering and leaving school. Where appropriate, the combination vaccine of tetanus and low-dose diphtheria may be administered, either as a primary course or as a booster for adults and children over the age of 10 years. In the United Kingdom, it is felt that an adult who has received five doses of tetanus vaccine does not require any reinforcing doses, except if a tetanus-prone injury has been sustained, at which time human tetanus immunoglobulin should also be administered. However, booster doses are recommended at 10-yearly intervals for travellers who may be inadvertently exposed to a risk and for whom the benefits of vaccination with tetanus vaccine clearly outweigh the risks of infection with both tetanus and possible blood-borne viruses as a result of the use of contaminated medical equipment in a foreign country.

Tick-borne Encephalitis

Travellers, specifically ramblers and those camping, are exposed to a risk of infection with tick-borne encephalitis when visiting the forested areas of central and eastern Europe and Scandinavia, particularly during the summer months.

The vaccine is administered intramuscularly as a primary course of two 0.5 ml injections given 4–12 weeks apart, which will provide protection for 1 year. A third dose is given 9–12 months after the second dose and confers immunity for 3 years. Booster doses are subsequently recommended at 3-yearly intervals for those at continued risk. Serious side-effects are uncommon. A specific immunoglobulin preparation is available for both preexposure and post-exposure use where appropriate. The vaccine is available in the United Kingdom on a named-patient basis only, and additional methods of personal protection should be afforded by the use of insect repellents and appropriate clothing.

Tuberculosis

The worldwide risk of tuberculosis has gained increased significance with the emergence of drug-resistant tuberculosis associated with the prevalence of HIV throughout the world. Such areas include Africa and the Indian subcontinent, Southeast Asia, Central and South America. Consequently, groups of travellers, including aid/health workers and expatriates living in close contact with the indigenous population in these areas for longer than a month, are at increased risk of exposure to tuberculosis. A recent study estimated the risk of acquiring infection as 7.9 per 1000 person-months of travel for health care professionals and 2.8 per 1000 person-months for all other long-term travellers.

There is no worldwide consensus regarding the recommendations for use of the BCG vaccine. Although given as a routine immunisation in some countries, others con-

sider immunisation only for those at high risk, including aid/health care workers and travellers undertaking a long stay in an endemic area. In the United States, for example, it has been determined that the overall risk for acquiring milliary tuberculosis by the total United States population is low, and therefore a national immunisation programme against tuberculosis has not been implemented. Alternative methods of prevention are used, including the interruption of transmission through the use of tuberculin skin testing for identification of cases and the subsequent appropriate administration of chemoprophylaxis. This policy was introduced following consideration that BCG is not immunogenic and it is associated with side-effects and loss of tuberculin skin test reactivity, so making interpretation of the test difficult if infection has truly occurred.

In the United Kingdom and other European countries, immunisation against tuberculosis is administered routinely following a negative tuberculin skin test, for children aged 14 years. The vaccine is given intradermally in the deltoid as a 0.1 ml dose, which provides protection against the milliary and meningeal forms of tuberculosis for approximately 10–15 years. This primary course provides protection within 6–8 weeks.

Immunisation with BCG should be administered with care as inadvertent subcutaneous administration may result rarely in the formation of an injection site abscess. Keloid scars are also not unusual and can be avoided by immunisation using both the correct site and technique. As BCG is a live vaccine, it may be given concurrently with other live vaccines or after a 3 week interval. Administration of simultaneous vaccines should be avoided in the same arm as BCG, so reducing the risk of regional lymphadenitis.

Tuberculin skin testing, used to determine the presence of immunity or active infection, should be performed prior to immunisation with BCG in order to avoid unnecessary repeat BCG immunisation and the subsequent development of a reaction if the individual is already immune. Reimmunisation with BCG should only be considered if the tuberculin skin test is negative and a BCG scar is not evident.

The reaction to tuberculin testing must be interpreted with caution because glandular fever, viral infections, live viral vaccines, immunosuppressive disease or treatment, and sarcoidosis may suppress it. If one of these is present at the time of the tuberculin test, the result of which is negative, the test should be repeated 3 weeks after recovery (using the other arm) before the administration of BCG, in order to avoid a hypersensitivity reaction. Other contraindications to the use of BCG include the presence of HIV infection, immunosuppression, pregnancy, fever and the presence of skin disease.

Several studies have demonstrated that booster doses of BCG do not provide additional protection and their protective efficacy for travel to endemic areas remains unknown; however, the risks of infection associated with travel to endemic countries have recently been demonstrated to be significant. This warrants a review of the most appropriate strategy of prevention for travellers, which will need to be country specific as national immunisation policies against tuberculosis differ. There has been considerable discussion regarding the administration of BCG vaccine and/or booster doses, or alternatively, the use of skin testing for travellers at risk of infection with *Mycobacterium tuberculosis*.

There are disadvantages associated with either approach. BCG vaccine may produce a false-positive skin test, thus interfering with the ability of the skin test to detect infection following travel. If booster doses of BCG are given, interpretation of the purified protein derivative (PPD) skin test must therefore be made with care. An alternative approach, followed in the United States, is that of undertaking skin testing both before and after travel. The pretravel skin test is used to establish the baseline immunological status of the traveller, and this may be supported by the use of two-step testing in which the skin test may be repeated in order to confirm the presence of a baseline negative result. The post-travel skin test should also be interpreted with caution as false-positives may occur owing to reactivation of previous infection with tuberculosis, to previous BCG vaccination or to the presence of active infection, which then necessitates active treatment. Two-step testing is therefore a valuable tool in assessing the post-travel skin test result; however, the disadvantage of this strategy is that of considerable inconvenience for travellers, in whom compliance may be difficult to achieve.

Another group of travellers to consider are immigrants, including infants, children and adults, to industrialised countries, who should receive a tuberculin skin test unless there is evidence of a BCG scar. Those whose response is positive should undergo further investigation to determine the presence of disease; those whose response is negative should be immunised with BCG as soon as possible. Infants born subsequently should receive BCG immunisation within a few days of birth. Such protocols should be followed because tuberculosis is once more becoming a public health concern, as demonstrated by an 80% increase in notified cases of tuberculosis in the United Kingdom during the past 10 years, mostly attributed to importation of disease.

Typhoid

Typhoid affects an estimated 30 million people per annum worldwide, resulting in approximately 600 000 deaths. The risk of infection to travellers is present throughout the world but particularly following travel to the Indian subcontinent, Asia, South and Central America and Africa where hygiene and sanitation is limited. The risk of infection to unprotected travellers residing in industrialised countries, and who visit India and North Africa, has been estimated as 300 per 100 000 per month of stay. However, for unprotected travellers visiting developing countries other than those previously mentioned, the incidence of infection declines tenfold. In the United

Kingdom there are approximately 200 notified cases per annum, of which 80% are associated with travel in the Indian Subcontinent. In comparison with the United States, 464 patients with typhoid were reported between 1975 and 1984, of whom 62% had travelled abroad. It can therefore be concluded that the incidence of typhoid infection in travellers is declining, due mostly to improvements in hygiene and sanitation in many countries throughout the world.

Typhoid vaccine is currently available in two formulations, oral and by injection. Immunisation with a single 0.5 ml dose for both children over the age of 18 months and adults, administered intramuscularly, provides 70% protection against infection, indicating that adjunct methods of protection, including strict observance of food and water precautions, are necessary. The vaccine is associated with a suboptimal response in infants under the age of 18 months as the polysaccharide vaccine is not T-cell dependent. A booster dose is required at 3-yearly intervals in the United Kingdom (2-yearly for the United States) for those at continued risk. The availability of polysaccharide vaccines has resulted in a decline in the reactogenicity of typhoid vaccine, although some vaccinees do experience pain at the site of injection, a slight fever and headache lasting for 24 h.

The live oral typhoid vaccine is administered as one capsule taken on 3 alternate days, i.e. days 1, 3 and 5, providing 62% protection against infection. The complete course of three capsules must be taken to provide a booster dose, at 3-yearly intervals; however, for those travellers at continued high risk of exposure to infection with typhoid, an annual booster course is recommended. The oral vaccine is well tolerated, with less reactogenicity, and is rarely associated with diarrhoea or vomiting. Its usefulness is complicated by the fact that it is licensed for use in children over the age of 6 years and adults, and there are theoretical concerns regarding its use when administered concurrently with antimalarial chemoprophylaxis or viral vaccines. Oral typhoid vaccine should not be given with mefloquine or antibiotics: the vaccine should be taken 12 h before or after mefloquine and more than 24 h after a dose of antibiotics. The standard contraindications to the use of live vaccines apply and the administration of live polio vaccine and oral typhoid vaccine should be separated by at least 3 weeks unless travel is to be undertaken at short notice, at which time oral typhoid may be administered before, simultaneously or after live polio vaccine. This is to avoid the potential of antibody response competition between the two oral vaccines, whose site of action within the intestinal mucosa is similar. The schedule of administration of the oral typhoid vaccine differs in the United States, where the vaccine is licensed for use as one capsule given as four doses every 2 days, with a booster given every 5 years by way of repeating the full course.

Overall, the currently available monovalent vaccines provide 60–80% protection against infection within 7 days of immunisation and travellers must therefore be advised about the observance of strict methods of personal, food and water hygiene as well.

The availability of a combination vaccine which provides dual protection against both hepatitis A and typhoid is of value to travellers to destinations where there is a risk of exposure to both food- and water-borne diseases (see above, Hepatitis A).

Varicella

Protection against varicella-zoster virus (VZV) infection through immunisation has been available since 1995 and this live attenuated vaccine is currently licensed for use in several countries, including the United States, although it is available on a named-patient basis only in the United Kingdom. The vaccine is administered subcutaneously as a single 0.5 ml dose to healthy children aged between 12 months and 12 years. It may also be administered as two 0.5 ml doses given 4–8 weeks apart to children over the age of 13 years and to adults. Seroconversion rates of 97% have been demonstrated in infants receiving one dose of vaccine, with consistently high levels of antibody present for up to 10 years following completion of the course. In those recipients over the age of 13 years, 78% seroconverted after the first dose, rising to 99% after completion of the course.

The vaccine is recommended routinely for all children aged 12–18 months, susceptible adolescents and adults, including high-risk occupational groups, e.g. health care workers, and nonpregnant women of childbearing age following determination of their immune status to VZV. Immunisation with varicella vaccine should also be considered for susceptible travellers, as confirmed by serological testing where appropriate. This applies particularly to those travelling to tropical countries, especially when close contact with the indigenous population is likely as varicella infection occurs predominantly in adolescents and adults, with significant morbidity and mortality in endemic countries. Recent immigrants from tropical to temperate climates may also be at risk of infection from the indigenous population to which they migrate. Consequently, if the same group return to their country of origin for a visit, they may inadvertently transmit varicella infection to those that they visit.

Yellow Fever

Areas of endemicity for yellow fever include sub-Saharan Africa and Central and South America, with yellow fever vaccination recommended for travel to these destinations. Many countries require evidence of vaccination by way of a certificate of vaccination from travellers arriving from, or who have been in transit through, endemic countries in order to restrict the potential of infection being imported into that country. The International Certificate of Vaccination for Yellow Fever is a requirement of the International Health Regulations of WHO and, as such, the vaccine can only be administered and the certificate

issued from designated yellow fever centres. It is valid for 10 years, beginning 10 days after the date of vaccination. There are circumstances in which administration of yellow fever vaccine is contraindicated for medical reasons, at which time an exemption certificate should be issued, which will then be accepted by the authorities.

Yellow fever vaccine, a live attenuated vaccine, is administered subcutaneously as a single 0.5 ml dose for children aged 9 months and over and adults. The risk of encephalitis following administration of yellow fever vaccine is greatest for those under 4 months old; if absolutely necessary, infants aged 4–9 months old who may be exposed to a high risk of infection can be vaccinated. Although a highly immunogenic vaccine which probably confers life-long immunity, a booster dose is required every 10 years for those at continued risk of exposure. As a live vaccine, its use is contraindicated in the immunosupressed, pregnancy and for those with a serious egg allergy or hypersensitivity to polymyxin and neomycin. It may be administered simultaneously with human normal immunoglobulin and the same guidance applies to the administration with other live vaccines.

The safety of immunisation with yellow fever vaccine has yet to be fully determined in asymptomatic HIV individuals. There are occasions when the risk of infection would appear to be unavoidable, at which time an exemption certificate may be provided, or, if absolutely necessary, vaccination may be given for those individuals with a CD4 count > 400 cells mm^{-3}. In these circumstances, immunisation may be less effective and protection should be afforded by other means, for example the use of insect repellent and appropriate clothing.

FURTHER READING

Ambrosch F, Wiedermann G, Andre FE et al. (1994) Clinical and immunological investigation of a new combined hepatitis A and hepatitis B vaccine. Journal of Medical Virology, 44, 452–456.

Anonymous (1998) World Health Organization's global programme for vaccines and immunisation: recommendations from the Scientific Advisory Group of Experts. Weekly Epidemiological Record, 37(73), 281–288.

Anonymous (2000) Influenza vaccine. Weekly Epidemiological record, 35, 281–288.

Anonymous (2000) Hepatitis A vaccines. Weekly Epidemiological Record, 5, 38–44.

Anonymous (2000) Human normal immunoglobulin: lack of availability for travellers. Communicable Disease Report Weekly, 10(34), 301.

Anonymous (2000) Typhoid vaccines. Weekly Epidemiological Record, 32(75), 257–264.

Bedford H and Elliman D (2000) Concerns about immunisation. BMJ, 320, 240–243.

Bock HL, Loscher T, Scheiermann et al. (1995) Accelerated schedule for hepatitis B immunisation. Journal of Travel Medicine, 2, 213–217.

Brown F, Dougan G, Hoey EM et al. (1993) Vaccine Design. Wiley, Chichester.

Centers for Disease Control (1988) Cholera vaccine: recommendations of the Advisory Committee on Immunisation Practices. *Morbidity and Mortality Weekly Report*, **37**(40), 617–618, 623–624.

Centers for Disease Control (1993) Inactivated Japanese encephalitis virus vaccine: recommendations of the Advisoty Committee on Immunisation. *Morbidity and Mortality Weekly Report* **42** (RR-1), 1–15.

Centers for Disease Control (1996) Prevention of varicella: recommendations of the Advisory Committee on Immunisation Practices. *Morbidity and Mortality Weekly Report*, **45** (RR-11).

Centers for Disease Control (1996) Prevention of plague: recommendations of the Advisory Committee on Immunisation Practices. *Morbidity and Mortality Weekly Report*, **45** (RR-14).

Centers for Disease Control (1999) Human Rabies Prevention USA: recommendations of the Advisory Committee on Immunisation Practices. *Morbidity and Mortality Weekly Report*, **48** (RR-1), 1–21.

Centers for Disease Control (1999) Prevention of varicella: updated recommendations of the Advisory Committee on Immunisation Practices. *Morbidity and Mortality Weekly Report*, **48** (RR-06), 1–5.

Centers for Disease Control (1999) Recommendations for the use of Lyme disease vaccine: Advisory Committee on Immunisation Practices. *Morbidity and Mortality Weekly Report*, **48** (RR-07), 1–17.

Centers for Disease Control (2000) Poliomyelitis prevention in the US: updated recommendations of the Advisory Committee on Immunisation Practices. *Morbidity and Mortality Weekly Report*, **48** (RR-5).

Cobelens FGJ, van Deutekom H, Draayer-Jansen IWE *et al.* (2000) Risk of infection with *Mycobacterium tuberculosis* in travellers to areas of high tuberculosis endemicity. *Lancet*, **356**, 461–465.

Department of Health *et al.* (1995) *Health Information for Overseas Travel*. Stationery Office, London.

Hutin YJF and Chen RT (1999) Injection safety: a global challenge. *Bulletin of the World Health Organization*, **77**, 787–788.

Kane M, Banatvala J, Da Villa G *et al.* (2000) Lifelong protection against hepatitis B and the need for boosters. *Lancet*, **355**, 561–565.

Lifson AR (2000) *Mycobacterium tuberculosis* infection in travel-

lers: tuberculosis comes home. *Lancet*, **356**, 442–443.

Pervikov Y (ed.) (2000) Dengue and Japanese encephalitis vaccines. *Vaccine*, **18** (suppl. 2).

Ryan CA, Hargett-Bean NT and Blake PA (1989) *Salmonella typhi* infections in the US 1975–84: increasing role of foreign travel. *Reviews in Infectious Disease*, **11**, 1–8.

Sagliocca L, Amoroso P, Stroffolini P *et al.* (1999) Efficacy of hepatitis A vaccine in prevention of secondary hepatitis A infection: a randomised trial. *Lancet*, **353**, 1136–1139.

Salisbury DM and Begg NT (1996) *Immunisation against Infectious Disease*. Stationery Office, London.

Sanchez JL and Taylor DN (1997) Cholera. Lancet, **349**, 1825–1830.

Scholtz M and Duclos P (2000) Immunisation safety: a global priority. *Bulletin of the World Health Organization*, **78**, 153–154.

Scottish Centre for Infection and Environmental Health (1999) Recommendations on hepatitisA immunisation for travellers. *SCIEH Weekly Report*, **33**, 173.

Steffen R (1993) Hepatitis A and hepatitis B: risks compared with other vaccine-preventable diseases and immunisation recommendations. *Vaccines*, **11**, 518–520.

WHO (2000) *International Travel and Health*. World Health Organisation, Geneva.

Zuckerman JN (1996) Non-respnse to hepatitis B vaccines and the kinetics of anti-HBs production. *Journal of Medical Virology*, **50**, 283–288.

Zuckerman JN and Steffen R (2000) Risks of hepatitis B in travellers as compared to immunisation status. *Journal of Travel Medicine*, **7**, 170–174.

Zuckerman JN, Dietrich M, Nothdurft HD *et al.* (2000) Rapid protection against hepatitis A and hepatitis B following an accelerated schedule of a combined hepatitis A/B vaccine. *Antiviral Therapy*, **5** (suppl. 1), 8.

ADDITIONAL RESOURCES

Centres for Disease Control and Prevention. *Travellers' Health. Health information for international travel.* www.cdc.gov

World Health Organisation. *International Travel and Health: Vaccination requirements and Health Advice.* www.who.int

12

Returned Travellers

Nicholas J. Beeching and Sharon B. Welby

Liverpool School of Tropical Medicine, Liverpool, UK

INTRODUCTION

The exponential growth of international travel means that health care workers regularly see patients who have recently travelled abroad or outside their local area of residence. A travel history is rarely elicited in most day-to-day consultations, leading to delay in considering and making a relevant diagnosis. The travel-related problem is often a minor cosmopolitan illness—we have probably all suffered from respiratory infections acquired while attending professional conferences, and international airline passengers routinely expect to have swollen feet and jet lag when they reach their destinations. However, the increasingly adventurous nature of many tourists and the continued emergence of new infection risks in all parts of the world make it essential that travel-related illness is both considered and managed appropriately.

The purpose of this chapter is to outline an approach to the diagnosis and management of travel-related disease, concentrating on infections imported from less economically advantaged areas of the world to the more affluent nations. The framework for this approach is careful history taking, relevant examination and investigation.

The travel 'expert' will need to have a detailed understanding of the health problems most likely to affect different groups of travellers, coupled with current knowledge of the illnesses prevalent in areas visited by the patient. Synthesis of this knowledge with the clinical presentation of the patient should enable a sensible syndromic differential diagnosis to be made, allowing for an appropriate management plan to be developed. Our aim is to highlight key decision points in these steps, using worked examples and illustrative tables and algorithms. The emphasis is on imported infections that are most 'important', either by virtue of being common and amenable to treatment, or because of their public health importance on the rare occasions that they are seen. Greater detail about individual infections is found in other chapters of this book or in major textbooks of infections and tropical medicine (see Further Reading).

Patients who are suspected in community practice of having a specific illness, such as malaria, HIV infection or imported parasitosis, will usually need to be referred to hospital or clinic-based specialists for further investigation and management. In these cases the priorities are to prevent immediate morbidity and mortality and to minimise any public health risks to the general population or to health care workers. In some groups of travellers, post-travel health screening may be appropriate in either a general practice setting or in specialist clinics, and we discuss issues relating to screening at the end of the chapter.

HISTORY

A precise and detailed travel history is essential. This should include questions about all previous international travel as well as the most recent trip, as valuable clues may be missed.

> Case History
> A 45-year-old man presented to the emergency room late in the evening with fever, dizziness and diarrhoea. He had returned from a 1 week holiday in Greece 6 days previously, and had visited India 6 months before. He had high fever, hypotension, mild renal failure and marked thrombocytopenia. His blood film was not examined until the following morning, when it showed 17% parasitaemia with *Plasmodium falciparum* malaria and treatment with quinine was started. Further questioning revealed that he had been working in West Africa for 2 months until he joined his wife in Greece.

Type of Traveller

The key initial questions to be asked when taking the travel history are summarised in Table 12.1. These can be

Principles and Practice of Travel Medicine. Edited by Jane N. Zuckerman.
© 2001 John Wiley & Sons Ltd.

Table 12.1 Initial questions for the travel history

When
- When did you last travel outside the country? Exact dates of departure and return
- When did you last travel away from home? When did you travel before that?
- When did you first get ill? Exact dates if possible

Where
- Where were you born?
- Where exactly did you go on this trip? Precise location, not just country or continent
- Where did you stop along the way?

Why
- Why did you go abroad? Business, tourism, visiting family, etc.

What
- What health problems did you already have before travel?
- What method of transport did you use?
- What did you do there? Risk activities—freshwater contact, etc.
- What precautions did you take before you went? List immunisations, etc.
- What precautions did you take while there? Quantify adherence to safe eating, safe sex, antimosquito measures

Who
- Who else went with you?
- Who else got ill?

modified depending on the type of traveller and the likely risk behaviour and possible exposure to disease. Short-term casual tourists to coastal Kenya are at risk of acquiring malaria even when taking chemoprophylaxis, but are less likely to acquire legionella infection, which is more typically associated with air-conditioned hotels in Spain, Turkey or other 'western' settings. The younger, adventurous overland traveller is more likely to be exposed to pathogens in the environment and to their vectors and to take risks with their diet, daily activities and interpersonal behaviour. For example, the incidence of hepatitis A is estimated to be 2–3/1000 in 'ordinary' travellers and 20/1000 in backpackers (Steffen et al., 1994). Expatriates working overseas have varying levels of access to preventive health care and often disregard advice they have received, especially about malaria prophylaxis. The risk of acquiring some infections also increases with the amount time spent overseas. Attack rates of malaria in British travellers to West Africa increased from 61/100 000 in those travelling for 1 week to 4899/100 000 in those travelling for 6–12 months (Phillips-Howard et al., 1990).

Immigrants present their own problems, which are discussed in greater detail in Chapter 28. Within this broad group there will be several subdivisions according to the reason for immigration. Refugees and other displaced persons are likely to import illnesses that are endemic within the communities from which they originate, and may also have been exposed to physical deprivation, abuse and overcrowding in reception camps during their travels. They may present with a combination of background endemic illness, as well as emerging or epidemic infection, often superimposed on a different cultural approach to health care usage and complicated by the psychosocial distress of the upheavals in their lives (Burnett and Peel, 2001). Other groups of immigrants often have a better established community base in their adopted country as well as maintaining links through several generations with their country of ethnic origin.

Members of these groups visiting relatives at 'home' are less likely to be aware of, or to take, preventive precautions advised for expatriate tourists or visitors (Phillips-Howard et al., 1990), but will have lost the immunity to endemic disease that is acquired by constant exposure. Illness in this group is relatively overrepresented in summary statistics of imported disease.

Individual host factors influence both susceptibility to disease and the mode of presentation. Patients should be asked about background illness, such as ischaemic heart disease, chronic respiratory illness, renal disease, immobility due to arthritis or other disability and prior psychiatric illness. Diabetes is thought to predispose the individual to many infections and is an important risk factor for acquiring melioidosis. Pregnant women are more likely to have recrudescence of malaria or to have more severe clinical illness due to malaria. Ill children present with less localising features of illness than adults and are more likely to have fever with gastrointestinal infections. Patients who have had a splenectomy are at increased risk of bacterial infections such as invasive pneumococcal disease, and blood parasites, particularly malaria and babesiosis. Pre-existing anaemia will exacerbate the presentation of many acute infections and sickle cell disease specifically carries risks of both pneumococcal disease and malaria, as well as crises induced by travelling to high altitude or by dehydration. Smoking increases the risk of pneumococcal infection, meningococcal disease and severe Legionnaires' disease. Excess alcohol consumption is associated with increased risk-taking in general, and particularly with a high risk of trauma, drowning incidents, and traffic accidents and increased sexual risk behaviour, while patients with cirrhotic liver disease have high morbidity from many bacterial infections and from viral infections causing hepatitis. Patients with immunosuppressive disorders, particularly HIV-related problems and those on chemotherapy for cancer or after transplants, are more susceptible to a wider variety of pathogens than the immunocompetent person.

Drugs and Vaccinations

A full immunisation history is essential as it will alter the approach to diagnosis in ill patients.

Case History
A 36-year-old man returned from the Ivory Coast to Germany with a febrile illness, jaundice and bleeding diathesis. He was initially thought to have Lassa fever and was nursed accordingly until his death. The cause of death was determined to be yellow fever, which had been thought unlikely as the patient had claimed, incorrectly, to have been immunised against yellow fever (Schmetzer, 1999).

Yellow fever vaccination is extremely effective, but cases continue to be imported to Europe and North America from both Africa and South America by travellers who have not been immunised. Active immunisations against hepatitis A and B are both more than 90% effective, whereas currently licensed vaccines against typhoid only have 70% or less protective efficacy. The effectiveness of antimosquito bite measures and antimalarial chemoprophylaxis is variable and highly dependent on adherence by travellers.

Concurrent medication for underlying illness may cause or exacerbate symptoms. For example, aspirin taken to prevent travel-related thrombosis may cause or worsen gastrointestinal bleeding, and diuretic therapy increases the dehydration associated with diarrhoeal illness. Mouth ulcers are common in patients taking proguanil; chloroquine can exacerbate psoriasis; prophylactic doxycycline is associated with vaginal thrush and with photosensitive rashes; and mefloquine use has been linked with various neuropsychiatric effects (Nosten and van Vugt, 1999).

Where Did the Patient Visit?

This must include the locality as well as the countries visited. While many infections are cosmopolitan, their prevalence within a given country may be very localised. British travellers to North America will not be exposed to infections such as plague, tularaemia, hantavirus infection, Colorado tick fever or coccidioidomycosis if they visit New York, although these are all possibilities if they have been camping out in some of the southern States. Malaria is a significant hazard for travellers to Kenya but should not be a problem for those who stay in Nairobi, and similarly tourists to Thailand are unlikely to acquire malaria in Bangkok but might be at risk in rural areas. The geographical distribution of the more common imported diseases is illustrated with cases in this chapter and in detail in other chapters in this book. Current information on established and emerging infections in different parts of the work is available from a number of websites (see Additional Resources).

Health care workers need to be aware of the geography of the patterns of drug resistance of organisms as well as the distribution of the pathogens themselves. Many gastrointestinal pathogens such as *Shigella* and *Salmonella* species acquired overseas are resistant to commonly used antimicrobials (Hart and Kariuki, 1998). *Salmonella typhi* from Asia and the Indian subcontinent and *Mycobacterium tuberculosis* from many countries exhibit multidrug resistance. Resistance of falciparum malaria to chloroquine is almost universal, while resistance to other antimalarials is more patchy in distribution (Chapter 8). Knowledge of these resistance patterns is essential when planning empirical therapy before the results of culture (and sometimes resistance testing) are available.

When Did They Travel and For How Long?

A precise history of timing of travel is essential for comparison with the known incubation periods of specific illnesses, some of which are summarised in Table 12.2.

In the clinic consultation, it is rarely as easy as one might expect to correlate exposure dates with illness in individual patients. In this situation, incubation periods are most useful for excluding illness. For example, malaria does not present in travellers less than 8 days after arriving in a malarious area. Viral haemorrhagic fever can safely be excluded in a patient who has had possible exposure, but has left an endemic area more than 21 days before the onset of symptoms. In epidemic situations or outbreaks clearly related to a point source, knowledge of precise travel and exposure times is very helpful, such as locating a patient within a known outbreak of Legionnaires' disease on a cruise ship or in a specific hotel, or identifying a person as being part of a point source outbreak of food-borne salmonellosis at a wedding reception on the other side of the country. Such examples emphasise both the use of the travel history to inform the diagnosis of the patient and the need for rapid notification of suspected and confirmed diagnoses to the appropriate public health authorities or surveillance scheme, so that patterns of illness and outbreaks can be recognised and disseminated back to the health care community.

At the other end of the scale, disease with long incubation periods may not be recognised as travel-related by either the patient or physician. Hepatitis B transmitted by tattoo during an overland trip through Asia might not cause illness until 6 months later. The increased risk of tuberculosis in immigrants persists for at least 5 years after arrival in Britain (Ormerod, 2000) and the clinical incubation period of symptomatic leprosy is several years. We have seen patients with colonic bleeding due to schistosomiasis presenting for the first time 10 years after travel to Africa. Some infections can persist for many years, such as strongyloidiasis, which we still see in ex-prisoners of war who worked over 50 years ago on the Thai–Burma railway during World War II (Gill and Bell, 1979; Archibald *et al.*, 1993). Knowledge of the biology of the pathogen can also be integrated with the detailed travel history to recognise the limitation of investigation at different phases of the illness.

Table 12.2   Sample incubation periods

Short (< 10 days)	Medium (10–21 days)	Long (> 21 days)	Very long
Amoebiasis (intestinal)	Amoebiasis	Amoebic liver abscess	AIDS/symptomatic HIV
Anthrax (pulmonary)	Arboviral infections (few)	Babesiosis	Amoebic liver abscess
Arboviral	Murray Valley fever	Bartonellosis	Chagas' disease
Japanese encephalitis	Encephalitis	Brucellosis	Leprosy
Dengue fever	St Louis	Cytomegalovirus	Leishmaniasis
Yellow fever	Tick-borne	Filariasis	Melioidosis
Babesiosis	Japanese	Hepatitis (A–E)	Neurocysticercosis
Bacterial meningitis	Babesiosis	HIV infection (acute)	Schistosomiasis
Brucellosis	Brucellosis	Infectious mononucleosis	Strongyloidiasis
Campylobacter enteritis	Cytomegalovirus	Leishmaniasis (visceral)	Tuberculosis
Diphtheria	Haemorrhagic fevers	Lyme disease	
Ehrlichiosis	Congo–Crimean	Malaria (all species)	
Fascioliasis (acute)	Lassa fever	Melioidosis	
Haemorrhagic fevers	Marburg/Ebola	Q fever	
Argentinian	Hepatitis A, E	Rabies	
Bolivian	Histoplasmosis	Schistosomiasis (acute)	
Lassa	Leptospirosis	Secondary syphilis	
Marburg/Ebola	Loeffler syndrome	Toxocariasis	
Congo–Crimean	Lyme disease	Trench fever	
Influenza	Malaria (all species)	Trypanosomiasis	
Legionnaires' disease	Measles	African	
Leptospirosis	Melioidosis	(*T. b. gambiense*)	
Loeffler syndrome	Monkeypox	American	
Lyme disease	Polio	Tuberculosis	
Malaria (unusual)	Psittacosis	Typhoid	
Melioidosis	Q fever		
Monkeypox	Rabies		
Necrotising enterocolitis	Toxocariasis		
Plague	Toxoplasmosis		
Poliomyelitis	Trichinosis		
Psittacosis	Trypanosomiasis		
Rabies	African		
Rat-bite fever	(*T. b. rhodesiense*)		
Relapsing fevers (borreliosis)	American		
Rotavirus	Typhoid		
Salmonella enterocolitis	Typhus		
Shigellosis	Flea-borne		
Streptococcal pharyngitis	Louse-borne		
Toxigenic *Eschérichia coli*	Mite-borne (scrub)		
Toxocariasis			
Trypanosomiasis (African, acute)			
Tularaemia			
Typhoid and paratyphoid			
Typhus			
African tick			
Flea-borne			
Louse-borne			
Mite-borne (scrub)			
Rocky mountain spotted fever			
Yersiniosis			

Case History

A 19-year-old student presented in Liverpool with a 4 week history of headache, fever and malaise, followed by a dry cough and a transient urticarial rash. He had fever and a peripheral eosinophil count of $2.4 \times 10^9 1^{-1}$ but appropriate examination of faeces and urine for parasites and schistosomal serology was negative. Acute schistosomiasis (Katayama fever) was diagnosed by the family practitioner, who was aware that the patient had been swimming in Lake Malawi 6 weeks previously with a group of students who had similar symptoms. We confirmed the clinical diagnosis and 6 weeks later his serology became positive, and scanty ova of *Schistosoma haematobium* were found.

Other students from the party had been investigated elsewhere in the country without a diagnosis being made, partly because the attending physicians failed to recognised that serology make take more than 2–3 months to become positive, and that conventional parasitological tests are negative during the acute phase of the illness.

Why Did They Travel and What Did They Do?

Some occupational groups are inevitably at greater risk of exposure to vectors and illness. Health care personnel are particularly prone to the risk of needlesticks and similar accidents, as well as dealing with patients with pathogens that can be spread by airborne droplets or by direct contact with body fluids and faeces. The difficulties in preserving high levels of risk avoidance in a rural hospital setting are all too common and emphasised by the tragic deaths of health care workers assisting patients with Ebola infection in Uganda or Congo–Crimean haemorrhagic fever in South Africa, the Middle East (Suleiman *et al.*, 1980) and Pakistan (Burney *et al.*, 1980). Tuberculosis has always been a problem for health care staff and remains a hazard for those working overseas in areas of high endemicity (Harries *et al.*, 1997).

Other groups, such as veterinarians and agricultural workers, will be at increased risk of zoonotic infections such as brucellosis, Q fever and anthrax through contact with animals. Forestry workers, construction workers and other project workers may venture into forested or other rural ecosystems and be at risk of arthropod-borne diseases such as trypanosomiasis, onchocerciasis, loiasis, filariasis, rickettsial infection, leishmaniasis and yellow fever.

Aid workers and others in refugee or school settings are at risk of acquiring diseases of overcrowding such as respiratory infections and meningococcal disease. Military personnel constitute a special group. Although they may have received adequate immunisation and advice on

Table 12.3 Specific exposures and tropical infections causing fever

Exposure	Infection or disease
Raw, undercooked or exotic foods	Enteric infections, hepatitis A or E, trichinosis
Drinking untreated water, milk, cheese	Salmonellosis, shigellosis, hepatitis, brucellosis
Freshwater swimming	Schistosomiasis, leptospirosis
Sexual contact	HIV, syphilis, hepatitis A or B, gonorrhoea, etc.
Insect bites	Malaria, dengue fever (mosquitoes); typhus, Crimean–Congo haemorrhagic fever, borreliosis, tularaemia (ticks); Chagas disease (reduviid bugs); African trypanosomiasis (tsetse flies)
Animal exposure/bites	Rabies, Q fever, tularaemia, borreliosis, viral haemorrhagic fevers, plague
Exposure to infected persons	Lassa, Marburg or Ebola viruses; hepatitis; typhoid; meningococcaemia

After Humar and Keystone (1996).

malaria prevention, the latter advice may not be heeded in difficult field conditions. Their activities may result in considerable exposure to a wide variety of soil-borne pathogens, for example hookworms and *Strongyloides* spp, as well as to arthropod-borne and food- and water-borne illnesses. Sexually transmitted diseases also continue to be a particular problem in military personnel and merchant seamen.

Table 12.3 summarises some of the typical risks associated with different patterns of exposure behaviour.

Sexual History

The importance of taking an appropriate sexual history from travellers cannot be overemphasised. This poses problems in the busy practice, clinic or hospital setting but it is essential to include such enquiries as a matter of routine. A suitable excuse needs to be found to exclude parents, partners or friends who accompany the patient while this part of the history is taken. People go on holiday to have fun, and for many this includes new sexual experiences, often associated with high-risk partners. This is particularly true for young adults. In one British study, 74% of male migrant tourism workers in a popular coastal resort had sex with tourists, almost half with more than four tourists, and only 40% of respondents had used a condom (Ford and Inman, 1992). Teenagers are just as busy when visiting other European destinations, particularly those associated with the dance-music scene. In a recent study performed in Ibiza, over a third of 846 young adults attending music venues had taken recreational drugs, and 58% of males and 50% of females had at least one new sexual partner during their 1–2 week stay. Twenty-six per cent did not use condoms and 23% had more than one sexual partner (Bellis *et al.*, 2000). We have observed similar risk behaviour in expeditioners and in long-term expatriates, often associated with high levels of alcohol use.

The risk of acquiring sexually transmitted infection abroad is very high and includes 'traditional' infections such as gonorrhoea (often multidrug resistant), syphilis, chancroid and lymphogranuloma venereum (Adler, 1997; Wang and Celum, 1999). The prevalence of HIV in sex workers in many cities and towns in India, Thailand and much of Africa exceeds 60% and is rapidly increasing in many other parts of the world, including the Eastern bloc countries, where syphilis is also reaching epidemic proportions (Tichonova *et al.*, 1997).

Rates of HIV infection in 2000 returning Dutch travellers were low (0.2%) in the late 1980s, despite considerable risk activity while overseas (Houweling and Coutinho, 1991) and compared with more than 1% in returning Belgian expatriate workers (Bonneux *et al.*, 1988) and 1.2% of heterosexual male travellers seen in London (Hawkes *et al.*, 1994). The improved recent Dutch figures may reflect improved attitudes to safe sex, with an increase in condom use to 67% of occasions by the 23% of Dutch expatriates who had sex with casual local partners while on overseas assignments (de Graaf *et al.*, 1997). In the UK, new heterosexual HIV infections have outnumbered those in homosexuals in both 1998 and 1999 and many of these infections are imported from overseas, either directly or indirectly.

HIV is the single most common imported lethal infection but modern management approaches are improving the prognosis. Patients who have been at risk of infection need appropriate counselling with a view to testing for HIV and sexually transmitted infections. This usually implies referral to a genitourinary medicine clinic for a full screen because sexually transmitted diseases may be asymptomatic in both men and women.

How Did They Go?

In addition to the behavioural and exposure risks already described in different groups of travellers, the mode of travel predisposes to specific medical problems. Immobility due to prolonged travel is likely to predispose to venous thrombosis and pulmonary embolism, especially in patients with pre-existing risk factors. It is possible that specific factors associated with air travel, such as low air pressure, hypoxia and dehydration, exacerbate this, but the evidence base is poor and few scientific data have been published to quantify such an increase in risk (Kesteven, 2000; Geroulakos, 2001). Venous thrombosis and pulmonary embolus should be considered in the differential diagnosis of recent travellers, particularly in those with leg pain, fever or dyspnoea.

In-flight medical emergencies affect about 1/11 000 passengers and comprise a full range of medical problems, some of which need further attention when the patient arrives, including the effects of overindulgence in alcohol (Beighton, 1967; Dowdall, 2000; Goodwin, 2000). Recirculation of air leads to sharing of pathogens, and the transmission of influenza (Klontz *et al.*, 1989) and tuberculosis between air passengers is recorded (Driver *et al.*, 1994; Kenyon *et al.*, 1996). Although the risk of tuberculosis transmission is low and is limited to passengers near to the index case, it generates considerable concern (Ormerod, 2000).

Passengers and crew on cruise ships are also exposed to conditions of crowding, and respiratory symptoms are the most common reason for consultation (29%) during cruises. Although tuberculosis transmission has not been reported in this setting, influenza A outbreaks are well described and in the last decade several serious outbreaks of Legionnaires' disease have been reported on cruise ships (Minooee and Rickman, 1999). Outbreaks of gastroenteritis are also commonly recorded, including bacterial infections caused by pathogens such as *Shigella* spp, *Salmonella* spp and *Vibrio* spp. More devastating are the frequently recorded explosive outbreaks of small round structured viruses, Norwalk and similar agents, particularly in an elderly population, although the majority of passengers so affected will be treated on ship and recover before returning to shore.

Expedition travel is less hazardous than one might expect. A recent questionnaire survey of 246 expedition leaders revealed only 835 medical incidents in 130 000 person-days of travel, of which 33% were gastrointestinal and 21% were 'general medical', including 23 cases of proven or suspected malaria, most of which were dealt with by local doctors (Anderson and Johnson, 2000). Of 206 expedition participants treated by a doctor, only 10 saw their general practitioner and only five needed to see a hospital doctor after their return to the UK.

The Patient Who Has Not Travelled

A key reason for identifying imported infection is to minimise the chance of onward transmission to the local population by appropriate treatment and isolation of the index case. One of the earliest examples of this was the 40 day (quarantine) period of detention offshore, introduced for ships arriving in Venice and Rhodes in 1377 to prevent the importation of plague. Similar detailed modern regulations exist for containment of specific pathogens that are rarely imported but are of public concern, such as the viral haemorrhagic fevers (Centers for Disease Control, 1995; Advisory Committee on Dangerous Pathogens, 1996). Travel histories of relatives and friends should always be considered when dealing with patients with a potentially infectious disease, particularly in groups such as students or immigrants who have frequent contact with international travellers.

Case History
A 24-year-old woman of Indian ethnic origin was admitted to hospital in Liverpool with 1 week of illness typical of acute viral hepatitis. She and her husband (also of Indian ethnic origin) had both been born and brought up in the UK. Her husband had returned from his first trip to India 2 months before, and had been managed at home with probable hepatitis starting 1 month before. She was confirmed as having hepatitis E, imported by her husband.

Hepatitis E is not a common diagnosis in Western countries unless the patient has travelled overseas (Schwartz et al., 1999). This case illustrates the importance of taking a good contact and travel history in all patients.

Travel histories should be relayed to diagnostic laboratories, so that the relevant tests are performed to diagnose exotic pathogens that might otherwise not be sought. This is also essential because of the potential risk of many pathogens to the laboratory workers themselves, including especially brucellosis, transmission of which is common in laboratories in endemic areas and is also a hazard when incorrectly identified samples are sent internationally (Pike, 1978; Luzzi et al., 1993). Apart from exposure to airborne pathogens such as brucellosis, laboratory workers are at special risk from inoculation accidents involving exotic pathogens, such as malaria, trypanosomiasis and leishmaniasis, which will require urgent specialist advice (Lettau, 1991). Failure to diagnose the index infection can lead to tragic consequences in health care workers involved in needlestick incidents.

Case History
A doctor in Sicily suffered a needlestick injury while attending a patient with fever imported from Africa. The patient's malaria was subsequently diagnosed and treated in London, but by then the doctor had died from undiagnosed malaria (Communicable Disease Report, 1997).

Exotic infections can travel with their vectors and the hazards of imported zoonotic infections have been highlighted by the recent epidemics of Rift Valley fever in the Yemen and Saudi Arabia, related to imported livestock (Arishi et al., 2000). Similar concerns accompany international movement of domestic pets; this is a particular issue for countries such as the UK that are currently rabies-free and whose regulations relating to pet movement are being relaxed, allowing exposure of animals to a variety of other infections as well as rabies, some of which have potential for spread to humans (Trees and Shaw, 1999). Exotic pathogens may be imported with other animals, such as psittacosis associated with a variety of

birds and salmonellosis with reptiles.

Insect vectors survive travel despite regulations designed to hinder them, such as spraying vehicles moving out of the trypanosome belt in Africa, or spraying aeroplanes to kill mosquitoes. So-called 'airport malaria' affecting nontravellers has been reported from several countries that do not usually have local malaria transmission (Gratz et al., 2000).

These imported hazards will only be considered by the health care worker who keeps an open mind and thinks laterally about the situation of the patient. This is not so easy in the growing number of cases of illness caused by pathogens imported with food, identification of which requires sophisticated public health surveillance mechanisms (Nichols, 2000).

THE PATIENT WITH FEVER

The majority of serious imported infections present with fever as the predominant or major symptom, and it is essential that a timely diagnosis is made in such patients (Humar and Keystone, 1996). The few published studies on the diagnostic outcome of imported fever cases are hospital-based and are therefore subject to considerable referral bias. One report from the Hospital for Tropical Diseases in 1986 (Bryceson, 1987) showed that 553 of 1084 adults admitted with imported infection had fever and that 42% of these had malaria. The findings of two recent studies (MacLean et al., 1994; Doherty et al., 1995) are summarised in Table 12.4, again showing that approximately 40% of patients had malaria and that cosmopolitan, nonspecific illness was the second most common diagnosis. In both series there is a large proportion of patients with no final diagnosis. Such reviews are helpful in emphasising the importance of malaria, but should be interpreted with caution. In the 1970s malaria was the most common imported infection recognised in children in the UK (Paget Stanfield and Reid, 1980) and Table 12.5 summarises the findings in two recent small hospital studies of British children with fever after travelling. The study from London (Klein and Millman, 1998) only included children who had travelled within the last month, so cases of vivax malaria presenting late would have been excluded, whereas the proportion of children with vivax malaria is higher in the Birmingham series (Riordan and Tarlow, 1998) because this includes any travel-related illness. Neither series includes children with malaria who were seen and managed by general practitioners or in the outpatient clinic, and other problems such as tuberculosis are probably underrepresented as the patients may have been seen in other clinics or managed as outpatients.

Malaria

It is essential to consider and exclude or treat malaria,

Table 12.4 Main causes of fever in adults admitted to hospital after returning from the tropics

Cause	Study 1[a] (n = 587) (%)	Study 2[b] (n = 195) (%)
Malaria	32	42
Undiagnosed	25	24.5
Respiratory infection	11	2.5
Diarrhoeal illness	4.5	6.5
Hepatitis	6	3
Dengue	2	6
Enteric fever	2	2

[a]MacLean et al. (1994).
[b]Doherty et al. (1995).

Table 12.5 Selected diagnoses in febrile children admitted to British hospitals after overseas travel

	Study 1[a] (n = 31)	Study 2[b] (n = 45)
Malaria		
vivax	1	10
falciparum	3	3
Respiratory infection		
lower	1	7
upper	1	7
Diarrhoea		
travellers'	0	6
bacterial	3	3
Hepatitis	1	6
Dengue	2	0
Typhoid	2	1
No diagnosis	14	3

[a]Klein and Millman (1998).
[b]Riordan and Tarlow (1998). Some children in this study had more than one cause of fever.

particularly as patients with falciparum malaria can deteriorate and develop severe complications within a few hours of presentation. In Britain, approximately 2000–2500 cases of malaria and 10–14 deaths are reported each year, a fatality rate of 1–2% in patients with falciparum malaria. Higher mortality rates have been reported in other countries (Kain et al., 1998). The number of tourists and expatriates who die overseas is not known. The majority of cases are imported by visitors and resident immigrants returning from a visit to their country of origin (Behrens and Curtis, 1993) and this pattern now predominates in other parts of Europe (Wetsteyn et al., 1997) and North America (Kain et al., 1998). Table 12.6 summarises the geographical origin of malaria reported in the UK in 1999; 16% of the patients were children, similar to earlier reports (Brabin and Ganley, 1997). An increasing proportion of cases in both adults

and children in Britain and North America are due to falciparum malaria, when compared to previous decades (Brabin and Ganley, 1997; Suh et al., 1999). Most, but not all, falciparum malaria is imported from Africa and any patient with fever from Africa must be assumed to have falciparum malaria until proven otherwise (Molyneux and Fox, 1993). However, it cannot be assumed that patients from the Indian subcontinent always have benign vivax malaria, as the following case report demonstrates.

Case History
A 62-year-old Indian businessman based in Mumbai (Bombay) developed a nonspecific fever 2 days after travelling to Europe. This failed to respond to paracetamol and antibiotics prescribed by two different doctors. Fourteen days after leaving home he presented in Liverpool with cerebral malaria, renal failure and 22% falciparum parasitaemia. This fatal infection was acquired during a visit to a rural area in India without taking chemoprophylaxis.

This unfortunate history also emphasises that it is not just expatriates who fail to recognise that they are at risk of catching malaria when they travel to endemic zones. The majority of patients who present with imported malaria have failed to take adequate chemoprophylaxis. Poor outcome is usually associated with delays in presentation by the patient, failure of the attending physician to consider the diagnosis, and delays in arranging for diagnostic tests and treatment (Kain et al., 1998).

The fever is of abrupt onset and is often mistaken for influenza, with headache, sweating, myalgia and in some cases paroxysms or rigors. Around 15% of malaria patients are afebrile at presentation or other symptoms may predominate, so that the diagnosis is not considered by the attending health care worker. In a recent audit in Liverpool, 31% of patients with falciparum malaria had diarrhoea as a prominent clinical feature, and in 16% of such cases malaria was not included in the admission differential diagnosis. Seventeen per cent had jaundice, which was sometimes ascribed to hepatitis rather than to malaria. Similar errors are commonly reported (Svenson et al., 1995; Kain et al., 1998) and emphasise the protean nature of malaria presentations (Table 12.7).

The timing of presentation of cases helps in the differential diagnosis of malaria. The majority of patients with falciparum malaria present within 6 weeks of leaving an endemic area, and over 90% present within 2 months (Kain et al., 1998). Patients taking chemoprophylaxis may have partial suppression of their parasitaemia, which both increases the clinical incubation period and hampers the laboratory diagnosis, as the lower degree of parasitaemia is more difficult to detect. Nevertheless, partial chemosuppression is better than none and probably reduces mortality in such patients (Lewis et al., 1992).

The benign malarias have a different spectrum of incu-

Table 12.6 Geographical source and type of malaria imported into the UK in 1999

	Africa	Asia	Other	Not given	Total
Plasmodium falciparum	1199	23	13	269	1504
Plasmodium vivax	59	232	19	64	374
Other species/mixed infections	124	8	0	35	167
Total	1382	263	32	368	2045

Reproduced by permission of the PHLS Malaria Reference Laboratory, London School of Hygiene & Tropical Medicine.

Table 12.7 Common errors in diagnosis and management of malaria

Delayed presentation by patient
Failure of health care worker to take a travel history
Failure of health care worker to consider malaria in symptomatic patient
Belief that chemoprophylaxis prevents all malaria
Belief that malaria is unlikely to be present if patient does not remember being bitten by mosquitoes
Belief that absence of splenomegaly excludes malaria
Belief that absence of regular fever pattern excludes malaria
Failure to recognise nonspecific clinical presentations of malaria
Failure to obtain good quality blood film diagnosis immediately (with species diagnosis)
Failure to obtain repeat films or use ancillary diagnostic tests if first films are negative
Failure to prescribe adequate and appropriate chemotherapy immediately
Failure to anticipate complications
Failure to treat complications
Failure to follow patient up after treatment

bation and must always be considered in a patient who has been to an endemic region within the last 2 years. Approximately a third of patients with vivax malaria present within 2 months of arrival, and another third do not develop symptoms until 6–12 months after leaving a malarious area. Ovale malaria, usually from West Africa, presents with similar delays. Late presentations of vivax or ovale malaria should not be overlooked in a febrile patient who has been successfully treated for falciparum malaria several months earlier, as chemosuppression will have been discontinued and the treatment for falciparum malaria will not have treated the hypnozoites (quiescent liver stages) of the benign malarias. *Plasmodium malariae* has the potential to relapse for years but is only found in a small proportion of imported cases. It is rare for patients with recurring 'fevers' years after return from the tropics to have malaria: other diagnoses should be sought for such patients.

The physical findings in malaria are nonspecific and malaria cannot be distinguished clinically from other illnesses. Jaundice and diarrhoea have already been mentioned. Rashes suggest other illnesses except in very rare cases of petechiae due to disseminated intravascular coagulopathy complicating falciparum malaria. The fever pattern of malaria, when present, is usually continuously elevated in falciparum infection. Parasite populations do not become synchronised (Chapter 8) until at least the second week of clinical illness in the benign malarias, so that it is unusual to see the classical 48 or 72 h pattern of fever produced by simultaneous lysis of erythrocytes and release of merozoites. Patients with malaria may have an enlarged liver, and splenomegaly is present in only a minority at presentation and has little positive or negative predictive diagnostic value.

The diagnosis of malaria can only be made by performing the appropriate laboratory tests.

Case History
A 55-year-old businessman consulted his general practitioner with fever 2 weeks after returning from a holiday in coastal Kenya. He took no prophylaxis as his daughter, an air stewardess, had told him that it would make him ill. The general practitioner sent a blood film to a local laboratory and did not receive their negative blood film report until 36 h later. The patient continued to be unwell and was sent into hospital after a further 3 days, by which time he had 2% parasitaemia with falciparum malaria. Expert review of the original blood films later confirmed the presence of falciparum malaria.

In this case the general practitioner had done well to consider malaria, but there was a failure to obtain results within a few hours and the diagnosis was missed by an inexperienced laboratory. In all cases in which malaria is a possibility, results of good quality blood tests must be obtained within half a working day at the most. In everyday practice, most family practitioners should refer such patients immediately to hospital for diagnosis, or to their regional specialist clinic if one is available.

Laboratory Diagnosis of Malaria

Malaria is conventionally diagnosed by examination of blood films for characteristic parasites within the erythrocytes. Thin blood films are routinely processed in most hospitals, but are not usually stained at the optimum pH for malaria diagnostics. Thin films are most valuable for confirming the species of parasite, especially in mixed infections, and for determining the degree of parasitaemia, but have low diagnostic sensitivity. In the tropics and in expert laboratories, examination of thick blood films is the preferred method because a larger volume of blood is examined in the film and sensitivity is improved. Few laboratories in western countries are proficient at this and numerous studies confirm that many diagnostic laboratories either cannot identify the species correctly (the usual problem) or fail to see parasites at all (Malaria Working Party, 1997; Kain et al., 1998). In imported malaria cases, the first blood films are positive in more than 95% of cases examined by experts (Kain et al., 1998) but may genuinely be negative, especially if the patient is taking partially effective chemosuppression and parasitaemia is very scanty. Patients with negative films should have a second film examined 12 h later, and possibly a third one 12 h after that if clinical suspicion continues. The timing of taking the specimen in relation to fever is not clinically important.

Thus the conventional management approach to a patient with 'fever ?malaria' is to admit to hospital for 24–48 h for observation, syndromic management and for blood films to rule out malaria as well as other investigations. Recent improvements in laboratory technology are revolutionising this approach and can be expected to improve diagnostic sensitivity and specificity of the first blood test. One approach has been to stain the buffy coat of centrifuged blood with acridine orange and to examine this for fluorescence in capillary tubes (quantitative buffy coat; QBC method). This is similar in sensitivity to thin-film examination but parasites cannot be speciated. Special equipment is needed and the method is technically demanding. More useful are the tests that are currently being developed for detection of malaria antigens (Chiodini, 1998). The first generation of tests have been based on detection of histidine-rich protein 2 (HRP-2) derived from *Plasmodium falciparum* (but not from other species). These tests ('ParaSight F, ICT, malaria Pf') have approximately the same or lower sensitivity compared with a thick blood film that is read by an expert, and can be used in field or clinic situations or in less expert laboratories as an ancillary to routine blood film diagnosis (Cropley et al., 2000). Problems include occasional false positivity, for example in patients with rheumatoid factor (Laferi et al., 1997), and the persistence of antigen for 1–2 weeks after successful treatment. This is useful for making a recent retrospective diagnosis but means the test cannot be used to monitor the success of treatment. Occasional false negative tests have been reported in patients with high parasitaemia rates (Risch et al., 2000), so blood films must always be examined as well.

Species of malaria other than falciparum are not detected by HRP-2-based tests, but alternative methods use the secretion of parasite species-specific lactic dehydrogenase (LDH) as a marker of active parasitaemia. The OptiMAL and similar tests are now well validated for the diagnosis of falciparum and vivax malaria and are being improved for the diagnosis of other species (Iqbal et al., 1999). LDH-based tests can be used to monitor the success of treatment, as they become negative at the same time as parasites disappear from blood films. They may also suffer from false positivity in the presence of rheumatoid factor (Grobusch et al., 1999). The dipstick methods have the great advantage that they are less prone to observer error than film interpretation in less experienced laboratories, but they are not yet simple enough for travellers to use for self-diagnosis in remote situations (Jelinek et al., 1999). The measurement of antibodies has no place in the routine diagnosis of patients with fever, but is used to make a retrospective diagnosis of recent malaria in previously nonimmune subjects, particularly in the context of detecting subclinical malaria infection in clinical trials or epidemiological studies. Polymerase chain reaction (PCR)-based tests are increasingly being used to monitor the quality of diagnostic laboratories (Kain et al., 1998; Iqbal et al., 1999; Rubio et al., 1999) or for epidemiological investigations of unusual situations such as the nosocomial transmission of malaria (Rubio et al., 1999), but are not yet generally used for clinical diagnosis or for monitoring therapy (Tham et al., 1999). New techniques, such as the use of automated counters to detect malaria pigment in whole blood specimens, may produce new methods for diagnosis in the future (Hanscheid et al., 2000). Table 12.8 summarises the use of these tests.

Other Causes of Fever

The emphasis so far has been on malaria and its laboratory diagnosis. Other causes of fever can be determined by a combination of history, examination and laboratory investigations. In practice the most useful aid is a precise history of exposure or risk behaviour, together with recognition of the overall clinical pattern of presentation, as many features of febrile illness overlap. Risk activities such as those in Table 12.3 suggest the diagnosis and can be combined with the incubation periods (Table 12.2) and groups of physical signs in Tables 12.9–12.11, and routine laboratory tests may yield further clues.

Case History
A 23-year-old woman developed high fever, headache, back pain and a generalised blanching erythematous rash 3 days after returning from rural Thailand. The clinical diagnosis of dengue was confirmed by detection of antibodies 2 weeks later.

This typical presentation of fever and rash with a short incubation period is highly suggestive of dengue fever, which is now widespread throughout Asia and South and Central America and the Caribbean, and is rapidly spreading through Africa (Gubler, 1999; Jelinek, 2000). Diagnosis is by PCR in the first week of illness and by

Table 12.8 Laboratory diagnosis of malaria

Method	Uses	Comments
Thin blood film	Routine use in Western laboratories	Insensitive
	Speciation; determination of parasitaemia	
Thick blood film	Routine in tropics	Requires experience
	Approximate parasitaemia; speciation	
Antimalarial antibodies	Retrospective diagnosis in returned travellers (e.g. trials)	Crossreactions. Not useful for acute diagnosis
Quantitative buffy coat (QBC)	Diagnosis in inexperienced laboratories	Insensitive. No speciation. Requires special equipment. Cost
Antigen detection based on histidine-rich protein 2 (HRP-2)	Current or recent falciparum malaria only. Useful in inexperienced laboratories	Only falciparum. Sensitivity equivalent to thick film. Stay positive for 1–2 weeks
Antigen detection based on lactate dehydrogenase (LDH)	Current malaria (species-specific). Useful in inexperienced laboratories. May alert laboratory to mixed infections	Will probably supplant HRP-2 based tests. Can also be used to monitor early success of therapy
Polymerase chain reaction (PCR)	Sensitive and species-specific; mainly for laboratory quality assurance	Not routinely available for diagnosis
Malaria pigment detection	Hypothetical method of automated counting	Speculative

Table 12.9 Common syndrome/disease associations with imported fever

Sore throat	Cough	Abdominal pain	Arthralgia/myalgia	Diarrhoea
Bacterial pharyngitis	Amoebiasis (hepatic)	Amoebiasis (intestinal)	Arboviruses	Amoebiasis (intestinal)
Diphtheria	Anthrax	Anthrax	Dengue	Anthrax
Glandular fever	Bacterial pneumonia	Campylobacter	Yellow fever	Campylobacter
HIV seroconversion	Filarial fever	enteritis	Babesiosis	enteritis
Lyme disease	TPE	Legionnaires' disease	Bartonellosis	HIV seroconversion
Poliomyelitis	Histoplasmosis	Malaria	Brucellosis	Legionnaires' disease
Psittacosis	Legionnaires' disease	Measles	Erythema nodosum	Malaria
Tularaemia	Leishmaniasis	Melioidosis	leprosum	Measles
Viral haemorrhagic	(visceral)	Plague	Hepatitis (viral)	Melioidosis
fever (Lassa)	Loeffler syndrome	Relapsing fevers	Histoplasmosis	Plague
Nonspecific viral upper	Malaria	Salmonellosis	HIV seroconversion	Relapsing fever
respiratory tract	Measles	Schistosomiasis (acute)	Legionnaires' disease	Salmonellosis
infection (URTI)	Melioidosis	Shigellosis	Leptospirosis	Schistosomiasis (acute)
	Plague	Typhoid in children	Lyme disease	Shigellosis
	Q fever	Viral haemorrhagic	Malaria	Typhoid in children
	Relapsing fever	fevers	Plague	Viral haemorrhagic
	Schistosomiasis (acute)	Yersiniosis	Poliomyelitis	fevers
	Toxocariasis		Q fever	Yersiniosis
	Trichinosis		Relapsing fevers	
	Tuberculosis		Secondary syphilis	
	Tularaemia		Toxoplasmosis	
	Typhoid and		Trichinosis	
	paratyphoid		Trypanosomiasis	
	Typhus		(African)	
	Viral haemorrhagic		Tularaemia	
	fevers		Typhoid and	
	Nonspecific viral		paratyphoid	
	URTIs		Typhus	
			Viral haemorrhagic	
			fevers	

TPE = tropical pulmonary eosinophilia.

serological tests thereafter (these may cross-react with antibodies from prior yellow fever immunisation).

Recovery can be prolonged. Haemorrhagic complications are unusual in primary attacks in nonimmune tourists (Chapter 6), but aspirin should not be used as an antipyretic in patients with possible dengue. Many other arbovirus infections have similar presenting syndromes, the diagnosis being suggested by geographical exposure and confirmed by serology.

Fever patterns are rarely useful at the bedside for differentiating the cause of illness, and the classical biphasic 'saddleback' fever of dengue is not often seen. Enteric fever (typhoid and paratyphoid) tends to cause a sustained fever but the 'classical' relative bradycardia is infrequent and is not diagnostic, as it may also be a feature of brucellosis and hepatitis.

Generalised rashes accompanying fever may be non-specific or suggest specific causes. A petechial rash is seen in meningococcal disease, a particular hazard for pilgrims to Mecca for the Hajj, and may accompany any septicaemic illness. Maculopapular rashes are seen with most rickettsial illnesses, a further clue to which is the presence of an eschar at the site of tick or mite bites in tick typhus or scrub typhus, respectively.

Case History

A middle-aged couple were admitted to hospital on return from a 2 week safari holiday in South Africa with identical symptoms of headache, malaise, fever, dry cough and tender maculopapular rash on their legs. Single eschars, consisting of a necrotic black central skin lesion surrounded by erythema, were found in both patients. The lesion in the woman was under her bra strap, and her husband's was located under the elastic of his underwear. Both patients later had positive serology for infection with *Rickettsia conorii* and responded promptly to doxycycline therapy, which was given as soon as the clinical diagnosis was made.

This is a typical presentation of tick typhus. The tick bite is not usually remembered by the patient, who may also have overlooked the eschar, which is sometimes located in the scalp, in which case regional lymphadenopathy may provide a clue to its presence.

Focal solitary skin lesions with fever raise the possibility of African trypanosomiasis, in which the initial tsetse fly bite at the site of the subsequent chancre is usually vividly recalled by the patient. Similar chancres (chagomas) may be seen at the site of bites by reduviid bugs that transmit *Trypanosoma cruzii* in South America. Lyme disease may present with focal or migrating erythema at the site of the initial tick bite, which is not always recalled.

Non-specific rashes accompany fever due to other infections, including rarities such as the viral haemorrhagic fevers (facial oedema is a clue in early Lassa fever) and

Table 12.10 Neurological syndrome/disease associations with imported fever

Fits	Meningitis/encephalitis
Arboviruses	Angiostrongyloidiasis
Japanese encephalitis	Anthrax
Bacterial meningitis	Arboviruses
Histoplasmosis	Dengue fever
Malaria	Japanese encephalitis
Rabies	West Nile fever
Shigellosis (children)	Yellow fever
Tetanus	Bacterial meningitis
Tuberculosis	Histoplasmosis
meningitis	HIV seroconversion
tuberculomata	Legionnaires' disease
	Leptospirosis
	Lyme disease
	Malaria
	Poliomyelitis
	Rabies
	Relapsing fevers
	Secondary syphilis
	Trypanosomiasis (African)
	Tuberculosis
	Typhoid and paratyphoid
	Typhus

African trypanosomiasis. The classical rose spots of typhoid are only seen transiently in pale-skinned patients in the second week of illness, and consist of blanching macules 2–3 mm in diameter. These should not be mistaken for the rash of secondary syphilis or disseminated gonococcaemia.

Lymphadenopathy is typically a feature of the 'glandular fever' group of infections, seen commonly in young adults, including infectious mononucleosis, cytomegalovirus and toxoplasmosis, and is also found in dengue fever, brucellosis and a wide variety of other infections (Table 12.11). Malaria does not cause lymphadenopathy. Acute HIV seroconversion illness is usually accompanied by lymphadenopathy (which is also common in chronic HIV infection) and this should always be part of the differential diagnosis.

Case History

A 32-year-old man was referred by his general practitioner with possible typhoid because of fever, headache, diarrhoea and a nonspecific pink maculopapular rash on his torso. He also had lymphadenopathy. He had returned 4 weeks previously from a visit to Thailand where he had unprotected sex. Initial HIV antibody tests were negative, although a blood test for HIV antigen was positive. His antibody tests became positive 6 weeks later.

All of the above features are common in HIV serocon-

Table 12.11 Possible association of physical signs with imported infections

Lymphadenopathy	Hepatomegaly	Splenomegaly	Jaundice
Arboviruses (Dengue)	Amoebiasis (hepatic)	Babesiosis	Cytomegalovirus
Bartonellosis	Babesiosis	Bartonellosis	Fascioliasis
Brucellosis	Bartonellosis	Brucellosis	Hepatitis (viral)
Cytomegalovirus	Brucelolosis	Cytomegalovirus	Leptospirosis
Diphtheria	Cytomegalovirus	Erythema nodosum leprosum	Malaria
Erythema nodosum leprosum	Dengue	Filarial fever (TPE)	Relapsing fevers
Filarial fever	Fascioliasis	Hepatitis (viral)	Toxoplasmosis
Histoplasmosis	Hepatitis (viral)	Histoplasmosis	Trypanosomiasis
HIV seroconversion	Histoplasmosis	HIV	African, acute
Infectious mononucleosis	HIV seroconversion	Leishmaniasis (visceral)	Typhoid and paratyphoid
Leishmaniasis (visceral)	Legionnaires' disease	Lyme disease	Typhus
Lyme diseae	Leishmaniasis (visceral)	Malaria	Yellow fever
Plague	Lyme disease	Melioidosis	
Psittacosis	Malaria	Psittacosis	
Q fever	Q fever	Q fever	
Schistosomiasis (acute)	Relapsing fevers	Relapsing fevers	
Secondary syphilis	Schistosomiasis (acute)	Salmonellosis	
Toxoplasmosis	Toxocariasis	Schistosomiasis (acute)	
Trichinosis	Trypanosomiasis	Toxoplasmosis	
Trypanosomiasis	African, acute	Trichinosis	
African, acute	America, acute	Trypanosomiasis	
American, acute	Tuberculosis	African, acute	
Tuberculosis	Typhus	American, acute	
Tularaemia		Tuberculosis	
Typhus		Tularaemia	
		Typhoid and paratyphoid	
		Typhus	

TPE = tropical pulmonary eosinophilia.

version illness, during which conventional HIV antibody detection tests are usually negative. The importance of the exposure history is self-evident.

Focal lymphadenopathy is usually associated with regional sepsis, most commonly infected skin wounds and arthropod bites, but rarities such a plague (exquisitely tender unilateral nodes or buboes) should also be considered, as well as more common illnesses such as tuberculosis.

Jaundice is a feature of many illnesses, including malaria, viral hepatitis, leptospirosis, the glandular fever group and arbovirus infections such as yellow fever.

Case History
A 33-year-old man developed headache, fever, myalgia and jaundice 10 days after white-water rafting in Thailand. He had meningism, jaundice, tender muscles, splenomegaly and mild renal failure. He had been immunised against hepatitis A and B before travel and serological tests subsequently confirmed infection with leptospirosis.

Leptospirosis is found worldwide and the history of exposure to freshwater is typical, particularly in Asia, where large epidemics affect the local population each year. In the absence of other focal features and specific exposure history, viral hepatitis should be considered as the cause of jaundice. Hepatitis A is still a hazard for nonimmunised travellers; hepatitis B and C are both transmitted by unsterile injections and infusions; and hepatitis B is a risk after unprotected sexual exposure. Water-borne hepatitis E is endemic and also causes sporadic epidemics in the Indian subcontinent, in much of adjacent Asia and in Mexico and is probably underrecognised in most other parts of the tropics. It should be suspected in jaundiced travellers to Asia who are immune to hepatitis A and have not been immersed in fresh water. Serological tests are essential to differentiate the causes of viral hepatitis, which are indistinguishable clinically (Chapter 6).

After malaria, respiratory infections are the most common causes of imported fever, with or without localising signs. Most are due to cosmopolitan infections, such as influenza and other respiratory viruses, or community-acquired pneumonia. Rare but important causes of pharyngitis include diphtheria (look for membrane) and Lassa fever (exposure in rural West Africa). It is impossible to distinguish the different causes of community-acquired pneumonia at the bedside, and the usual conventional diagnostic tests should be employed, including convalescent serological tests several weeks after the onset of illness.

Of particular importance to travellers is the increasing prevalence of multi-drug resistant *Streptococcus pneumoniae* in many countries, including most of the Far East, Papua New Guinea, South Africa and Spain, so that therapy with penicillin is inappropriate for travellers from these areas. Legionella infection imported to the UK is typically associated with travel to Mediterranean resorts and with cruises, or contaminated air conditioners or showers in hotels. Surveillance suggests that approximately a quarter of legionella infections are associated with recent travel (Anonymous, 1997). The older patient who smokes and drinks alcohol to excess is most likely to develop severe disease; he or she is also most likely to have delayed antibody seroconversion, so that serological tests may not become positive until 6–8 weeks after onset of illness. Other clues to atypical pneumonia pathogens include contact with animals for Q fever (splenomegaly, thrombocytopenia) and tularaemia (lymphadenopathy) and with psittacine birds (psittacosis).

Hantavirus infections transmitted by rodent contact, such as *sin nombre* virus, are increasingly being recognised as causes of severe atypical pneumonia in visitors to rural areas of the USA or South America (Doyle *et al.*, 1998).

A nonproductive cough is found in typhoid fever and in brucellosis, often without radiographic abnormality. Fever with wheezy cough or asthmatic presentation is a feature of filarial tropical pulmonary eosinophilia (TPE) and of the migratory phase of immature stages of many nematode and trematode infections, including the hookworms, roundworms and schistosomes. In these situations, eosinophilia will suggest the diagnosis (see below, Eosinophilia).

Haemoptysis suggests tuberculosis (or tumour) but travellers who have eaten raw crustacea in the Far East, West Africa or South America may have paragonimiasis, which can be mistaken radiologically for tuberculosis and is diagnosed by looking for characteristic ova in sputum.

Imported infections may produce a variety of neurological or psychiatric syndromes. In addition to the usual bacterial pathogens causing meningitis, infections such as brucellosis, leptospirosis, rickettsial illness and arboviruses frequently have a meningoencephalitic element. Drowsiness, meningism, focal neurological signs or progression to coma are all features of malaria, which must always be excluded, as must trypanosomiasis in travellers who have visited Africa. Transient psychological problems are common in travellers and are often associated with alcohol or drug misuse or rapid translocation between cultures. Rabies should be considered in patients who behave abnormally and may have had exposure to animals in the tropics, even if they do not remember the bite or lick.

Case History
A 47-year-old Indian seaman was admitted with fever and rigors for 4 days, accompanied by headache and mild diarrhoea. He had a high fever and developed right shoulder-tip pain the next day, when he was observed to have a tender enlarged liver with a right basal pleural effusion. His blood count showed neutrophilia, and ultrasound confirmed the presence of a large abscess in the right lobe of the liver. Liver function tests were normal and amoebic serology was strongly positive. He responded rapidly to metronidazole.

This typical history emphasises the need to re-examine patients carefully and to consider amoebic liver abscess in occult fever. The presence or absence of diarrhoea or of trophozoites or cysts of *Entamoeba histolytica* in the faeces is of no diagnostic value, but neutrophilia is supportive and serology is usually positive at presentation.

In the absence of the above syndromes, physical examination should exclude other organ-based infections, including mundane sinusitis and ear infections. Focal signs may be diagnostic.

Diarrhoeal illness is common while travelling (von Sonnenburg *et al.*, 2000) but is self-limiting in the majority of cases (Chapter 10). The usual bacterial and viral causes are implicated and enterotoxigenic *Escherichia coli* is overrepresented in travellers with diarrhoea on their return home (Svenungsson *et al.*, 2000). Cholera is rarely imported by travellers, partly because of the lack of risk to travellers while overseas and mainly because the incubation period is so short that most patients need medical treatment before repatriation. Diarrhoea is a feature of many of the febrile infections already described and is more likely to cause fever in children than in adults. Children with enteric fever are also more likely to have diarrhoea than adults. Diarrhoea with blood, fever and systemic illness is usually due to *Campylobacter*, *Shigella* or *Salmonella* spp, but the recent traveller with bloody diarrhoea (dysentery) and without much general illness may have amoebiasis. This is confirmed by examination of unpreserved faeces (the 'hot stool') or rectal scrapings within 20–30 min for active trophozoites of *Entamoeba histolytica* containing ingested erythrocytes. If these infections are excluded, the patient will need a further work-up including lower bowel endoscopy to exclude underlying gastrointestinal disease or chronic tropical conditions such as schistosomiasis. Watery diarrhoea caused by Cyclospora infections is also diagnosed by faecal microscopy, and is suggested by a history of travel to known endemic areas such as Nepal or Peru. Co-trimoxazole is effective treatment, with ciprofloxacin as an alternative.

In about 3% of cases, travel-related diarrhoea lasts for more than 14 days (DuPont and Capsuto, 1996). Patients need a full work-up to exclude underlying immunosuppression, especially HIV, and adequate faecal tests for bacterial and parasitic (protozoan) parasites. *Giardia lam-*

blia is the most common culprit, typically causing explosive steatorrhoic diarrhoea in the mornings and often associated with 'eggy burps'. Untreated, the patient can develop significant malabsorption. Parasitological diagnosis may be difficult and many physicians opt for empirical therapy with agents such as tinidazole or metronidazole. Failure to respond to therapy may represent drug resistance (Zaat *et al.*, 1997) but is more likely to be due to failure to take the medication (ask the patient), or to transient lactase deficiency (exclude all lactose-containing food and drink for 1 week) or to reinfection by other family members. If all the above have been excluded, second-line drugs such as mepacrine or paromomycin may be needed.

Apart from the exclusion of underlying gastrointestinal disease, schistosomiasis or postinfectious irritable bowel syndrome, tropical sprue must be considered. The aetiology of tropical sprue is unknown and it causes persistent small bowel diarrhoea and malabsorption and requires a full expert diagnostic work-up. Treatment with tetracyclines, folic acid and vitamin B_{12} is effective (DuPont and Capsuto, 1996).

Investigation of fever

Baseline investigations include full blood count, including differential white count and platelet count, serum electrolytes and liver function tests, blood cultures and malaria films. Urinalysis and cultures of urine and stool should be sent and a sample of serum stored for possible serological testing. The need for chest X-ray and other focal imaging, such as ultrasound of the liver, may be suggested by clinical findings. As indicated in the cases already presented, the potential list of serological tests and other investigations can be extensive but practitioners should resist the temptation to order everything just because the patient has travelled to an exotic country. Special examinations include microscopy of cerebrospinal fluid for trypanosomiasis, bone marrow culture for partially treated typhoid or brucellosis, or bone marrow for microscopical examination for visceral leishmaniasis.

The initial emphasis should be on excluding malaria and infections of chest, urine or gastrointestinal tract before focusing on the most likely exotic diagnosis if these investigations prove negative. Convalescent serology taken at least 2 weeks later is often needed to make a retrospective diagnosis if this is thought to be important after the patient has recovered.

The small risk of transmission of infection to health care workers should always be kept in mind and appropriate infection control precautions should be taken. For patients with suspected diphtheria or with a possible viral haemorrhagic fever, more stringent isolation is needed and immediate advice should be obtained from public health specialists as well as from infectious disease experts (Centers for Disease Control, 1995; Advisory Committee on Dangerous Pathogens, 1996).

Blood films for malaria can also be used to exclude borreliosis, filariasis, babesiosis and African trypanosomiasis. Neutropenia is an inconsistent finding in malaria, in viral infections and in typhoid and must be interpreted with caution, as the normal neutrophil and platelet counts are lower in patients of African ethnic origin than Caucasians (Bain, 1996). Neutrophilia usually suggests a pyogenic bacterial infection but is also seen in malaria, and eosinophilia suggests a helminth infection or atopy. Thrombocytopenia is present in the majority of both benign and falciparum malaria infections and may alert the microscopist to the presence of parasitaemia, but it is also found with dengue, brucellosis and many viral infections. A combination of thrombocytopenia ($<$ $150 \times 10^9 \mathrm{l}^{-1}$) and raised bilirubin ($> 18 \mu\mathrm{mol}\,\mathrm{l}^{-1}$) was found to have a positive predictive value of 95% and specificity of 98%, but a low sensitivity in diagnosing malaria in one study in London (Doherty *et al.*, 1995). However, this combination was only found in 36 of the 82 patients with malaria, limiting the diagnostic usefulness to a small proportion of patients. Hypoglycaemia may also suggest malaria or African trypanosomiasis. Liver function abnormalities are rarely of specific diagnostic value but are helpful in assessing disease severity.

Treatment

A sequential approach to the diagnosis and treatment of the patient with imported fever is summarised in Figure 12.1. For details of specific treatment of most infections, the relevant chapters in this book should be consulted. The pharmacological management of malaria and its complications are described in full in Chapter 8 and in a recent useful publication (World Health Organization, 2000).

A few principles guide malaria treatment, once the diagnosis has been confirmed. Treatment should cover falciparum malaria unless there is a confident expert laboratory diagnosis of another *Plasmodium* species. Patients with falciparum malaria should usually be treated as inpatients for at least the first 24–48 h in western settings, unless they are recent immigrants (with partial immunity) with very mild infections. Therapy is usually initiated via the parenteral route in severe or complicated falciparum malaria, one of the definitions of which includes hyperparasitaemia, and the level of parasitaemia must always be measured. Although the World Health Organization defines hyperparasitaemia as a parasite rate $> 5\%$, the majority of tropical specialists use a pragmatic cut-off level of 2% parasitaemia to indicate increased clinical risk in nonimmune travellers with imported malaria. Children and pregnant women are particularly likely to experience hypoglycaemia as a complication of falciparum malaria. This may be exacerbated by quinine therapy, and blood glucose levels should be monitored before and during treatment. Parenteral quinine remains the mainstay of British treatment regimens and it is essential that this (or quinidine) is available in western hospitals. Parasite rates should be estimated at

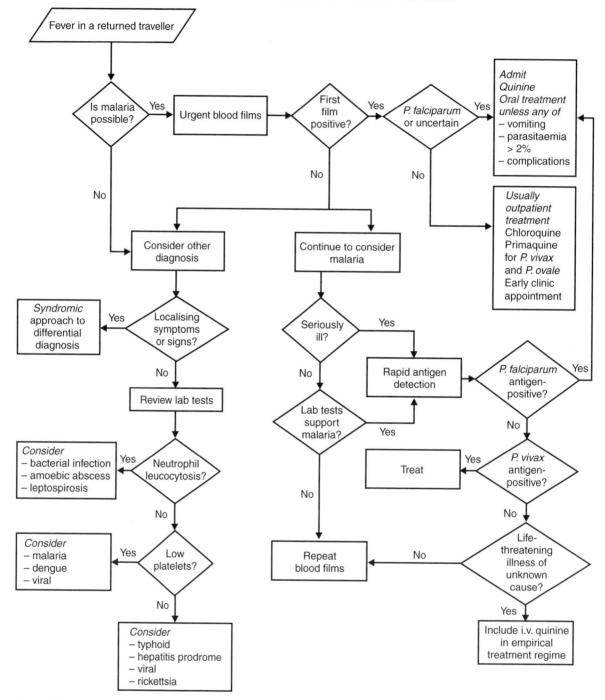

Figure 12.1 Algorithm for diagnosis of fever in the returned traveller. (Modified from Jacobs, *Journal of Royal Society of Medicine*, 2000, **93**: 124–8, and reproduced with permission)

least daily until negative and the patient must be followed up early after discharge to detect recrudescence due to resistance or inadequate treatment. Concurrent infections, particularly bacteraemia (Berkley *et al.*, 1999), should be considered in severe malaria, with a low threshold for introducing broad-spectrum antibiotics pending the results of blood cultures. Careful attention should be paid to fluid balance and monitoring renal, hepatic, neurological and respiratory function, and ill patients should be managed in a high dependency or intensive care setting. The role of exchange transfusion or erythrocytapheresis in reducing morbidity or mortality remains controversial in the absence of any controlled trials, and is favoured in some centres but not in Liverpool (Macallan *et al.*, 1999; Pasvol and Jacobs, 1999).

Less severe cases of falciparum malaria can be managed with oral quinine, mefloquine, co-artemether or atovaquone plus proguanil (Malarone) (Anonymous, 2000). Patients with benign malarias can be managed, often as outpatients, with chloroquine (the above agents are also effective), which is followed by primaquine to eradicate the hypnozoite stages of vivax and ovale malaria to prevent late relapse. Resistance to both agents is present in the Pacific 'Chesson' strain of vivax (Murphy *et al.*, 1993) and is increasingly seen in vivax malaria imported from other areas, including India (Whitby, 1997); however, treatment should be started with chloroquine even if resistant vivax is suspected, and can be switched later if there is no response.

SKIN DISEASE

The most common dermatological problems in travellers are caused by overexposure to sun and insect bites (Hay, 1993; Caumes *et al.*, 1995). A variety of hypersensitivity reactions can follow arthropod bites and these, together with complicating staphylococcal and streptococcal infections, are common reasons for travellers to consult their family doctor after return. Suntans will also make dermatophyte infections such as pityriasis versicolor more obvious to the patient.

Cutaneous larva migrans is frequently seen in the clinic.

Case History

A young British couple had been for their honeymoon in the Caribbean. One week after their return, both developed multiple red serpiginous raised lesions on their legs and abdomen. Both had been lying on the sand to sunbathe. The rash persisted for a week until treatment with albendazole.

The tracks are caused by animal hookworms that invade skin in contact with sand or soil contaminated by cat or dog faeces. This common problem can be avoided by wearing shoes and not lying directly on the sand (use the sunlounger) or by choosing the part of the beach that is regularly cleaned by tidal action (Bouchaud *et al.*, 2000; Caumes, 2000). Treatment of single lesions can be performed by applying a topical paste of tiabendazole but this is rarely available and a short course of albendazole or ivermectin is very effective.

Other invasive parasitic skin diseases are described in the section on eosinophilia, below. The most frequent delayed skin lesion seen in travellers is cutaneous leishmaniasis, particularly in people who have travelled in rural or forested areas of South and Central America or in the Indian subcontinent, although the cutaneous leishmaniases have a widespread geographical distribution (Chapter 8). The rash typically starts as a papule that enlarges and ulcerates with indurated edges. The lesion slowly expands over weeks and is usually relatively painless unless there is bacterial superinfection. Lesions are usually on the face or peripheral parts of the limbs that have been exposed to sandfly bites, and may be single or multiple. There is often local lymphadenopathy and careful examination may reveal smaller nodules proximal to the main lesion. Most patients present within 6 months of exposure. There is no systemic upset and patients are often treated unsuccessfully for suspected staphylococcal infection before referral to a specialist clinic for investigation. Diagnosis is made by aspirating material from the active edge of the lesion or by making an impression smear from the lesion and staining with Giemsa for amastigotes. Special culture media are needed to grow the organism and species-specific PCR is a quicker and more sensitive method of confirming the diagnosis (Noyes *et al.*, 1998). Infections with *Leishmania tropica* from India and the Middle East do not usually need specific treatment, but *L. braziliense* lesions should be treated by specialists with parenteral antimonial agents because of the small risk of mucocutaneous dissemination (Hepburn *et al.*, 1993; Aronson *et al.*, 1998). *L. braziliense* lesions cannot be distinguished clinically from those caused by *L. mexicana* and other Central and South American species.

Myiasis is a frequent problem in travellers to Africa. The tumbu fly, *Cordylobia anthropophaga*, lays its eggs on clothes and the larvae from these directly invade the skin, producing lesions resembling a staphylococcal boil. At the centre of these the tip of the larva can be seen to wriggle. Treatment is by suffocating the larva with topical petroleum jelly, then careful removal with forceps as it extrudes itself to obtain air. Travellers to South and Central America may acquire more invasive cutaneous myiasis due to larvae of *Cochliomyia homnivorax* or *Dermatobia hominis*. These larvae have lateral spines that make removal more difficult, often requiring minor surgery under local or even general anaesthetic. The 'jiggers flea', *Tunga penetrans*, frequently infects the feet of people who walk barefoot in the tropics. The female flea, full of eggs, grows to cause a nodule, from which it can be carefully shelled out with a toothpick or needle. Care should be taken not to rupture the flea, which could lead to local bacterial infection.

Table 12.12 Selected parasitic infections and eosinophilia in travellers

Parasite/disease	Clinical clues
Nematodes	
Ascaris lumbricoides	Visible worms in faeces; Loeffler
Hookworms	Anaemia; Loeffler
Strongyloides spp	Diarrhoea; larva currens rash
Trichuris trichiura	Diarrhoea (bloody)
Loa loa	Travel history; visible worm in eye; Calabar swelling
Mansonella perstans	Travel history
Onchocerca volvulus	Travel history; eye symptoms; rash; nodules
Wuchereria bancrofti	Travel history; sometimes
Brugia malayi	tropical pulmonary eosinophilia; rarely chyluria, elephantiasis, etc.
Nonhuman hookworms	Rash of cutaneous larva migrans
Trematodes	
Schistosoma spp	Travel history and freshwater exposure; Katayama fever; haematuria or blood in faeces
Fasciola hepatica	Travel history; tender enlarged liver
Clonorchis spp ⎱ *Opisthorcis* spp ⎰	Travel history; cholangitis-like presentation
Paragonimus spp	Travel history and food history; haemoptysis

EOSINOPHILIA

A raised eosinophilia count usually suggests a helminth infection in returned travellers. Although the traditional definition of eosinophilia is an absolute count $> 0.44 \times 10^9 \, l^{-1}$ (Wolfe, 1999), many clinicians use a cut-off level of $> 0.5 \times 10^9 \, l^{-1}$ in working practice (Gyawali and Whitty, 2000). This level of eosinophilia is used for travellers returning from the tropics, but no normal ranges have been published for those who live in the tropics long-term.

Up to 10% of the travelling population have atopic conditions, such as eczema or asthma, which cause a raised eosinophil count, and some medications such as nonsteroidal anti-inflammatory agents also cause a raised count. A wide variety of nematode and trematode infections produce eosinophilia, particularly during the migratory phases of larvae through the body (Table 12.12). Some of these, such as hookworms, roundworms and *Strongyloides* spp are universally distributed in the tropics, while other parasitic infections will be suggested by the specific travel history of the patient and by the symptoms and physical findings.

Asymptomatic schistosomiasis is a common imported

cause of eosinophilia: a history of immersion in fresh water in Africa, the Middle East or in much of the Far East or South America should always be sought. Only a minority of patients recall having 'swimmer's itch' 24–48 h after bathing in infected water, caused by the initial penetration of skin by the schistosomule. As the earlier case report illustrated, acute schistosomiasis may cause symptoms in nonimmune travellers 3–8 weeks later as the larvae begin to mature and to excrete eggs, which elicit an eosinophilic response. Patients experience fever, transient urticarial rashes, headache, a dry cough and malaise (Katayama fever) (Colebunders *et al.*, 1998). Hepatosplenomegaly is occasionally found and transitory nonspecific infiltrates may be seen on chest X-ray (Cooke *et al.*, 1999). High levels of eosinophilia ($> 1 \times 10^9 \, l^{-1}$) are common at this stage but specific diagnostic tests are usually negative. The condition settles and the patient may then remain asymptomatic or subsequently develop haematuria, alteration in colour and/or consistency of semen (McKenna *et al.*, 1997), or blood in the faeces. By this stage, serological tests and microscopy of terminal urine specimens, filtered urine collections (*Schistosoma haematobium*) and stool or rectal snips (*S. japonicum*, *S. mansoni*) should be positive (Whitty *et al.*, 2000a). Treatment with praziquantel during the acute state has no effect on migrating schistosomules and we repeat the treatment 3 months later. The role of a short course of steroids in Katayama fever is unproven but they are often used for patients who are ill enough to merit treatment in hospital (Harries and Cook, 1987). Haematuria requires further investigation and follow-up for possible complications. Patients with schistosomiasis can be treated as outpatients and should be followed up to confirm parasitological cure. This is important as ectopic egg deposition may cause crippling transverse myelitis later on if the patient is not cured (Blanchard *et al.*, 1993). The enzyme-linked immunosorbent assay (ELISA) titre often rises initially and can take several years to become negative. This reduces its usefulness for diagnosis of new infection after repeated exposures during subsequent travels.

Schistosomiasis is the most common cause of eosinophilia in travellers from Africa seen in our clinic or in London. The next most common systemic cause is filarial infections. Onchocerciasis is still a major problem in West Africa, the Yemen and in Central and South America (Chapter 8). Patients are often asymptomatic or present years after exposure with itchy skin. Occasionally nodules containing adult worms can be found, and fundoscopy should always be performed to detect choroidoretinitis, which leads to blindness. Diagnosis is usually confirmed by examining skin snips for motile larvae. Treatment with diethylcarbamazine (DEC) is invariably followed by an allergic reaction (the Mazzotti reaction) which can be severe enough to cause hypotensive collapse in heavily infected patients. It can be used to confirm the diagnosis in skin-snip negative patients by giving a small dose of DEC. This reaction is much less common following the current treatment of choice which is ivermectin, but expatriates should still be treated under hospital supervision.

Loa loa infection is relatively common in people who have visited West Africa, some of whom may complain of transient oedematous swellings of the limbs (Calabar swelling). Patients occasionally notice the larvae migrating under the conjunctiva of the eye, where they are readily visible to the health care worker. Patients with *L. loa* should always be investigated with skin snips to exclude coexistent onchocerciasis, especially if they are to be treated with DEC, when pretreatment with steroids is used by some (Churchill *et al.*, 1996). Ivermectin or possibly albendazole are now the treatments of choice and heavy filarial loads may need to be reduced by plasmapharesis prior to chemotherapy.

Other blood and lymphatic filariases have a more widespread distribution in the tropics and are common causes of eosinophilia in Asia and the Pacific region, as well as in Africa and South and Central America. Infections are usually asymptomatic but the early phase of infection is characterised by wheezing, dyspnoea, cough, fever and fatigue, with widespread shadowing on the chest X-ray (tropical pulmonary eosinophilia). Eosinophil levels are very high ($> 3 \times 10^9 1^{-1}$) but microfilariae are not found in the blood. Serological tests (ELISA) for filariasis are positive. Symptoms may require relief with a short course of steroids. This condition is less commonly seen in travellers after their return, when filariasis is usually asymptomatic. Emergence of the microfilariae of *Wuchereria bancrofti* into the bloodstream is nocturnal and they are most easily found in blood taken at midnight. Daytime blood samples are positive if the patient is given a single dose of DEC 1 h beforehand. Other filarial infections do not usually have nocturnal periodicity and can routinely be detected in daytime blood films. Treatment is with DEC, ivermectin or albendazole.

After excluding schistosomiasis and filarial infections, the most common imported causes of eosinophilia are intestinal nematode infections such as hookworm infection, trichuriasis and strongyloidiasis. *Trichuris trichuria* is often asymptomatic but heavy infections can cause bloody diarrhoea and even rectal prolapse in young children. Patients with hookworm may have abdominal pain but anaemia is only caused by heavy infections, especially in malnourished children.

Tapeworm infections of the gut are often associated with moderate eosinophilia but are not common in returned travellers. They are diagnosed by finding proglottids in stool which are visible to the naked eye. Treatment is with praziquantel. Hydatid cysts rarely cause a raised eosinophil count unless they have ruptured or leaked. Ascaris and hookworms can also cause transient parasitic pneumonitis (Loeffler syndrome) during the pulmonary larval migration phase. This is less severe than tropical pulmonary eosinophilia, from which it can be distinguished by negative filarial ELISA tests, and blood films for microfilariae are also negative. Eosinophilia can also accompany cutaneous larva migrans caused by nonhu-

man hookworm larvae or the transient rash (ground itch) that is occasionally seen in nonimmune travellers following skin penetration by larvae of human hookworms. These rashes should be distinguished from the 'larva currens' rash of *Strongyloides stercoralis* infection, which can persist for decades by autoreinfection.

Intestinal nematodes can usually be identified by stool microscopy but this is often negative in *Strongyloides* infections, for which special culture methods are needed, together with specific ELISA tests on serum. Strongyloidiasis should be excluded in patients who are about to undergo chemosuppressive therapy, and who have travelled or were born in the tropics or subtropics, because of the risk of fatal hyperinfection syndrome.

Case History

A 45-year-old Nigerian presented to our clinic 10 years after leaving West Africa with chronic nonbloody diarrhoea and weight loss. On direct questioning he admitted to occasional rashes that consisted of a linear urticarial track moving rapidly across his abdomen for 24–48 h. He had high eosinophilia, a positive serum ELISA for *Strongyloides*, and positive charcoal culture of faeces for the characteristic larvae of *S. stercoralis*. His symptoms resolved after treatment with ivermectin.

Patients in whom the above infections have been excluded as causes of eosinophilia may harbour fluke infections from ingestion of raw foods and a careful history should be sought about dietary habits while travelling. Consumption of contaminated salads or cress is associated with fascioliasis, particularly in the Middle East. Patients experience painful hepatomegaly and fever during the migratory phase, with alarming findings on ultrasound of holes in the liver resembling peliosis hepatis. Serological tests may be helpful, as the characteristic ova may be difficult to find in stools. Patients who have eaten raw fish, crabs or other freshwater crustacea in the Far East may acquire clonorchiasis or paragonimiasis, producing cholangitis and haemoptysis, respectively. Ingestion of frogs in the Far East can transmit gnathostomiasis, characterised by solitary swellings, often on the face, which persist for days to weeks. Ingestion of slugs or snails (usually inadvertently in salads) in much of the Pacific region can result in eosinophilic meningitis. This presents acutely with fluctuating focal neurological signs and meningitis, with eosinophils in peripheral blood and cerebrospinal fluid. Eosinophils are occasionally seen in the cerebrospinal fluid of patients with neurocysticercosis, which may cause epilepsy years after acquiring *Taenia solium* after ingestion of pork. Subcutaneous nodules may be present and calcified cysts can be visualised in plain X-ray films of the thighs. Computed tomography or magnetic resonance imaging of the head confirm the diagnosis. Trichinosis and visceral larva migrans (toxocariasis) are cosmopolitan infections that should be con-

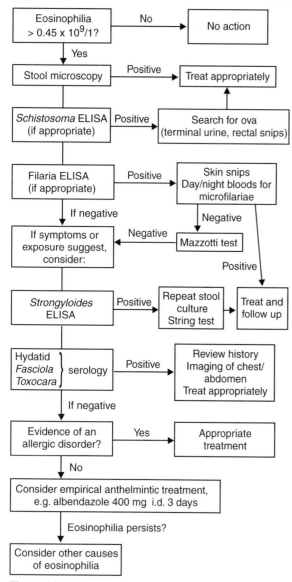

Figure 12.2 Approach to diagnosis of eosinophilia in returned travellers. (Modified from Churchill *et al.*, 1993, with permission)

sidered in the differential diagnosis of eosinophilia but are not specifically associated with travel.

The investigation of eosinophilia may be a protracted process, a useful scheme for which is summarised in Figure 12.2. Simple investigations, including examination of at least two faecal specimens for ova and larvae, and blood for microfilariae, should precede more focused serological and parasitological tests of skin snips, sputum and duodenal samples. The exposure history or clinical picture may also suggest the need for specific tests such as imaging of the liver. If these fail to provide a diagnosis, treatment with a broad-spectrum agent, such as albendazole, with follow-up to establish resolution of

eosinophilia is usually adequate. Alternatively, the patient can be observed for 2–3 months and a repeat stool examination performed to detect parasites that have completed their development and are now excreting ova. It should be remembered that the absence of eosinophilia does not exclude helminth and cestode infections, which should be investigated as in Fig 12.2 if there is clinical suspicion for other reasons.

POST-TRAVEL CHECK

Post-travel checks are frequently requested by travellers, although their usefulness remains controversial. These travellers usually fall into three groups: those concerned about specific risk exposures; those who have had unexplained illness in the tropics; and those who have been abroad but are otherwise well. The first two groups have had a risk exposure or an illness for which diagnosis and treatment could prevent possible future health problems, and further investigation is usually recommended. This includes patients at risk of relapse or late complications of incompletely treated malaria, borreliosis, amoebiasis, schistosomiasis, giardiasis and the filariases. The importance of sexually transmitted diseases has already been discussed. The third group may have unknowingly had a risk exposure while living under local conditions for a prolonged period of time, and it may be worthwhile screening them for subclinical tropical infections; however, there is no evidence that screening asymptomatic long-term (usually considered more than 6 months) travellers is cost-effective.

Another category of asymptomatic patients who might benefit from screening include specific occupational groups such as food handlers or nursery workers who may have acquired infections that could be transmitted to others. The principles of screening individual travellers are somewhat different from instituting a public health-oriented screening programme for specific groups of people such as immigrants, refugees or other displaced persons, or for children arriving from overseas for adoption (Okereke and Gelletlie, 1999). In these groups the spectrum of illnesses that are screened for are different and focused more on transmissible diseases such as tuberculosis and hepatitis B, for which specific prevention measures are available.

Some studies have described the prevalence of tropical infections in asymptomatic travellers and one study has compared the cost-effectiveness of using different diagnostic screening strategies on asymptomatic travellers.

Prevalence of Tropical Diseases in Asymptomatic Returning Travellers

In 1029 British travellers (age range 8 months to 74 years) who had recently returned from the tropics (staying for 3 months to 45 years) and requested screening in London, one in four had an abnormality. Stool microscopy was positive for ova and cysts in 186/995 (19%); 67/852 (8%) had eosinophilia and in this group a parasitological cause was found in 26 (39%). Schistosomal serology was positive in 72/676 (11%) (Carroll et al., 1993). In a Dutch study, tropical diseases were diagnosed in 99/253 (39%) asymptomatic children returning from the tropics, of whom 58 (23%) had giardiasis and 19 (8%) had schistosomiasis (Brouwer et al., 1999). In Montreal, 1605 asymptomatic expatriates were screened and a parasitological diagnosis was found in 225 (17%) (Libman et al., 1993). An Australian study found that, of 221 travellers who visited East Africa, 117 (53%) considered themselves at risk for schistosomiasis and 10 (9%) were positive on subsequent testing (Hipgrave et al., 1997).

Consequences of Not Detecting and Treating Parasites

The potential of untreated schistosomiasis or strongyloidiasis to cause serious problems has already been discussed. If HIV infection remains undetected the traveller will not benefit from chemoprophylaxis against opportunistic infections, or from specific antiretroviral therapy, and will be at risk of passing infection on to others. The consequences of untreated filariasis in the ordinary traveller is unclear and probably not significant. The majority of other intestinal parasites will eventually die without causing any harm to the host, and many feel that routine comprehensive travel screens of the asymptomatic patient are inappropriate for these reasons (Conlon and Peto, 1993). Moreover, screening will not reliably detect significant infections such as malaria and may lull the patient into a false sense of security. Some have suggested that the main value of screening asymptomatic travellers is to inform the travel specialist about the health problems prevailing in different destinations, so that preventive advice for future travellers can be improved (Ellis, 1993). Meanwhile, the cost-effectiveness of routine post-travel screening has not been proven (Genton and Gehri, 1999).

Screening Methods

Nevertheless, it is common practice to offer screening to travellers that request it and a structured approach is required. A full travel and risk history should be taken. The extra information gained from a thorough physical examination is limited (Whitty et al., 2000b). A full blood count should be examined, looking particularly for eosinophilia, together with stool microscopy for ova, cysts and parasites and specific culture for Strongyloides spp (but not for bacterial pathogens). The predictive diagnostic value of eosinophilia is reduced by its nonspecific nature, so that a large number of investigations may be required. In our own experience and that of others (Libman, 1993), an eosinophil count $> 1 \times 10^9 \, l^{-1}$ is predic-

Table 12.13 Some travel-related infections which may exclude the traveller from donating blood, either because of geographical exposure or past infection

African trypanosomiasis
American trypanosomiasis
Hepatitis B
Hepatitis C
HIV
HTLV-I/II
Malaria
New variant Creutzfeldt–Jakob disease
Visceral leishmaniasis

tive of a parasitic infection in 40–50% of cases.

Patients who may have been exposed to schistosomiasis should be screened at least 3 months after departure. This is also a convenient time for discussion of HIV testing, as HIV seroconversion is likely to have occurred by then. If the tests are negative but there is strong concern, repeat screening at 6 months may be required for either of these infections. Other serological tests are of variable availability and cost, and we try to keep these to a minimum. However, adequate stool examination requires at least two, and ideally three, faecal specimens taken on different occasions (patients need specific instructions not to split one specimen three ways). This is time-consuming and expensive, but a study of 1605 asymptomatic travellers showed that, in a Canadian setting, a combination of serological tests and up to three faecal examinations was more effective and cheaper than the combination of faecal microscopy and an eosinophil count for diagnosing schistosomiasis, filariasis and strongyloidiasis (89% versus 61%, respectively) (Libman et al., 1993).

Whatever the specific combination of tests used, patients who test negative need to be warned about the possibility of late appearance of malaria if they have been to a malarious area. They may need to be warned that travel to or residence in some parts of the world may be sufficient to bar them from being blood donors, even if they have no signs of past or current infection (Table 12.13).

Finally, screening should explore noninfectious and situational problems, particularly in the 'worried well' or anxious patient. Reverse culture shock is a genuine problem for many travellers returning to their former western environment, and the health care worker should be attuned to the possibility of significant social or psychiatric problems (Lankester, 2000). This should be an integral part of the 'post-travel check', which, if it is to be performed at all, should not just be reduced to a couple of laboratory tests. In this context, family practice-based screening is likely to provide a more suitable environment than many busy hospital clinics. If for nothing else, the post-travel check-up should be seen as an opportunity for promoting healthy, safe behaviour next time the traveller ventures overseas.

Treatment versus Screening

Alternative strategies are now being used to treat immigrant populations in some settings, based on the total costs (actual and projected) to the health care system. A study of refugees in New York concluded that presumptive treatment of all immigrants at risk for parasitosis with a broad-spectrum anthelmintic, such as albendazole, was cheaper and more effective than screening and treating, or waiting until clinical symptoms developed before treating. This policy prevented death and hospitalisation as well as saving money in the model used (Muennig *et al.*, 1999). Similar considerations have now been extended to justify routine treatment of refugees for undiagnosed malaria as well as for intestinal parasites (Miller *et al.*, 2000). This approach has not been widely adopted in the UK or other countries and is not generally suitable for individual returning travellers. It may have a role in special situations, for example empirical treatment of groups of travellers exposed to schistosomiasis by freshwater bathing in Africa, but the balance of risks and costs in this type of setting has not been modelled.

ACKNOWLEDGEMENTS

We thank our colleagues Mike Beadsworth, David Lalloo and George Wyatt for comments on earlier manuscripts for this chapter.

REFERENCES

Adler MW (1997) Sun, sex and responsibility. *Journal of the Royal College of Physicians*, London, **31**, 425–433.

Advisory Committee on Dangerous Pathogens for Department of Health (1996) *Management and Control of Viral Haemorrhagic Fevers*. Stationery Office, London.

Anderson SR and Johnson CJH (2000) Expedition health and safety: a risk assessment. *Journal of the Royal Society of Medicine*, **93**, 557–562.

Anonymous (1997) Legionnaire's disease in Europe, 1997. *Weekly Epidemiological Record*, **73**, 257–261.

Anonymous (2000) Malarone™ for malaria treatment and prophylaxis.
http//www.cdc.gov/travel/disease/malaria/malarone.htm

Archibald LK, Beeching NJ, Gill GV *et al.* (1993) Albendazole is effective treatment for chronic strongyloidiasis. *Quarterly Journal of Medicine*, **86**, 191–195.

Arishi H, Ageel A, Rahman MA *et al.* (2000) Outbreak of Rift Valley fever—Saudi Arabia, August–October, 2000. *Morbidity and Mortality Weekly Report*, **49**(40), 905–908.
http://www.cdc.gov/mmwr/preview/mmwrhtml/mm4940a1.htm

Aronson NE, Wortmann GW, Johnson SC *et al.* (1998) Safety and efficacy of intravenous sodium stibogluconate in the treatment of leishmaniasis: recent US military experience. *Clinical Infectious Diseases*, **27**, 1457–1464.

Bain BJ (1996) Ethnic and sex differences in the total and differential white cell count and platelet count. *Journal of Clinical Pathology*, **49**, 664–666.

Behrens RH and Curtis CF (1993) Malaria in travellers: epidemiology and prevention. *British Medical Bulletin*, **49**, 363–381.

Beighton PH (1967) Medical hazards of air travel. *Practitioner*, **198**, 668–672.

Bellis MA, Hale G, Bennett A *et al.* (2000) Ibiza uncovered: changes in substance use and sexual behaviour amongst young people visiting an international night-life resort. *International Journal of Drug Policy*, **11**, 235–244.

Berkley J, Mwarumba S, Bramham K *et al.* (1999) Bacteraemia complicating severe malaria in children. *Transactions of the Royal Society of Tropical Medicine and Hygiene*, **93**, 283–296.

Blanchard TJ, Milne LM, Pollock R *et al.* (1993) Early chemotherapy of imported neuroschistosomiasis. *Lancet*, **341**, 959.

Bonneux L, van der Stuyft P, Taelman H *et al.* (1988) Risk factors for infection with human immunodeficiency virus among European expatriates in Africa. *BMJ*, **297**, 581–584.

Bouchaud O, Houzé S, Schiemann R *et al.* (2000) Cutaneous larva migrans in travellers: a prospective study, with assessment of therapy with ivermectin. *Clinical Infectious Diseases*, **31**, 493–498.

Brabin BJ and Ganley Y (1997) Imported malaria in children in the UK. *Archives of Diseases in Childhood*, **77**, 76–81.

Brouwer M, Tolboom JJM and Hardeman JHJ (1999) Routine screening of children returning home from the tropics: retrospective study. *BMJ*, **318**, 568–569.

Bryceson ADM (1987) Imported fevers. *Advanced Medicine*, **23**, 336–343.

Burnett A and Peel M (2001) Health needs of asylum seekers and refugees. *BMJ*, **322**, 544–547.

Burney MI, Ghafoor A, Saleen M *et al.* (1980) Nosocomial outbreak of viral hemorrhagic fever caused by Crimean hemorrhagic fever—Congo virus in Pakistan, January 1976. *American Journal of Tropical Medicine and Hygiene*, **29**, 941–947.

Carroll B, Dow C, Snashall D *et al.* (1993) Post-tropical screening; how useful is it? *BMJ*, **307**, 541–542.

Caumes E (2000) Treatment of cutaneous larva migrans. *Clinical Infectious Diseases*, **30**, 811–814.

Caumes E, Carrière J, Guermonprez G *et al.* (1995) Dermatoses associated with travel to tropical countries: a prospective study of the diagnosis and management of patients presenting to a tropical disease unit. *Clinical Infectious Diseases*, **20**, 542–548.

Centers for Disease Control (1995) Update: management of patients with suspected viral hemorrhagic fever—United States. *MMWR*, **44**(25), 475–479.

Chiodini PL (1998) Non-microscopic methods for diagnosing malaria. *Lancet*, **351**, 80–81.

Churchill DR, Chiodini PL and McAdam KPWJ (1993) Screening the returned traveller. *British Medical Bulletin*, **49**, 465–474.

Churchill DR, Morris C, Fakoya A *et al.* (1996) Clinical and laboratory features of patients with loiasis (*Loa loa* filariasis) in the UK. *Journal of Infection*, **33**, 103–109.

Colebunders R, Verstraeten T, van Gompel A *et al.* (1998) Acute schistosomiasis in travellers returning from Mali. *Journal of Travel Medicine*, **2**, 235–238.

Communicable Disease Report (1997) Needlestick malaria with tragic consequences. *Communicable Disease Report Weekly*, **7**(28).

Conlon CP and Peto T (1993) Post-tropical screening (letter). *BMJ*, **307**, 1008.

Cooke GS, Lalvani A, Gleeson FV *et al.* (1999) Acute pulmonary scchistosomiasis in travelers returning from Lake Malawi, sub-Saharan Africa. *Clinical Infectious Diseases*, 29, 836–839.

Cropley IM, Lockwood DNJ, Mack D *et al.* (2000) Rapid diagnosis of falciparum malaria by using the ParaSight F test in travellers returning to the United Kingdom: prospective study. *BMJ*, **321**, 484–485.

de Graaf R, van Zessen G, Houweling H *et al.* (1997) Sexual risk of HIV infection among expatriates posted in AIDS endemic areas. *AIDS*, **11**, 1173–1181.

Doherty JF, Grant AD and Bryceson ADM (1995) Fever as the presenting complaint of travellers returning from the tropics. *Quarterly Journal of Medicine*, **88**, 277–281.

Dowdall N (2000) 'Is there a doctor in the aircraft?' Top 10 in-flight medical emergencies. *BMJ*, **321**, 1336–1337.

Doyle TJ, Bryan RT and Peters CT (1998) Viral hemorrhagic fevers and hantavirus infections in the Americas. *Infectious Disease Clinics of North America*, **12**, 95–110.

Driver CR, Valway SE, Morgan WM *et al.* (1994) Transmission of *Mycobacterium tuberculosis* associated with air travel. *JAMA*, **272**, 1031–1035.

DuPont HL and Capsuto EG (1996) Persistent diarrhea in travellers. *Clinical Infectious Diseases*, **22**, 124–128.

Ellis CJ (1993) Post-tropical screening (letter). *BMJ*, **307**, 1008.

Ford N and Inman M (1992) Safer sex in tourist resorts. *World Health Forum*, **13**, 77–80.

Genton B and Gehri M (1999) Routine screening of children returning home from the tropics (letter). *BMJ*, **319**, 121.

Geroulakos G (2001) The risk of venous thromboembolism from air travel. *BMJ*, **322**, 188.

Gill GV and Bell DR (1979) *Strongyloides stercoralis* infection in former Far East prisoners of war. *BMJ*, **12**, 572–574.

Goodwin T (2000) In-flight medical emergencies: an over-view. *BMJ*, **321**, 1338–1341.

Gratz NG, Steffen R and Cocksedge W (2000) Why aircraft disinfection? *Bulletin of the World Health Organization*, **78**, 995–1003.

Grobusch MP, Alpermann U, Schwenke S *et al.* (1999) False-positive rapid tests for malaria in patients with rheumatoid factor. *Lancet*, **353**, 297.

Gubler D (1999) Dengue and dengue hemorrhagic fever. *Clinical Microbiological Reviews*, **11**, 480–496.

Gyawali P and Whitty CJM (2000) Investigating eosinophilia in patients returned from the tropics. *Hospital Medicine*, **62**, 25–28.

Hanscheid T, Valadas E and Grobusch MP (2000) Automated malaria diagnosis using pigment detection. *Parasitology Today*, **16**, 549–551.

Harries AD and Cook GC (1987) Acute schistosomiasis (Katayama fever): clinical deterioration after chemotherapy. *Journal of Infection*, **14**, 159–161.

Harries AD, Maher D and Nunn P (1997) Practical and affordable measures for the protection of health care workers from tuberculosis in low-income countries. *Bulletin of the World Health Organisation*, **35**, 477–489.

Hart CA and Kariuki S (1998) Antimicrobial resistance in developing countries. *BMJ*, **317**, 647–650.

Hawkes S, Hart GJ, Johnson AM *et al.* (1994) Risk behaviour and HIV prevalence in international travellers. *AIDS*, **8**, 247–252.

Hay RJ (1993) Skin disease. *British Medical Bulletin*, **49**, 440–453.

Hepburn NC, Tidman MJ and Hunter JAA (1993) Cutaneous leishmaniasis in British troops from Belize. *British Journal of Dermatology*, **128**, 63–68.

Hipgrave DB, Leydon JA, Walker J and Biggs IBA (1997) Schistosomiasis in Australian travellers to Africa. *Medical Journal of Australia*, **166**, 294–297.

Houweling H and Coutinho RA (1991) Risk of HIV infection among Dutch expatriates in sub-Saharan Africa. *International Journal of STD and AIDS*, **2**, 252–257.

Humar A and Keystone J (1996) Evaluating fever in travellers returning from tropical countries. *BMJ*, **312**, 953–956.

Iqbal J, Sher A, Hira PR *et al.* (1999) Comparison of the Opti-MAL test with PCR for diagnosis of malaria in immigrants. *Journal of Clinical Microbiology*, **37**, 3644–3646.

Jelinek T (2000) Dengue fever in international travellers. *Clinical Infectious Diseases*, **31**, 144–147.

Jelinek T, Amsler L, Grobusch MP *et al.* (1999) Self-use of rapid tests for malaria diagnosis by tourists. *Lancet*, **354**, 1609.

Kain KC, Harrington MA, Tennyson S *et al.* (1998) Imported malaria: prospective analysis of problems in diagnosis and management. *Clinical Infectious Diseases*, **27**, 142–149.

Kenyon TA, Valway SE, Ihle WW *et al.* (1996) Transmission of multi-drug resistant *Mycobacterium tuberculosis* during a long airplane flight. *New England Journal of Medicine*, **334**, 933–938.

Kesteven PLJ (2000) Traveller's thrombosis. *Thorax*, **55** (suppl. 1), S32–S36.

Klein JL and Millman GC (1998) Prospective, hospital based study of fever in children in the United Kingdom who had recently spent time in the tropics. *BMJ*, **316**, 1425–1426.

Klontz KC, Hynes NA, Gunn RA *et al.* (1989) An outbreak of influenza A/Taiwan/1/89 (H1N1) infections at a naval base and its association with airplane travel. *American Journal of Epidemiology*, **129**, 341–348.

Laferi H, Kandel K and Pichler H (1997) False positive dipstick test for malaria. *New England Journal of Medicine*, **337**, 1635–1636.

Lankester T (2000) Health screening and psychological considerations in the returned traveller. In *Travel Medicine and Migrant Health* (eds C Lockie, E Walker, L Calver *et al.*), pp 443–452. Churchill Livingstone, Edinburgh.

Lettau LA (1991). Nosocomial transmission and infection control aspects of parasitic and ectoparasitic diseases Part II. Blood tissue parasites. *Infection Control and Hospital Epidemiology*, **12**, 111–121.

Lewis SJ, Davidson RN, Ross EJ *et al.* (1992) Severity of imported falciparum malaria: effect of taking antimalarial prophylaxis. *BMJ*, **305**, 741–743.

Libman MD, MacLean JD and Gyorkos TW (1993) Screening for schistosomiasis, filariasis and strongyloidiasis among expatriates returning from the tropics. *Clinical Infectious Diseases*, **17**, 353–359.

Luzzi GA, Brindle R, Sockett PN *et al.* (1993) Brucellosis: imported and laboratory-acquired cases, and an overview of treatment trials. *Transactions of the Royal Society of Tropical Medicine and Hygiene*, **87**, 138–141.

Macallan DC, Pocock M, Bishop E *et al.* (1999) Automated erythrocytapheresis in the treatment of severe falciparum malaria. *Journal of Infection*, **39**, 233–236.

McKenna G, Shousboe M and Paltridge G (1997) Subjective change in ejaculate as symptom of infection with *Schistosoma haematobium* in travellers. *BMJ*, **315**, 1000–1001.

MacLean JD, Lalonde RG and Ward R (1994) Fever from the tropics. *Travel Medicine Advisor*, **5**, 27.1–27.14.

Malaria Working Party of the General Haematology Task Force of the British Committee for Standards in Haematology (1997) The laboratory diagnosis of malaria. *Clinical Laboratory Haematology*, **19**, 165–170.

Miller JM, Boyd HA, Ostrowski SR *et al.* (2000) Malaria, intestinal parasites and schistosomiasis among Barawan Somali refugees resettling to the United States: a strategy to reduce morbidity and decrease the risk of imported infections. *Ameri-*

can Journal of Tropical Medicine and Hygiene, **62**, 115–121.

Minooee A and Rickman LS (1999) Infectious diseases on cruise ships. *Clinical Infectious Diseases*, **29**, 737–744.

Molyneux M and Fox R (1993) Diagnosis and treatment of malaria in Britain. *BMJ*, **155**, 861–868.

Muennig P, Pallin D, Sell RL *et al.* (1999) The cost effectiveness of strategies for the treatment of intestinal parasites in immigrants. *New England Journal of Medicine*, **340**, 773–779.

Murphy GS, Purnomo HB, Andersen EM *et al.* (1993) Vivax malaria resistant to treatment and prophylaxis with chloroquine. *Lancet*, **341**, 96–100.

Nichols GL (2000) Food-borne protozoa. *British Medical Bulletin*, **56**, 209–235.

Nosten F and van Vugt M (1999) Neuropsychiatric adverse effects of mefloquine. What do we know and what should we do? *CNS Drugs*, **1**, 1–8.

Noyes HA, Reyburn H, Bailey JW *et al.* (1998) A nested-PCR-based schizodeme method for identifying *Leishmania* kinetoplast minicircle classes directly from clinical samples and its application to the study of the epidemiology of *Leishmania tropica* in Pakistan. *Journal of Clinical Microbiology*, **36**, 2877–2881.

Okereke E and Gelletlie R (1999) Routine screening of children returning home from the tropics (letter). *BMJ*, **319**, 121–122.

Ormerod P (2000) Tuberculosis and travel. *Hospital Medicine*, **61**, 171–173.

Paget Stanfield J and Reid D (1980) Imported infections in children. *Journal of the Royal College of Physicians of London*, **14**, 232–237.

Pasvol G and Jacobs M (1999) What is the future for exchange transfusion for falciparum malaria? *Journal of Infection*, **39**, 183–184.

Phillips-Howard PA, Radalowicz A, Mitchell J *et al.* (1990) Risk of malaria in British residents returning from malarious areas. *BMJ*, **300**, 499–504.

Pike RM (1978) Past and present hazards of working with infectious agents. *Archives of Pathology and Laboratory Medicine*, **102**, 333–336.

Riordan FAI and Tarlow MJ (1998) Imported infections in East Birmingham children. *Postgraduate Medical Journal*, **74**, 36–37.

Risch L, Bader M, Huber AR (2000) Self-use of rapid tests for malaria diagnosis. *Lancet*, **355**, 237.

Rubio JM, Benito A, Berzosa PJ *et al.* (1999) Usefulness of seminested multiplex PCR in surveillance of imported malaria in Spain. *Journal of Clinical Microbiology*, **37**, 3260–3264.

Schmetzer O (1999) Hemorraghic fever ? Germany ex Cote D'Ivoire. ProMED Mail, 6 Aug. http://www.healthnet.org/programs/promed.html

Schwartz E, Jenks NP, van Damme P *et al.* (1999) Hepatitis E virus infection in travellers. *Clinical Infectious Diseases*, **29**, 1312–1314.

Steffen R, Kane MA, Shapiro CN *et al.* (1994) Epdemiology and prevention of hepatitis A in travellers. *JAMA*, **272**, 885–889.

Suh KN, Kozarsky PE and Keystone JS (1999) Evaluation of fever in the returned traveller. *Medical Clinics of North America*, **83**, 997–1017.

Suleiman MN, Muscat-Baron JM, Harries JR *et al.* (1980) Congo–Crimean haemorrhagic fever in Dubai. *Lancet*, **ii**, 939–941.

Svenson JE, MacLean JD, Gyorkos TW *et al.* (1995) Imported malaria: clinical presentation and examination of symptomatic travellers. *Archives of Internal Medicine*, **155**, 861–868.

Svenungsson B, Lagergren Å, Ekwall E *et al.* (2000) Enteropathogens in adult patients with diarrhoea and healthy control subjects: a 1-year prospective study in a Swedish clinic for infectious diseases. *Clinical Infectious Diseases*, **30**, 770–778.

Tham JM, Hee Lee S, Tan TMC *et al.* (1999) Detection and species determination of malaria parasites by PCR: comparison with microscopy and with Parasight-F and ICT malaria Pf tests in a clinical environment. *Journal of Clinical Microbiology*, **37**, 1269–1273.

Tichonova L, Borisenko K, Ward H *et al.* (1997) Epidemics of syphilis in the Russian Federation: trends, origins, and priorities for control. *Lancet*, **350**, 210–213.

Trees A and Shaw S (1999) Imported disease in small animals. In *Practice* (*Journal of Veterinary Postgraduate Clinical Study*), October, 482–491.

von Sonnenburg F, Turnieporth N, Waiyaki P *et al.* (2000) Risk of aetiology of diarrhoea at various tourist destinations. *Lancet*, **356**, 133–134.

Wang CC and Celum CL (1999) Global risk of sexually transmitted diseases. *Medical Clinics of North America*, **83**, 975–995.

Wetsteyn JCFM, Kaer PA and van Gool T (1997) The changing pattern of imported malaria in the Academic Medical Centre, Amsterdam. *Journal of Travel Medicine*, **4**, 171–175.

Whitby M (1997) Drug resistant *Plasmodium vivax* malaria. *Journal of Antimicrobial Chemotherapy*, **40**, 749–752.

Whitty CJM, Mabey DC, Armstrong M *et al.* (2000a). Presentation and outcome of 1107 cases of schistosomiasis from African diagnosed in a non-endemic country. *Transactions of the Royal Society of Tropical Medicine and Hygiene*, **94**, 531–534.

Whitty CJM, Carroll B, Armstrong M *et al.* (2000b) Utility of history, examination and laboratory tests in screening those returning to Europe from the tropics for parasitic infection. *Tropical Medicine and International Health*, **5**, 818–823.

Wolfe MS (1999) Eosinophilia in the returned traveller. *Medical Clinics of North America*, **83**, 1019–1032.

World Health Organization (2000) Severe falciparum malaria. *Transactions of the Royal Society of Tropical Medicine and Hygiene*, **94** (suppl. 1), 1–90.

Zaat JOM, Mark TG and Assendelft WJJ (1997) A systematic review on the treatment of giardiasis. *Tropical Medicine and International Health*, **2**, 63–82.

FURTHER READING

Armstrong D and Cohen J (1999) *Infectious Diseases*, Mosby, London.

Cook GC (1996) *Manson's Tropical Diseases*, 20th edn. WB Saunders, London.

DuPont HL and Steffen R (1997) *Textbook of Travel Medicine and Health*. Decker, Hamilton.

Feigin RD and Cherry JD (1998) *Textbook of Pediatric Infectious Diseases*, 4th edn. WB Saunders, Philadephia.

Gilles HM and Wallace P (1995) *Colour Atlas of Tropical Medicine and Parasitology*, 4th edn. Mosby-Wolfe, London.

Guerrant RL, Walker DH and Weller PF (1999) *Tropical Infectious Diseases: Principles, Pathogens and Practice*. Churchill Livingstone, Philadelphia.

Hunter GW and Strickland GT (2000) *Hunter's Tropical Medicine and Emerging Infectious Diseases*, 8th edn. WB Saunders, Philadelphia.

Lockie C, Walker E, Calvert L *et al.* (2000) *Travel Medicine and Migrant Health*. Churchill Livingstone, Edinburgh.

Mandell GL, Bennett JE and Dolin R (2000) *Mandell, Douglas and Bennett's Principles and Practice of Infectious Diseases*, 5th edn. Churchill Livingstone, Philadelphia.

Wilson ME (1991) *A World Guide to Infections: Disease, Distribution Diagnosis.* Oxford University Press, New York.

ADDITIONAL RESOURCES

English Language Websites Giving Useful Geographically-oriented Medical Information

Australian Travel Medicine and Vaccination Centres.
http://www.tmvc.com.au/about1.html
Australian comprehensive travel information and health alerts.

British Foreign Office Travel Warnings.
http://193.114.50.10/travel/countryadvice.asp
Country specific safety information.

Centers for Disease Control (CDC) Travellers' Health.
http://www.cdc.gov/travel/
Regional specific database for recommended immunisations and malaria prevention. Also includes international outbreaks.

European Surveillance.
http://www.euroserv.org/
Weekly and monthly European surveillance information.

International Society of Travel Medicine.
http://www.istm.org/index.html
Current news and conference information. Listing of travel clinics worldwide. Electronic interaction of health care professionals via Travelmed forum.

International Travel and Health (WHO)
http://www.who.int/ith/english/index.htm
Country specific yellow fever requirements and malaria recommendations. Updated annually.

Outbreak Information (WHO).
http://www.who.int/disease-outbreak-news/
Regular reports on WHO-confirmed outbreaks of international importance.

ProMED Mail.
http://www.promedmail.org/pls/promed/promed.home
Regular unconfirmed reports on international outbreaks. A programme of the International Society for Infectious Diseases.

Scottish Centre for Infection and Environmental Health (SCIEH).
http://www.show.scot.nhs.uk/scieh/
Country specific database for recommended immunisations and malaria prevention regularly updated with international outbreak information (£40.00 per annum outside Scotland)

Travel Health Online Shoreline.
http://www.tripprep.com/
American information giving country-specific immunisation and malaria advice, safety information and listings of medical providers overseas.

US State Department Travel Warnings
http://travel.state.gov/travel_warnings.html
US State Department travel warnings and consular information sheets.

Weekly Epidemiological Record (WHO).
http://www.who.int/wer/
Weekly report on infections from WHO.

World Health Organization (WHO)
http://www.who.int/
Good information source for worldwide communicable and noncommunicable disease.

Section IV

Hazards of Air and Sea Travel

13

Aviation Medicine

Michael Bagshaw

British Airways Health Services, Harmondsworth, UK

INTRODUCTION

Aviation medicine is a branch of occupational medicine which has developed from human needs to adapt to the inherently hostile environment of the air. It is a wide-ranging discipline, encompassing physiological and psychological aspects of fitness to fly, and the human factors facets of flight safety are recognised as an important component of flight crew training. The normal physiology of the human body when in flight can be influenced by altitude, changes in pressure, temperature, acceleration and sensory perception. This chapter is concerned only with those areas of aviation medicine applicable to travel medicine. For fuller consideration of the wider discipline, the reader is referred to more comprehensive texts (Campbell and Bagshaw, 1999; Ernsting *et al.*, 1999).

Commercial air travel is a comfortable, speedy and safe means of transport and is now accepted as a part of everyday life for many people in the developed world. It is affordable and accessible to almost all sectors of the population, and it is easy to forget that the individual is travelling in a potentially physiologically hostile environment.

THE ATMOSPHERE

Composition

The atmosphere surrounds the earth and forms an elastic layer of air composed of a mixture of gases and water vapour. The most abundant gases are nitrogen (78%) and oxygen (21%), with the remaining 1% being argon, carbon dioxide, neon, hydrogen and ozone. The proportions remain constant up to the tropopause (approximately 36 000 feet (11 000 m)). The pressure at sea level in the standard atmosphere is 760 mmHg and this falls to half (380 mmHg) at 18 000 feet (5500 m), where the ambient temperature is about −20°C.

The Physical Gas Laws

Since air is a mixture of gases which exert pressure, have measurable mass and can be compressed, it is subject to certain established laws governing reaction to changes in pressure, temperature, volume and density. A basic knowledge of these gas laws helps in understanding how the human body reacts to the aviation environment.

Boyle's law states that:

providing the temperature is constant, the volume of a gas is inversely proportional to its pressure.

This means that when the pressure increases, the volume decreases and, conversely, when the pressure decreases, the volume increases. Boyle's law explains some of the effects of altitude on the gas-containing cavities of the human body during flight. For example, as altitude increases, gas contained within the middle ear, sinuses and gut will expand, sometimes with painful results.

Charles's law states that:

the volume of a fixed mass of gas held at a constant pressure varies directly with absolute temperature.

A feature of gas expansion is that equal volumes of different gases expand by the same amount when heated to the same temperature, so another way of stating Charles's law is that volume of a fixed mass of gas at constant pressure is directly proportional to its absolute temperature.

The gas laws of Boyle and Charles can be summarised in the equation:

$$pv/T = \text{constant},$$

where p = pressure, v = volume, T = absolute temperature. This is known as the gas equation, or general gas law, and it applies even when there is a change in all three variables—pressure, volume and temperature.

Principles and Practice of Travel Medicine. Edited by Jane N. Zuckerman.
© 2001 John Wiley & Sons Ltd.

Dalton's law states that:

the total pressure of the gas mixture is equal to the sum of its partial pressures.

This means that the proportion of oxygen remains 21% throughout the atmosphere, irrespective of the total atmospheric pressure at that particular altitude.

Finally, *Henry's law* states that:

at equilibrium the amount of gas dissolved in a liquid is proportional to the gas pressure.

This means that the amount of gas in solution varies directly with the pressure of that gas. In aviation, this is relevant in that, as altitude is increased and atmospheric pressure reduces, gases such as nitrogen will come out of solution in the body tissues. At high altitude this can lead to decompression sickness.

OXYGEN REQUIREMENTS AT ALTITUDE

Respiration and Circulation

Respiration is essentially the process by which some organisms (humans, for example) liberate energy to maintain the processes of life by oxidation of food. For convenience it may be divided into three phases:

1. The exchange of gases between body and atmosphere.
2. The carriage of gases to and from the reservoir (the lungs) and the site of oxidation (the tissue cells).
3. The actual oxidative process at cellular level, liberating energy.

Aviation can profoundly affect the first two, but has little or no effect upon the third.

Gaseous Exchange

The oxygen used in the energy liberation is obtained from atmospheric air. This enters the body via the nasopharynx and passes down the trachea into one of the lungs via the appropriate bronchus and bronchioles, ending in an alveolus, millions of which form the lungs.

The mechanism of the gas flow is simple. The lungs, which communicate fully with the atmosphere, lie in the thoracic cavity, which is bounded by the rib cage and diaphragm. As the thorax is a closed cavity, any change in its volume causes a corresponding change in lung volume. Inspiration is the act of diaphragm contraction and elevation of the ribs using the intercostal muscles, thereby increasing lung volume and drawing in air (an active process). Expiration is a reverse of this process, relaxing the diaphragm and intercostal muscles, decreasing the lung volume and driving out air (a passive process). The rate and depth of respiration are controlled by the metabolic demands of the tissues in their need for oxygen and elimination of the waste products carbon dioxide and water vapour. These can vary enormously, depending on

the state of activity of the body. At rest, each breath involves about half a litre of air, and the cycle occurs 12–15 times a minute.

As stated previously the atmospheric air ends in the alveolae or air sacs. An alveolus is a very thin-walled structure, covered with a complex of capillaries or small blood vessels, which brings the blood within the closest possible apposition to the lung air. Here diffusion takes place; oxygen from the lung air diffuses across the thin barrier of alveolar and blood vessel walls to enter the blood, and the waste products of cellular respiration carried by the blood to the lung diffuse from the blood into the air sac.

Carriage of Gases

Oxygen diffusing across the alveolar wall into the closely apposed blood is carried to its ultimate destination in chemical combination with haemoglobin, a component of the red blood cell (erythrocyte). A very small proportion of oxygen is carried in physical solution. The circulatory path is as follows:

1. Blood leaves the lungs and returns to the left side of the heart, from where it is pumped in arteries to the tissues of the body.
2. Here oxygen diffuses into the cells and is used in the oxidative processes. Energy is released, with the consequent production of carbon dioxide and water.
3. These waste products thence diffuse back into the bloodstream and are ultimately carried back to the right side of the heart via the venous system.
4. From here the blood is pumped to the lungs, where gaseous exchange occurs in the alveoli.

Despite the embolic inference of the description it must be understood that the whole is one continuous flowing process. The path of oxygen to the tissues and that of carbon dioxide from the tissues may be summarised as follows:

- *Oxygen pathway in the body*: atmosphere → trachea → bronchi → alveoli → blood → tissue.
- *Carbon dioxide pathway in the body*: tissue → blood → alveoli → bronchi → trachea → atmosphere.

Control of Respiration

We have seen that the rate and depth of breathing is controlled by the metabolic demands of the tissues. The fundamental controlling factor is the partial pressure of carbon dioxide (Pco_2) in the blood perfusing the respiratory centre in the brain. This is extremely sensitive to small changes in the carbon dioxide tension in the blood, and continuously adjusts the breathing rate to maintain this tension at a normal level. The receptors in the respiratory centre are also sensitive to the acidity of the arterial blood. Another set of chemoreceptors is located in the carotid arteries and these also respond to changes in the tension of carbon dioxide in the arterial blood by influencing the breathing rate. In addition, these carotid receptors are very sensitive to reduction in arterial oxygen tension.

Composition of Alveolar Air

As can be appreciated from the above, the composition of alveolar air differs from that of atmospheric air due to the constant diffusion of gases to and from the alveolus and the blood. The difference may be visualised as follows:

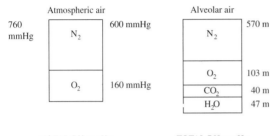

(Note: diagramatic representations not to scale)

While the total pressure is the same, the composition is different. Unlike the ambient atmospheric air, alveolar air includes water vapour and carbon dioxide generated by the body, which remains as a constant, provided the respiratory rate remains constant and the body at rest. As the total pressure has remained the same, to accommodate the water vapour and carbon dioxide the pressures of oxygen and nitrogen must be reduced. The levels shown are found in the healthy young individual at sea level, and may be regarded as the ideal.

While the above is the ideal, from common experience it may be observed that human beings' apparent efficiency deteriorates but little during ascent from sea level. Despite a fall in atmospheric pressure and consequent reduction in oxygen pressure in the lung, they remain reasonably efficient to an altitude of about 10 000 feet (3000 m). An analysis of lung gases at this altitude can be represented thus:

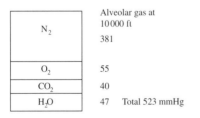

(Note: diagramatic representation not to scale)

Above 10 000 feet (3000 m), however, the oxygen tension falls below a critical level and deterioration in performance becomes obvious.

To prevent this deterioration when flying, a method has to be found of augmenting the oxygen content of the respired air such that, by gradual displacement of nitrogen, the alveolar oxygen tension is not allowed to fall below the ideal level of 103 mmHg. This can be done by supplying oxygen from a source through a mask to the subject's respiratory tract with increasing concentration, such that the inspired mixture has the correct amount of oxygen to give a partial pressure of oxygen of 103 mmHg in the lung. An alternative method is to pressurise the aircraft cabin with engine-bleed air to give an effective altitude of less than 10 000 feet (3000 m).

Clearly the ideal situation of breathing through a mask has a limit; sooner or later the ever-increasing concentration of oxygen necessary to supplement the inspired air will mean that to maintain the ideal value in the lungs it will be necessary for the individual to breath 100% oxygen. It can be calculated that this will occur at the altitude where the barometric pressure equals the alveolar oxygen pressure of 103 mmHg plus the pressure of water vapour (47 mmHg) and the pressure of alveolar carbon dioxide (40 mmHg) (which, of course, remain constant). The altitude in feet at which this will happen is the altitude at which the barometric pressure is 190 mmHg, which coincides with 33 700 feet (10 250 m) in the standard atmosphere. This can be visualised as follows:

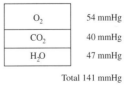

Therefore an individual breathing 100% oxygen at 33 700 feet has the same oxygen tension in the lung as when breathing air at sea level. Any ascent above this level will clearly lower the oxygen tension in the lung below 103 mmHg, the accepted ideal. However, an individual breathing air can ascend to an altitude of approximately 10 000 feet (3000 m), i.e. a lung oxygen tension of 55 mmHg, without serious deterioration in performance. Therefore the limiting altitude for 100% oxygen need not be 33 700 feet (10 250 m) but that altitude which coincides with an alveolar oxygen pressure of 55 mmHg. This may be deduced from the simple addition of:

O_2	54 mmHg
CO_2	40 mmHg
H_2O	47 mmHg

Total 141 mmHg

which is the atmospheric pressure at 40 000 feet (12 000 m). Therefore, 40 000 feet (12 000 m) is clearly the maximum altitude that can be considered acceptable for

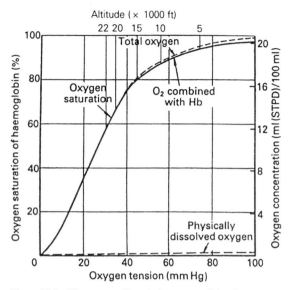

Figure 13.1   The oxygen dissociation curve of blood

exposure of aviators, even breathing 100% oxygen. Exposures above this need to achieve the 40 000 feet (12 000 m) lung picture irrespective of altitude, and this is achieved by actually pressurising the gas in the respiratory tract. This process is known as pressure breathing and is beyond the scope of this discussion.

The Oxygen Dissociation Curve

The ability of the normal healthy individual to function efficiently up to an altitude of approximately 10 000 feet (3000 m) is explained by the relationship between the oxygen saturation of haemoglobin and oxygen tension. Ascent to an altitude of 10 000 feet (3000 m) produces a fall in the partial pressure of oxygen in the alveoli but only a slight fall in the percentage saturation of haemoglobin with oxygen. However, once altitude rises above 10 000 feet (3000 m) the percentage saturation of haemoglobin falls quickly, resulting in the condition of hypoxia. In fact, above 8000 feet (2400 m) the effects of lack of oxygen will begin to appear and a decrease in the individual's ability to perform complex tasks and a reduction in night vision can be measured.

Figure 13.1 shows the oxygen dissociation curve of blood, with the concentrations of physically dissolved and chemically combined oxygen being shown separately. The curve illustrated is the average for a fit young adult. The actual shape of the curve will be influenced by factors such as age, state of health, tobacco abuse and ambient temperature.

Summary of Oxygen Requirements

- 0–10 000 feet (0–3000 m): air
- 10 000–33 700 feet (3000–10 250 m): increasing oxygen concentration
- 33 700–40 000 feet (10 250–12 000 m): 100% oxygen
- 40 000 feet (12 000 m) and above: 100% oxygen under pressure.

HYPOXIA AND HYPERVENTILATION

Hypoxia

This is the term used to denote the body condition when the oxygen available to the tissues is insufficient to meet their needs. We have seen that this condition will become obviously manifest when the partial pressure of oxygen in the lungs falls below about 55 mmHg. The tissues of the body become deprived, each becomes less efficient, but by far the most sensitive and susceptible is the brain. Consequently the first symptoms experienced by the hypoxic individual will be those resulting from brain inefficiency. The symptoms are in general terms similar in everybody, but have minor variations in individuals.

The classical symptoms of hypoxia may be summarised as follows:

1. *Personality change.* This is the initial stage of hypoxia. It is characterised by a change in the person's outlook, and his or her normal inhibitive forces of common sense tend to be diminished.
2. *Impaired judgement.* Loss of self-criticism, euphoria or depression. This stage can be particularly dangerous for aircrew, as, far from realising something is wrong, the aircrew member may well be led into a false state of well-being, which may lead on to a careless, carefree attitude, with reckless behaviour.
3. *Mental and muscular incoordination.* This is the stage of finding difficulty in 'thinking straight'. Constructive, progressive, logical thought processes become difficult, while coordinated muscular movements , such as clear speech or writing, become impaired.
4. *Sensory loss.* Concomitantly, inputs to the body via the sense organs are also diminished, thus such things as vision, hearing and the sense of touch become impaired.
5. *Memory impairment.* A classical symptom of hypoxia is impairment of recall for recent events, and is in the main due to difficulty in structuring thought. Obviously this is a most important effect for aircrew to be aware of as an unimpaired memory is imperative for recall of vital actions necessary to remedy the situation by previously taught emergency drills. Fortunately this is a fairly late symptom, and provided the aircrew member has absorbed previous training, he or she should have spotted the predicament before this potentially catastrophic stage is reached.

6. *Loss of consciousness.* Following memory loss, impairment of consciousness followed by loss of consciousness supervenes, leading ultimately to death.

The above are symptoms experienced or felt. Other signs are directly observable. These are:

1. *Cyanosis.* This is due to low oxygen concentration in the blood. As a consequence the complexion takes on a bluish hue, the skin becoming dusky, and fingernails and lips in particular become blue, similar to the colour of the hands on a cold day.
2. *Hyperventilation.* Low oxygen tension in the blood will lead to 'air hunger', manifested by deeper breathing. There may be other causes of deeper breathing, but above 10 000 feet the probability of hypoxia as a cause of hyperventilation should always be considered.

Factors Increasing Susceptibility to Hypoxia

- *Exercise.* Any increase in physical activity will increase oxygen consumption.
- *Cold.* Cold will induce an increase in the body metabolism, thus increasing oxygen consumption.
- *Ill health.* Any illness or intercurrent infection will probably induce increased need for oxygen, thereby lowering the threshold for hypoxia.
- *Fatigue.* While fatigue may not increase the need for oxygen, the threshold for hypoxia is lowered.
- *Drugs.* The dulling of the senses induced by some drugs, in particular cold cures and the lowering of one's well-being following alcohol consumption, no doubt lowers the tolerance to hypoxia.
- *Smoking.* Carbon monoxide, as produced by smoking, has a much greater affinity for haemoglobin than oxygen. Thus less oxygen is carried, increasing susceptibility to hypoxia.

Hyperventilation

Hyperventilation may be defined as breathing in excess of the metabolic needs of the body. As a consequence the level of carbon dioxide in the blood is lowered, while by definition it is not being replaced by carbon dioxide produced as a result of metabolic processes.

It can be seen from this definition that a man breathing heavily following exertion has increased his metabolism. He needs more oxygen and has produced more carbon dioxide. Consequently the rate and depth of breathing is not in excess of his needs. Conversely an individual breathing in excess without accompanying activity cannot take in extra oxygen, and does not produce extra carbon dioxide. The excessive breathing will remove carbon dioxide from the bloodstream faster than metabolic production, thereby lowering blood carbon dioxide level, leading to a change in blood acidity. This will lead to symptoms which in themselves can be alarming.

Factors that Induce Hyperventilation

- *Stress.* In circumstances that threaten the perceived well-being of an individual, certain reactions take place in the body which prepare it for physical activity, anticipating its struggle for survival. In the past this meant either fighting or fleeing. In either case great muscular activity would take place, consuming more oxygen and producing more carbon dioxide. Therefore, part of this preparatory reaction entails deeper breathing. However, should the extra physical activity not take place, the extra carbon dioxide will not be produced and the increased breathing would be in excess of the body needs, i.e. hyperventilation would occur.
- *Pressure breathing.* Breathing oxygen under pressure (a situation which may happen due to loss of pressure at altitudes greater than 40 000 feet (12 000 m), as explained above) may, due to its unfamiliarity in the untrained, stimulate excessive breathing. (Note that this is not particularly relevant when considering travel medicine, but is included for the sake of completeness of causes of hyperventilation.)
- *Hypoxia.* Whereas the normal stimulation for the waxing and waning of respiration is the level of blood carbon dioxide, any significant fall in the availability of oxygen will override this and hypoxia immediately stimulates both rate and depth of breathing. This in turn obviously lowers the blood carbon dioxide, precipitating symptoms of hyperventilation.
- *Vibration.* Whenever whole body vibration is experienced, respiration is stimulated, and if severe enough results in hyperventilation symptoms.

Symptoms

The symptoms of hyperventilation are classical and may be summarised as follows:

- *Dizziness.* Shortly after the onset of hyperventilation it is common for most people to experience a giddy or dizzy sensation.
- *Tingling.* Tingling of the extremities (hands, feet) or face may be felt.
- *Visual disturbances.* Many people experience a clouding or dimming of vision, perhaps accompanied by palpitations and hot flushes, which in turn generates further anxiety.
- *Disturbed consciousness.* It is possible in a severe attack for the symptoms to progress to clouding of consciousness and ultimately loss of consciousness; however, this is followed by immediate recovery as the respiratory rate returns to normal.

EFFECTS OF REDUCED ATMOSPHERIC PRESSURE

By Boyle's law the pressure of any gas is inversely related to its volume, providing the temperature remains constant. Hence, in aviation, where the body temperature remains essentially constant, when we ascend to altitude gas trapped anywhere in the body will tend to expand as altitude increases and atmospheric pressure decreases. The problems thus produced are known as 'trapped gas dysbarism'.

In addition, gas which is dissolved in the tissues and body fluids at sea-level pressures may come out of solution in the form of bubbles as the pressure reduces with altitude, in accordance with Henry's law. The problems associated with this phenomenon are known as 'evolved gas dysbarism' and the gas of concern is nitrogen. When these nitrogen bubbles form in the tissues they give rise to a condition known as decompression sickness.

Trapped Gas Dysbarism

The body cavities that contain gas are as follows:

Middle ear. Many air travellers are familiar with what happens when they cannot clear their ears as a result of a common cold. The mechanism of this disturbance, known as otic barotrauma, may be explained as follows.

The eustachian tube connects the middle-ear cavity with the nose. It permits the passage of air in and out of the middle-ear cavity, thus preventing distortion of the eardrum during changes in ambient pressure. The normal state of the tube is collapsed, similar to a bicycle tyre inner tube which is not inflated, where the lower half of the tube passes through the soft tissues behind the nose. During ascent, the expanding air in the middle-ear cavity escapes easily down the tube. On descent, however, the increasing pressure may cause difficulty with re-entry of air to the middle ear due to swollen mucous membranes and congestion around the opening of the tube behind the nose. Normally, the tube can be opened voluntarily by certain manoeuvres such as yawning or swallowing. In the event of congestion of membranes lining the nose and throat, the lining of the tube becomes swollen and may not open. The unequal pressures so produced cause the eardrum to be drawn inwards, resulting in pain, deafness and possible dizziness and disorientation. In the worst case, the eardrum may perforate. Ideally one should not fly with a cold or other forms of upper respiratory congestion, such as hay fever. If travel is essential, frequent steam inhalation on the days preceding travel plus the judicious use of a nasal decongestant spray (e.g. oxymetazoline or xylometazoline) may prevent the development of barotrauma.

Sinuses. The sinuses are cavities in the bones of the face which open into the nose. They are situated above the eyes, in the cheeks and at the back of the nose. Like the middle ear, no problems are usually encountered on ascent, but on descent, if their openings into the nose become blocked by a cold or catarrh preventing air entry, the relative vacuum created in the cavities will cause damage to their lining membranes. This leads to inflammation and bleeding within the sinus cavities, which may produce pain, often severe, and frequently nose bleeding. This condition of pressure effect on the sinuses is known as sinus barotrauma.

Gut. Ascent to 18 000 feet (5500 m) from ground level halves the atmospheric pressure and therefore doubles the volume of gas trapped in the stomach and in the intestines. Normally this is voided quite easily but occasionally, when ascent is fairly rapid, it can cause discomfort or pain. Avoidance of gas-forming foods, such as curries, beans, etc., can minimise these effects.

Teeth. Any tooth that has been filled recently has a small quantity of air trapped underneath the filling. Usually, this air escapes around the edge of the filling when its owner goes to altitude. Occasionally, however, the air does not escape and, on ascent, it causes pressure on the nerve of the tooth, resulting in pain. Similar pain can be caused by gas produced in dental decay. This is known as aerodontalgia.

Lungs. If a sudden decompression is rapid enough and over a big enough pressure range, damage to the lungs is theoretically possible. Such high rates of pressure change could occur when a large defect is suddenly produced in a high-differential pressure cabin. However, in an aircraft with a cabin altitude of 8000 feet (2400 m), decompression resulting from the loss of a window, even at very high altitude, has not been known to cause lung damage.

Decompression Sickness

Decompression sickness is a condition that can arise as a result of exposure of the body to reduced atmospheric pressure either in an aircraft or in a decompression chamber. It is rare below 25 000 feet (7600 m), but the incidence and onset increases rapidly above this altitude.

Causes

The human body is saturated with nitrogen, which is in solution in tissues and body fluids, at a partial pressure of gas equal to that of the surrounding atmosphere. When the ambient pressure is lowered, the nitrogen tends to come out of solution. The formation of nitrogen bubbles thus released from solution is generally accepted as the cause of decompression sickness.

The following factors increase susceptibility to decompression sickness:

• *Altitude.* Decompression sickness rarely occurs below

18 000 feet (5500 m) cabin altitude, is unlikely below 25 000 feet (7600 m), and the incidence increases with altitude above this level.

- *Duration of exposure.* The longer the exposure, the greater the number of individuals affected by decompression sickness.
- *Re-exposure.* Re-exposure to altitude, within 48 h, increases susceptibility to decompression sickness.
- *Exercise.* Exercise while at altitude is one of the most important factors influencing susceptibility to this condition. There is also evidence that preflight exercise may increase the incidence of decompression sickness.
- *Temperature.* Cold may increase the incidence of decompression sickness.
- *Age.* There is an increased incidence of decompression sickness with age: each decade roughly doubles the susceptibility.
- *Obesity.* Fat, having a relatively high nitrogen content, predisposes obese individuals to decompression sickness.
- *Individual susceptibility.* Certain individuals are more susceptible than others in comparable circumstances, and this susceptibility varies from day to day.
- *Subaqua swimming.* Swimming underwater exposes the body to an increased ambient pressure (atmospheric pressure plus the pressure of water, which varies with depth). If air is breathed underwater, nitrogen will enter the body until the partial pressure of nitrogen equals the ambient pressure. Flying, even at low cabin altitudes, after subaqua swimming is very likely to result in decompression sickness. This increased susceptibility lasts for up to 48 h, and it is recommended that flying should be avoided for at least 12 h following exposure to a pressure of up to 2 atmospheres absolute (33 feet (10 m) of sea water), as in subaqua swimming, and at least 24 h when exposure exceeds 2 atmospheres.
- *Hypoxia.* Coexistent hypoxia makes an individual more prone to the symptoms of decompression sickness.
- *Fatigue.*
- *Ill health.*
- *Recent alcohol intake.* This can increase significantly the likelihood of decompression sickness.

Symptoms

The symptoms of decompression sickness may be summarised as follows.

Bends. The 'bends' is pain arising in and around certain joints in the limbs. The most common sites are the upper part of the arm near the shoulder, the wrists, the elbow, the knee and the ankle. It may start as a mild ache in one or more of these areas, progressing to a deep severe pain spreading up and down the affected limb. It can eventually give rise to clumsiness, weakness and complete disablement of the limb. Rubbing or moving the limb makes the condition worse. On descent, symptoms usually pass off but will recur immediately on reascent.

Creeps. This is a transient, mild, itching or tingling feeling, usually of the thigh and trunk. A blotchy red rash may sometimes accompany the condition. In itself it is not a serious condition, but it indicates the presence of decompression sickness.

Chokes. This is a name used to describe respiratory symptoms, which may be preceded by 'bends' pain. It is characterised by a burning feeling in the chest with pain on breathing in, often accompanied by severe bouts of dry coughing. In spite of the name, there is no respiratory obstruction and no danger, therefore, of choking. Although rare, the condition must be treated seriously and descent should be initiated immediately, to avoid serious complications. The individual should receive expert medical care as soon as possible.

Nervous system symptoms. Symptoms of decompression sickness arising from the central nervous system are very varied and may take the form of a temporary loss of areas in the visual field, inability to concentrate or weakness and paralysis of a limb. The last symptom is the origin of the diver's name of 'staggers'.

Decompression collapse. This is a serious condition which may be primary, secondary or postdecompression. Primary collapse occurs with little or no warning. There is a feeling of apprehension, pallor of the skin and a cold sweat, which may be followed by a faint. Secondary collapse is similar, but is preceded by some other form of decompression sickness, usually chokes or severe bends. This is the commonest form of collapse. Postdecompression collapse occurs after return to ground level, usually within 4 h, but it can occur after many hours. It may be preceded by headache, nausea or a feeling of malaise. Decompression collapse is uncommon but, should it occur, it must be treated as a medical emergency. If it occurs in flight, land as quickly as possible and seek urgent specialist assistance and immediate transfer to a hyperbaric chamber facility.

Treatment

The actions to take in the event of decompression sickness arising in flight are as follows:

1. Descend as low as possible initially.
2. Land as soon as possible, i.e. divert to nearest airfield.
3. Put the patient on 100% oxygen, having checked the oxygen system is connected.
4. Keep the patient at rest and warm.
5. Radio for medical advice and ask for medical assistance to be available on landing.

CABIN PRESSURISATION

The sections on hypoxia and decompression sickness have shown the need for protection from these hazards. In passenger-carrying aircraft these problems are overcome by pressurising the aircraft cabin.

Environmental Requirements of a Pressure Cabin

The physiological ideal for a pressure cabin would be to pressurise it to sea level, but this would require an extremely strong, and consequently very heavy and complex, cabin or fuselage structure. This is incompatible with the need to carry a large number of passengers, baggage and freight over long distances. Aircraft are therefore designed with cabin differential pressures that are a compromise between the physiological ideal and the economic realities of the aircraft's role and performance.

In general, pressure cabins fall into two broad categories, low- and high-differential cabins. The advantage of a high cabin differential is that it protects the occupants of the cabin from any serious effects of hypoxia without having to use personal breathing equipment, and there is no risk of decompression sickness at the cabin altitudes maintained [commonly 6000–8000 feet (1800–2400 m)]. Passenger-carrying aircraft normally have high-differential cabins. These aircraft must be able to operate at high altitudes for long periods and they are able to carry the weight of pressurisation equipment which is necessary. A low-differential cabin is usually found in military aircraft in which the crew use personal oxygen equipment routinely. When pressurising aircraft cabins the following factors must be controlled:

- Pressure
- Relative humidity
- Mass flow
- Volume flow
- Temperature.

If these factors are adequately controlled, the problems of cabin conditioning, i.e. temperature and ventilation, are also taken care of.

In modern passenger aircraft, it is normal for 50% of the cabin air to be recirculated. This recirculated air is passed through high-efficiency particulate filters (HEPA filters), which remove bacteria and viral particles. The benefits of recirculating air are an increase in relative humidity and a reduction in ozone levels, as well as reduction in uncomfortable drafts of fresh air. Flow rates of fresh air in passenger aircraft cabins are designed to exceed the minima laid down for indoor rooms by the American Society of Heating, Refrigeration and Air-conditioning Engineers (ASHRAE). This rate is 5 cubic feet (142 litres) per minute per person, which ensures that carbon dioxide levels remain below 5000 parts per million by volume. Most modern airliners achieve flow rates of approximately double this value.

Methods of Pressurisation

A pressure cabin is built strong enough to withstand its maximum intended pressure differential, plus an element for safety, and is sealed to meet regulatory standards for leak rates. Pressurisation is then achieved by tapping air from a suitable stage of the engine compressor, cooling it and ducting it into the cabin. In some aircraft, a separate engine-driven compressor is used. The differential pressure level is then set by controlling the inflow of compressor air together with a fine control for regulating the rate of escape of air from the cabin by means of a barometrically operated outflow valve. The cabin altitude is usually allowed to increase with aircraft altitude until a cabin altitude of between 5000 and 8000 feet (1500 and 2000 m) is reached. Barometric control of the outflow valve then maintains the cabin at that altitude until the maximum differential pressure for that aircraft cabin is achieved. If the aircraft continues to climb, the maximum differential bleed valve control takes over; the maximum differential pressure is maintained and the cabin altitude increases, maintaining that differential over ambient atmospheric pressure. In reality, it is rare for a commercial airliner to exceed a cabin altitude of 8000 feet (2400 m) during normal operation.

There are other methods of pressurising cabins. For example, space vehicles carry their own source of pressurisation, which may be 100% oxygen (stored in liquid form) or a mixture of oxygen and an inert gas. It is advantageous to use an oxygen–inert gas mixture for reasons of safety. Because a space vehicle is a closed environment, there has to be a system for absorbing carbon dioxide, something that is not necessary in a passenger airliner.

Loss of Cabin Pressure

Loss of cabin pressure can vary from a slow leak, due to some minor mechanical problem such as a faulty door seal, to a rapid or even explosive decompression due to a rupture of the cabin wall or loss of one or more windows. The occurrence of a rapid decompression is readily indicated by a loud noise due to the sudden release of pressure. The compressed air within the cabin 'roars' out of the defect at a velocity near the speed of sound until the cabin pressure reaches that of the surrounding atmosphere. As this air leaves the cabin, so the remaining gas expands, causing the temperature of the air within the cabin to drop to its dewpoint and water condenses out as a mist, which can be so dense that it interferes with the occupants' vision. The loud noise plus misting has led crews to believe that their aircraft is severely damaged and on fire. In the case of a slow leak, there is no such dramatic indication. The first sign is likely to be the sound of a cabin pressurisation failure warning device, the illumination of the appropriate warning light or a cabin altimeter indication, depending upon the aircraft instrumentation.

Possible causes of loss of cabin pressure are:

- Compressor failure
- Malfunction of the control system
- Pressure leakage; especially around doors
- Window blowout
- Structural failure.

Aerodynamic Suck

In the case of a rapid decompression resulting from a defect in the cabin wall rather than a failure of the pressurisation system, the final cabin altitude may exceed the actual pressure altitude of the aircraft. This is due to the flow of air over the defect, which tends to suck the residual air out of the cabin (aerodynamic suction effect), except in cases where the defect faces directly into the airstream. The magnitude of this effect varies with the aircraft type, the position of the defect in relation to the atmospheric airstream, and the aircraft's altitude and speed. In the worst case the height discrepancy could be such that the cabin altitude is many thousands of feet above the aircraft pressure altitude. This can, therefore, be an important phenomenon because of the effect it can have on the aircraft occupants and whether or not their personal emergency oxygen equipment has the performance necessary to prevent hypoxia at the resulting cabin altitude.

Effects of Rapid Decompression

The effects of loss of cabin pressure are dependent upon:

- The altitude at which the decompression takes place and the presence or absence of aerodynamic suck
- The pressure differential at the time of failure
- The size of the hole permitting loss of pressure and therefore the duration of the decompression
- The volume of the pressurised compartment.

The possible physiological effects, dependent on the factors above, are:

- Pressure change effects on ears, sinuses, lungs and gut. Of these, only rapid expansion of trapped gas in the gut is usually of any significance, as in the other sites the expansion is normally counterbalanced by the rate of leakage from the body. Rapid distension of the gut can lead to a faint as a result of vagal inhibition.
- Hypoxia, particularly in high-differential cabins where the crew and passengers are not wearing oxygen equipment at the time of decompression.
- Decompression sickness, if there is any need to continue the flight at cabin altitudes above 25 000 feet (7600 m).
- Cold, depending upon the size and position of the defect in the cabin.
- Difficulty in communication: depending upon the size

and position of the defect there may be considerable wind noise, which interferes with communication between crew members.

The pressure cabin is an essential part of the modern high-performance aircraft, without which it would not have any useful high-altitude capability. Without pressurisation, aircrew and passengers would only be able to carry out high-altitude flying by the continuous use of personal oxygen equipment, which of course would not be acceptable for the transport of fare-paying passengers.

SLEEP AND FATIGUE

Sleep is essential for restoring the normal balance between the different parts of the central nervous system. During sleep, the body's physical functions are rested and some renewal takes place; sympathetic nervous activity decreases and the muscular tone becomes almost nil; the arterial blood pressure falls, the pulse rate decreases, the blood vessels in the skin dilate and the overall basal metabolic rate of the body falls by up to 20%. On average, most humans need physiologically about 8 h of sleep per night; however, in modern society most adults report an average of 7–7.5 h sleep per night, with 75% reporting daytime sleepiness (Rosekind et al., 1994).

Sleep loss can be acute or cumulative. In an acute situation, sleep loss can occur either totally or as a partial loss. It can accumulate over time into what is referred to as 'sleep debt'. As little as 2 h of sleep loss can result in impairment of performance and levels of alertness. Sleep loss leads to increased reaction time, reduced vigilance, cognitive slowing, memory problems, time-on-task decrements and optimum response decrements. It has also been shown that performance variability increases with sleep loss.

Physiology of Sleep

Sleep can be divided into five stages: stages 1 to 4 and rapid eye movement (REM) sleep. Stage 1 is a transitional phase between waking and sleeping and this normally lasts around 10 min as an individual falls asleep. Sleep then becomes deeper, with 15 min in stage 2 sleep and a further 15 min in stage 3 sleep before moving into stage 4. Approximately 90 min after sleep onset, REM sleep will occur. The cycle of REM sleep and stages 1–4 sleep repeats during the course of the night in 90 min cycles, each succeeding cycle containing greater amounts of REM sleep. An 8 h sleep period will typically contain about 4–5 bouts of REM sleep. Most stage 4 sleep happens early in the night. It is thought that stages 1–4 sleep is related to body restoration, whereas REM sleep may be related to strengthening and organising memory. When learning new tasks, an increased proportion of REM sleep is seen.

The need to operate commercial airliners worldwide

for 24 h each day inevitably leads to the problems of unsocial and irregular hours, time zone (transmeridian), climatic and cultural changes, sleep disturbances, and alterations to circadian rhythms. Fatigue is the main danger for flight crew, as a decline in performance is likely to accompany it. The economic and operational requirements of an airline must be balanced against these undesirable factors, but good aircrew scheduling has been developed to minimise the effects on health, morale and safety.

For passengers travelling by air, the effects of sleep loss and fatigue are likely to be less critical than for aircrew. However, when important business decisions have to be taken after a long journey it is essential that the traveller has some understanding of the nature of sleep and fatigue so that the effects of sleep loss and circadian disruption can be minimised.

Scheduling

For flight crew, there are statutory constraints on scheduling. These constraints include limitations on the maximum flying duty period, minimum rest periods, maximum scheduled duty hours, and minimum cumulative off-duty periods. In the United Kingdom proposed flight schedules have to be submitted by the airline management to the Flight Times Limitation Board of the Civil Aviation Authority before their introduction. Other countries have similar limitations, and within such frameworks airlines operate schedules that are further restricted by the need to meet the needs of passengers and to comply with night flying bans, peak hour saturation, and political influences on route planning. In addition, flight time limitations usually reflect conditions acceptable to industrial bodies rather than to medical advisers. The commercial need to keep aircraft flying, and so earning revenue, and the requirements of engineering schedules for airframe and engine inspection and checks are also relevant considerations.

Transmeridian Travel

The endogenous circadian system, in which over 50 physiological and psychological rhythms have now been identified, is known to be affected by many environmental factors. These include local clock hour, light and dark, and temperature, although many of the rhythms continue in the absence of such cues, albeit usually with a slightly prolonged periodicity. The environmental factors facilitate entertainment or phasing of the rhythms and are known as synchronisers or 'Zeitgebers' (time givers). Travel across time zones outstrips the ability of synchronisers to entrain rhythms and desynchronisation occurs. This is responsible for the syndrome known as jet lag, as circadian rhythms need a finite period to become re-entrained to local time (usually estimated at about 1 day per time zone crossed). Westward travel is generally considered to be better tolerated than eastward, possibly because the endogenous system, with a natural periodicity in most individuals of about 25 h, is more able to adapt to the longer 'day' encountered during westward flight.

The aetiology of the effects of jet lag—sleep disturbances, disruption of the other body functions such as feeding and bowel habit, general discomfort, and reduced psychomotor efficiency—has been the subject of much investigation. This has largely concentrated on underlying hormonal variations, but for aircrew and business travellers the important changes are those associated with performance levels. Ability at many mental skills, including vigilance, choice reaction time, and simulator performance, rises to a peak during the day between 12.00 and 21.00, with a dip during the afternoon, and then falls to a minimum between 0300 and 0600. Results of memory tests peak in the morning and then fall steadily.

Sleepiness and Fatigue

There are two principal components of sleepiness or fatigue:

- Physiological sleepiness or fatigue—this is a requirement like hunger or thirst and can only be reversed by sleep.
- Subjective sleepiness or fatigue—this is an individual's perception of his or her sleepiness but it may be affected by other factors. It may be difficult for an individual to subjectively assess his or her own alertness, with a tendency to report a greater level of alertness than is actually the case.

Factors affecting sleepiness include:

- Prior sleep and wakefulness
- Circadian phase leading to:
    increased sleepiness in the early hours of the morning and during the afternoon
    decreased performance in the early hours of the morning
- Age (the amount of nocturnal sleep required reduces after the age of 50)
- Alcohol (reduces the quality of sleep)
- Work and environmental conditions.

Prevention and Management of Fatigue

Individuals have different needs and react differently to sleep loss. Therefore each individual must apply recommendations to suit his or her particular circumstances.

Sleep Scheduling

- At home the best possible sleep should be obtained before a trip.

- On a trip, as much sleep per 24 h should be obtained as would be at home.
- Feelings should be trusted: if the individual feels sleepy and circumstances permit, then he or she should sleep; however, if the individual wakes spontaneously and cannot get back to sleep in about 15–30 min, then he or she should get up out of bed.

Good Sleep Habits

- A regular presleep routine should be developed.
- Sleep time should be kept protected.
- The individual should avoid going to bed hungry, but should not eat or drink heavily before going to bed.
- Alcohol or caffeine should be avoided before bedtime.

An optimum dark, quiet and comfortable sleep environment is important. A healthy lifestyle with regular exercise should be maintained, which seems to help with the first stages of sleep. Caffeine consumption may be used to increase alertness. A cup of coffee usually takes about 15–30 min to become effective, and the effect lasts for between 3 and 4 h. A balanced diet, including drinking plenty of fluids, can also prevent the onset of fatigue.

Bright light (more than 2500 lux), used at the appropriate time in the circadian cycle, can help to reset the circadian clock. After flying east, the traveller should be exposed to evening light with respect to body time, but morning light avoided. Conversely, when travelling west, morning light should be sought and evening light avoided. This makes the best use of the natural Zeitgebers in resetting the body clock.

When used appropriately, certain drugs can help in the short term to resynchronise the sleep cycle after time zone crossing. Temazepam is a short-acting benzodiazepine that is rapidly cleared from the body. Many people find this drug helpful in promoting sleep and, used for 2–3 days after travel, it can assist in resetting the sleep cycle. Melatonin is a substance secreted by the pineal gland with a rhythm linked to the light–dark cycle through the suprachiasmatic nucleus. It is available in tablet form and has been used by many people in an attempt to assist sleep; however, the timing of administration to match the late evening part of the pineal circadian cycle is critical. Also, despite being a natural substance, the long-term side-effects are not fully understood, particularly those affecting reproductive function and cardiac activity. It therefore does not have a pharmaceutical licence for general use. Although alcohol is widely used as an aid to sleep, it is a nonselective nervous system depressant and is effectively a drug. Although alcohol may induce sleep, REM sleep is considerably reduced and early waking is likely. It is therefore not appropriate to use alcohol in this manner.

It should be remembered that there is no simple or single solution for combating the effects of sleep loss and jet lag. The individual has to discover what helps him or her, and evolve the appropriate strategies to suit his or her particular needs.

MOTION SICKNESS

Motion sickness is a condition characterised primarily by nausea, vomiting, pallor and sweating, which occurs when humans are exposed to real or apparent motion stimuli with which they are unfamiliar and hence unadapted. It is a generic term that embraces sea sickness, air sickness, car sickness, swing sickness, simulator sickness, ski sickness, camel sickness, space sickness, etc.—all various forms of the same malady named after the provocative environment or vehicle. Despite the diversity of the causal environment, the essential characteristics of a provocative stimulus and the response of the afflicted individual are common to all these conditions, hence the use of the general term motion sickness. Nevertheless, it must be acknowledged that the term motion sickness is, in certain respects, a misnomer. First, because symptoms characteristic of the condition can be evoked as much by the absence of expected motion as by the presence of unfamiliar motion, such as in simulator sickness and Cinerama sickness. Secondly, the word 'sickness' carries the connotation of being affected with disease and tends to obscure the fact that motion sickness is a quite normal response of the healthy individual, without organic or functional disorder, when exposed for sufficient length of time to unfamiliar motion of sufficient severity. Indeed, under severe stimulus conditions, it is the absence rather than the presence of symptoms that is indicative of true pathology, for only those individuals who lack a functional vestibular system are truly immune (Miller and Graybiel, 1970).

Symptoms and Signs

Typically, the development of motion sickness follows an orderly sequence, the time scale being determined by the intensity of the stimulus and the susceptibility of the individual. The earliest symptom is usually epigastric discomfort, which is normally described as stomach awareness. Should the provocative motion continue, well-being usually deteriorates quite quickly, with the appearance of nausea of increasing severity. At the same time, facial pallor may be observed and the individual begins to sweat, the sweating usually being confined to those areas of skin where thermal sweating rather than emotional sweating occurs. This is followed by the so-called avalanche phenomenon, with increased salivation, feelings of bodily warmth, light-headedness and, not infrequently, quite severe depression and apathy. By this stage vomiting is usually not far away, although there are some individuals who remain severely nauseated for long periods and do not obtain the transitory relief that many people report following the act of vomiting.

Apart from these characteristic features of motion sickness, other signs and symptoms are frequently, although more variably, reported. In the early stages, increased salivation, belching and flatulence are commonly associated with the development of nausea, and hyperventilation is frequently observed. Headache is another variable prodromal symptom and complaints of tightness round the forehead or of a buzzing in the head are not uncommon. Another symptom commonly associated with exposure to unfamiliar motion is drowsiness, and, typically, feelings of lethargy and somnolence persist for many hours after withdrawal of the provocative stimulus and nausea has abated. The soporific effect of repeated motion stimulus on infants has long been recognised and it may be that the drowsiness observed in the adult when exposed to appropriate motion is a manifestation of the same mechanism, although this is conjecture.

Incidence

Motion sickness is a normal response to an abnormal environment. Thus, individuals who are unadapted to a particular type of motion are all likely to suffer from the disability if the motion is of sufficient intensity and the period of exposure is sufficiently prolonged. Of course there are wide differences in individual susceptibility, although in severe sea states, sickness rates as high as 99% have been recorded (Bles *et al.*, 1984). Nonetheless, in less provocative environments a proportion of the population at risk do not succumb. Although many of the factors that determine individual susceptibility have been identified, and the nature of evocative motions recognised, it is still not yet possible to predict with certainty the incidence of sickness in a given population, even when exposed to a motion stimulus that can be defined. This has caused severe problems with the space programme, where the incidence of sickness is in excess of 50%, despite very careful screening of the astronaut population (Homick *et al.*, 1984). Similarly, it has proved difficult to predict susceptibility in applicants for military aircrew training and an absence of sea sickness or swing sickness does not confer immunity from air sickness. Conversely, a susceptibility to these stimuli does not imply that an individual will in turn necessarily suffer from air sickness.

Air sickness in passenger transport aircraft is nowadays a relatively rare occurrence, the incidence being of the order of 0.4–1.0% (Benson, 1988). This is largely due to the fact that large jet transports are able to fly above the turbulent weather and a smooth ride is the norm. The incidence is higher in small light aircraft, particularly among passengers unfamiliar with this form of travel.

Aetiology

An explanation of the causation of motion sickness must include the fact that it can be induced not only by motion in which the individual experiences changing linear and angular accelerations but also by purely visual stimuli without a changing force environment (as in simulators or Cinerama). Furthermore, it must account for the phenomenon of adaptation to the provocative motion, as well as the sickness that can occur when the individual returns to a normal motion environment after having adapted to an atypical one (an example being land sickness on disembarking after a few days at sea).

Undoubtedly the vestibular apparatus plays a significant role in the condition because, as has been known for more than half a century, individuals without vestibular function do not get motion sickness. Nonetheless, the theory that motion sickness is due to vestibular overstimulation alone does not account for the fact that sickness may not be induced at quite strong motion stimuli (for example, vertical oscillation at frequencies above 0.5–1.0 Hz), yet weaker stimuli (for example head movement during turns) are highly provocative. Nor does it account for the visually induced forms of motion sickness or the characteristic adaptive phenomenon (Benson, 1988).

The most satisfactory explanation is still provided by Reason's neural mismatch theory which views motion sickness not as an isolated vestibular phenomenon but as the response of the body to discordant motion cues (Reason, 1978). In all the situations where motion sickness is provoked, the information transmitted by the eyes, the vestibular system and other sensory receptors is at variance with the information the individual expects, from past experience, to receive. It is postulated that within the central nervous system there is some form of store or memory and with it a comparator, where signals from the sensory receptors and neural store are correlated. If the signals to the sense organs stimulated by the motion agree with the stored association, there is no mismatch and all is well. However, when the input signals do not agree with the expected (stored) information, then a mismatch signal is generated. This has two effects. One is to modify the store so that a new association of cues is elaborated (the store is rearranged); the other is to initiate the sequence of neurovegetative responses which characterise the motion sickness syndrome. Both these responses depend on the duration and intensity of the mismatch signal. A sustained strong mismatch signal is likely to provoke sickness and concurrently a significant rearrangement of the store. Conversely, a weak mismatch signal, provided it is sustained, can allow rearrangement or adaptation to occur without engendering nausea.

In the human's normal typical environment, usually natural movement on the ground, the inputs from the sensory receptors accord with the expected signals. On transfer to a new or atypical motion environment, such as riding a camel or flying in an aeroplane, the comparator signals differ appreciably from those coming from the visual and/or vestibular receptors, because the stored information remains appropriate to the typical conditions. With continued exposure, the contents of the neural store are slowly modified so that the intensity of the mismatch signal decreases as the expected signal comes to agree with the sensory input appropriate to the new atypical environment. Thus there is no longer any mismatch. At this stage, the individual may be considered to have adapted to the atypical motion environment, and the symptoms of motion sickness will disappear.

On return to the normal or typical motion environment a mismatch again occurs and this may provoke symptoms similar to those experienced on initial transfer to the atypical environment. This mismatch arises because the expected signals are still appropriate to the atypical environment. The store has now to be rearranged to make it compatible once again with the sensory input. In general this phase of adaptation proceeds more quickly than the initial adaptation to the atypical environment, because the correlations established by long experience are more easily retrieved than new ones can be acquired. By the same argument, should the individual return to the atypical environment, adaptation is likely to be a more rapid process than on first exposure, because the store can be rearranged with the aid of retained stimulus patterns acquired during previous exposures to the atypical environment. If transfer from one specific motion environment to another is frequent, than a stage is reached where the neural store can be modified quite rapidly, so that the mismatch signal is short-lived or of insufficient strength to engender motion sickness.

Unfortunately, this neural mismatch theory does not explain why motion sickness should take the particular form that it does, nor indeed why motion sickness should occur at all. However, the theory is a unifying concept and gives us a basis from which to begin to try and explain it.

Provocative Stimulus

The neural mismatch theory implies that there is dissonance between the incoming sensory signals and those expected by the neural store. Basically, two sensory systems are involved: the visual system and the vestibular system. The vestibular system is further divided into the angular acceleration receptor system, which is the ampullary receptors of the semicircular canals, and the linear acceleration or force environment receptor system of the utricular and saccular maculae, usually referred to as the otolith organs. Other mechanoreceptors are also stimulated by the changes in the force environment, but in general they act synergistically with the macula receptors and need not be considered separately. The motion cue mismatch can be specified according to the sensory system involved:

- Visual–vestibular mismatch
- Canal–otolith mismatch.

These can be further subdivided into type 1 conflict, when both systems concurrently signal contradicting or uncorrelated information, and type 2, when one system signals information in the absence of the expected signal from the other system (Benson, 1988).

Individual Susceptibility

There are wide differences between individuals in their susceptibility. It used to be thought that a person who is prone to sickness in one motion environment is also likely to suffer when exposed to other types of provocative motion, but, as already indicated, experience shows this not to be so. However, susceptibility does appear to be a relatively stable and enduring characteristic of the individual, even though it can be modified by environmental and experimental factors.

An attempt was made to correlate for the Spacelab 1 astronauts their preflight motion sickness susceptibility test scores with their inflight susceptibility (Homick *et al.*, 1984). Little correlation was apparent, although an important finding from Spacelab 1 was that motion sickness was not experienced after return to earth. Therefore the astronauts seemed less susceptible postflight than preflight to several forms of provocative vestibular stimulation.

Effect of Age

Susceptibility changes with age, sickness rarely occurring before the age of 2. In childhood, the incidence of sickness increases markedly to reach a peak at puberty (10–13 years) and thereafter susceptibility declines rapidly between the 12th and 21st years. Motion sickness is not a geriatric problem, being quite rare above the age of 50 years (Benson, 1988). The mechanism underlying the large changes in age susceptibility is not understood, although it is tempting to ascribe the phenomenon to long-term adaptation. It may also be due to a reduction in general neural sensitivity, which is part of the normal ageing process.

Alcohol

It is known that alcohol induces nystagmus. Positional alcohol nystagmus appears in two phases. The first appears within 30 min of alcohol intake and shows nystagmus, with the fast component beating to the right if the subject is in the right lateral position and vice versa. This phase lasts about 3–4 h and is followed by an intermediate period in which no nystagmus is observed. The second phase begins 5–6 h after the consumption of alcohol and the direction of movement is reversed, in that the fast component beats to the left when the subject is on the right side. The duration of the second phase and the intensity of both phases are related to the maximal blood alcohol concentration, and hence to the amount of alcohol consumed. This second phase always persists for several hours after all alcohol has disappeared from the blood.

It is thought that when alcohol diffuses from the blood into the endolymph of the semicircular canals it does not become evenly distributed. It is less dense than water and so creates a light spot at the ampulla, because the concentration of blood vessels there means that most of the diffusion occurs in this region. If the canal is then orientated appropriately to gravity, this light spot will tend to rise, causing the fluid to move as it would if the head were turning. This leads to nystagmus. The second phase can be explained as follows. When alcohol starts to diffuse back out of the endolymph, the area around the ampulla becomes free of alcohol fastest and this creates a relatively heavy spot, which in turn causes a reversal of the direction of the nystagmus fast beat. This effect on the endolymph causes an increased vestibular sensitivity and hence the finding of motion sickness in susceptible individuals following minimal alcohol intake.

Receptivity, Adaptability and Retentivity

Receptivity refers to the way in which the individual processes a stimulus within the nervous system. It is suggested that a person who has high receptivity transduces the sensory stimulus more effectively, and that it evokes a more powerful subjective experience than in a person of low receptivity. Hence, according to the mismatch theory, the receptive has a more intense mismatch signal and is therefore more likely to suffer from motion sickness than the nonreceptive when exposed to provocative motion.

Adaptability describes the rate at which the individual adapts to an atypical motion environment or, in more general terms, adjusts to the conditions of sensory rearrangement. Those who adapt slowly suffer more severe symptoms and require a longer period for adjustment to the motion than the fast adaptors. It follows that slow adaptors are more susceptible to motion sickness than the fast adaptors, but this does not mean that slow adapters are also receptives, and it has been shown that these two factors are in fact unrelated.

One factor remains. This is the manner in which adaptation is retained between exposures to the provocative motion. Poor retention of adaptation is illustrated by the flying individual who is troubled by motion sickness when flights are separated by several days, but is symptom-free when able to fly regularly with not more than a few days between flights. The individual with the better retention is not so afflicted, such that, once having adapted to the provocative motion of a particular flight environment, he or she remains free even when flights are quite spasmodic.

Anxiety and Neurotic Reactions

Nausea and vomiting are not common symptoms of fear and anxiety, although it is often assumed that anxiety coexisting with provocative motion increases susceptibility to motion sickness. However, there is little firm evidence to support this assumption, although it is important to recognise that neurotic reactions may be manifest

by sickness in those environments where motion sickness occurs. In the airborne environment, anxiety does not produce motion sickness, but it can be the prime cause of 'sickness in the air', which is a separate condition often associated with phobic anxiety.

Prevention and Treatment

As always, prevention is better than cure. Having understood some of the aetiology it is now fairly obvious that the head movements should be reduced to a minimum and discordant visual cues (such as reading during the journey with the head down) should be minimised. Alcohol should be avoided in the 24 h prior to flight and during the flight itself, particularly if there is any suggestion that the individual may be susceptible to motion sickness.

Drugs

A number of drugs have been shown to be of value in reducing the incidence of motion sickness, or attenuating symptoms of those suffering from the disability. However, as ever, no pharmacologically active agent is entirely specific and they all have side-effects. No drug can prevent the occurrence of motion sickness in every member of a population at risk. Drugs currently available for the treatment of motion sickness include antihistamines, phenothiazines or atropine derivatives. The exact mode of action of many of these drugs is not fully understood, other than a so-called vestibular sedative action.

Receptors for some antimotion sickness drugs are unevenly distributed in the vestibular nuclei, where they apparently modulate, but do not relay, primary sensory inputs. It is thought that a dynamic balance exists between muscarinic cholinergic-activated brainstem neurons, which initiate motion sickness, and noradrenaline (norepinephrine)-activated brainstem neurons, which act against motion sickness development. The action of dopamine and its function in sensory switching in the basal ganglia is thought to be the most likely mechanism of action.

Hyoscine hydrobromide (available in the UK as Kwells) is still the most effective drug in most of the population and has the advantage of a relatively short duration of action. This is an advantage in aviation, but in the marine world it can be a disadvantage. At sea the favoured drug is cinnarizine (sold in the UK as Stugeron) because it has a long half-life and is effective for a day's sailing. It has calcium antagonistic properties and appears to exert a significant depressant effect on the vestibular nuclei, possibly by antagonising the stimulated influx of calcium ions from the endolymph into the vestibular sensory cells. Unfortunately it can cause drowsiness, due to its antihistamine activity.

Calcium antagonists are potent blockers of neurotransmitter release in the brain and it has been a chance finding that nifedipine (Adalat) has reduced motion sickness, possibly by antagonising the influx of calcium ions into vestibular cells. However, this finding has failed to be reliably repeated under experimental conditions (J.R.R. Stott, personal communication, 1990).

Adaptation

The most potent therapeutic measure, at least in the long term, is adaptation to the provocative motion through repeated exposure. This is nature's own cure and is obviously the preferred method of preventing sickness, particularly for aircrew who cannot fly when under the influence of antimotion sickness drugs.

Since 1966, the Royal Air Force has run a programme for the treatment and desensitisation of military aircrew suffering from motion sickness. The programme involves graduated exposure to provocative motion, both on the ground and in the air. The success rate measured by the number of treated aircrew who successfully complete flying training is in excess of 85% (Bagshaw and Stott, 1985), and similar desensitisation programmes are now in routine use for military aircrew throughout the world.

PASSENGER HEALTH

With an understanding of the basic principles of aviation medicine, it can be seen that flying as a passenger should be no problem for the fit, healthy and mobile individual. But for the passenger with certain pre-existing conditions or developing an acute medical problem in flight, the cabin environment may exacerbate the situation. We have seen that modern commercial airliners fly with a cabin altitude of between 4000 and 8000 feet (1200 and 2400 m) when at cruising altitude, which means a reduction in ambient pressure of the order of 20% compared with sea level and a consequent reduction in blood oxygen saturation of about 10%. The cabin air is relatively dry, and the limited room available in the nonpremium cabin may be a factor to be considered.

Inflight medical problems can result from the exacerbation of a pre-existing medical condition, or can be an acute event occurring in a previously fit individual. Although the main problems relate to the physiological effects of hypoxia and expansion of trapped gases, it should be remembered that the complex airport environment can be stressful and challenging to the passenger, leading to problems before even getting airborne.

Although passengers with medical needs require medical clearance from the airline, passengers with disabilities do not. However, disabled passengers do need to notify the requirement for special needs, such as wheelchair assistance or assignment of seats with lifting armrests, and this should be done at the time of booking.

Preflight Assessment and Medical Clearance

The objectives of medical clearance are to provide advice to passengers and their medical attendants on fitness to fly, and to prevent delays and diversions to the flight as a result of deterioration in the passenger's well-being. It depends upon self-declaration by the passenger, and upon the attending physician having an awareness of the flight environment and how this might affect the patient's condition. Most major airlines provide services for those passengers requiring extra help, and most have a medical adviser to assess the fitness for travel of those with medical needs (Bagshaw and Byrne, 1999). Individual airlines work to their own guidelines, but these are generally based on those published by the Aerospace Medical Association (Air Transport Medicine Committee, 1996) on fitness for travel. The International Air Transport Association (IATA) publishes a recommended Medical Information Form (MEDIF) for use by member airlines. The MEDIF should be completed by the passenger's medical attendant and passed to the airline at the time of booking to ensure timely medical clearance.

Medical clearance is required when:

- Fitness to travel is in doubt as a result of recent illness, hospitalisation, injury, surgery or instability of an acute or chronic medical condition.
- Special services are required, e.g. oxygen, stretcher or authority to carry or use accompanying medical equipment such as a ventilator or a nebuliser.

Medical clearance is *not* required for carriage of an invalid passenger outside these categories, although special needs (such as a wheelchair) must be notified to the airline at the time of booking. Cabin crew members are unable to provide individual special assistance to invalid passengers beyond the provision of normal inflight service. Passengers who are unable to look after their own personal needs during flight (such as toiletting or feeding) will be asked to travel with an accompanying adult who can assist. It is vital that passengers remember to carry with them any essential medication, and not pack it in the baggage checked in for the hold.

Deterioration on holiday or on a business trip of a previously stable condition, such as asthma, diabetes or epilepsy, or accidental trauma can often give rise to the need for medical clearance for the return journey. A stretcher may be required, together with medical support, and this can incur considerable cost. It is thus important for all travellers to have adequate travel insurance, which includes provision for the use of a specialist repatriation company to provide the necessary medical support where necessary.

Assessment Criteria

In determining the passenger's fitness to fly, a basic knowledge of aviation physiology and physics can be applied to the pathology. Any trapped gas will expand in volume by up to 30% during flight, and consideration must be given to the effects of the relative hypoxia encountered at a cabin altitude of 8000 feet (2400 m) above mean sea level. The altitude of the destination airport may also need to be taken into account in deciding the fitness of an individual to undertake a particular journey.

Particular evaluation may be necessary for cardiovascular disease (e.g. angina pectoris, congestive heart failure, myocardial infarction), deep venous thrombosis, respiratory disease (e.g. asthma, chronic obstructive airways disease, emphysema), surgical conditions, cerebrovascular accident, epilepsy, psychiatric illness, diabetes and infectious disease.

The passenger's exercise tolerance can provide a useful guide on fitness to fly; if unable to walk a distance greater than about 50 metres without developing dyspnoea, there is a risk that the passenger will be unable to tolerate the relative hypoxia of the pressurised cabin. More specific guidance can be gained from knowledge of the passenger's blood gas levels and haemoglobin value.

Table 13.1 shows the guidelines recommended by one international carrier. This list is not exhaustive, and it should be remembered that individual cases might require individual assessment by the attending physician.

The prolonged period of immobility associated with long haul flying can be a risk for those individuals predisposed to develop deep venous thrombosis (DVT). Although many airlines promote lower limb exercise via the inflight magazine and encourage mobility within the cabin, those passengers known to be vulnerable to DVT should seek guidance from their attending physician on the use of compression stockings and/or anticoagulants. There is currently no evidence that flying, *per se*, is a risk factor for the development of DVT.

As well as the effect of the condition upon the sick passenger, account must be taken of the effect or potential effect on other passengers or crew members. It is obvious that an individual should not fly during the infectious stage of a contagious disease, although any risk of transmission of infection in the cabin is usually confined to those passengers seated near to the infected passenger (the 'index case'). Recirculated cabin air is passed through HEPA filters that remove bacteria and viral particles, reducing the risk of infection via air circulation. Any risk is due to person-to-person droplet spread, as in any situation where people sit in close proximity. The determination of infective periods is defined by the American Public Health Association (Benenson, 1990). Most states have strict rules with respect to infectious passengers entering the country; in the UK, the port health authority have strict disembarkation rules for an aircraft which is carrying a passenger suspected of having an infectious disease.

Considerations of Physical Disability or Immobility

As well as the reduction in ambient pressure and the relative hypoxia, it is important to consider the physical constraints of the passenger cabin. A passenger with a disability must not impede the free egress of the cabin occupants in case of emergency evacuation. There is limited leg space in an economy class seat and a passenger with an above-knee leg plaster or an ankylosed knee or hip may simply not fit in the available space. The long period of immobility in an uncomfortable position must be taken into account, and it is imperative to ensure adequate pain control for the duration of the journey, particularly following surgery or trauma. Even in the premium class cabins with more available leg room, there are limits on space. To avoid impeding emergency egress, immobilised or disabled passengers cannot be seated adjacent to emergency exits, despite the availability of increased leg room at many of these positions. Similarly, a plastered leg cannot be stretched into the aisle because of the conflict with safety regulations. There is limited space in aircraft toilet compartments and, if assistance is necessary, a travelling companion is required.

The complexities of the airport environment should not be underestimated, and must be considered during the assessment of fitness to fly. The formalities of check-in and departure procedures are demanding and can be stressful, and this can be compounded by illness and disability as well as by language difficulties or jet lag. The operational effect of the use of equipment such as wheelchairs, ambulances and stretchers must be taken into account, and the possibility of aircraft delays or diversion to another airport must be considered. It may be necessary to change aircraft and transit between terminals during the course of a long journey, and landside medical facilities will not be available to a transiting passenger. At London's Heathrow Airport, for example, transfer traffic accounts for more than 40% of all passengers.

There is often a long distance between the check-in desk and the boarding gate. Not all flights depart from or arrive to jetties, and it may be necessary to climb up or down stairs and board transfer coaches. It is thus important for the passenger to specify the level of assistance required when booking facilities such as wheelchairs.

Stretchers

All equipment used on board a commercial aircraft must comply with the safety and compatibility requirements of both the regulatory authority and the airline. This applies to a stretcher, which must be securely fixed in the cabin, must not impede normal or emergency egress, and must provide adequate restraint for the sick passenger. There is an assessment and approval system for all aircraft equipment and the airline itself will normally provide a suitably approved stretcher.

A qualified attendant, whether nurse or doctor, must be responsible for all care and attention to the passenger throughout the journey. Any supporting equipment such as a ventilator must be approved by the airline. Consideration must be given to factors such as disposal of biohazardous waste, and the effect on other passengers and crew members of carrying the sick passenger. Pre- and

Table 13.1 Guidelines for medical clearance

Category	Do not accept	Remarks
Cardiovascular disorders	Uncomplicated myocardial infarction within 7 days	Myocardial infarction less than 21 days requires MEDIF assessment
	Uncontrolled heart failure	
	Open heart surgery within 10 days	This includes CABG and valve surgery MEDIF assessment required up to 21 days postoperatively Transpositions, ASD/VSD, transplants etc. will require discussion with airline medical advisor

	Angioplasty:
	  no stenting 3 days
	  with stenting 5 days	

Circulatory disorders	Active thrombophlebitis of lower limbs	
	Bleeding/clotting conditions	Recently commenced anticoagulation therapy requires assessment
Blood disorders	Hb less than $7.5\,\mathrm{g\,dl^{-1}}$	MEDIF assessment required for Hb less than $10\,\mathrm{g\,dl^{-1}}$
	History of sickling crisis within 10 days	
Respiratory disorders	Pneumothorax which is not fully inflated, or within 14 days after full inflation	
	Major chest surgery within 10 days	MEDIF assessment required up to 21 days postsurgery
	If breathless after walking 50 metres on ground, or on continuous oxygen therapy on ground	Consider mobility and all aspects of total journey, interlining, etc.
Gastrointestinal disorders	General surgery within 10 days	Laparoscopic investigation may travel after 24 h if all gas absorbed. Laparoscopic surgery requires MEDIF up to 10 days
	GI tract bleeding within 24 h	MEDIF required up to 10 days
CNS disorders	Stroke, including subarachnoid haemorrhage, within 3 days	Consider mobility/oxygenation aspects. MEDIF up to 10 days
	Epileptic fit (grand mal) within 24 h	Petit mal or minor twitching—common sense prevails
	Brain surgery within 10 days	Cranium must be free from air
ENT disorders	Otitis media and sinusitis	
	Middle-ear surgery within 10 days	
	Tonsillectomy within 1 week	
	Wired jaw, unless escorted and with wire cutters	If fitted with self quick-release wiring may be acceptable without escort
Eye disorders	Penetrating eye injury/intraocular surgery within 1 week	If gas in globe, total absorption necessary—may be up to 6 weeks, specialist check necessary
Psychiatric disorders	Unless escorted, with appropriate medication carried by escort, competent to administer such	MEDIF required. Medical, nursing or highly competent companion/relative escort
Pregnancy	After end of 36th week for single uncomplicated	Passenger advised to carry medical certificate
	After end of 32nd week for multiple uncomplicated	
Neonates	Within 48 h	Accept after 48 h if no complications present
Infectious disease	If in infective stage	As defined by American Public Health Association (Benenson, 1990)
Terminal illness	Until individual case assessed by airline medical advisor	Individual case assessment
Decompression	Symptomatic cases (bends, staggers, etc.) within 10 days	May need diving or aviation physician advice
Scuba diving	Within 24 h	
Fractures in plaster	Within 48 h unless splint bivalved	Extent, site and type of plaster may allow relaxation of guidelines. Exercise caution with fibreglass casts
Burns	Consult airline medical advisor	

Table 13.2 Supplementary oxygen product of one airline

- Oxygen can be delivered via various systems: cylinders, aircraft portable oxygen units or, on B747-400/B777, therapeutic ring main
- Cylinders can be present at flow rates of 2 or $4 \, \mathrm{l \, min^{-1}}$. Ring main 4 or $8 \, \mathrm{l \, min^{-1}}$. (A passenger requiring $8 \, \mathrm{l \, min^{-1}}$ would not generally be considered fit to fly)
- $2 \, \mathrm{l \, min^{-1}}$ provides approximately 23%; $4 \, \mathrm{l \, min^{-1}}$ provides approximately 40%

- *Cylinders*

Dumpy	530 litres	Medium	$= 2 \, \mathrm{l \, min^{-1}}$ lasts 4.24 h
		High	$= 4 \, \mathrm{l \, min^{-1}}$ lasts 2.12 h
Invalid set × 2 cylinders, each 170 litres	340 litres	Medium	$= 2 \, \mathrm{l \, min^{-1}}$ lasts 2.50 h
		High	$= 4 \, \mathrm{l \, min^{-1}}$ lasts 1.25 h
Invalid set × 2 cylinders, each 120 litres	240 litres	Medium	$= 2 \, \mathrm{l \, min^{-1}}$ lasts 2.00 h
		High	$= 4 \, \mathrm{l \, min^{-1}}$ lasts 1.00 h

- *Masks*
  Adult Hudson mask and tubing is supplied. Any alternative mask must be provided by the passenger

---

postflight ground handling of the stretcher requires arrangement in advance of the flight.

Airlines generally prefer stretcher cases to be arranged by a specialist medical assistance or repatriation company because of the potential practical and organisational difficulties inherent in the operation. There are cases when it is more appropriate for the sick passenger to be carried in a specialist air ambulance.

Oxygen

In addition to the main gaseous system, all commercial aircraft carry an emergency oxygen supply for use in the event of failure of the pressurisation system or during emergencies such as fire or smoke in the cabin. The passenger supply is delivered via drop-down masks from chemical generators or an emergency reservoir, and the crew supply is from oxygen bottles strategically located within the cabin. This emergency supply has a limited duration. Sufficient first-aid oxygen bottles are carried to allow the delivery of oxygen to a passenger in case of a medical emergency inflight, but there is insufficient to provide a premeditated supply for a passenger requiring it continuously throughout a journey. If a passenger has a condition requiring continuous ('scheduled') oxygen for a journey, this needs prenotification to the airline at the time of booking the ticket. Most airlines make a charge to contribute to the cost of its provision.

It is not permissible for the passenger to use his or her own oxygen system in flight. As we have already seen, all

Table 13.3 Inflight medical incidents reported in 1 year by a major airline (total 2522 incidents in 34 million passengers)

Incident type	No.	%
Gastrointestinal system	563	22.3
Cardiovascular system	551	21.8
Central nervous system	392	15.5
Musculoskeletal system/skin	337	13.4
Respiratory system	256	10.2
Urogenital system	82	3.3
Metabolic system	64	2.5
Otorhinolaryngology (ENT)	34	1.4
Miscellaneous	243	9.6

equipment used on board must meet regulatory standards; the specification for aviation oxygen is higher than that for normal medical oxygen in terms of permissible water content (to prevent freezing of valves and regulators at high altitude). The supplementary or scheduled oxygen provided for use by the sick passenger may be delivered from gaseous bottles, or it may be delivered on some aircraft by tapping into the ring-main system. Some carriers provide molecular sieve concentrators, although these can be expensive to service and maintain. Those airlines that do provide oxygen usually do so only in flight; if oxygen is required on the ground, e.g. at an airport of transit, the passenger is probably unfit to fly.

Table 13.2 describes the supplementary (scheduled) oxygen product available from one international carrier.

Inflight Medical Emergencies

An inflight medical emergency is defined as a medical occurrence requiring the assistance of the cabin crew. It may or may not involve the use of medical equipment or drugs, and may or may not involve a request for assistance from a medical professional travelling as a passenger on the flight. Thus it can be something as simple as a headache, or a vasovagal episode, or something major such as a myocardial infarction or impending childbirth.

The incidence is comparatively low, although the media impact of an event can be significant. One major international airline recently reported 3022 incidents occurring in something over 34 million passengers carried in 1 year (Bagshaw, 1996). The breakdown of these incidents into generalised causes is shown in Table 13.3. The top six inflight emergency medical conditions reported by the same airline are shown in Table 13.4.

Any acute medical condition occurring during the course of a flight can be alarming for the passenger and crew due to the remoteness of the environment. The cabin crew receive training in advanced first aid and basic life support and the use of the emergency medical equipment carried on board the aircraft. Many airlines give training in excess of the regulatory requirement, particularly when an extended range of medical equipment is carried.

Table 13.4 Six most common inflight medical incidents reported in 1 year by a major airline (total 2522 incidents in 34 million passengers)

Incident	No.	%
Faint	377	14.9
Diarrhoea	291	11.5
Head injury	158	6.3
Vomiting	153	6.1
Collapse	136	5.4
Asthma	124	4.9

Good Samaritans

Although the crew are trained to handle common medical emergencies, in serious cases they may request assistance from a medical professional travelling as a passenger. Such assisting professionals are referred to as Good Samaritans. Cabin crew members attempt to establish the bona fides of medical professionals offering to assist, but much has to be taken on trust.

The international nature of air travel can lead to complications in terms of professional qualification and certification, specialist knowledge and professional liability. An aircraft in flight is subject to the laws of the state in which it is registered, although when not moving under its own power (i.e. stationary at the airport) it is subject to the local law. In some countries it is a statutory requirement for a medical professional to offer assistance to a sick or injured person (e.g. France), whereas in other states no such law exists (e.g. UK or USA). Some countries (e.g. USA) have enacted a Good Samaritan law, whereby an assisting professional delivering emergency medical care within the bounds of his or her competence is not liable for prosecution for negligence. In the UK, the major medical defence insurance companies provide indemnity for their members acting as Good Samaritans. Some airlines provide full indemnity for medical professionals assisting in response to a request from the crew, whereas other airlines take the view that a professional relationship is established between the sick passenger and the Good Samaritan and any liability lies within that relationship. To the end of 1999, there is no record of any action for negligence or professional malpractice arising out of a Good Samaritan act on board a commercial airliner.

Recognition by the airline of the assistance given by the Good Samaritan is complicated by the special nature of the relationship between the professional, the patient and the airline. Indemnity, whether provided by the airline or the professional's defence organisation, depends upon the fact that a Good Samaritan act is performed. If a professional fee is claimed or offered, the relationship moves away from being that of a Good Samaritan act to one of a professional interaction with an acceptance of clinical responsibility. This implies that the professional is suitably trained, qualified and experienced to diagnose, treat and follow up the particular case, and the Good Samaritan indemnity provision no longer applies.

Airlines are always grateful for assistance willingly offered by medical professionals travelling as passengers, particularly when the costs and inconvenience of an unscheduled diversion are avoided. There is no standard industry response, but the expression of gratitude can vary from a quick word of thanks from the cabin crew to a free first-class ticket sent from the office of the airline chief executive. In practice, most airlines provide an immediate reward, such as a bottle of champagne, followed up with a letter of thanks. As already discussed, for reasons of indemnity it is inappropriate to pay a full professional fee to the Good Samaritan.

Follow-up of the passenger after disembarkation is frequently difficult, because he or she is no longer in the care of the airline and becomes the responsibility of the receiving hospital or medical practitioner.

Aircraft Medical Diversion

Responsibility for the conduct of the flight rests with the aircraft captain, who makes the final decision as to whether or not an immediate unscheduled landing or diversion is required for the well-being of a sick passenger. The captain has to take into account operational factors as well as the medical condition of such a passenger. In practice, it is rarely possible to land immediately because, even if a suitable airport is in the immediate vicinity, the aircraft has to descend from cruising altitude, possibly jettison fuel to reduce to landing weight, and then fly the approach procedure to land. Consideration has to be given to the availability of appropriate medical facilities, and in many cases, it is of greater benefit for the sick passenger to continue to the scheduled destination where the advantage of appropriate facilities will outweigh the risks of continuing the flight.

Operational factors to be considered include the suitability of an airport to receive the particular aircraft type. The runway must be of sufficient length and load-bearing capacity, the terminal must be able to accommodate the number of passengers on the flight, and if the crew go out of duty time, there must be sufficient hotel accommodation to allow an overnight stay of crew and passengers. The cost to the airline may be substantial, including the knock-on effects of aircraft and crew unavailability for the next scheduled sector, as well as the direct airport and fuel costs of the diversion. In making the decision whether or not to divert, the captain will take advice from all sources. If a Good Samaritan is assisting, he or she has an important role to play, perhaps in radio consultation with the airline medical adviser.

Telemedicine

Many airlines use an air-to-ground link which allows the captain and/or the Good Samaritan to confer with the airline medical adviser on the diagnosis, treatment and prognosis for the sick passenger (Bagshaw, 1996). The airline operations department is also involved in the decision-making process. Some airlines maintain a worldwide database of medical facilities available at or near the major airports; others subscribe to a third-party provider giving access to immediate medical advice and assistance with arranging emergency medical care for the sick passenger at the diversion airport.

The link from the aircraft is made using either high-frequency radio communication (HF) or a satellite communication system (satcom). Satcom is installed in newer long-range aircraft, and is gradually replacing HF as the industry norm for long-range communication. HF utilises the Heavyside-Appleton layer of the upper atmosphere to 'skip' radio waves around the curvature of the globe. This layer moves diurnally and HF propagation is also sensitive to atmospheric conditions. There are areas of the world where HF contact cannot be established, and these vary from day to day or hour by hour. This means that occasionally it is not possible to establish an air-to-ground voice link, or, if it is established, contact can be lost for several minutes. Satcom does not suffer from these limitations and usually provides clear and unbroken communication links.

Digitisation and telephone transmission of physiological parameters is a well-established practice; for example, in the remote highlands and islands of Scotland, a consultant obstetrician in a main hospital is able to monitor the antenatal progress of pregnant patients by the digital transmission of routine tocograms from outlying clinics to the hospital. In many parts of the world, ECG data can be digitised and transmitted via a telephone modem for interpretation by a consultant cardiologist at a specialist centre. An aircraft cabin at 37 000 feet (11 250 m) can be considered a remote location in terms of availability of medical support, and the digital technology used in satcom is similar to that used in modern ground-to-ground communication. The advent of satcom has enabled the development of air-to-ground transmission of physiological parameters to assist in diagnosis. Pulse oximetry and ECG are examples of data that can assist the medical adviser to give appropriate advice to the aircraft captain, although the cost–benefit analysis has to be weighed very carefully.

Aircraft Emergency Medical Equipment

National regulatory authorities stipulate the minimum scale and standard of all equipment to be carried on aircraft operating under their jurisdiction. This includes emergency medical equipment. Although these standards stipulate the minimum requirement, in practice many airlines carry considerably more equipment. Table 13.5 gives the minimum standard of equipment to be carried by aircraft registered in the USA, while Table 13.6 gives the standard determined by the European Joint Aviation Authorities for aircraft registered in European states.

In determining the type and quantity of equipment and drugs to include in the medical kits, the airline must obviously fulfil the statutory requirements laid down by the regulatory authority. Other factors to be considered are:

- *Route structure and stage lengths flown.* Different countries of the world vary in their regulations on what might be imported and exported, particularly in terms of drugs. For example, it is illegal to import morphine derivatives into the USA, even if securely locked in a medical kit.
- *Passenger expectations.* Premier class business passengers from the developed world expect a higher standard of care and medical provision than passengers travelling on a relatively inexpensive package holiday flight.
- *Training of cabin crew.* The crew must have a knowledge and understanding of the kit contents, for use by themselves or in assisting a Good Samaritan. They must be proficient in first aid, resuscitation and basic life support.
- *Differences in medical cultures.* Ideally, the kit contents should be familiar to any Good Samaritan irrespective of nationality or training. Some authorities require information and drug names to be given in more than one language.
- *Equipment and drugs appropriate for likely medical emergencies.* It is important to audit the incidence and outcome of inflight medical emergencies and maintain a review of the kit content. This review should also take account of changes in medical practice.
- *Space and weight.* The medical equipment must be accessible, but securely stowed. Some airlines divide the equipment and drugs between basic first-aid kits, which are readily accessible on the catering trolleys, and a more comprehensive emergency medical kit that is sealed and stowed with other emergency equipment. Space and weight are always at a premium within the cabin, and the medical kits must be as light and compact as possible.
- *Shelf life and replenishment.* A tracking system for each kit must be in place to ensure that contents have not exceeded their designated shelf life. Similarly, after use of a kit, there has to be a procedure for replenishment. In practice, the aircraft can depart if the kit contents meet the statutory minimum, even though drugs or equipment have been used from the nonstatutory part of the kit. Many airlines subcontract the tracking and replenishment to a specialist medical supply company.

Resuscitation Equipment

Although basic cardiopulmonary resuscitation (CPR) techniques are an essential part of cabin crew training, the outcome of an inflight cardiac event may be improved if appropriate resuscitation equipment is available. This can range from a simple mouth-to-mouth face guard, to a resuscitation bag and mask and airway, to an endo-

Table 13.5   Federal Aviation Regulations (USA) part 121

First-aid kits

Approved first-aid kits required by §121.309 must meet the following specifications and requirements:

(1) Each first-aid kit must be dust and moisture proof, and contain only materials that either meet Federal Specification GG-K-291a, as revised, or are approved

(2) Required first-aid kits must be distributed as evenly as practicable throughout the aircraft and be readily accessible to the cabin flight attendants

(3) The minimum number of first-aid kits required is set forth in the following table

No. of passenger seats	No. of first-aid kits
0–50	1
51–150	2
151–250	3
More than 250	4

(4) Except as provided in paragraph (5), each first-aid kit must contain at least the following or other approved contents:

Contents	Quantity		
Adhesive bandage compresses, 10-inch	16	Burn compound, $\frac{1}{8}$-ounce or an equivalent of other burn remedy	6
Antiseptic swabs	20	Arm splint, noninflatable	1
Ammonia inhalants	16	Leg splint, noninflatable	1
Bandage compresses, 4-inch	8	Roller bandage, 4-inch	4
Triangular bandage compresses, 10-inch	5	Adhesive tape, 1-inch standard roll	2
		Bandage scissors	1

(5) Arm and leg splints which do not fit within a first-aid kit may be stowed in a readily accessible location that is as near as practicable to the kit

Emergency medical kits

The approved emergency medical kit required by §121.309 for passenger flights must meet the following specifications and requirements:

(1) Approved emergency medical equipment shall be stored securely as as to keep it free from dust, moisture, and damaging temperatures

(2) One approved emergency medical kit shall be provided for each aircraft during each passenger flight and shall be located so as to be readily accessible to crew members

(3) The approved emergency medical kit must contain, as a minimum, the following appropriately maintained contents in the specified quantities

Contents	Quantity		
Sphygmomanometer	1	Nitroglycerin tablets	10
Stethoscope	1	Basic instructions for use of the drugs in the kit	
Airways, oropharyngeal (3 sizes)	3	Oral antihistamine	
Syringes (sizes necessary to administer required drugs)	4	Non-narcotic analgesic	
		Aspirin	
Needles (sizes necessary to administer required drugs)	6	Atropine	
		Bronchodilator inhaler	
50 percent Dextrose injection, 50 ml	1	Lidocaine and saline	
		IV administration kit with connectors	
Epinephrine (Noradrenaline) 1:1000, single dose ampoule or equivalent	2	AMBU bag (to assist respiration following defibrillation)	
Diphenhydramine HCl injection, single-dose ampoule or equivalent	2	CPR masks	
		Latex gloves	

Table 13.6 European Joint Aviation Requirements: JAR-OPS 1, subpart L

First-aid kits
The following should be included in the first-aid kits:
Bandages (unspecified)
Burns dressings (unspecified)
Wound dressings, large and small
Adhesive tape, safety pins and scissors
Small adhesive dressings
Antiseptic wound cleaner
Adhesive wound closures
Adhesive tape
Disposable resuscitation aid
Simple analgesic e.g. paracetamol
Antiemetic e.g. cinnarizine
Nasal decongestant
First-aid handbook
Splints, suitable for upper and lower limbs
Gastrointestinal antacid
Antidiarrhoeal medication, e.g. Loperamide
Ground/air visual signal code for use by survivors
Disposable gloves

A list of contents in at least two languages (English and one other). This should include information on the effects and side-effects of drugs carried

Note: An eye irrigator while not required to be carried in the first-aid kit should, where possible, be available for use on the ground

In addition, for aeroplanes with more than nine passenger seats installed, an emergency medical kit must be carried

Emergency medical kit (additional, for aircraft with more than nine passenger seats)
The following should be included in the emergency medical kit:
Sphygmomanometer—nonmercury
Stethoscope
Syringes and needles
Oropharyngeal airways (2 sizes)
Tourniquet
Coronary vasodilator, e.g. nitroglycerine
Antispasmodic, e.g. hyoscine
Noradrenaline (epinephrine) 1 : 1000
Adrenocortical steroid, e.g. hydrocortisone
Major analgesic, e.g. nalbuphine
Diuretic, e.g. frusemide
Antihistamine, e.g. diphenhydramine hydrochloride
Sedative/anticonvulsant, e.g. diazepam
Medication for hypoglycaemia, e.g. hypertonic glucose
Antiemetic, e.g. metoclopramide
Atropine
Digoxin
Uterine contractant, e.g. ergometrine/oxytocin
Disposable gloves
Bronchial dilator—including an injectable form
Needle disposal box
Catheter

A list of contents in at least two languages (English and one other). This should include information on the effects and side-effects of drugs carried

tracheal tube and laryngoscope, to an automatic advisory external defibrillator (AED). The decision on the scale of equipment to be carried has to take account of the same parameters used in determining the content of the emergency medical kits (see above). In addition, a cost–benefit analysis has to balance the cost of acquisition, maintenance and training against the probability of need and the expectation of the travelling public. Indeed, the decision will often be influenced by commercial considerations as much as medical, as seen in the debate on carriage of

AEDs on commercial aircraft.

The European Resuscitation Committee and the American Heart Association endorse the concept of early defibrillation as the standard of care for a cardiac event both in and out of the hospital setting. However, the protocol includes early transfer to an intensive care facility for continuing monitoring and treatment, which is not always possible in the flight environment. Despite this inability to complete the resuscitation chain, it is becoming increasingly common for commercial aircraft to be equipped with AEDs and for the cabin crew to be trained in their use. This is partly driven by public expectation. Experience of those airlines which carry AEDs indicates that there may be benefits to the airline operation as well as to the passenger. Some types of AED have a cardiac monitoring facility, and this can be of benefit in reaching the decision on whether or not to divert. For example, there is no point in initiating a diversion if the monitor shows asystole, or if it confirms that the chest pain is unlikely to be cardiac in origin. Lives have been saved by the use of AEDs on aircraft and diversions have been avoided, so it could be argued that the cost–benefit analysis is weighted in favour of carrying AEDs as part of the aircraft medical equipment. Nonetheless, it is important that unrealistic expectations are not raised. An aircraft cabin is not an intensive care unit and the AED forms only a part of the first-aid and resuscitation equipment.

Death in Flight

Death in flight is a cause of distress to everybody concerned. The number of people who travel on domestic and foreign airlines each year is approximately 1 billion, so the laws of chance suggest that there is a risk that some of those travellers may reach the end of their natural life during the course of a flight. One major airline reported 10 deaths in flight during a year in which it carried over 34 million passengers (Bagshaw, 1996). A major aim of preflight medical clearance is to reduce the chance of an acute medical event and the risk of death in flight.

Death can legally be confirmed only by a registered medical practitioner. If a doctor is not present on board the aircraft, and in the absence of an AED or monitor, or of the telemetry of an ECG, cabin crew may continue resuscitation attempts until the aircraft lands. Death can then be confirmed by the receiving physician. If a doctor is in attendance on board, or confirmation of asystole is given by an AED or telemetry, the captain is required to record the event, including details of time of death and the geographical coordinates where death occurred. Medical diversion is not appropriate once death has been confirmed, and may only complicate matters for the next of kin.

The regulations for the procedure to be followed on landing vary greatly between countries. Indeed, when landing in certain states police may detain the cabin crew while investigations into the circumstances of the death on board are investigated. This can take several days, or even weeks, and so it may be advisable to avoid the suggestion that the passenger has died during the flight. In the UK, the police must be notified and the event will be reported to the Civil Aviation Authority and to the coroner.

The storage and disposition of the body in the aircraft for the remainder of the flight can cause difficulties. There is inevitable distress for the cabin crew, the accompanying relatives and for fellow passengers. In some cases, it is appropriate to leave the body in the seat covered with a blanket. In other cases, it may be more appropriate to leave the body on the floor of a galley covered with a blanket, particularly if there have been resuscitation attempts. It may not be appropriate to store the body in a toilet compartment, despite the apparent attraction of this option. The cubicle is small, and there may be difficulties in removing the body at the end of the flight, particularly if rigor mortis has occurred. Each case must be considered individually.

Many airlines have in place a procedure for the follow-up of crew members involved in a distressing event, such as an on-board death. This can be valuable in avoiding long-term post-traumatic stress disorder, and also in reinforcing the training which the crew member has undergone.

Birth in Flight

This is a happier event for all concerned, but not without risks to the mother and baby. For this reason, many airlines refuse to carry women in the later stages of pregnancy, typically after the 36th week for a single uncomplicated pregnancy or the 32nd week for a multiple pregnancy. One major airline reports an average of one inflight births per year, out of a total of more than 34 million passengers carried (Bagshaw, 1996).

Cabin crew receive training in assisting childbirth, and in most countries a delivery pack is a statutory component of the inflight emergency medical equipment.

CONCLUSION

The passenger cabin of a commercial airliner is designed to carry the maximum number of passengers in safety and comfort, within the constraints of cost-effectiveness. It is incompatible with providing the facilities of an ambulance, an emergency room, an intensive care unit, a delivery suite or a mortuary. The ease and accessibility of air travel to a population of changing demographics inevitably means that there are those who wish to fly who may not cope with the hostile physical environment of the airport, or the hostile physiological environment of the pressurised passenger cabin. It is important for medical professionals to be aware of the relevant factors, and for unrealistic public expectations to be avoided.

Most airlines have a medical adviser who may be consulted prior to flight to discuss the implications for a particular passenger. Such preflight notification can prevent the development of an inflight medical emergency, which is hazardous to the passenger concerned, inconvenient to fellow passengers and expensive for the airline. For those with disability, but not a medical problem, preflight notification of special needs and assistance will reduce the stress of the journey and enhance the standard of service delivered by the airline. The importance of adequate medical insurance cover for all travellers cannot be overemphasised.

Finally, as with all things in commercial aviation, there is a continuing audit of activity and an ongoing risk-benefit analysis. The industry is under constant evolution, and is now truly global in its activity. Application of basic physics and physiology, and an understanding of how this may affect underlying pathology, will minimise the medical risks to the travelling public.

REFERENCES

Air Transport Medicine Committee, Aerospace Medical Association (1996) Medical guidelines for air travel. *Aviation Space and Environmental Medicine*, **67**, B1–B16.

Bagshaw M (1996) Telemedicine in British Airways. *Journal of Telemedicine and Telecare*, **2**, 36–38.

Bagshaw M and Byrne NJ (1999). La santé des passagers. *Urgence Pratique*, **36**, 37–43.

Bagshaw M and Stott JRR (1985) The desensitisation of chronically motion sick aircrew in the Royal Air Force. *Aviation Space and Environmental Medicine*, **56**, 1144–1151.

Benenson AS (ed.) (1990) *Control of Communicable Diseases in Man*. American Public Health Association, Washington DC.

Benson AJ (1988) Aetiology of motion sickness. In *Aviation Medicine*, (eds J. Ernsting and PF King), 2nd edn, pp. 323–329. Butterworths, London.

Bles W, de Jong HAA and Oosterveld WJ (1984) Prediction of seasickness susceptibility. In *Motion Sickness: Mechanisms, Prediction, Prevention and Treatment*. Conference Proceedings 372, **27**, 1–6. AGARD/NATO, Neuilly sur Seine.

Campbell RD and Bagshaw M (1999) *Human Performance and Limitations in Aviation*, 2nd edn. Blackwell Science, Oxford.

Ernsting J, Nicholson AN and Rainford DJ (1999). *Aviation Medicine*, 3rd edn. Butterworth-Heinemann, London.

Homick JL, Reschke MF and Vanderploeg JM (1984) Space adaptation syndrome: incidence and operational implications for the Space Transportation System programme. In *Motion Sickness: Mechanisms, Prediction, Prevention and Treatment*. Conference Proceedings 372, **36**, 1-6. AGARD/NATO, Neuilly sur Seine.

Miller AD and Graybiel A (1970). The semicircular canals as a primary etiological factor in motion sickness. In *4th Symposium on the Role of the Vestibular Organs in Space Exploration*, SP-187, pp 69–82. NASA, Washington.

Reason JT (1978) Motion sickness adaptation: a neural mismatch model. *Journal of the Royal Society of Medicine*, **71**, 819–829.

Rosekind MR, Gander PH, Connell LJ *et al.* (1994) Alertness management in flight operations. *NASA Technical Memorandum*, DOT/FAA/RD-93/18.

FURTHER READING

McNeill EL (1983) *Airborne Care of the Ill or Injured*. Springer-Verlag, New York.

Martin T and Rodenberg HD (1996) *Aeromedical Transportation: A Clinical Guide*. Avebury, London.

14

Aviation Psychology

Robert Bor, Justin Parker and Linda Papadopoulos

London Guildhall University, London, UK

INTRODUCTION

Aviation psychology is concerned with safe, efficient and comfortable air travel, with an emphasis on the role of human factors. The origins of aviation psychology can probably be traced back to early experimental studies of human vigilance, system design, person–machine design problems, pilot performance and related human factors problems among air crew during World War II, both in the UK and the USA. Aircrew flew combat missions under extreme levels of physical and emotional stress and had to be carefully selected and trained to cope with the unique and specific challenges of their job. The growth in commercial aviation after the war, together with rapid advances in the speed and distances covered by jet-powered aircraft made air travel more accessible and revolutionised transportation and communication. A secondary effect has been on human relationships: air travel has changed how we relate to people because almost any destination in the world can be reached in under 24 h.

Human beings have not evolved naturally to fly and there are countless obstacles or physical 'evolution barriers' to our position or motion senses, as well as our capacity for processing information, that are apparent to both the novice air traveller as well as to the most seasoned pilot. We remain a species that is best designed and equipped to be self-propelling at a few miles per hour in two dimensions under the conditions of terrestrial gravity (Reason, 1974). Remarkable achievements in engineering have made air travel both possible and highly accessible within the span of a single lifetime. Various penalties are exacted, however, when evolutionary barriers to motion are exceeded. The most common include motion sickness, jet lag and increased arousal and stress at different stages of flight. For flight crew, there may be additional problems relating to judgement, decision making, perception and concentration, among others. Air travel often brings us into close contact with strangers, and an understanding of the social psychology of behaviour within groups (among passengers) and teams (among crew) is relevant.

The principal focus of recent published literature in the field of aviation psychology has been on the selection, training and performance of pilots, air traffic controllers and ground engineers. Emerging problems, such as the advent of larger commercial aircraft flying greater distances nonstop, disruptive passengers and an increasing awareness of how human factors play a role in aircraft accidents and survivability of these, have broadened the focus for and agenda of aviation psychologists. This chapter provides an overview of how psychological research and theories have contributed to an understanding of how air travel disrupts human relationships and behaviour, as well as bodily functions and systems.

MODERN AIR TRAVEL

Air travel has never been so accessible. A billion people worldwide will soon make at least one plane trip per year. Unfortunately, the dream of flight, nurtured by Leonardo da Vinci, the Wright brothers, and others, is sometimes tarnished by stress. Less than three decades ago, air travel was exciting, attracted a small number of the elite and wealthy passengers, was dangerous, an adventure, and enabled people to travel at greater speeds than ever before. Passengers were pampered and obedient. The advent of large commercial carriers in the 1960s in an industry of mass air transportation and cheap, accessible flights has irreversibly changed all of this. Airline advertisements continue to raise expectations among air travellers because the product being promoted is still perceived as glamorous. Disappointment sets in when expectations are not met, and high levels of stress may be one outcome of this.

Stress may begin long before passengers set out for the airport. Making travel arrangements, preparing to leave home and saying 'goodbye' to family, friends or colleagues can increase stress and distress. Frequent air travel may also disrupt relationships. Psychologists have studied relationship dynamics both among aircrew and passengers, and examined attachment patterns in 'intermittent spouse' relationships. Attachment behaviour in adults (e.g. avoidance, anxiety) and symptoms of emotional distress (e.g. insomnia, isolation, feeling upset) were found to be affected by relationship status, length and strength, with anxiously attached partners displaying or suffering greater distress (Fraley and Shaver, 1998). Crowds at airports or the close proximity of fellow travellers on board aircraft, coupled with noise, apprehension about travel, fatigue, hunger, emotional arousal due to separation from a loved one and language and communication difficulties, can test even the most resilient and healthiest travellers.

Most passengers have expectations about travel, and these may be built around punctuality, quality of service, or amenities available at airports or on board aircraft. There are times when these expectations are not met, due to delays or poor levels of service. These may be predictable but no less annoying as a result. Passengers react differently to stress. Some resort to alcohol ingestion to relieve boredom, anxiety or irritation. Others become militant about what they believe to be their 'rights' and may become insistent or hostile towards ground staff or cabin crew. Still others resort to taking medication to reduce anxiety or induce sleep. Each of these coping strategies may, however, further aggravate the situation and increase stress. Many passengers have a fear of flying and psychological treatment for them is both readily available and effective.

FEAR OF FLYING

Relative to other phobias, a fear of flying affects a large proportion of the population, and up to 20% of airline passengers at any one time (Foreman and Borrill, 1994). Similar to other phobias, a fear of flying is unlikely to disappear without treatment, as, each time the patient avoids flying, the phobia is likely to become more entrenched and the symptoms more severe. Patients may ask their doctor or nurse to treat the phobia medically and therefore provide a medical solution to what is essentially a psychological problem with physiological manifestations. This section describes a psychological approach to the treatment of fear of flying.

Patients who present with a fear of flying may identify flight anxiety directly when they request treatment for flight phobia. Alternatively a fear of flying may be demonstrated through indirect consequences of the symptoms, which may impinge on other aspects of their lives, for example where it causes difficulties in relationships, inhibits career progression or through incidence of so-called 'air rage' as a result of excessive alcohol use (Bor, 1999). A fear of flying should not be lightly dismissed by health care professionals, as the effects can wreak havoc in people's lives and the fear may also be indicative of a more general anxiety disorder (Bor et al., 2001a).

Flight phobics may present to health care professionals with symptoms that initially indicate a simple association between anxiety and the experience of flying. However, certain features of a fear of flying must be considered and

these are most relevant in the assessment stage. Flight phobia differs from other 'simple' phobias in that it is considered to be a constellation of four fundamental fears: that of heights, crashing, instability and confinement. Around 46% of travellers with a fear of flying also have other phobias: 33% of these travellers commonly present with agoraphobia and 25% with claustrophobia (Dean and Whitaker, 1980). In addition, other events and factors in the patient's life that cause stress, such as relationship problems or redundancy, can increase their susceptibility to anxiety (Doctor et al., 1990).

Health care professionals should ensure that they make a full assessment of the patient's situation in general, as well as obtaining specific information relevant to the implementation of systematic desensitisation treatments. Information of general relevance may include:

- Psychological history of the traveller and family. Given that most phobias can be acquired through vicarious learning and modelling, the behaviour of primary carers in relation to the fear stimuli should be identified, as well as the coping strategies that they commonly employ.
- Personality factors. Individuals who have a high degree of emotional reactivity are more at risk of acquiring phobias. As such, introverts have been shown to be more prone to conditioning and may acquire fear of flying more quickly or to a greater degree.
- Psychiatric factors. Particular attention should be paid to travellers who have a psychiatric diagnosis. For example, treatment of patient with a borderline personality disorder for fear of flying must include very close monitoring for progress and relapse. An evaluation of the patient's emotional stability and level of cognitive functioning must be made prior to treatment.
- Standardised tests can provide accurate information about the nature and degree of the fear of flying. The Flight Anxiety Situations questionnaire (Van Gerwen et al., 1999) determines the degree of anxiety experienced in different situations associated with air travel. The Flight Anxiety Modality questionnaire (Van Gerwen et al., 1999) differentiates between cognitive and somatic symptoms of the fear of flying.
- The reasons why the traveller is seeking treatment at this particular time can provide a useful indication of the anxiety components specific to the individual's fear of flying.

When making a behavioural assessment for systematic desensitisation treatment, information should be obtained that relate to the following areas (Cautela and Upper, 1977):

- Identification of target behaviours to be changed and the maintaining factors.
- Ascertaining the patient's social and personal resources, as well as their coping skills. The aim is to capitalise on useful strategies and, where appropriate, to introduce more appropriate skills. Factors that may limit and/or inhibit treatment can also be identified.

- Identification of interventions most likely to be adopted by the patient according to his or her particular circumstances.

Flight phobic travellers may require a 'package' of treatments, where the emphasis may or may not be on their fears about flying and may address other external factors. All treatments should, however, be directed towards improving the traveller's ability to manage anticipatory anxiety as well as those fears encountered at airports and on board the aircraft.

The most widely accepted psychological explanation for the acquisition of fear of flying comes from the classical conditioning paradigm. Anxiety is considered to be a response that is learned when a 'danger signal' is perceived. The 'danger signal' is previously paired with a situation which naturally produces a negative reaction, through direct exposure, modelling or vicarious learning. The individual behaves, by means of a process of operant conditioning, to either reduce anxiety levels or achieve a state of safety. The fear of flying, in common with most phobias, is viewed as a form of aversive conditioning, maintained by avoidance behaviours.

People who suffer from a fear of flying commonly present with number of symptoms that are either related to their thoughts, behaviour, physiology or social circumstances (McIntosh, 1989). These symptoms can occur at any stage, from anticipating the journey to the airport to returning home. Individuals with flight phobia frequently have negative thoughts associated with the air travel and have a tendency to amplify, or 'catastrophise' the level of threat posed by certain aspects of flying. They experience anxiety symptoms when they anticipate the flight or are unable to avoid a flight. The physical symptoms of flight anxiety include breathlessness, sweating, palpitations and tension. Flight phobics invariably become preoccupied with ways to avoid flying when faced with the prospect of air travel; they actively plan alternatives and seek to minimise the likelihood of having to take the trip. This can have significant consequences for the individual's personal and professional lives; for example, avoidance may prevent them progressing in their career or lead to problems in their relationships when planning the family's holiday.

Psychological interventions are designed to introduce new information about the situation with the aim of increasing individuals' perception of their ability to cope or altering their appraisal of the situation as threatening. Treatments designed to increase individuals' ability to cope are usually aimed at their physiological reactions to the situation and include relaxation training, thought-stopping and stress inoculation training. Interventions designed to decrease the appraisal of threat are most commonly directed towards travellers' thoughts about flying and their behaviours. A reduction in threat appraisal might be achieved by providing information about the flying experience, exposure to air travel (actual or imagined) and through cognitive restructuring of travellers' beliefs about flying.

Interventions aimed at re-evaluating the perceived threat have the additional psychological benefit of helping to maintain the individual's perception of effective coping with feared situations in general, which is referred to as 'self-efficacy' (Bandura, 1977). This improves the patient's confidence and sense of control over critical factors in the feared situation. Control is a particularly important factor in flight phobias as travellers tend to place control over the situation externally (Borrill and Foreman, 1996) and this is frequently associated with stress (Lazarus and Folkman, 1984). In the case of fear of flying, control may relate to the person's physiological symptoms, actions and/or thoughts. When treating a person with a fear of flying, it is important to address the traveller's self-efficacy, because his or her perception of the general level of coping may reduce the degree of stress experienced as a result of any of the component phobias.

Treatment for a flight phobia is also directed at helping to facilitate the traveller's reappraisal of the threat of those aspects of flying that evoke anxiety. This is achieved through three main interventions: (1) education about the physical principles of flight and the process by which the aircrew control the aircraft; (2) experiential learning through participating in the simulated or actual flight situations; and (3) training in techniques to manage physiological symptoms of anxiety.

The most commonly used intervention is systematic desensitisation, developed by Wolpe (1958); it is based upon the principle of reciprocal inhibition where a response, which is incompatible with anxiety, is evoked at the time when the fear reaction ordinarily occurs. Most treatments use relaxation training to evoke a calm response to substitute for the anxiety reaction. Treatments using systematic desensitisation tend to follow a standard protocol. Firstly, the patient is counselled about relaxation techniques; this is followed by the creation of an anxiety hierarchy and then by systematic desensitisation proper (Wolpe, 1958). The intervention may include either direct exposure, by asking the traveller to experience the situation 'live', or indirect exposure, where the traveller is asked to picture the feared situation using guided imagery techniques.

The anxiety hierarchy is developed by first asking patients to describe different situations, associated with the phobia, which evoke an anxiety response. The degree to which the person is able to imagine a situation can also be determined at this point, to indicate whether or not exposure techniques will be effective. By writing these situations on index cards, the patient can then organise the cards according to how much each situation is rated as anxiety provoking on a scale of 1 to 100 (where 100 denotes extreme anxiety). The patient is asked to provide between 15 and 20 situations, which may include, for example, leaving a partner, going through passport control, waiting at the departure gate and entering the aircraft. At this stage, it is important to ensure that those antecedents that evoke anxiety are explicit and the descriptions of the stimuli are realistic.

During desensitisation proper, patients are first helped

to achieve a state of deep relaxation and then asked to imagine the scene that produces the least anxiety, and themselves within it, for 20 s. It is important to ensure that the patient is given the opportunity to signal when anxiety levels become intolerable: a situation that evokes a lower level of fear should be used or the period of exposure should be reduced. When the situation no longer evokes anxiety, the patient then addresses the next situation. This process is repeated until the patient has been exposed successfully to all the situations in the hierarchy without the fear reaction being evoked. The total length of treatment can depend on the number of situations identified by the patient and any factors that may interfere with the treatment process, such as external life stressors or personality factors. All treatments should aim ultimately to include 'live' exposure to the feared situation, adopting the same strategy for desensitisation as with exposure using imagination.

As is common with many other interventions for psychological problems, treatment can be enhanced with the use of selected medication, such as beta-blockers (McIntosh, 1989). This can be of particular importance when the traveller's physiological reaction is so intense that it prevents the psychological treatment from having any effect. Medication can also be effective in complementing anxiety management and relaxation techniques, allowing the traveller to inhibit the avoidance response and gain new information to re-evaluate the situation as nonthreatening.

The efficacy of treatment programmes for fear of flying have been examined to determine whether the successes that are reported within treatment are maintained over time, and whether different treatment components between programmes are more likely to predict lasting change in the traveller's anxiety levels (Doctor *et al.*, 1990). Programmes that include behavioural interventions, such as systematic desensitisation, have an overall success rate of 88%, while the success of nonbehavioural programmes fall dramatically to 18% of treated travellers. Long-term explorative psychoanalytic therapy has not been shown to be effective in the treatment of a fear of flying.

An important distinction arises between cognitive-behavioural treatment programmes that have used direct *in vivo* exposure compared with those only using exposure. Treatment involving direct exposure showed a significant reduction in anxiety levels over time (Roberts, 1989). However, if the programme only requires travellers to imagine the feared situation, then the reduction in fear achieved during treatment does not transfer to the actual flight, and consequently patients tend to have a higher relapse rate.

In summary, health care professionals are increasingly likely to encounter patients who present with flight phobia or related anxieties that arise from inappropriate coping or avoidance. Assessment of the fear of flying is a crucial stage in the treatment, particularly with regard to the multicomponent nature of flight phobias. Treatments may usually require a 'battery' of interventions to address these aspects of the phobia, as well as those difficulties arising from the symptoms. An awareness of the psychosocial implications of flight anxiety is important and care should be taken to address the effects of the symptoms on the patient's broader situation, particularly in their professional and personal lives.

PASSENGER BEHAVIOUR

The quality of the travel experience has significant implications not only for the psychological well-being of passengers and crew but also for onboard safety. The increase in accessibility of air travel through cheaper and more frequent flights has meant that there are an ever-increasing number of passengers. The aviation industry has had to invest large resources in maintaining levels of safety while remaining competitive. Aviation psychologists have been at the forefront of initiatives designed to improve safety. These include training in teamwork for multicrew operations (commonly termed 'crew resource management'), helping to develop 'hardware' and systems to reduce error, and improving the design and layout of the aircraft cabin in order to enhance safety. Contributing to an understanding of passenger behaviour has been an important addition to this.

Research into passenger behaviour has, until recently, been overlooked because it was assumed that all passengers are compliant with and adaptive to the unique demands of air travel; however, the increase in the frequency and severity of disruptive passenger incidents, including recent deaths, has challenged this belief. The safety implications of passenger behaviour have thus assumed greater significance and have come to dominate the aviation psychology agenda.

There are a number of factors that impinge upon the traveller, each of which may directly or indirectly influence passenger behaviour (Lazarus and Folkman, 1984). These factors include the quality of the travel experience and the traveller's ability to cope with potential stressors during the journey. For those who find managing the travel experience more difficult, lack of effective coping is manifest in behaviours akin to the 'fight or flight' response found in animals. The response is one directed towards either escape or attack in relation to the threatening situation. The lack of 'escape' or avoidance possibilities on board an aircraft has resulted in 'fight' reactions of aggression associated with high anxiety levels. One consequence of this has been an increase the incidence of threats to flight safety, and in particular to crew and other passengers. While it has always been accepted that a small proportion of passengers who have psychiatric problems may become disruptive on board aircraft, a sense of entitlement, resentment of the authority of crew and stress associated with modern air travel appear to trigger aggression in a wider group of passengers (Bor, 1999; Bor *et al.*, 2001b).

An air traveller's ability to manage relationships with other passengers is a crucial part of the travel experience, particularly where individual space is compromised. This is especially relevant among air passengers who are likely to come into close contact with people from other cultures. Passengers are required to respond flexibly to the interpersonal dynamics of heterogeneous groups and to manage differences in communication. When passengers have a reduced capacity to cope, due to a lack of skills, knowledge, empathy or high levels of stress, their behaviour can inadvertently exacerbate their own stress. This may lead to anxious and fractious relationships with others. Many passengers resort to using alcohol in order to cope with boredom and stress. The overuse of alcohol to manage stress has been linked in some cases to so-called 'air rage'.

Passengers' behaviour during flight is directly linked to stress that they experience in their life generally, as well as to the extent of emotional arousal associated with travel and attachment dynamics. Passengers who experience difficulties at work, in their relationships or with their physical health may be more prone to stress when flying and potentially more emotionally charged or aggressive. Frequent flyers are not necessarily immune from stress and results from surveys of business travellers suggest a direct relationship between severity of stress and frequency of trips abroad.

In flight, the traveller has to contend with a number of stressors that may determine how they manage the journey. Beginning with queues for checking-in, to long walks to the departure lounge and air bridge, the traveller has to negotiate crowds, which may be particularly difficult for those unfamiliar with the 'terrain' of large modern airports. Once on board the aircraft, the passenger may feel the need to compete for the armrest or overhead locker space. Airline passengers also have to contend with a physical environment that differs significantly from that experienced in other forms of travel. The lowered air pressure in the cabin is associated with mild hypoxia that results in a reduction in cognitive performance (Dension et al., 1966). The air in the cabin is 'recycled' during the flight and mixed with the outside air which also results in lower humidity (Edwards and Edwards, 1990), and this can lead to an increase in the stress and irritability of passengers, especially for those on long-haul flights.

The layout of the cabin and seating can also add to levels of stress, particularly in the economy area, where conditions may be more cramped. The increased seating density in economy class results in a greater propensity for 'crowd behaviour' such as deindividuation, where passengers may become more disinhibited, believing their actions to be 'anonymous' within a group. The physical effects of being in cramped seating for extended periods can lead to health problems, such as deep vein thrombosis, commonly referred to as 'economy class syndrome'. Environmental conditions associated with noise and vibration add to the stress and may lead to irritability.

Flight crew work under the same environmental conditions and they are also affected by the unique conditions aboard the aircraft. The stress this places on crew may impact upon passengers and simple customer relations incidents may lead to increased conflict between passengers and crew. The strained relationship between passengers and crew has been suggested as contributing to the increase incidence of 'air rage' (Bor, 1999). Fatigue and sleep deprivation are additional factors that may affect personal well-being and crew–passenger relations.

PASSENGER SAFETY

An understanding of passenger behaviour is important in relation to flight safety, and survivability of air accidents.

As a result of improved safety measures that have been implemented over the years, the number of air accidents has decreased. However, this has not been accompanied by a corresponding decrease in the number of passengers who survive accidents or incidents (Muir and Marrison, 1989). The actions of passengers on flights where an accident takes place is a crucial factor in determining the degree to which they are injured and the number of fatalities that occur. This is pertinent given the fact that 90% of passengers survive the initial impact in an accident where death is not inevitable (Muir and Marrison, 1989) and the majority of the fatalities occur in the post-impact period. The number of fatalities at this point is explained four main factors: (1) the physical features of the aircraft; (2) the level of competence of the crew and rescue services; (3) the environmental conditions both inside and outside the aircraft; and (4) the behaviour of individual passengers and the group.

The likelihood that a passenger will live in a survivable accident is largely determined by his or her behaviour in the postimpact period. The passenger's response to the accident situation can include one or a number of behaviours. The most usual of these is fear, particularly preimpact and in the postimpact period where the conditions pose a threat to life. This is commonly accompanied by anxiety associated with identifying and implementing the best strategy to maintain life. These physiological reactions can lead to a variety of behaviours that can either maximise or minimise the passenger's chance of survival. Behaviours that interfere with the passengers ability effectively to manage the postimpact situation include disorientation, depersonalisation, panic, behavioural inaction and affiliate behaviour, that of searching out familiar objects or people.

Interaction between the aircrew and the passengers can be crucial in guiding passenger behaviour to maximise the opportunity for survival in the event of an accident. Cabin crew must inspire the confidence of passengers with respect to their safety. This may have a negative consequence, in that passengers may abdicate responsibility for their own safety to the crew, which may in turn encourage behavioural inaction. In addition, during an accident the relationship between the cabin crew and passengers changes dramatically. Cabin crew must quickly take charge of the passengers to guide them to safety, rather than being at their service. This sudden shift in roles can be confusing for both passengers and crew.

The impact of crew behaviour on air safety has been strongest in the flight deck. As safety measures on the aircraft systems have become progressively more complex, the cause of air accidents has been increasingly attributed to pilot error. Approximately two-thirds of all air accidents are considered to be caused by 'pilot error'. 'Pilot error' is defined as errors that occur due to a failure in the flight deck appropriately to manage the flight resources but does not include errors associated with the improper use of the controls.

Crew behaviour can be strongly determined by the 'culture' of the flight deck, which is often highly structured and hierarchical. For example, subordinate crew members are reluctant to challenge the captain about a decision. The impact of this culture can be exacerbated by the fact that there are a small number of individuals who are required to execute a large number of complex tasks. In this environment, group processes that take place can mean that individual personalities can play a pivotal role in the overall performance.

Research suggests that most air accidents that are attributed to 'pilot error' result from a breakdown in crew coordination, where crews who make a large number of errors are characterised by having a lower quality of communication, interaction and integration. The quality of communication is of particular relevance and crews who regularly share flight status information, as well as confirm information given, were found to make the least errors. However, crews who made a large number of performance errors tended to communicate in a way that was ambiguous, irritable, uncomfortable or involved a high degree of disagreement amongst the crew members (Foushee and Manos, 1981).

Flight crew behaviour has been addressed by airlines through the implementation of 'cockpit resource management training', including developing effective communication procedures, and through the restructuring of tasks to ensure that the crew work together for these to be carried out. Aviation psychologists play an important role in aircrew training by facilitating the improvement of interactions on the flight deck, as well as between the flight deck and the cabin crew.

JET LAG

Jet lag (technically called 'circadian desynchronisation') is now used commonly to describe the disruption that occurs to one's sleeping pattern when travelling on long-haul flights. Air travel can produce a wide range of discomforts that may be physical or psychological in nature, or both. To the seasoned traveller these discomforts may be a familiar inconvenience, whereas for the uninitiated they can be an unpleasant surprise. Of all the problems associated with long distance air travel, jet lag is possibly the most distressing and unwelcome, as it does not disappear on arrival. Indeed, it may take some days to recover

from jet lag, and, in certain cases, up to 2 weeks. The effects may prevent the air traveller from enjoying the start of a holiday, getting down to planned business, or adjusting to regular routines upon return home. A change in the times of waking and sleeping cause the traveller's 'internal clock' to no longer be synchronised with that of the country of arrival.

The body uses cycles or internal rhythms that are regulated by the release of hormones and include a hormone to lower its temperature in preparation for sleep. The body temperature starts falling at around midnight and is at its lowest level at around 4 a.m. It then rises again at around 10 a.m. and remains reasonably constant for the rest of the day. Other changes that occur as a result of the body clock are a fall in blood pressure during the night, and the slowing of breathing and digestion.

As jet lag is closely associated with daylight changes as the passenger moves across time zones, the effect is more marked for those travelling in an easterly direction and on longer journeys. The symptoms can be both intense and long-lasting and can be cumulative for frequent travellers. Commonly, air passengers experience extreme fatigue accompanied by insomnia, loss of appetite, depression, irritability, poor concentration, physical pains and aches, and reduced physical and mental performance. The severity of jet lag is mediated by a number of factors, including the number of time zones crossed, direction of travel, age, gender and frequency of flights.

Strategies to minimise jet lag include efforts to synchronise the traveller's body clock with the time zone of the destination country by adjusting their sleeping, eating and socialising habits. Travellers should be encouraged to adjust routines to the new time zone before the trip, which may include eating early or going to bed later for a few days before the journey. For trips where the arrival time is early morning, strategies to induce sleep are especially important and include creating the right conditions by reducing noise and light, relaxation techniques and, if necessary, short-term medication. Travellers can also use short 'naps' to gain sleep but the length of these must depend upon the duration of the visit to the destination country, as naps over 4 h can 'reset' the 'internal clock' to local time. Alternatively, air travellers who arrive in the daytime may use different strategies to make themselves more alert, which may include brief exercise or a high protein meal to boost energy levels.

Strategies for minimising general discomfort include wearing appropriate clothing, eating light food and avoiding caffeine/alcohol/carbonated drinks. The stress associated with physical discomfort is particularly relevant on board aircraft, given the restrictions on space and mobility. Air travellers should be encouraged to develop appropriate exercise programmes, which may focus on particular areas, such as the upper back. Passengers should take opportunities to take regular strolls around the cabin and to employ stretching techniques.

IMPACT OF TRAVEL ON RELATIONSHIPS

The negative effects of travelling on the nontravelling partner and family members also have a significant impact on the level of stress experienced by the passenger. Air travellers should be encouraged to develop strategies for managing their relationships with those close to them, particularly relating to explicit communication regarding the trip and the effect it has for all parties. Passengers should also be encouraged to be creative about using the trip as a way to enhance their relationships, such as providing opportunities to express feelings and to explore individual goals of family members. Strategies for managing stress in relationships also include placing the trip in the context of family life by ensuring sufficient warning is given and the reason for the journey is clear (Persaud, 1999).

Passengers who have been abroad for extended periods may find returning home a stressful experience and as demanding as arriving in any 'new' unfamiliar environment, a phenomenon referred to as 'reverse culture shock'. Homesickness can also lead to emotional arousal. This may be characterised by obsessional thoughts about home and negative thoughts about the new environment, accompanied by low mood. Travellers should acknowledge their nostalgia and develop skills to ensure that they achieve appropriate social support. They should, however, endeavour to create involvement with and a degree of commitment to the new environment, and should engage in physical activity. Travellers should ensure that they develop an awareness of likely 'high-risk' situations that are likely to evoke feelings of homesickness (van Tilburg et al., 1996). Similarly, travellers who return from long periods abroad often feel a longing for the country they have left, causing significant levels of stress. Travellers experiencing 're-entry shock' often benefit from those strategies applicable to homesickness and should address adjustment reactions.

Stress associated with travel may produce negative consequences socially, psychologically and physically; these can often depend on the individual's ability to 'buffer' stress. Passengers can improve their capacity to manage stress associated with their journey by adopting a proactive stance. Travellers can increase the level of control they have within a threatening situation by either maximising their coping strategies or improving the quality of the existing strategies. The first stage of improving coping, and reducing stress, is for the traveller to identify, in as much detail as possible, those specific parts of the flight that evoke fear. This allows interventions to be appropriately targeted and 'threats' to be distinguished from one another, which is particularly useful given the complex nature of flight phobias. Air travellers should be helped to identify those strategies that are already used and to determine how effective they are at dealing with the stress associated with the situation. They should also be encouraged to develop new coping strategies between journeys and to put these into practice during the next trip. New strategies should be evaluated with the view of improving their effectiveness.

RISK-TAKING BEHAVIOUR AMONG TRAVELLERS

Most of this chapter deals with passengers on board aircraft. This short section deviates slightly from this context to consider some of the risks to the traveller in a foreign environment and how these may arise. Behavioural scientists who work in public health settings are concerned with disease prevention and treatment compliance. Surveys of travel clinic attendees repeatedly confirm that travellers worry about becoming unwell while abroad, due to eating certain foods or drinking contaminated water. Although the effects of such contamination may be unpleasant, they are rarely life threatening and it is usually possible to reduce the risk of gastrointestinal illness while abroad. Research carried out among returning travellers has demonstrated that, unfortunately, a significant proportion of travellers fail to take the necessary precautions or heed the advice given by experts and are unnecessarily exposed to other, and potentially more serious, medical conditions. This also happens in spite of their knowledge and awareness of the risks. Three common examples are:

- Contracting malaria by not taking prophylaxis or completing the full course of treatment
- Exposure to sexually transmitted infections, including HIV, through unprotected intercourse with a partner abroad
- Sunburn (and the increased risk of skin cancer) after not adequately protecting exposed skin.

Although these are different health problems, the common thread of risk-taking among some travellers links them. There are several possible explanations why travellers might take unnecessary risks:

1. In terms of sexual risks, some people make judgements about the degree of risk to which they believe they will be exposed according to the physical appearance of their partner(s). Health care professionals sometimes hear patients returning from abroad state: 'he looked too healthy to be infected', or 'she was too good looking a type to be ill'. Of course, these beliefs are unreliable because sexual infections can be transmitted irrespective of the age or appearance of the person, who may be infected but free of obvious symptoms. The theory of cognitive dissonance (Festinger, 1957) suggests that that we are prone to making up explanations to fit with our beliefs rather than objective facts. A further example of this strategy to manage dissonance is the smoker who says that the risk to health of smoking is manageable because only a small proportion of smokers contract cancer.

2. When people are away from home and their usual

routine, different decisions may be reached about the acceptability of certain risks. For example, someone may choose to have a brief extramarital sexual relationship while on a business trip because he or she believes that it poses no significant threat or risk to the relationship with the regular partner. Similarly, having to take medication to prevent malaria may be equated with ill health. This belief may conflict with the sense of fun and relaxation normally associated with recreation and being on holiday. This may be further exacerbated by some of the unpleasant effects of taking antimalaria prophylaxis. Some travellers may also argue that, as they did not detect any mosquito bites on their body, they could not have contracted malaria, thereby justifying their decision not to take prophylaxis. There are attendant risks to gambling behaviour of this kind.

3. Prevention of some health problems is often associated with having to give up something enjoyable, exposure to something unpleasant or the inconvenience of having to take measures to prevent exposure to infection. In the case of sexual risk, this may necessitate the use of condoms, while, to prevent malaria, a course of medication may need to be completed for the duration of the period of exposure to infection and for several weeks thereafter. Each of these situations is associated with having to weigh up relative risk and the possibility of the inconvenience of behavioural change.

Health care professionals who work with travellers should inform them of the risks and encourage behavioural change where appropriate. Intentions are a reasonable prediction of behaviour. Young, single men travelling abroad with friends are at greatest risk of health care problems for two reasons. Firstly, they may intend to take sexual and other risks while abroad. Secondly, the group may influence the individual and his intentions (for example, to tan responsibly or to take condoms when planning a night out). Cofactors, such as alcohol use, may further influence risk-taking behaviour. Counselling of travellers should therefore include some discussion about how they intend to manage different risks, using a range of possible scenarios, and rehearsal of possible situations, linking these to both beliefs and actions.

GIVING ADVICE TO THE TRAVELLER

The role of the health care professional is crucial in informing air travellers about the necessary precautions they should take before their flight to manage the stress associated with their journey. The greatest risk to the traveller's health is noncompliance with advice given by the health professional (Noble, 1997). Compliance can be reduced if the advice given to travellers is incomplete or conflicts with information obtained from other sources.

Compliance with advice is reduced when travellers find the information complex or confusing. Eliciting feedback about the traveller's understanding of the information offered therefore provides an opportunity to clarify and elaborate on advice. The delivery of advice given by health care professionals can improve compliance if a number of rules are followed (Noble, 1997):

- Avoid using jargon.
- Ensure that both you and the traveller agree on what advice is required and which aspects are most important.
- Ensure any written information you give is understandable.
- Emphasise the relevance of the advice but be aware that the traveller's anxiety levels may interfere with the ability to retain information (Noble, 1997).
- Complex information should be made simple and concrete and possibly be introduced over a number of consultations.
- Discuss the risks of noncompliance with the traveller.
- After the trip, try to obtain information about the nature and extent of compliance with health advice.

Taking the opportunity to discuss information before the trip and compliance after the trip allows the health professional to assess the degree to which the individual's personal, family or cultural beliefs are compatible with the advice given. This permits the health professional to tailor future travel advice by framing information differently or by using motivational interviewing techniques, such as cost–reward assessments, to improve the travellers compliance with health advice.

CONCLUSION

Modern air travel is both complex and stressful and places considerable psychological demands on passengers and crew. Psychologists have played a significant role in improving safety in the airline industry, in training flight crew in teamwork and in understanding passenger behaviour. Safe and efficient air travel is a team effort and requires close cooperation between crew, ground staff, operators and passengers. Aviation psychology has contributed an understanding to what happens to individuals, teams and large groups when confronted with the unique and specific demands of air travel. The increase in stress associated with modern air travel means that this understanding will be in greater demand in the foreseeable future.

REFERENCES

Bandura A (1977) Self-efficacy: toward a unifying theory of behaviour change. *Psychological Review*, **84**, 191–215.

Bor R (1999) Unruly passenger behaviour and in-flight violence: a psychological perspective. *Travel Medicine International*, **17**, 5–10.

Bor R, Parker J and Papadopoulos L (2001a) Brief, solution-focused initial treatment sessions for clients with a fear of flying. *British Travel Health Association Journal* (in press).

Bor R, Russell M, Parker J *et al.* (2001b) Survey of the world's airlines about managing disruptive passengers. *International Civil Aviation Organisation Journal*, **56**, 21–30.

Borrill J and Foreman E (1996) Understanding cognitive change: a qualitative study of cognitive-behavioural therapy on fear of flying. *Clinical Psychology and Psychotherapy*, **3**, 62–75.

Cautela J and Upper D (1977) Behavioral analysis, assessment and diagnosis. In *Perspectives in Behavior Therapy* (ed. D. Upper), pp 3–27. Behaviordelia, Kalamazoo MI.

Dean R and Whitaker K (1980) Fear of flying: impact on US air travel industry. *Journal of Travel Research*, **21**, 7–17.

Denison D, Ledwith F and Poulton E (1966) Complex reaction times at simulated cabin altitudes of 5000 feet and 8000 feet. *Aerospace Medicine*, **37**, 1010–1013.

Doctor R, McVarish C and Boone R (1990) Long-term behavioral treatment effects for the fear of flying. *Phobia Practice and Research Journal*, **3**, 33–42.

Edwards M and Edwards E (1990) *The Aircraft Cabin: Managing the Human Factors*. Gower Technical, Brookfield VT.

Festinger L (1957) *Theory of Cognitive Dissonance*. Stanford University Press, Stanford CA.

Foushee H and Manos K (1981) Information transfer within the cockpit: problems in intracockpit communications. In *Information Transfer Problems in the Aviation System* (eds CE Billings and ES Cheaney), NASA Report No. TP-1875, NTIS No. N81-31162. NASA-Ames Research Center, Moffett Field CA.

Foreman EI and Borrill J (1994) The freedom to fly: a long-term follow-up of three cases of fear of flying. *Journal of Travel Medicine*, **1** 30–35.

Fraley R and Shaver P (1998) Airport Separations: a naturalistic study of adult attachment dynamics in separating couples. *Journal of Personality and Social Psychology*, **75**, 1198–1121.

Lazarus R and Folkman S (1984) The concept of coping. In *Stress and Coping* (eds. A Monat and R. Lazarus), 3rd edn, pp 189–206. Columbia University Press, New York.

McIntosh I (1989) Flying phobias. *Travel Medicine International*, 112–115.

Muir H and Marrison C (1989) Human factors in cabin safety. *Aerospace*, **April**, 18–22.

Noble L (1997) Communicating risks to the traveller. *Travel Medicine International*, **15**, 111–115.

Persaud R (1999) When will I see you again? *Business Traveller*, **March**, 50–52.

Reason J (1974) *Man in Motion: The Psychology of Travel*. Walker, New York.

Roberts R (1989) Passenger fear of flying: behavioural treatment with extensive *in-vivo* exposure and group support. *Aviation, Space and Environmental Medicine*, **60**, 342–348.

Van Gerwen L, Spinhoven P, Van Dyck R. *et al.* (1999) Construction and psychometric characteristics of two self-report questionnaires for the assessment of fear of flying. *Psychological Assessment*, **11**, 146–158.

Van Tilburg M, Vingerhoets A and van Heck G (1996) Homesickness: a review of the literature. *Psychological Medicine*, **26**, 899–912.

Wolpe J (1958) *Psychotherapy by Reciprocal Inhibition*. Stanford University Press, Stanford CA.

15

Altitude and Expedition Medicine

David R. Murdoch

Canterbury Health Laboratories, Christchurch, New Zealand

Andrew J. Pollard

BC Research Institute for Children's and Women's Health, Vancouver, Canada

J. Simon R. Gibbs

National Heart and Lung Institute at Imperial College School of Science, Technology and Medicine, London, UK

INTRODUCTION

Over the past few decades there has been an increase in the number of travellers visiting high-altitude areas and other remote regions of the world. Increased accessibility, development and promotion of wilderness destinations, and the popularity of adventure tourism, has meant that many people are visiting areas that were previously the domain of mountaineers and others with specialised skills. Some of these visitors also have borderline health. Improved air and ground transportation has resulted in access within hours to days to high-altitude areas that could previously only be reached by a long walk over several weeks. As a consequence many high-altitude travellers have barely enough (or inadequate) time to acclimatise and are at risk of altitude illness. Unfortunately, some die of altitude-related problems.

Health care professionals are often asked about the prevention and treatment of altitude illness, and to advise about whether pre-existing diseases will be adversely affected by high-altitude exposure. It is essential that those who regularly give predeparture advice to travellers are familiar with the major health hazards at high altitude, especially as death can be prevented and morbidity minimised by following some simple recommendations.

THE HIGH-ALTITUDE ENVIRONMENT

Barometric pressure falls with increasing altitude, and is accompanied by a corresponding fall in partial pressure of oxygen (Figure 15.1). Hypoxia is the main cause of high-altitude illness. As examples, the air around Denver (1610 m) has 83%, Mexico City (2350 m) 75%, La Paz, Bolivia (3625 m) 65%, and the summit of Mount Everest (8848 m) 31% of sea-level oxygen. Barometric pressure, and hence partial pressure of oxygen, varies slightly with latitude (higher for a given altitude near the equator than at the poles) and season (higher in summer than winter). In terms of human physiology, the following definitions are commonly used:

- *Intermediate altitude (1500–2500 m).* Exercise performance is decreased, ventilation is increased, but arterial oxygen saturation remains above 90%. Altitude illness is possible, but uncommon.
- *High altitude (2500–3500 m).* Altitude illness becomes common following rapid ascent to over 2500 m.
- *Very high altitude (3500–5800 m).* Arterial oxygen saturation falls below 90%, and extreme hypoxaemia can occur during exercise and sleep.
- *Extreme altitude (>5800 m).* Progressive physiological deterioration occurs because successful acclimatisation cannot be achieved. Permanent human habitation is impossible.

Approximately one-half of the world's countries have at least one point higher than 2500 m. The main high-altitude destinations for travellers are the Rocky Mountains, the Himalaya, Tibetan Plateau, the Andes, European Alps, and the mountains of East Africa. In addition, there are many high-altitude travel destinations elsewhere, the elevation of which may not be widely appreciated. Such areas include parts of Hawaii, the Canary Islands, Indonesia, Papua New Guinea, Japan, New Zealand, and Antarctica.

Principles and Practice of Travel Medicine. Edited by Jane N. Zuckerman.
© 2001 John Wiley & Sons Ltd.

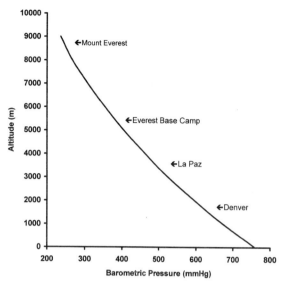

Figure 15.1 Change in barometric pressure with increasing altitude

ACCLIMATISATION

Acclimatisation is the process by which individuals adjust to the hypoxia of high altitude. The physiological changes that comprise the acclimatisation process serve to maintain intracellular oxygen tension in the face of a decrease in inspired oxygen tension. An increase in ventilation is probably the most important component of this process.

The hypoxic ventilatory response (HVR) is a carotid body reflex that responds rapidly to changes in arterial oxygenation. HVR may be genetically determined, and this may at least partially explain individual variation in rates of acclimatisation. Respiratory alkalosis initially limits increased ventilation, but this is eventually compensated by renal excretion of bicarbonate. Erythropoietin secretion is increased within hours of ascent to high altitude, resulting in an increase in red cell mass over the ensuing days to weeks. Although this may permit optimal oxygen transport to tissues, it contributes little to initial acclimatisation. Central blood volume also increases with ascent due to peripheral venous constriction, and, through antidiuretic hormone (ADH) suppression, induces a diuresis. Haemoconcentration and diuresis are healthy responses to altitude exposure; fluid retention and antidiuresis are associated with altitude illness. Heart rate increases on ascent to high altitude and, as the limit of acclimatisation is approached at extreme altitude, resting and maximum heart rates converge.

The absence of altitude illness and improved sleep signal successful acclimatisation. Although there is considerable interpersonal variation in the ability to acclimatise, very few people cannot acclimatise given sufficient time. Acclimatisation is maintained for a relatively short period of time following descent to low altitude. For reascent to the same altitude, it probably lasts at least 1 week.

ALTITUDE ILLNESS

Altitude illness is a collective term that encompasses the major conditions caused directly by hypobaric hypoxia. These conditions are classified as acute mountain sickness (AMS), high-altitude cerebral oedema (HACE), and high-altitude pulmonary oedema (HAPE). As discussed below, AMS and HACE probably represent different ends of a severity spectrum, and share a common pathophysiology. Another condition, chronic mountain sickness, affects only certain permanent high-altitude residents, and will not be discussed here.

ACUTE MOUNTAIN SICKNESS

AMS is the most common type of altitude illness. While it is a relatively benign illness, it can cause major disruptions to travel plans. More importantly, the presence of AMS indicates that acclimatisation is incomplete and that the traveller is at risk of developing life-threatening altitude illness (HACE or HAPE) should they continue to ascend with symptoms.

Rate of ascent and height attained are two of the most important risk factors for AMS. Approximately 25% of visitors who ascend rapidly to altitudes between 2000 and 3000 m in Colorado experience AMS (Honigman et al., 1993). On the major trekking routes in Nepal, about 50% of people who hike to altitudes above 4000 m over 5 or more days develop AMS (Hackett et al., 1976; Murdoch, 1995a). Rapid transit by motorised transport to altitudes above 3500 m is a particular risk. A survey of 116 tourists who flew directly to a hotel at an elevation of 3860 m in Nepal revealed that 84% developed AMS (Murdoch, 1995b). Tourists flying to high-altitude cities such as Lhasa (3658 m), Leh (3514 m), La Paz (3625 m), and Cuzco (3415 m) are likely to have a similar high incidence of AMS.

Individual susceptibility is another risk factor for AMS. Some people readily develop AMS on ascent to high altitude, while others are able to ascend rapidly without difficulty. This pattern tends to be repeated with further journeys to high altitude. Several techniques have been used to predict who is likely to develop AMS, but their clinical usefulness needs to be evaluated further. Measurement of cardiac and respiratory responses to hypoxia in a physiology laboratory may have some predictive value but are impractical in clinical practice.

It is generally thought that both sexes are equally susceptible to AMS, although several studies have shown that women have a higher incidence compared with men. There does not appear to be any relationship with age, and children are probably no more susceptible than

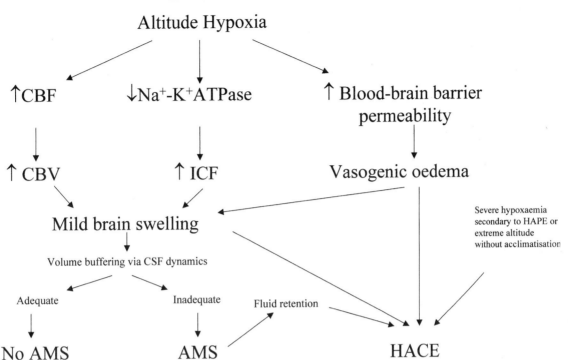

Figure 15.2 A schema of the pathophysiology of AMS and HACE. The primary mechanism of AMS/HACE is vasogenic oedema, but increased blood volume and intracellular fluid volume will contribute to the altered brain compliance and increase in intracranial pressure as illness progresses. Mild oedema remains asymptomatic if CSF volumetric buffering is successful. Once AMS develops, fluid retention aggravates oedema formation. CBF = cerebral blood flow; CBV = cerebral blood volume; ICF = intracellular fluid. (Adapted from Hackett, 1999, by permission of the Wilderness Medical Society)

adults (Yaron *et al.*, 1998). Exertion may be a risk factor for AMS, but lack of physical fitness is not. Whether dehydration increases the risk of AMS is unclear.

Clinical Features

The diagnosis of AMS relies on a recent ascent to high altitude, and the presence of characteristic symptoms. A typical scenario is the development of headache following rapid ascent to a new altitude, accompanied by some or all of nausea, vomiting, anorexia, lassitude, and dizziness. Symptoms of AMS typically start a few hours (often 1–6 h) after arrival, but are frequently first noticed the next morning. Headache is the cardinal symptom, but lacks specific features. It can be bifrontal, or occipital, is often made worse by bending and the Valsalva manoeuvre, and may be severe. Although most AMS case definitions require the presence of headache, a minority of people with AMS describe an unusual feeling or tightness in the head rather than true pain. People with AMS are frequently irritable and uninterested in ongoing activities. Although often accompanied by tiredness, many people complain of difficulty sleeping, which may be at least partly due to the headache.

The most common physical finding in AMS is a rather apathetic, uninterested facial expression. Other signs are generally lacking. Localised crackles may be heard in the lung fields and fluid accumulation may be evident as peripheral and periorbital oedema. The latter is more common in women and may occur at high altitude in the absence of AMS. Blood pressure and heart rate are usually within normal limits. Body temperature may be elevated, especially with more severe AMS.

The nonspecific nature of symptoms and paucity of physical findings may make it difficult to differentiate AMS from other conditions such as migraine, alcoholic hangover, and some acute viral infections. If symptoms accompany a recent gain in altitude it is usually safer to assume the person has AMS, as the consequences of misdiagnosing this condition are serious.

Pathophysiology

The aetiology of AMS is incompletely understood. The most likely hypothesis is that AMS is due to mild cerebral oedema, and that AMS and HACE share a common pathophysiology, each representing a different end of a spectrum of severity (Figure 15.2). Support for this theory comes from several quarters. Symptoms of AMS are consistent with a pathological process involving the central nervous system, namely headache, dizziness, gastrointestinal upset (nausea, vomiting, and anorexia), and sleep disturbance. AMS/HACE-like syndromes in a sheep model are associated with brain swelling and raised intracranial pressure. Neuroimaging studies in humans have also demonstrated brain swelling in AMS, although this also occurs on ascent to high altitude in the absence of AMS. An interesting hypothesis is that susceptibility to AMS may relate to the 'tightness' of the brain within the cranial vault (Hackett, 1999). Variations in cranial anatomy may make some people less able to accommodate brain swelling through cerebrospinal fluid (CSF) dynamics, and thus more susceptible to AMS.

Prevention

Graded Ascent

The best way to avoid AMS is to ascend slowly to allow sufficient time for acclimatisation to occur. Unfortunately, no single ascent schedule is suitable for all people and settings. One recommendation that has been used along the major trekking routes in Nepal advises that, when above 3000 m, each night should be spent on average no higher than 300 m above the previous, and compulsory rest days should be incorporated every 1000 m or every 2–3 days. Several comments need to be made about this recommendation. First, a reduction in the incidence of AMS and death rate among trekkers was observed in the Mount Everest region following introduction of this recommendation. Second, even among those who follow this recommendation, approximately 50% still develop AMS. Comparable figures for HACE and HAPE are lacking, and it is possible that the impact of this guideline is greater for these serious conditions. A moderate risk of AMS may be tolerated if the incidence of HACE and HAPE (and death) is low. Third, this formula emphasises sleeping altitudes. Hypoxic stress is greatest during the night because of lower ventilation during sleep, which may be made worse by periodic breathing which is common above 2500 m. Finally, this schedule works well in Nepal where satisfying itineraries can be built around it. In many other areas of the world a daily ascent rate of 300 m is painfully slow, such that few people would adhere to it.

For most people a daily average ascent rate of 400 m is likely to be sufficient to allow acclimatisation, while minimising the risk of HACE and HAPE, and some people will be able to safely ascend at a rate of 600 m day^{-1}.

The following should serve as a guideline for advising travellers about ascent rates at high altitude:

1. Abrupt ascent to sleeping elevations > 3000 m should be avoided, if possible.
2. At least one night spent at an intermediate elevation (1500–2500 m) will aid acclimatisation.
3. If rapid ascent to > 3000 m is unavoidable (e.g. flying to La Paz or Lhasa), travellers should allow sufficient time for acclimatisation after arrival by avoiding exertion and ascending no higher for several days. Drug prophylaxis may also be appropriate in this situation (see below).
4. If there is an established safe ascent itinerary recommended for a given destination, this should be followed. Ideally, there should be sufficient time in the itinerary to permit an ascent rate of 300–400 m day^{-1} above 3000 m.
5. Travellers who know from previous experience that they are susceptible to AMS may need to ascend at a rate slower than that recommended.
6. Spare days should always be built into the itinerary so that unplanned rest days can be taken as needed.
7. Travellers should be familiar with the symptoms of AMS, and should observe closely for the development of AMS in themselves and their companions. Ascent to a higher sleeping altitude should not occur while experiencing symptoms of AMS.

Drug Prophylaxis

Individuals who are susceptible to AMS or who are to undertake a large rapid ascent may benefit from drug prophylaxis. Outside this setting, the use of drugs is discretionary and controversial.

Acetazolamide is the drug of choice for the prevention of AMS. The drug inhibits the enzyme carbonic anhydrase, reducing renal reabsorption of bicarbonate. This causes a bicarbonate diuresis and metabolic acidosis, thereby stimulating ventilation and mimicking the process of ventilatory acclimatisation. In addition, the drug's diuretic action counteracts the fluid retention of AMS. Several placebo-controlled trials have demonstrated the effectiveness of acetazolamide for the prevention of AMS (Reid et al., 1994). As acetazolamide genuinely aids acclimatisation, concerns about masking serious illness are unwarranted. The standard dosage recommendation is 250 mg twice daily, although many anecdotal reports suggest that 125 mg twice daily is also effective. Alternatively, a single daily dose of the 500 mg slow-release formulation can be used. For prophylaxis, acetazolamide should be started at least 1 day before ascent, and continued until about 2 days after maximum ascent is reached.

Anyone prescribed acetazolamide should be warned about potential side-effects, which are common, but generally mild in nature. Mild diuresis and paraesthesiae tend to diminish with continued use, and carbonated beverages may taste flat. Other side-effects include nausea, drowsiness and headache. Most of these side-effects result from the uptake of the drug in the central nervous system (CNS); related drugs with little CNS penetration, such as benzolamide, prevent AMS and have fewer side-effects, but are not generally available. Acetazolamide is a sulfa drug and carries the usual precautions about hypersensitivity.

Dexamethasone is an alternative to acetazolamide for AMS chemoprophylaxis, but is less effective (Reid et al.,

1994), and is generally reserved for situations when acetazolamide is contraindicated. The mechanism of action is unknown but, unlike acetazolamide, dexamethasone does not aid acclimatisation. Doses of 4 mg every 8–12 h are usually recommended, starting the day prior to ascent. Aspirin has also been used prophylactically to prevent high-altitude headache.

Treatment

The presence of AMS symptoms indicate that additional time is required for acclimatisation. They also serve as a warning that more serious, potentially life-threatening, complications may occur if ascent continues before adequate acclimatisation has been achieved.

The principles of treatment of AMS are as follows:

1. Stop further ascent.
2. Descend if there is no improvement or if symptoms worsen.
3. Descend immediately if any signs or symptoms of cerebral or pulmonary oedema develop.

For mild AMS, rest at the same altitude may be all that is required to ameliorate symptoms. Symptomatic treatment with analgesics (paracetamol, aspirin, or other non-steroidal anti-inflammatory agents) and antiemetics may be beneficial. Preliminary evidence suggests that sumatriptan may relieve high-altitude headache, but this needs to be studied further. Acetazolamide (250 mg every 8–12 h) relieves symptoms and improves arterial oxygenation in established AMS (Grissom et al., 1992). Dexamethasone (4 mg every 6 h) relieves symptoms of AMS effectively, but symptoms can recur with abrupt discontinuation of the drug (Ferrazzini et al., 1987; Hackett et al., 1988). It is usually reserved for the treatment of moderate to severe AMS.

Descent is the only definitive treatment for all forms of altitude illness. If symptoms of AMS persist or worsen, or if there is any doubt, descent is indicated. Descent should be immediate if there is any suggestion of cerebral or pulmonary oedema, as deterioration can occur rapidly. Descent of 500–1000 m can be very effective at ameliorating symptoms. Oxygen relieves effectively symptoms of AMS, but is rarely available in the field. The combination of descent and oxygen is the optimal therapy.

Portable hyperbaric chambers are fabric bags that can be pressurised using a hand or foot pump to simulate descent. When available, these devices may be used to facilitate descent or for treatment when descent is impossible. In controlled studies, portable hyperbaric chambers relieve symptoms of AMS and improve arterial oxygenation, but the beneficial effects usually disappear within 12 h (Bärtsch et al., 1993).

HIGH-ALTITUDE CEREBRAL OEDEMA

HACE is a rare, life-threatening form of altitude illness. It probably shares the same underlying pathophysiology with AMS, and most people with HACE have had preceding symptoms of AMS. HACE occurs at altitudes above 2500 m, but is much more common above 4000 m. The incidence of HACE is difficult to estimate amongst high-altitude travellers because the number of exposed individuals is ill defined. An epidemiological study among the Indian military found that as many as 1–2% of those ascending to an altitude of 4500 m developed HACE (Singh et al., 1969) and a study of trekkers in Nepal found an incidence of 1.8% (Hackett et al., 1976).

Risk factors for HACE are probably the same as for AMS. Some individuals may be susceptible to HACE and will develop recurrent symptoms on reascent to altitude; however, previous episodes of HACE do not necessarily imply that a further episode will develop on reascent.

Pathophysiology

The precise mechanism of HACE remains unknown. However, increased cerebral blood flow and capillary leakage of fluid occur, resulting in an increase in cerebral blood volume and parenchymal volume (interstitial oedema), respectively (Hackett, 1999; Hackett et al., 1998) (Figure 15.2). Neural cell swelling may also occur. The swelling and subsequent compression within the cranial vault result in the clinical features of HACE. The development and severity of HACE probably relates to individual factors such as the relative tightness of the brain in the vault, pressure buffering capacity of the CSF spaces and cerebral vascular responses to hypoxia. Cerebral oedema is likely to be initially vasogenic (leakage of fluid and protein from capillaries across the blood–brain barrier) in origin as it affects primarily white matter and rapidly resolves following treatment of early HACE (Hackett et al., 1998). The mechanism of this capillary leakiness remains unknown but may be linked to high capillary pressures causing vessel wall stress, or various substances, released in response to hypoxia, that are active on the endothelium, including histamine, arachidonic acid, bradykinin, nitric oxide and vascular endothelial growth factor (VEGF) (Severinghaus, 1995). Neural cell swelling probably also occurs either as a primary phenomenon or secondary to vasogenic oedema.

Clinical and Pathological Features

HACE is usually, but not always, preceded by AMS and is frequently associated with signs of HAPE. Unsteadiness of gait and altered mental status are clear warning signs. Ataxia is often the first sign to appear and can be tested for by asking the person to walk heel-to-toe in a straight line. Unless there is a good alternative explanation, anyone who performs poorly in this test at high altitude should be regarded as having HACE. Mental status changes can be subtle at first, with altered behaviour and/or confusion, but will progress to loss of consciousness and coma. Other signs that may be present include nuchal rigidity, extensor plantar responses, cranial nerve palsies, hemiparesis, hyperreflexia and clonus. Retinal haemorrhages are apparent on fundoscopy in many patients, but this may also be a 'normal' finding in up to one-third of individuals at 5000 m. Papilloedema is common.

If lumbar puncture can be performed, it will typically demonstrate raised CSF pressure and normal biochemical and cellular findings. Cerebral oedema may be demonstrated on both computed tomography and magnetic resonance imaging (Hackett *et al.*, 1998). In the latter, white matter oedema particularly affecting the corpus callosum has been noted. Postmortem examination of the brain reveals cerebral oedema, thromboses in the cerebral venous sinuses, subarachnoid haemorrhage and parenchymal petechial haemorrhages (Dickinson *et al.*, 1983). Spongiosis is prominent in the white matter.

Progression to coma and death occurs over a few hours but may take as long as several days in untreated cases. After descent, symptoms often resolve rapidly, but may persist for days or weeks. Ataxia persists longer than other symptoms of HACE and may still be evident months after apparent recovery. Neurological sequelae are rare in survivors, but may occur particularly after prolonged coma or delayed treatment.

Prevention

As HACE and AMS probably share a common pathophysiology, the previous discussion about AMS prevention applies to HACE as well. In individuals with recurrent HACE, reascent to the altitude where illness occurred should only be undertaken with extreme caution, if at all.

Treatment

Descent should always begin as soon as HACE is recognised. The immediate practical difficulty in a remote mountain area is how to evacuate physically the individual with HACE. The use of adjunctive measures described below may improve the clinical condition of the patient so that they can walk and facilitate descent. When possible an individual should be carried by his companions, porters, animals or preferably by motorised transport. In most remote areas, motorised land or air transport are not immediately available, but descent should not be delayed while awaiting a vehicle. Evacuation should continue to as low an altitude as is possible and symptoms have resolved. Individuals with severe HACE should ideally be evacuated to hospital at low altitude.

Dexamethasone and oxygen (if available) should be used to treat HACE as an adjunct to descent. Dexamethasone (8 mg followed by 4 mg 6-hourly) probably improves HACE. Treatment in a portable hyperbaric chamber may bring a temporary improvement in clinical status by improving oxygenation and facilitate descent. Some have also recommended the use of acetazolamide as a treatment for HACE but there are no data on its effectiveness. Others have advocated the use of frusemide, but concerns over excessive diuresis and plasma volume contraction have limited its use.

HIGH-ALTITUDE PULMONARY OEDEMA

HAPE is a potentially life-threatening form of noncardiogenic pulmonary oedema which occurs at altitudes above 2500 m. It is uncommon compared to AMS. The prevalence depends mainly on individual susceptibility and on the rate of ascent. HAPE-prone individuals fall into five groups:

1. *Susceptible individuals* who are apparently healthy and who have a past history of one or more episodes of HAPE. Episodes are precipitated by rapid ascent, strenuous exercise and cold. In these subjects, episodes tend to recur at about the same altitude. The rate of recurrence for each individual is about 60–70%. The severity of recurrent attacks is unpredictable.
2. Idiosyncratically in those with a *recent inflammatory illness* such as a viral infection. This occurs especially in children during and following upper respiratory tract infections.
3. *Anybody who ascends rapidly and high enough* is prone. For example, unacclimatised individuals who use air transportation to reach very high altitude and immediately start a rapid ascent without hope of acclimatisation may achieve this. Vigorous young men are at most risk possibly because they climb fastest.
4. Individuals with *obstruction, congenital hypoplasia or absence of a pulmonary artery*. They are very likely to develop HAPE.
5. *High-altitude residents* are not immune. They may develop 're-entry' HAPE on return to high altitude after a sojourn of 3 or more days at low altitude. They are not considered further here.

Pathophysiology

The mechanism of HAPE is uncertain. It is clear that pulmonary hypertension precedes the formation of pulmonary oedema (Bärtsch *et al.*, 1991) and appears to be crucial for its pathogenesis. Compared with control subjects at sea level, HAPE-susceptible subjects have a higher pulmonary artery pressure (although still within normal limits) due to increased pulmonary vascular resistance and a marked pulmonary hypertensive response to exercise. At altitude the pulmonary hypertension is caused by a brisk hypoxic pulmonary vasoconstrictor response in HAPE-susceptible subjects. Vasodilators which lower pulmonary artery pressure have been shown to prevent (Bärtsch *et al.*, 1991) and attenuate the formation of oedema (Oelz *et al.*, 1989), with associated improvement in symptoms and gas exchange.

Since vasoconstriction of the pulmonary circulation ought to reduce capillary pressure and prevent pulmonary oedema, Hultgren (1978) proposed that pulmonary vasoconstriction might be uneven throughout the vascular bed. Evidence for this came from animal studies and the chest radiographic appearance of patchy nonuniform oedema at high altitude. In humans there is wide variation in the amount of pulmonary vasoconstriction and this may be determined by the amount of muscle in the distal arteries. Hultgren (1978) described this as the concept of overperfusion: the patchy vasoconstriction of the small pulmonary arteries causes underperfusion of some areas of the lungs and overperfusion of others. Pulmonary oedema develops in the overperfused areas as a result of high pulmonary capillary pressure, which may result in fluid and red cells leaking between capillary endothelial cells into the alveolar space (stress capillary failure) (West and Mathieu-Costello, 1995) or through cells via transcellular channels.

This mechanism of hydrostatic pulmonary oedema is corroborated by the predisposition of patients with congenital anomalies of the pulmonary arteries and those with acquired obstruction of the pulmonary circulation to HAPE. These patients share a markedly reduced capacity of their pulmonary circulation which may cause capillary overperfusion more readily.

Studies of subjects suffering from pulmonary oedema have also suggested a further mechanism. Bronchoalveolar lavage fluid taken during HAPE has shown evidence of an inflammatory response (Schoene et al., 1986), although these data cannot determine whether this is cause or effect. Studies of children with HAPE in the Rockies have also shown evidence for intercurrent respiratory tract infections, and animal studies have demonstrated that respiratory syncytial virus infection leads to pulmonary oedema in hypoxia. Thus inflammation in the presence of hypoxia may be the cause of pulmonary capillary leak in some cases.

One further factor in the pathogenesis of HAPE may be a failure of fluid clearance from the alveoli. Hypoxia inhibits transepithelial salt and water reabsorption in vitro but its clinical significance is yet to be established.

Clinical Features

The onset of HAPE is usually after one or two nights at a new altitude on ascent, but can very occasionally occur within a few hours of arrival. HAPE rarely occurs after 5 days at the same altitude.

HAPE is frequently preceded by symptoms of AMS (see above). The main symptoms of HAPE are breathlessness and cough. Breathlessness first becomes noticeable on exercise and progresses to orthopnoea and breathlessness at rest. Cough is initially dry and may progress to the production of white then pink frothy sputum associated with gurgling in the chest. Subjects may also describe chest tightness or pain.

Physical signs include sinus tachycardia, pyrexia (not usually exceeding 38.5 °C), tachypnoea, central cyanosis, and inspiratory crackles in the chest that may be highly localised despite the widespread oedema. In severe cases the patient may develop concomitant cerebral oedema with signs as described above.

Where medical facilities are available, a chest radiograph should be performed to confirm the diagnosis. This may show patchy pulmonary oedema, although as the disease progresses this becomes confluent. Arterial blood gases reveal pronounced hypoxia with little abnormality of the P_{CO_2}.

Differential Diagnosis

In its early stage HAPE may be mistaken for AMS. As symptoms develop, chest infection is a common misdiagnosis. In addition the differential diagnosis includes high-altitude cough (a benign but irritating dry cough), pulmonary embolism or infarction, acute myocardial infarction and heart failure.

Prognosis and Mortality

Following recovery clinical sequelae are rare. Untreated the mortality is up to 50%, although this can be considerably reduced by recognition of the illness early in its course and provision of prompt treatment.

Prevention

Individuals susceptible to HAPE cannot be reliably identified prospectively at sea level, either clinically or by routine clinical investigations. Exposure to high altitude simulated in a barochamber or hypoxia chamber for several days is limited to research laboratories. Nevertheless, HAPE is preventable. Subjects with known susceptibility to HAPE should understand that high-altitude ascent may expose them to a life-threatening situation.

Avoidance of a hasty ascent and gaining altitude slowly are the cornerstone of prevention. This may even be effective in subjects known to be susceptible. Above 2500 m subjects may ascend up to 350 m per day in sleeping altitude provided they have no symptoms of AMS. Subjects must be advised never ascend to a higher sleeping altitude with symptoms. If symptoms of AMS persist for more than a day they should descend. During acclimatisation vigorous exercise should be avoided.

Nifedipine MR 20 mg orally t.d.s. is effective when the rate of ascent must be faster than is desirable in subjects known to be susceptible (Bärtsch et al., 1991). Side-effects are not normally a significant problem at this dose. Nifedipine should be continued until the subject descends to an altitude to which they are well acclimatised or below 3000 m. Nifedipine will not prevent symptoms of AMS. The role of acetazolamide in preventing HAPE is unclear at present. Subjects should also be advised to avoid alcohol and sleeping tablets, which may potentially worsen hypoxia and exacerbate dehydration.

The risk of an individual developing HAPE associated with an inflammatory illness is unknown. At the very least attention should be paid to the recommended rate of ascent. Patients known to have congenital absence or hypoplasia of a pulmonary artery, or acquired obstruction of a pulmonary artery, are at high risk of developing HAPE, sometimes at relatively low altitude. It is not clear whether any of the preventive measures described above will be effective and these patients should be advised not to go to high altitude.

Where doubt exists about the management of HAPE-susceptible individuals an opinion should be sought from a physician experienced in high-altitude medicine.

Treatment

The treatment of HAPE is urgent as delay may result in further deterioration. The aim of treatment is to improve oxygenation and hence reduce pulmonary artery pressure. Exactly how this achieved depends on the local facilities.

The sick patient should be sat up, kept warm and given oxygen. In remote places the patient should descend at least 1000 m in altitude immediately. In severe cases evacuation by air to low altitude should be undertaken if possible but the logistics of organising evacuation should not result in a delay in descent. Where the patient cannot descend or is significantly unwell they should be given nifedipine MR 20 mg orally q.d.s. in an attempt to relieve symptoms and facilitate urgent descent. Sublingual nifedipine 5–10 mg may be administered where a rapid effect is needed or the patient is vomiting, but is prone to cause hypotension. If nifedipine is not available then a portable hyperbaric bag may be used to improve oxygenation temporarily and facilitate descent. The patient should not be placed supine in the portable hyperbaric bag as this may compromise oxygenation further.

Where proper medical facilities are available, oxygen should be administered to maintain arterial oxygen saturation > 90% and the patient encouraged to rest. They should be reviewed regularly but may require several days treatment. If an oxygen saturation > 90% can be achieved with no more than 4 litres oxygen per minute then descent may be avoided and no further treatment may be required.

Expiratory positive airway pressure achieved using a special mask is theoretically useful but the increased work of breathing and the difficulty of using the device do not recommend it as effective therapy.

Unlike cardiogenic pulmonary oedema, HAPE is associated with relative intravascular volume depletion, and diuretics, nitrates, opiates and alcohol should be avoided.

OTHER ALTITUDE-RELATED CONDITIONS

Peripheral Oedema

Swelling of the extremities and face is common at high altitude, and is more common in females than males. Although the presence of peripheral oedema should raise suspicion of altitude illness, it does occur in the absence of AMS. Treatment is usually unnecessary.

Sleep Disturbance

Sleep disturbance is very common at high altitude. There is a decrease in both deep and rapid eye movement (REM) sleep, with frequent arousals. Some of these arousals are due to periodic breathing (Cheyne–Stokes respirations), which is surprisingly common at high altitude, and does not appear to be related to AMS. Some people are unaware that they have periodic breathing, while others wake in a panicked state following an apnoeic episode, thinking that they are being suffocated. A low dose of acetazolamide (125–250 mg) taken before bedtime is effective in relieving periodic breathing and maintaining arterial oxygen saturation during sleep. The use of benzodiazepines to facilitate sleep at high altitude has been generally discouraged because of the theoretical risks of respiratory depression. However, recent preliminary data suggest that short-acting benzodiazepines are actually associated with improved nocturnal oxygen saturation, although this needs to be confirmed.

Retinopathy

High-altitude retinopathy (HAR) is characterised by disc hyperaemia, tortuosity and dilatation of retinal veins, and retinal hemorrhages. These changes are seen in about 30–50% of people at 5000 m, and are even more common at higher elevations. Retinal haemorrhages are usually asymptomatic, unless involving the macula, and resolve spontaneously in 10–14 days. Whether the presence of HAR is a warning sign for altitude illness is unclear.

Other Neurological Disorders

In addition to AMS, HACE, and high-altitude retinopathy, several other syndromes have been described at high altitude in the absence of concomitant altitude illness. The sudden appearance of focal neurological deficits in previously healthy high-altitude travellers has been described on many occasions. The aetiology in most cases remains obscure. Cerebral thromboembolism has been clearly documented in a few cases, and others appear migrainous in origin. Regardless of aetiology, immediate descent, administration of oxygen and dexamethasone (if available), and evacuation to a hospital are indicated. A thorough neurological examination should also be performed before further ascent to high altitude.

Thrombosis

Cerebral and peripheral venous thrombosis and pulmonary embolism have been reported in high-altitude travellers, but usually after exposure to extreme altitudes (> 5500 m). Polycythaemia, increased blood viscosity, dehydration, cold, and inactivity (e.g. tent-bound in bad weather) are thought to be risk factors.

Cough and Infections

A dry, hacking cough and sore throat are common occurrences at high altitude. Among trekkers to Mount Everest base camp, 42% developed cough (half of these producing sputum) and 39% had sore throat (Murdoch, 1995a). Most cases probably do not have an infectious aetiology, but are the result of increased ventilation, breathing cold dry air, and increased cough receptor sensitivity. The cough may be severe enough to cause rib fractures. Sucking hard candies, breathing steam, and placing a silk balaclava or similar material across the nose and mouth may relieve symptoms.

Many travellers have noted that infections are common at high altitude and are slow to resolve. The presence of a respiratory infection may increase the risk for altitude illness. This association appears to be true for viral respiratory tract infections and the development of HAPE in children (Durmowicz et al., 1997).

SPECIAL CONSIDERATIONS FOR ALTITUDE TRAVEL

Children

Children are probably no more susceptible to high-altitude illnesses than individuals of other ages. However, altitude illness may be difficult to identify because young children do not report the very subjective symptoms of these syndromes, resulting in the possibility of a delay in recognition and treatment. An international consensus statement concerning ascent to high altitude with children has considered this issue in detail (Pollard et al., 2001).

There is some suggestion that there may be an increased risk of sudden infant death syndrome (SIDS) in communities living at altitude. Furthermore, more prolonged exposure to high altitude (> 1 month) in infancy risks the development of subacute infantile mountain sickness (SIMS). SIMS is right heart failure secondary to pulmonary hypertension (caused by hypoxia) and occurs in up to 1% of infants residing over 3000 m for more than 1 month (Sui et al., 1988).

Heart Disease

Ascent to high altitude is associated with activation of the sympathetic nervous system and an increase in heart rate, cardiac output and blood pressure, which return to sea-level values by 3 months. In addition, hypoxic pulmonary vasoconstriction results in pulmonary hypertension. The physiological stress of hypoxia and cold has important implications for patients with coronary artery disease, who may experience new or worse angina, hypertension which may be harder to control, and heart failure and pulmonary vascular disease which may deteriorate. Risks can be minimised with appropriate medical advice.

Hypertension

Uncontrolled hypertension is a contraindication to ascent to high altitude as it will be exacerbated by hypoxia. Hypertension must be controlled prior to travel, the ideal level being below 140/85.

Coronary Artery Disease

In myocardial ischaemia the balance between myocardial oxygen supply and demand is disturbed. Hypoxaemia in the presence of coronary stenoses would be expected to reduce oxygen supply to the myocardium and worsen ischaemia. Sympathetic activation also worsens myocardial ischaemia as a consequence of increased cardiac work and coronary vasoconstriction in regions of abnormal endothelial vasomotor control (Hultgren, 1997; Levine et al., 1997). The increased work of breathing probably has a minor effect but respiratory alkalosis produced by hyperventilation may also cause coronary vasoconstriction.

Patients with coronary artery disease may experience an increase in symptoms. Nevertheless, neither acute ECG changes of myocardial ischaemia at rest (Yaron et al., 1995; Levine et al., 1997) nor symptomatic deterioration (Yaron et al., 1995) have been reported in patients aged over 65 years with coronary artery disease who visited 2500 m for 5 days.

Exercise studies in patients with coronary artery disease have shown decreased exercise tolerance and earlier appearance of angina and ST segment changes on the ECG. Acute exposure to 2500 m is associated with a small but significant reduction in the work required to provoke myocardial ischaemia (Levine et al., 1997). This is induced at a lower level of myocardial oxygen demand than at sea level. These studies suggest that the acute effects of hypoxia are due mainly to increased cardiac work and do not appear to be directly related to myocardial hypoxia

Patients with uncomplicated chronic stable angina in Canadian Cardiovascular Society (CCS) classes I and II are at low risk. Patients with more severe, but stable, angina (CCS III and IV) require review by their physician and, if they ascend to altitude, may require an increase in medications to control symptoms. Unstable angina and recent myocardial infarction are contraindications to ascent. Old myocardial infarction is only a problem when there is significant angina, left ventricular dysfunction or arrhythmias. These patients should undergo medical examination prior to travel.

Patients ascending above 2500 m should be warned to expect an increase in their anginal symptoms and to minimise exercise during the first 4 days on arrival at high altitude. They should plan for a slower rate of ascent than normal. They should take a fresh supply of glyceryl trinitrate with them. It has been suggested that if a patient can reach stage 3 of the Bruce treadmill protocol (> 6 min) without discomfort, that patient will be able to tolerate an altitude of 4270 m without discomfort (Hultgren, 1997). The predictive value of pretravel exercise testing in acute hypoxia is not established.

Heart Failure

Normal myocardial performance is not affected by altitudes up to the summit of Mount Everest. Patients with coronary artery disease with mild to moderately impaired left ventricular function without residual ischaemia have good tolerance to exposure to an altitude of 2500 m (Erdmann et al., 1998). Acute or decompensated heart failure is a contraindication to ascent. Patients in New York Heart Association (NYHA) class I and II may travel provided they are medically stable and their baseline Pao_2 is > 70 mm Hg. Patients in NYHA class III or IV must be medically stable and should be discouraged from ascent above 2500 m.

Arrhythmias

Arrhythmias may be precipitated by sympathetic activation, and respiratory alkalosis which may reduce serum potassium. No change has been detected in arrhythmic substrate in hypoxia as detected by signal averaged ECGs (Levine et al., 1997). Single premature ventricular complexes during exercise do increase modestly with acute exposure to 2500 m without an increase in repetitive forms and it is unlikely that moderate altitude exposure substantially alters the risk of life-threatening arrhythmias in patients with coronary disease.

Patients with uncontrolled ventricular or supraventricular arrhythmias should not ascend to high altitude. Frequent or high-grade ventricular ectopy is also a contraindication to ascent above 2500 m.

Congenital Heart Disease

Congenital heart disease encompasses a wide range of conditions whose natural history and response to hypoxia may be altered by surgery. In general, conditions associated with cyanosis and/or pulmonary vascular disease may deteriorate significantly above 2500 m. Some patients with right ventricular disease are intolerant of the extra load placed on the ventricle by the pulmonary hypertensive response to hypoxia. Anomalies of the pulmonary circulation may precipitate HAPE (see above, High-altitude Pulmonary Oedema). Coarctation of the aorta may cause cerebral hypertension and precipitate HACE. Patients with coarctation of the aorta should not ascend to altitude unless their coarctation has been repaired and shown to be relieved, and hypertension is well controlled below 140/85. Particular care should be taken to avoid dehydration in cyanosed patients because of the risk of thrombosis. Many patients with congenital heart disease will require a specialist opinion prior to ascent.

Respiratory Disease

Asthma

Although theoretically the cold, dry, hypoxic mountain environment should worsen bronchoconstriction, there is little evidence of deterioration in practice. Asthmatics often find that they have less trouble at high altitude and this is likely to be related to the absence of allergens in the air and the reduced air density. They may also be helped by the increased sympathetic drive and production of corticosteroids at altitude.

Patients should not ascend to altitude unless their asthma is stable. Travellers to remote places should take an emergency supply of steroids with them in case of deterioration.

Chronic Obstructive Pulmonary Disease

A small fall in Pao_2 results in a large fall in arterial oxygen saturation in these patients because their Pao_2 falls on the steep slope of the oxygen dissociation curve. These patients will notice significant deterioration in their breathlessness on ascent to altitude. AMS prophylaxis with acetazolamide may worsen breathlessness by increasing ventilation.

Lung function should be optimised and stable prior to ascent to altitude. Administration of gas mixtures containing oxygen levels the patient will encounter in the field may be used to assess gas exchange and risk in the lung function laboratory. A chest infection is more serious at high altitude than at sea level and patients should carry an emergency supply of steroids and antibiotics.

Ventilatory Failure

Patients with sleep apnoea, kyphoscoliosis and disorders of the chest wall including the respiratory muscles may be unable to increase ventilation in response to hypoxia.

This problem will worsen ventilatory failure particularly at night. A specialist opinion may be required.

Sickle Cell Disease

People with sickle cell disease or sickle thalassaemia are at risk for sickle crises at altitudes over 2000 m and, consequently, should avoid ascent to high altitude. The risk for those with sickle cell trait is less, although splenic infarction has been reported in this group while exercising at altitude.

Diabetes Mellitus

The major challenges to diabetic control at high altitude are the increased energy expenditure compared with sea-level activity, and the risk of intercurrent illnesses. Close attention to glucose level is essential, although this may be complicated by inaccurate and inconsistent performance of some blood glucose meters above 2000 m.

Pregnancy

Few data exist on the risks to pregnant women and their fetuses from brief visits to high altitude. Intrauterine growth retardation, pregnancy-induced hypertension, and neonatal hyperbilirubinaemia are complications associated with permanent high-altitude residents. Until further data are available, it is prudent to advise pregnant women to avoid prolonged exposures to altitudes over 3000 m.

Radial Keratotomy

Exposure of the cornea to hypoxia causes swelling and changes in corneal topography. For persons who have had radial keratotomy, the swelling of the hypoxic cornea is not uniform, and this results in significant visual changes. In contrast, significant refractive changes are not noted in people who have had LASIK surgery (laser-assisted in situ keratomileusis) following corneal hypoxia.

Contraception

There has been concern about the risk of thrombosis while taking the oral contraceptive pill at high altitude, especially given the presence of other prothrombotic factors at altitude, such as polycythaemia and dehydration. There is currently no evidence to support an increased risk.

EXPEDITION MEDICINE

Commercial expeditions provide travellers with ready access to all types of adventure. Expedition travel may involve transport by varying means to remote areas, and usually exposure to environmental extremes such as high altitude, heat or cold. Most expeditions will have an experienced group leader, and many will have an expedition physician.

Pre-expedition Planning

A key component of expedition planning is to ensure that potential medical problems during the expedition are anticipated. The expedition doctor or medical advisor can achieve this aim through helping travellers make a rational decision about whether to participate in the expedition, ensuring that general health recommendations (e.g. immunisations) are followed, educating travellers about potential health hazards that may be encountered, and emergency management planning *before* the expedition.

Immunisations and the Health Check

Specific medical advice for the travel destination should be sought and immunisations and antimalarial prophylaxis recommended as appropriate. Pre-existing medical problems are best discussed confidentially prior to the expedition, by such means as of a health questionnaire. Specific health advice about medical problems may need to be given, depending on the type of expedition to be undertaken. Occasionally, the physician may need to recommend that the traveller should not participate in the expedition for medical reasons. Information about existing medical problems will be important in planning the medical kit. Dental problems frequently surface during remote expeditions and dental health should be checked prior to travel.

Education

On expeditions to remote areas, the most common medical problems encountered will be minor injuries and intercurrent illnesses, including travellers' diarrhoea. Education about basic hygiene and safe preparation of food and water will contribute to the health of the expedition and may prevent some episodes of gastroenteritis. Expedition members should be encouraged to attend a basic first-aid course that will empower the team to manage most minor injuries effectively and reduce the workload of the expedition doctor.

Specific education about health problems may be required for particular expeditions. For example, high-altitude expeditions will benefit from pre-expedition discussion of altitude-related illness, frostbite, hypothermia, snowblindness and traumatic injuries. It is also essential to emphasise from the outset that medical problems that develop during the course of the expedition should be

Table 15.1   An example of an expedition medical kit

Indication	Uses and comments	Examples or class of drug
Allergy	Asthma, hayfever and anaphylaxis	Adrenaline (epinephrine)
		Oral antihistamines
		Inhaled and injectable steroids
		Inhaled Beta-2 agonist
Altitude illness	AMS, HAPE, HACE (see details in text)	Acetazolamide
		Dexamethasone
		Nifedipine
		Oxygen
		Portable hyperbaric chamber
Anaesthesia	Nerve blocks, local and general anaesthesia (avoid general anaesthesia at altitude where possible)	Local anaesthetic
		Ketamine
Analgesia	Minor and major pain: altitude headache, trauma, etc.	Paracetamol
		Diclofenac
		Codeine phosphate
		Opiate
		Naloxone
Cardiac conditions	Angina, myocardial infarction and heart failure	Aspirin
		Loop diuretic
		Sublingual nitrate
Dermatological conditions	Burns, sunburn, pruritus, eczema	Sunblock cream
		Silver sulfadiazine cream
		Oral antihistamine
		Topical steroids
		Moisturising cream
		Anusol
Diabetes mellitus	Hyper- and hypoglycaemia	Insulin and glucagon
Ear and Nose and throat	Nasal congestion, sinusitis and allergy; sore throat	Nasal decongestant
		Oral antihistamine
		Steroid nasal spray
		Anti-inflammatory mouth gel
		Throat lozenges
Gastointestinal problems	Gastroenteritis, gastritis, peptic ulcer	Antimotility agent
		Antacid
		Oral rehydration powder
		Antiemetic
Infections	Travellers' diarrhoea and persistent infectious diarrhoea, pneumonia, otitis, urinary tract infections, skin infections, severe infections, scabies, superficial fungal infections	A variety of oral and parenteral antibiotics
		Topical antifungals
Malaria	If travelling to or through a malarious area	Antimalarials for prophylaxis and treatment
Ophthalmic problems	Ophthalmic infections, snowblindness and eye examination	Topical anaesthetic agent
		Chloramphenicol eye drops
		1% cyclopentolate
		Fluorescein
Psychiatric and sleep disturbance	Anxiety, psychosis and insomnia	Antipsychotic agent
		Benzodiazepine (anxiolytic and hypnotic)
Diagnostic Equipment		Stethoscope, sphygmomanometer, pulse oximeter, otoscope, ophthalmoscope, BM stix, thermometer, spirometer
Dressings		A variety of dressings and bandages, eye pads, gloves, tape
Intravenous equipment	For use in remote areas or where the sterility of local equipment cannot be quaranteed	A variety of needles, syringes, i.v. cannulas, and consider fluids
Surgical equipment	Minor and major trauma, pneumothorax, bladder drainage, nasogastric fluids. Depends on the expertise of the expedition members	Chest drain, Heimlich valve, scalpel blade, suture material, needle holders, surgical needles, Foley catheter, nasogastric tube

immediately brought to the attention of the expedition leader. Many expedition participants will keep their symptoms to themselves for fear that their ill health may jeopardise the itinerary for other participants. This has been a problem with trekking groups at high altitude, when group members keep ascending with symptoms of AMS, often with disastrous consequences. This may be the reason for the increased risk of dying from altitude illness among members of organised expeditions than individual trekkers in Nepal (Shlim and Gallie, 1992). Practical education about mountain safety, survival techniques, and avalanche rescue from a qualified mountain guide may facilitate rescue of a casualty on a mountain expedition.

Managing Illness or Injury on the Expedition

Any medical or surgical emergency or traumatic injury can occur on an expedition and initial management should follow basic first-aid principles. The ability of the team or the expedition doctor to manage specific conditions effectively thereafter often has more to do with the geographic situation than with specific training or availability of medical equipment. The key to managing unanticipated illness or injuries is improvisation. Pre-expedition planning of how an emergency should be handled organisationally can greatly relieve the stress of the situation in the field.

Evacuation

Occasionally an expedition will have to deal with serious illness, injury or death. In a remote setting, emergency management is usually little more than first aid, and the doctor's primary role may be the organisation of a rapid evacuation to safety. Careful evacuation planning requires consideration of the local geography and communications to arrange evacuation. The method of evacuation must be considered in advance and usually involves more than one mode of transport. Air evacuation is expensive and adequate insurance should be arranged in advance to cover helicopter evacuation (if available) and repatriation expenses.

Medical Kits

The size and contents of the expedition medical kit are determined by the size and duration of the expedition, the remoteness of the destination, the medical knowledge of the team, the pre-existing medical conditions of the team members, the cost of the kit and the mode of transport. The expedition team should be encouraged to provide their own individual basic first-aid kits for management of minor injuries (cuts, abrasions and blisters), and to carry insect repellent, sunblock cream and simple analgesics. Each individual should also have a method of

water purification (such as iodine) and antimalarials if required.

On many small expeditions little more than a personal medical kit is required. On larger expeditions a central base camp medical kit and other smaller group kits may be required in different locations so that basic equipment and drugs are easily accessible. All medical kits should include clear instructions for use of each drug.

For high-altitude expeditions dexamethasone and nifedipine should be easily available for treatment of HACE and HAPE, respectively, and it may be appropriate for these to be carried by each individual to facilitate descent in an emergency. A portable hyperbaric chamber is useful to facilitate descent of a member of a trekking group who becomes unwell and should be available as part of the base camp medical kit, but it is not practical to carry a pressure bag high on the mountain. Oxygen is a useful item of medical equipment for initial treatment of altitude illness at base camp and to facilitate descent by relieving symptoms. Oxygen is not usually carried high on the mountain because of weight considerations, unless the climb involves extreme altitude and supplementary oxygen is to be used for climbing.

Medical kits will necessarily have to be tailored to suit individual expeditions but some suggestions for an expedition medical kit are outlined in Table 15.1.

REFERENCES

Bärtsch P, Maggiorini M, Ritter M et al. (1991) Prevention of high-altitude pulmonary edema by nifedipine. New England Journal of Medicine, **325**, 1284–1289.

Bärtsch P, Merki B, Hofstetter D et al. (1993) Treatment of acute mountain sickness by simulated descent: a randomised controlled trial. British Medical Journal, **306**, 1098–1101.

Dickinson J, Heath D, Gosney J et al. (1983) Altitude-related deaths in seven trekkers in the Himalayas. Thorax, **38**, 646–656.

Durmowicz AG, Noordeweir E, Nicholas R et al. (1997) Inflammatory processes may predispose children to high altitude pulmonary edema. Journal of Pediatrics, **130**, 838–840.

Erdmann J, Sun KT, Masar P et al. (1998) Effects of exposure to altitude on men with coronary artery disease and impaired left ventricular function. American Journal of Cardiology, **81**, 266–270.

Ferrazzini G, Maggiorini M, Kriemler S et al. (1987) Successful treatment of acute mountain sickness with dexamethasone. British Medical Journal, **294**, 1380–1382.

Grissom CK, Roach RC, Sarnquist FH et al. (1992) Acetazolamide in the treatment of acute mountain sickness: efficacy and effect on gas exchange. Annals of Internal Medicine, **116**, 461–465.

Hackett PH (1999) The cerebral etiology of high-altitude cerebral edema and acute mountain sickness. Wilderness and Environmental Medicine, **10**, 97–109.

Hackett PH, Rennie D and Levine HD (1976) The incidence, importance, and prophylaxis of acute mountain sickness. Lancet, **ii**, 1149–1154.

Hackett PH, Roach RC, Wood RA et al. (1988) Dexamethasone for prevention and treatment of acute mountain sickness. Aviation, Space and Environmental Medicine, **59**, 950–954.

Hackett PH, Yarnell PR, Hill R *et al.* (1998) High altitude cerebral edema evaluated with magnetic resonance imaging: clinical correlation and pathophysiology. *Journal of the American Medical Association*, **280**, 1920–1925.

Honingman B, Theis MK, Koziol-McLain J *et al.* (1993) Acute mountain sickness in a general tourist population at moderate altitudes. *Annals of Internal Medicine*, **118**, 587–592.

Hultgren HN (1978) High altitude pulmonary edema. In *Lung Water and Solute Exchange* (ed. NC Staub), pp 437–469. Dekker, New York.

Hultgren HN (1997) High altitude pulmonary edema: hemodynamic aspects. *International Journal of Sports Medicine*, **18**, 20–25.

Levine BD, Zuckerman JH and de Filippi CR (1997) Effect of high-altitude exposure in the elderly: the Tenth Mountain Division study. *Circulation*, **96**, 1224–1232.

Murdoch DR (1995a) Symptoms of infection and altitude illness among hikers in the Mount Everest region of Nepal. *Aviation, Space and Environmental Medicine*, **66**, 148–151.

Murdoch DR (1995b) Altitude illness among tourists flying to 3740 m elevation in the Nepal Himalayas. *Journal of Travel Medicine*, **2**, 255–256.

Oelz O, Maggiorini M, Ritter M *et al.* (1989) Nifedipine for high altitude pulmonary oedema. *Lancet*, **ii**, 1241–1244.

Pollard AJ, Niermeyer S, Barry P *et al.* (2001) Children at high altitude: an international consensus statement by an ad hoc committee of the International Society for Mountain Medicine, March 12th 2001. *High Altitude Medicine and Biology* (in press).

Reid LD, Carter KA and Ellsworth A (1994) Acetazolamide or dexamethasone for prevention of acute mountain sickness: a meta-analysis. *Journal of Wilderness Medicine*, **5**, 34–48.

Schoene RB, Hackett PH, Henderson WR *et al.* (1986) High altitude pulmonary edema. Characteristics of lung lavage fluid. *Journal of the American Medical Association*, **256**, 63–69.

Severinghaus JW (1995) Hypothetical roles of angiogenesis, osmotic swelling and ischemia in high altitude cerebral edema. *Journal of Applied Physiology*, **79**, 375–379.

Shlim DR and Gallie J. (1992) The causes of death among trekkers in Nepal. *International Journal of Sports Medicine*, **13** (suppl.), S74–76.

Singh I, Khanna PK, Srivastava MC *et al.* (1969) Acute mountain sickness. *New England Journal of Medicine*, **280**, 175–184.

Sui GJ, Liu YH, Cheng XS *et al.* (1988) Subacute infantile mountain sickness. *Journal of Pathology*, **155**, 161–170.

West JB and Mathieu-Costello O (1995) Vulnerability of pulmonary capillaries in heart disease. *Circulation*, **92**, 622–631.

Yaron M, Hultgren HN and Alexander JK (1995) Low risk of myocardial ischemia in the elderly visiting moderate altitude. *Wilderness and Environmental Medicine*, **6**, 20–28.

Yaron M, Waldman N, Niermeyer S *et al.* (1998) The diagnosis of acute mountain sickness in preverbal children. *Archives of Pediatric and Adolescent Medicine*, **152**, 683–687.

16

Diving Medicine

Peter J. Benton

Institute of Naval Medicine, Gosport, UK

INTRODUCTION

Recreational diving is becoming an increasingly common sporting activity, with some 80 000 qualified recreational divers in the UK alone. It is estimated that each diver averages approximately 25 dives per year, giving a figure of some 2 million recreational dives completed per annum. With the increase in travel to more distant resorts, often resorts where a combination of clear warm water and colourful marine life make entry into the subaquatic world enticing, many of these qualified divers travel abroad to dive. As well as qualified divers, an increasing number of individuals travel abroad with the specific aim of learning to dive or are attracted by dive shops and schools who visit resort hotels offering dive training. Each year some 20–25 of these divers return to the UK with residual symptoms of diving-related incidents that require recompression therapy. These divers constitute approximately 10% of the 150–200 divers who are treated for decompression illness in the UK each year.

PHYSICAL ASPECTS OF THE UNDERWATER ENVIRONMENT

The human animal, unlike marine mammals such as the whale, has evolved to live and work on land and as such is poorly adapted to life in water. Water and air are very different media. Water, a fluid, is dense ($1000 \, \text{kg m}^{-3}$) whereas air, a gas, has a density of only $1.29 \, \text{kg m}^{-3}$. This vast difference in densities affects the performance of the human diver in many ways.

Vision

The human eye is designed to operate with a low-density medium, air, in contact with the cornea. If this is replaced by water then refraction of light at the water–cornea boundary occurs, with resultant distortion. Use of a diver's facemask, by placing a pocket of air in front of the eye, avoids this problem; however, refraction will still occur at the interface between the water and the glass faceplate. This results in images appearing closer to the diver and enlarged by approximately 30%. The diving mask also restricts the diver's field of view.

Water absorbs light and even in the clearest water only about 20% of the light at the surface penetrates to a depth of 10 m. At a depth of 85 m this is reduced to approximately 1%. The absorption of light is not equally distributed across the visible spectrum (red and orange light are absorbed most readily), with the result that colours are distorted at depth. Even at shallow depths true colours will only be seen if artificial light sources are provided. The figures quoted are all based on the assumption that the water is clear and the water surface is flat. Even small waves will result in light being reflected from the surface and hence less light penetrating to depth. Often, especially following storms, large quantities of silt will be suspended in the water, which will further absorb light and may restrict the diver's vision to a few inches/centimetres or less.

Hearing

In common with the eye, the human ear is designed to operate in air. The middle ear is designed to compensate for the impedance mismatch that exists between the low-density, low-impedance medium that usually surrounds the head, air, and the head itself, which is a high-density, high-impedance medium. The diver, by flooding the outer ear, effectively cuts out the middle ear, with hearing in water being primarily by bone conduction. The middle ear not only operates as an impedance matching device but also as an amplifier, the result being that by bypassing this amplifier hearing acuity in water is reduced by between 20 and 30 dB. Even if the outer ear is kept dry, as the diver descends the pressure and hence the density of the breathing gas increases. The function of the middle ear is affected by this increase in gas density, which acts as a damper to the middle-ear amplifier, the result being that

Principles and Practice of Travel Medicine. Edited by Jane N. Zuckerman.
© 2001 John Wiley & Sons Ltd.

with increased depth there is a proportional increase in loss of hearing acuity of up to 30 dB.

Distortion of speech also occurs as the density of breathing gas alters with depth; with helium–oxygen mixtures this distortion can be so great as to make speech indecipherable. In recreational diving this is rarely a problem, as not only are helium–oxygen mixtures only used by a small number of 'technical' divers but also recreational divers rarely use in-water communication devices.

Thermal

Water is an excellent conductor of heat, with the result that a diver immersed in water will lose or gain heat far more rapidly than the diver would in air of the same temperature. To counter this heat loss it is necessary for the diver to wear special clothing, usually a wet or dry suit. Such diving suits are bulky, and in the case of wet suits, need to be tight fitting in order to reduce to a minimum the amount of water that can enter. The diver's mobility, both on land and in the water, can be severely restricted by such a suit. Another problem is that the wearing of a suit with such excellent insulative properties prior to the dive may, in a warm environment, lead to heat stress.

The gas the diver breathes will also result in heat loss. This is because the inspired gas is usually relatively cold, both because the supply cylinder is immersed in water and also because of the cooling associated with the expansion of gas that takes place within the diver's breathing apparatus. This cool air gains heat from the diver, and on exhalation heat is lost. With increased depth the density, and hence mass, of exhaled gas increases, which in turn leads to increased heat loss. The excess heat lost in this way when breathing air is of little significance. However, when oxyhelium mixtures are breathed, because helium has a thermal conductivity six times that of nitrogen, the heat loss can become highly significant. For this reason, in the commercial sector, when oxyhelium is used for deep dives (below 150 m) the inspired gas has to be prewarmed.

PRESSURE EFFECTS

Because the density of water is so much greater than that of air, the diver only has to descend a small distance to encounter a significant increase in pressure. Whereas it is necessary to ascend 5486 m to reduce ambient pressure to 0.5 atmospheres (50.7 kPa), the diver has only to descend 5 m to increase pressure from 1 atmosphere (101.3 kPa) to 1.5 atmospheres (152 kPa). Unlike air, which is compressible, water as a liquid is incompressible and so the increase in pressure with increasing depth is proportional. For each and every 10 m a diver descends, the pressure exerted on the diver's body increases by 1 atmosphere (101.3 kPa). This increase in pressure results in the vol-

ume of gas in the body's air spaces (lungs, sinus cavities, middle ear, bowel, caried teeth) to decrease in accordance with Boyle's law, which states:

If the temperature remains constant, the volume of a fixed mass of gas is inversely proportional to the absolute pressure.

The effect of this change in volume of a fixed mass of gas with increasing depth within the lung is illustrated in Figure 16.1. As can be seen, although the breath-hold diver starts with lungs inflated to total lung capacity (TLC), with increasing depth the volume of gas within the lungs decreases as the ambient pressure increases. If the dive is to sufficient depth, 30–40 m, to compress the air in the diver's lungs to a volume less than the residual volume, then in theory damage should occur to the lungs: compression barotrauma. In practice during such dives up to a litre of blood is pooled within the lung vasculature and great veins of the thorax. When combined with the remaining volume of air within the lungs this permits breath-hold dives far below the theoretical maximum. The current world record for a breath-hold dive is 160 m, set in 2000 by Pipin Ferraras.

Pulmonary Barotrauma

The diver who uses breathing apparatus is supplied with gas at the same pressure as the surroundings. If the diver should ascend too rapidly, or breath hold during the ascent, this gas will expand, resulting in pulmonary overinflation and hence lung rupture. The lungs are fragile and require an over pressure of only 10–13 kPa to rupture (Malhotra and Wright, 1961). In water, that equates to less than 1 metre and so lung rupture can occur while using diving breathing apparatus in the shallow end of a swimming pool (Benton et al., 1996). If lung rupture should occur during diving, the extra-alveolar gas will be at the same pressure as the water surrounding the diver. During ascent the ambient pressure will decrease and the extra-alveolar gas will expand in volume. Following lung rupture air may pass to one, or all, of three areas:

1. *The pleural space*. Extra-alveolar air entering the pleural space will result in the formation of a pneumothorax. The air within such a pneumothorax will be at ambient pressure and, in accordance with Boyle's law, will expand during ascent. Thus, a pneumothorax in which one lung has collapsed by 50% will, if it occurs at a depth of 30 m, expand in volume fourfold during the diver's ascent to the surface. Such a fourfold increase will result in the collapse of both lungs and severe cardiac embarrassment.

2. *The interstitial tissues*. Extra-alveolar air entering the interstitial tissues will pass to the mediastinum and usually track upwards into the neck. Interstitial emphysema may be completely asymptomatic, only being detected by chest X-ray or palpation. Mediastinal emphysema may produce retrosternal pain, often worse on inspiration, while on occasions the diver may become aware of a

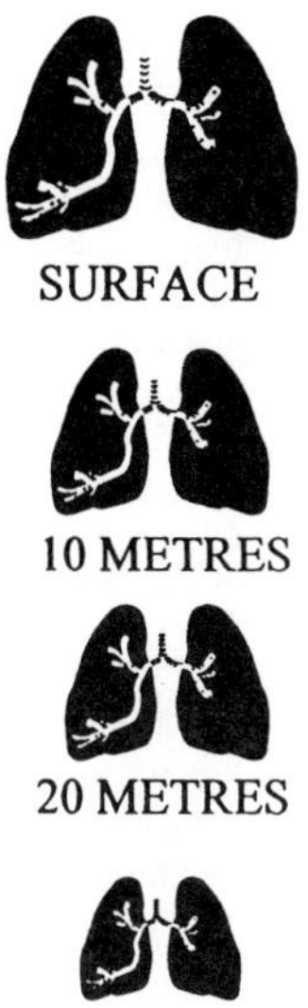

	Lung Volume	Pressure (atmospheres)	pO_2	pN_2
SURFACE	100%	1 (101kPa)	0.21 (21.2kPa)	0.79 (79.8 kPa)
10 METRES	50%	2 (202 kPa)	0.42 (42.4kPa)	1.58 (159.6 kPa)
20 METRES	33%	3 (303 kPa)	0.63 (63.6kPa)	2.37 (239.4 kPa)
30 METRES	25%	4 (404 kPa)	0.84 (84.8kPa)	3.16 (319.2 kPa)

Figure 16.1   Change in lung volume of breath-hold diver, Po_2 and PN_2 with increasing depth

change in tone of voice or a tight feeling in the neck. Specific treatment is rarely required, although administration of oxygen will speed the resorption of the gas. Rarely precordial gas may be palpable, which may be associated with crepitus synchronous with the pulse, the Hamman sign.

3. *Pulmonary vasculature.* Extra-alveolar gas entering the pulmonary vasculature will result in arterial gas emboli. Not only may such arterial gas emboli obstruct blood vessels but also the very presence of these bubbles in contact with the vessel walls may damage the delicate endothelial lining, with subsequent leakage of fluid into the surrounding tissues. Symptoms following such an insult range from minor neurological changes to rapid loss of consciousness and death.

Inert Gas Absorption

The concentration of the inert gas nitrogen in arterial blood is approximately the same as the concentration of nitrogen in the air we breathe. At sea level, where the partial pressure of the nitrogen (PiN_2) in the air we breathe is 79 kPa, the PN_2 in arterial blood will also be approximately 79 kPa. During a dive, the ambient pressure surrounding the diver increases, and so too will the partial pressures of the component gases of the gas breathed by the diver (Figure 16.1). If the diver is breathing air, then as the PiN_2 of the air breathed increases so will the alveolar PN_2 and hence pulmonary capillary PN_2. This nitrogen-loaded blood will travel throughout the body and the nitrogen will pass down the concentration gradient from the arterial blood to the surrounding tissues. In time the PN_2 of the tissues will equilibrate with

that of the arterial blood, and hence air breathed, and so the tissues become saturated with nitrogen. Tissues with a good blood supply, such as the brain and spinal cord, will rapidly become saturated with nitrogen, while tissues with a relatively poor blood supply (cartilage and bone) may take 24 h or more to become fully saturated with nitrogen. If the diver breaths a helium–oxygen mixture, the same principles apply with the inert gas, in this case helium, equilibrating with the body tissues. The dynamics of tissue gas exchange are highly complex and beyond the scope of this text. Further details of this complicated, and as yet not fully understood process, can be found in the specialist texts listed under Further Reading.

As the diver ascends, the inert gas absorbed during the dive will move in the opposite direction, from the tissues into the blood, where it is carried to the lungs and exhaled. If the ascent, and hence decompression, is in accordance with recognised diving tables this process of 'off-gassing' will occur in a controlled manner, and the inert tension gas within the tissues will not reach a sufficient level of supersaturation for bubbles to form. However, if the rate of decompression is such that supersaturation does occur, then bubbles will form within both blood and body tissues. Even when such bubbles form, the human body is capable of tolerating a certain bubble load. Bubbles in venous blood, for example, are efficiently removed from the circulation by the lungs, with numerous studies demonstrating the presence of such 'venous gas emboli' in asymptomatic divers. Although the lungs are excellent filters of gas bubbles, this capacity is finite and if the bubble burden is such that this is exceeded, bubbles may transit the lungs and enter the arterial circulation, where they form arterial gas emboli.

Patent Foramen Ovale

In approximately 25–30% of the normal adult population this relic of the fetal circulation remains patent and usually results in no ill effects. However, it does offer a possible route for venous gas bubbles to bypass the pulmonary filter and consequently, along with other right-to-left shunts, has the potential to promote the arterialisation of otherwise relatively harmless venous bubbles. Although routine screening of divers for patent foramen ovale is not performed, if an individual should be found to have a patent foramen ovale with significant right-to-left shunting during the normal cardiac cycle, he or she should be advised not to dive.

Decompression Illness

As well as forming in blood, bubbles may form in any tissue within the body. In some tissues (such as adipose tissue) they may form without causing overt disease; however, other tissues, particularly nervous tissue, are much more sensitive and the presence of even a small number of gas bubbles may result in abnormal tissue function. The precise mechanisms by which bubbles provoke tissue dysfunction is not fully understood but possibly include the physical disruption of tissue architecture, interruption of tissue microcirculation and derangement of tissue biochemical activity at the tissue–bubble interface.

One obvious mechanism is that they physically obstruct small blood vessels and thereby cause tissue ischaemia. The behaviour of bubbles in the cerebral circulation has been studied extensively and, although the obstruction of blood vessels occurs as soon as bubbles arrive in the brain, this effect appears to be short-lived. Cerebral blood vessels respond to the presence of bubbles by dilating and thus allowing the bubbles to move on (Francis and Gorman, 1993).

It is now thought that much of the illness that results from bubble embolism of the brain is due to the consequences of traumatic injury to the delicate endothelial lining of cerebral blood vessels, which in places may be stripped away from the vessel wall. This results not only in a breakdown of the blood–brain barrier, and the consequential leaking of potentially harmful blood constituents into the brain, but also, by exposing blood components such as white blood cells and platelets to the damaged blood vessel wall, promotion of a tissue reaction to the injury. Ironically, it is the physical and biochemical consequences of this process that may actually result in a further deterioration of cerebral blood flow and function.

Although it is recognised that tissue bubbles may arise from two fundamentally different processes (pulmonary barotrauma and/or inert gas release), it is often difficult, in individual cases, to be certain of the origins of the disease-provoking gas. Indeed, with respect to some organ systems, such as the ear and lungs, it may occasionally be difficult to distinguish between a bubble-induced condition and the results of barotrauma.

Table 16.1 Effects of nitrogen narcosis with depth when breathing air

Depth (m)	Symptoms
30–60	Light headedness, euphoria, loss of fine discrimination
60–90	Poor judgement and reasoning, slowed reflexes, peripheral paraesthesiae, overconfidence
90–120	Progressive depression of the sensoria, hallucinations, amnesia
>120	Loss of consciousness

Consequently, it is now recognised that, for practical purposes, the distinction between the conditions that used to be known as decompression sickness and arterial gas embolism was artificial. As a result, the term decompression illness, which encompasses both mechanisms, is being increasingly used.

GAS TOXICITY

With increased depth, and hence ambient pressure, the partial pressures of the component gases breathed by the diver increase. This section will discuss briefly the problems associated with exposure to nitrogen, oxygen, carbon dioxide and helium at increased partial pressures.

Nitrogen Narcosis

Nitrogen, when breathed at raised partial pressure, has an anaesthetic effect and produces narcosis. The symptoms and signs of nitrogen narcosis are similar to those of drunkenness, except that there is no 'hangover'. With increased narcosis comes a demonstrable decrease in diver performance and hence ability to respond to any emergency situation. On ascent and reduction in P_{N_2} the effects rapidly wear off, the danger of nitrogen narcosis being not from the narcotic effect itself but that the narcosed diver may act inappropriately and hence sustain an injury or drown while so impaired. Although there is variation in individual susceptibility to nitrogen narcosis and some degree of habituation to the effects of narcosis from frequent exposure, all divers will be impaired to some degree. Some drugs, particularly alcohol and sedatives, may have an effect additive to the narcosis and should not be taken prior to diving. The degree of impairment with increasing depth is illustrated in Table 16.1.

Because of the effects of nitrogen narcosis, professional divers in the UK are limited to a maximum depth of 50 m breathing air. Most recreational dive organisations recommend a similar, or shallower, depth limit. Other gases also have a narcotic effect, the narcotic potency being proportional to their lipid solubility. Of the gases which are used in diving, the order of potency is: nitrogen > hydrogen > helium.

Oxygen Toxicity

Although essential for life, oxygen is an extremely reactive element that is controlled within well-defined limits in the body. Exposure to raised partial pressures of oxygen will result in toxicity, the type and severity of which will be determined by both duration of exposure and partial pressure. For divers, the two most important toxic effects of oxygen are its effects on the lungs and on the central nervous system (CNS).

• *CNS oxygen toxicity.* Exposure to a raised partial pressure of oxygen may result in a variety of symptoms, including lip twitching, dizziness, anxiety, nausea, tinnitus, tunnel vision, a choking sensation, difficulty breathing, tremor and convulsion. There is no fixed oxygen exposure at which CNS oxygen toxicity becomes apparent, with susceptibility varying both between individuals and within the same person from day to day. However, CNS oxygen toxicity is uncommon if the $P_{i}o_2$ of the breathing gas is kept below 140 kPa. This equates to the $P_{i}o_2$ of air when breathed at 60 m or of 100% oxygen breathed at a depth of 4 m. The danger to the diver who breathes a gas mixture with a high $P_{i}o_2$ is that the first sign of CNS oxygen toxicity may be a convulsion, which, when it occurs underwater, often results in drowning as the diver releases the mouthpiece.

• *Pulmonary oxygen toxicity.* Prolonged exposure to over 50% oxygen at the surface (50 kPa) has long been known to affect adversely pulmonary function. Divers may be exposed to a $P_{i}o_2$ significantly in excess of this and in some individuals the first symptoms of pulmonary oxygen toxicity may develop within 3 h of breathing oxygen at a $P_{i}o_2$ of 200 kPa. Symptoms and signs often start with a tickling sensation in the throat, which is worse on inspiration and which may provoke coughing. After a few hours of continued oxygen exposure, the tickle is gradually replaced by a sensation of substernal burning, and coughing becomes uncontrollable. Shortness of breath eventually prevents even mild exertion. There are often few physical signs associated with pulmonary oxygen toxicity in its early stages; however, progress of the condition can be monitored by measurement of the vital capacity, which decreases with oxygen exposure, a 10% decrease in vital capacity occurring after about 10 h exposure to a $P_{i}o_2$ of 200 kPa.

The pathological changes noted in the human lung exposed to raised partial pressures of oxygen comprise two phases, an early exudative phase followed by a proliferative phase. During the exudative phase there is alveolar oedema, intra-alveolar haemorrhage, fibrinous exudate and generalised congestion of the lung. This phase merges into the proliferative phase, which is characterised by marked thickening of alveolar and interlobular septa, with marked proliferation of fibroblasts, early fibrosis and alveolar cell hyperplasia. Such extreme changes are highly unlikely to occur during conventional diving exposures but may occur during prolonged hyperbaric oxygen therapy. In extreme cases, despite breathing gas with a high partial pressure of oxygen, the patient may become hypoxic as a result of the thickened alveolar walls and reduction in diffusing capacity.

Carbon Dioxide

The compressed air, or other gas, breathed by a diver should contain little if any carbon dioxide. However, due to a combination of increased work of breathing associated with immersion, the 'dead space' of the breathing apparatus and the increased density of the gas, the end-tidal carbon dioxide of a diver breathing air, may exceed 8.5 kPa. Indeed, at depths in excess of 40 m, even with the most efficient breathing apparatus, a diver breathing a dense gas such as air and who is working hard may easily exceed this level. Divers using 'rebreathers' may also encounter a high level of carbon dioxide. These 'rebreathers' utilise a carbon dioxide absorbent, such as sodium or lithium hydroxide, which if exhausted or incorrectly packed will result in the diver being exposed to high levels of carbon dioxide.

Symptoms of hypercapnia include dyspnoea, dizziness, nausea, headache, anxiety, sweating, palpitations, neuromuscular twitching, convulsions and loss of consciousness. When the $P_{i}o_2$ exceeds 50 kPa, which equates to 15 m breathing air, the dyspnoea associated with hypercapnia may not be as severe. If the diver is breathing hard due to heavy exertion, he or she might receive little warning of hypercapnia, become confused and even slightly euphoric, before losing consciousness. Without doubt, some of the fatalities associated with deep air dives in recent years have been due in part to hypercapnia. Symptoms, with the exception of a severe throbbing headache, rapidly resolve once the diver reaches fresh air on the surface.

Helium

Gas mixtures containing helium are used for deep dives (below 50 m) as helium does not have the narcotic effect of nitrogen. For such deep dives the divers use either heliox (a helium–oxygen mixture) or trimix (a helium–nitrogen–oxygen mixture). The precise proportions of gas used will depend upon the depth dived to, and will be chosen to keep the P_{O_2} at maximum depth below 141 kPa, and, in the case of trimix, the P_{N_2} at a level that does not incur an unacceptable level of narcosis.

FITNESS TO DIVE

To enter the underwater environment, which by its nature is hostile to air-breathing humans, it is essential that the diver is both physically and medically fit. Professional divers within the UK are required to undergo regular medical examinations by doctors who have specialist knowledge of diving medicine and physiology. This is not so for many recreational divers who, unless they wish to join the British Sub-Aqua Club, which requires a medical examination, may have to do nothing more than complete a simple medical screening questionnaire. In view of the fact that the underwater environment does not distinguish between those who dive for pleasure and those who dive for employment, it is difficult to justify the total lack of competent medical screening for recreational divers.

Physical fitness is important, especially for the diver who plans to dive in northern European waters where the combination of tidal flow, cold, and the heavy equipment and thermal protection required to survive in such an environment makes such diving physically demanding. In tropical waters, although diving may appear to be less demanding physically, the divers may still be required to exert themselves entering and exiting the water carrying heavy equipment and also if required to rescue another diver.

Medical conditions that often create problems include asthma, chest trauma, diabetes mellitus, head injury, epilepsy, cardiovascular disease and decompression illness. Each of these conditions and their implications with regard to diving will be discussed.

Asthma

Normal lung function is required by all divers, both to enable them to achieve adequate work capacity and to ensure that their lungs can accommodate the pressure and volume changes that occur during diving. Failure to accommodate these changes in pressure and volume can result in lung rupture, which may manifest as interstitial emphysema, pneumothorax or arterial gas embolism. Whereas interstitial emphysema may be no more than uncomfortable, the development of a pneumothorax or arterial gas embolism in a diver can be life threatening. Individuals with asthma are known to be at increased risk of lung rupture (Light, 1994), even under normobaric conditions: 5.4% of a group of 479 children admitted during an asthmatic episode were noted to have pneumomediastinum on chest X-ray (Eggleston et al., 1974).

Asthmatics also frequently have impaired exercise tolerance and it is important to note that many of the factors that are known to precipitate asthma in susceptible individuals are to be found in the underwater environment. The most important factors include breathing cold dry air, extreme exercise, increased inspiratory effort, anxiety and saline inhalation. Although many people perceive diving to involve gently drifting effortlessly in clear blue water, the reality, especially in northern European waters and where commercial or military diving is concerned, is very different. Each year the Duty Diving Medical Officers at the Institute of Naval Medicine receive calls describing 'well-controlled' asthmatics who, when diving in cold water, have become disorientated, anxious, short of breath and finally developed frank bronchospasm at depth, resulting in a rapid panic ascent to the surface. Upon arrival at the surface some of these individuals are unconscious, having suffered lung rupture and arterial

gas embolism. Experience of such situations is the reason why even 'well-controlled' asthmatics are considered unfit to dive, both by the United Kingdom Health and Safety Executive (HSE) and the Royal Navy.

Within the recreational diving community certain dive organisations will permit 'well-controlled' asthmatics to dive, 'well-controlled' being defined as follows:

- Mild symptoms
- Stable with only infrequent and predictable episodes
- No requirement for regular use of bronchodilators
- Normal exercise capacity
- No exercise-induced symptoms
- Inhaled prophylactic steroid or cromoglycate therapy only
- Can tolerate use of breathing apparatus.

However, it must be remembered that lung function can decline slowly over a period of time without the asthmatic being aware of this; in such cases an asthmatic diver may decide, especially when subject to peer pressure, that he or she is fit when in fact that is not the case. In view of this, plus the diver's exposure to provocative factors and the difficulty in ensuring that an individual is 'well controlled' and genuinely asymptomatic at the commencement of a dive, many diving medicine specialists find this a difficult policy to accept (Elliott, 1995).

Chest Trauma

Major chest trauma may result in scarring of the lung parenchyma and/or pleura. In extreme cases the chest wall itself may be so deformed as to prevent normal inspiration and expiration. Less severe trauma may be manifest only as a traumatic pneumothorax that may or may not require formal aspiration or drainage. A history of a pneumothorax, be it spontaneous or traumatic, used to be considered to be an absolute contraindication to diving, the logic being that the lung had, in the case of a spontaneous pneumothorax, demonstrated a 'weakness' and, in the case of a traumatic pneumothorax, been 'weakened' by the injury. The 'weakened' lung being at greater risk of subsequent rupture, the consequences should this occur underwater would be catastrophic, with any pneumothorax occurring at depth rapidly expanding as the diver ascended.

With the development of ever more sophisticated investigative techniques it has, however, become apparent that many individuals who have suffered a pneumothorax, be it spontaneous or traumatic, have no detectable evidence of lung abnormality or function. In the absence of any 'weakness' it would appear that these individuals should be at no more risk of recurrence than a member of the general population. Furthermore, epidemiological studies reveal that the risk of recurrence following a spontaneous pneumothorax, although between 20 and 40% (Light, 1994; Lippert et al., 1991; Voge and Anthracite, 1986) in the first 1–2 years, drops to a rate similar to that of the general population by 4–5 years. In the case of a traumatic pneumothorax, recurrence is extremely uncommon provided that there is no residual pathology. This knowledge has lead to a revision in the advice given to divers who experience pneumothorax. Current advice, which is based upon a study of a group of 257 divers and submariners who have experienced both traumatic and spontaneous pneumothoraces (Denison and Francis, 1999), is that, provided there is no evidence of lung pathology, individuals who have suffered a spontaneous pneumothorax may return to diving after 4 recurrence-free years.

In the case of traumatic pneumothorax the individual may return to diving after 3 months, once again provided that there is no evidence of pathology. To determine whether or not there is any residual pathology all such individuals require full pulmonary function testing, including measurement of maximum inspiratory and expiratory flow–volume loops, absolute lung volumes by whole body plethysmography and transfer factor, as well as high resolution computed tomography (CT) of their lungs. CT subjects the individual to a significant exposure to ionising radiation and should only be contemplated if he or she wishes to return to diving. Ongoing review of the 257 cases who have returned to diving supports the view that the risk of recurrence is extremely low, with only one case suffering a recurrence of lung rupture.

Diabetes Mellitus

Diabetes mellitus is a complex condition that may lead to the development of a wide variety of both acute and chronic complications. Of the acute complications, hypoglycaemia, with the possibility of sudden loss of consciousness underwater, is of greatest concern. Loss of consciousness underwater, from whatever cause, often leads to the death of the unconscious diver and, not infrequently, that of the diver's buddy, who is faced with the difficult task of attempting a rescue. Hypoglycaemia can also lead to the development of an acute confusional state, which has led to diabetic drivers driving the wrong way down motorways and causing serious accidents. Such a confusional state in the diabetic diver could conceivably, especially if accentuated by nitrogen narcosis, result in the diver making decisions that could have fatal consequences to both diver and buddy. Few fatalities involving diabetic divers have been reported, perhaps the most well known example being that of a diver who died only a few feet from safety while exploring the Huautla Cave system, Mexico in 1994. Although this incident occurred during that which many may consider an extreme dive, the diver was vastly experienced and presumably a 'well-controlled' diabetic.

As well as the acute problems facing the diabetic diver, there is also the question of possible diagnostic confusion. Cases are known of diabetic divers being treated for 'diabetic comas', then subsequently being discovered to be suffering from acute neurological decompression illness (DCI). The resultant delay in treatment often results in poor response to recompression therapy. Sensory and motor neuropathies are not uncommon among diabetics and, if not known to the examining doctor, could lead to confusion following a diving incident. Finally, many diabetics have subclinical small vessel disease. This may not only increase the probability of an ischaemic event occurring during in-water exertion, but could also theoretically result in impaired inert gas exchange with a possible altered risk of DCI.

Research is ongoing, especially within the recreational diving organisations, to identify and develop techniques by which diabetic divers can dive 'safely', with certain recreational diving organisations permitting 'well-controlled' diabetics to dive. Techniques include ensuring that diabetic divers start the dive with slightly elevated blood sugar levels and that they carry glucose (contained within a squeezy tube) throughout the dive. This enables divers to correct any hypoglycaemic episode they might notice during the dive, or if they should be called upon to perform any unplanned hard work. Such techniques, although possibly acceptable in the recreational environment where the individual can freely choose whether or not to dive, do not translate well to either the military or commercial environment. Furthermore, these techniques make no allowance for the chronic problems that face the diabetic diver. Diving is a very strenuous task, often performed in cold, demanding conditions, and so even in diabetics who have never experienced symptomatic hypoglycaemia there can be no guarantee that they will not become hypoglycaemic while diving. Current Royal Navy and HSE medical standards prohibit diabetic divers who require medication to control their diabetes, be it insulin or an oral hypoglycaemic, from diving.

Head Injury

Head injuries account for 5% of the referrals to the Undersea Medicine Division at the Institute of Naval Medicine for an opinion regarding fitness to dive. The concerns with head injuries are twofold: first, to ensure that the individual has recovered fully, with normal cognitive function and no residual neurological deficit; and, second, to determine the risk of post-traumatic epilepsy. Epilepsy, whether idiopathic or post-traumatic, is an absolute contraindication to diving as sudden loss of consciousness while diving can have catastrophic effects. Formal assessment of return to normal cognitive function is usually only required following very severe head injuries, in which case formal neuropsychological testing is required. In the majority of cases simple testing of mental function is sufficient, with the primary focus being the assessment of risk of post-traumatic epilepsy.

A head injury is considered to be severe if any of the following are or have been present:

1. Loss of consciousness for more than 30 min
2. Evidence of residual focal neurological sequelae
3. A period of post-traumatic amnesia of more than 1 h

4. Any period of prograde amnesia
5. Depressed skull fracture with or without loss of consciousness.

Some 5% of patients admitted to hospital after a severe head injury have a seizure within the first week, with an additional 5% suffering seizures at a later date. With time, the risk of seizure after a head injury appears to decrease, eventually reaching a level not dissimilar to that of a member of the general population (> 1% per annum) (Marsden, 1988). The Medical Commission on Accident Prevention, in providing advice on return to driving after head injury, permit group II drivers to recommence driving if specialist assessment has determined the risk of post-traumatic epilepsy to have fallen below 2%. For divers, where there is the additional factor of exposure to raised partial pressures of oxygen, which may increase the risk of seizure, return to diving can be considered once the risk of post-traumatic epilepsy has fallen below 1%.

Cardiovascular Disease

Diving is a very strenuous activity and, as such, any cardiovascular disorder that results in impairment of exercise capacity should be considered as a contraindication to diving. This includes ischaemic heart disease, cardiomyopathies and valvular stenosis, all of which may impair exercise tolerance. Conduction disorders such as the Wolff–Parkinson–White syndrome may predispose an individual to dysrrythmias, which may in turn precipitate in-water loss of consciousness, already discussed as an absolute contraindication to diving.

An unusual condition that has been noted among divers is that of immersion pulmonary oedema. The precise mechanism of causation of this condition, in which the diver develops pulmonary oedema while immersed, is unknown, although mild hypertension, cold immersion, exercise, raised Pio_2 and beta blockers have all been suggested as possible provocative agents. Whatever the precise mechanism, once a diver has experienced immersion pulmonary oedema the condition usually recurs on subsequent dives, often with increasing severity. Because of the possible connection with hypertension, it is probably unwise for an individual with hypertension, unless very mild and only requiring diuretics, to dive. The use of beta blockers by divers is certainly to be discouraged.

Decompression Illness

Each year some 200–250 divers are treated for decompression illness in the UK. Of these, 75% make a full recovery following treatment but some 25%, despite treatment, are left with a residual deficit, which may range from a minor area of sensory loss to a full-blown paraplegia. Just as the first question asked by most injured motorcyclists admitted to an orthopaedic ward is 'When can I ride again?', the first question asked by most divers

on leaving the recompression chamber is 'When can I dive again?'. For those divers with major residual problems the appropriate advice is probably never (Elliott, 1990).

The majority of divers who appear to have made a full clinical recovery may, however, return to diving once their body has fully recovered from the insult. The difficulty is that, although the diver may have recovered to the extent that no deficit is detectable on clinical examination, postmortem studies of divers with a history of DCI who died from nondive-related causes (Palmer et al., 1987) have revealed 'silent' central nervous system damage. Neuropsychological screening (Elliott and Moon, 1993) of divers with a history of DCI has also revealed evidence suggestive of abnormal cognitive function in some groups of divers who, on careful clinical examination, appeared to have made a full recovery. In one study (Sutherland et al., 1993), this abnormal function persisted in some divers in excess of 12 months postincident. This evidence suggests it may be wise for all divers who suffer DCI, including those who have made a full clinical recovery, to consider never diving again.

For those who do wish to return to diving and who have made a complete recovery, current recommendations are that a period of at least 4 weeks (DMAC, 1994) should elapse before diving. However, the development of increasingly sophisticated examination techniques, including magnetic resonance imaging, electrophysiological studies, and postmortem studies in the very small number of cases where the diver has died due to a nondive-related course shortly after treatment for DCI, raise the suspicion that subtle changes are present in the central nervous systems of divers who appear to have fully recovered. This knowledge has led to some hyperbaric medicine centres advising individuals not to dive for at least 2–3 months and to consider giving up diving altogether.

Medication

When considering whether or not a particular drug is compatible with diving it is first essential to ask why the drug is being taken, as in most cases the condition for which the drug is being taken will disqualify the individual from diving. Where this is not the case, consideration must be given to the mechanism by which the drug works and any possible side-effects. Drugs that impair exercise tolerance or produce drowsiness are obviously incompatible with diving, while drugs that may have side-effects such as neuropathies and arthropathy should probably be avoided because of possible diagnostic confusion with DCI if such symptoms should first occur after a dive. Finally, it must be remembered that many drugs have very complex structures that might be affected, and hence have altered function, by exposure to raised ambient pressure and partial pressures of oxygen. In summary, few drugs are compatible with diving.

Malarial Prophylaxis

In the case of malarial prohylaxis it is essential that the individual is both protected from malaria and also that the drug, or drug combination, taken does not impair fitness to dive. Some of the reported side-effects of mefloquine (Larium), which include motor and sensory neuropathies, ataxia, anxiety and panic attacks, are without question incompatible with safe diving. The current advice of the Diving Medical Advisory Committee (DMAC, 1998) is that, if mefloquine is the drug of choice for a particular area, at least three doses, over a period of 2–3 weeks, should be taken prior to diving. If side-effects have not developed within this time, it is highly unlikely that they will, and so it is safe to dive. An individual who has previously taken mefloquine without side-effects may dive immediately.

CLINICAL FEATURES

The bends, more correctly termed decompression illness, are just one of a variety of diving-related disorders. Divers may also drown or suffer hypothermia, despite using breathing apparatus and wearing very effective thermal protection. Drowning and hypothermia are, however, hazards common to all water sports and as such will not be dealt with in this section. Diving-related disorders can be divided into two major categories: conditions that do not require recompression therapy, and those that do.

Conditions that do not require recompression therapy

Middle ear barotrauma. Middle ear barotrauma may occur during descent if the diver is unable to equalise the air pressure within the middle-ear cavity with that of the water pressure in the external auditory meatus. For pressure equalisation to occur the eustachian tube must be patent. However, the pharyngeal two-thirds of the eustachian tube is formed from cartilage and is buried within the mucosal folds of the pharynx. This acts as a very effective flap valve that prevents reflux of food and saliva into the middle ear on swallowing. Unfortunately, as the pressure of the air in the pharynx increases during the diver's descent, this flap valve can be forced shut, making it impossible to equalise the pressure in the middle ear even with the most forceful Valsalva manoeuvre. This results in the tympanic membrane bulging inwards due to the excess water pressure in the external auditory meatus, when compared to the air pressure in the middle ear.

The tympanic membrane can only withstand a relatively small pressure imbalance before becoming traumatised and eventually rupturing. The mucosal lining of the middle-ear cavity is also traumatised by exposure to this relative vacuum and becomes oedematous and haemorrhagic. As the drum bulges inwards and the mucosal lining swells, the diver will first experience a feeling of fullness, followed by pain of increasing intensity up until the point where the drum ruptures and allows water to enter. To prevent this from occurring, the diver must ensure that the pressure difference between the pharynx and the eustachian tube never reaches the point where the cartilaginous portion of the tube collapses. This is achieved by performing frequent swallowing, yawning, jaw movements or gentle Valsalva manoeuvres against a closed nose and mouth, but not glottis, during descent.

Middle ear barotrauma of descent is classified into six grades:

Grade 0:   Symptoms without signs
Grade 1:   Injection of the tympanic membrane, especially along the handle of the malleus
Grade 2:   Injection plus slight haemorrhage within the substance of the tympanic membrane
Grade 3:   Gross haemorrhage within the substance of the tympanic membrane
Grade 4:   Free blood in the middle ear as evidenced by blueness and bulging
Grade 5:   Perforation of the tympanic membrane.

Barotrauma resulting simply in rupture of the tympanic membrane usually results in no permanent loss of hearing, as in most cases the tympanic membrane heals rapidly with minimal scarring. More extensive scarring may lead to some slight conductive hearing loss but this is quite uncommon. Less common than simple rupture of the tympanic membrane is dislocation of the ossicles, which can occur if attempts are made forcibly to equalise pressure between middle- and outer-ear cavities during the diver's descent. Such dislocation will result in a conductive hearing loss as the middle-ear amplifier can no longer function. Prompt surgical reduction will result in almost complete restoration of function in most cases.

Middle-ear barotrauma, grades 0–2, will usually resolve rapidly within a few days. Grades 3 and 4 barotrauma may take 7–10 days to resolve, while the diver with grade 5 barotrauma should not dive until the tympanic membrane has healed fully, a process that may take 4–6 weeks. Active intervention is rarely required, although simple analgesics and decongestants may ease the discomfort. Middle-ear barotrauma is often accompanied by slight conductive hearing loss: this is temporary and rarely more than 20 dB. If the hearing loss persists, is greater than 20 dB or is accompanied by tinnitus and/or vertigo, the possibility of ossicular chain disruption or inner-ear barotrauma must be considered. In all such cases the diver must be referred to an ENT specialist as a matter of urgency, as prompt surgical intervention is essential if permanent hearing loss is not to occur.

Inner-ear barotrauma. Inner-ear barotrauma may occur during descent if a diver tries to equalise middle-ear pressure by a forcible Valsalva manoeuvre. This has the effect of raising intracranial pressure, the increased pressure being transmitted via a patent cochlea aqueduct to the inner ear. Animal studies have revealed that this pressure wave may reach 120 mmHg (16 kPa), which is sufficient to rupture the round window. The resulting leak of perilymph will produce a range of symptoms, including tinnitus, sensorineural deafness and vertigo. Symptoms may become apparent while the diver is still in the water but, if the leak is small, may not present until some time after the diver has left the water. Inner-ear barotrauma requires urgent referral to an ENT department for assessment, and possible exploration and repair of the ruptured round window. It is essential to consider inner-ear barotrauma in any diver who presents complaining of having difficulty clearing the ears and who has deafness and a normal-looking drum. Inner-ear barotrauma or even ossicular dislocation, both of which require an urgent ENT referral, may be the cause. Of interest is the fact that the round windows of many diving marine mammals are protected by a layer of fibrous tissue that strengthens the membrane and hence reduces the risk of rupture.

Alternobaric vertigo.   Alternobaric vertigo occurs when the pressure, usually during ascent but occasionally during descent, in one middle-ear cavity differs from that in the opposite ear due to unequal rates of middle-ear pressure equalisation. This can result in unequal stimulation of the inner ear via the round and oval windows and marked vertigo. The vertigo is short-lived and resolves spontaneously.

Caloric vertigo.   Caloric vertigo occurs when cold water enters one ear canal while the other is still full of relatively warm air, or water trapped by the diver's hood or by ear wax. This condition usually occurs during descent and can produce a marked, but transient, vertigo.

Middle-ear oxygen absorption syndrome.   During a long dive using either oxygen, or a nitrox mix with a high percentage of oxygen, gas with a high percentage of oxygen will enter the middle-ear cavity. Following such a dive the oxygen is slowly absorbed and metabolised by the tissues of the middle ear, and if the eustachian tube does not open spontaneously a negative pressure relative to ambient may develop. Symptoms, which include a mild discomfort and hearing loss in one or both ears plus, occasionally, a sense of pressure and a moist, crackling sensation, may not become apparent for some hours after completion of the dive. A fluid level (serous otitis media) may be seen in the middle ear on otoscopy. Middle-ear oxygen absorption syndrome is difficult to avoid but does not usually pose a significant problem because the symptoms are generally minor. Attempts at equalising the pressure in the middle ear using a Valsalva manoeuvre are usually successful, although occasionally a decongestant may be required.

Otitis externa (swimmer's ear).   Repeated immersion breaks down the skin that lines the external ear canal, allowing the bacteria and fungi that are normally present to multiply. This is a condition that most commonly occurs during saturation diving, although frequent immersion of the ears for any reason, such as an intensive diving course or holiday, can promote the condition. Swimmer's ear can be prevented by use of 8% aluminium acetate solution applied after each wet dive. This solution is bacteriostatic and astringent. Three or four drops of the solution should be poured into each ear in turn and left for a *minimum* of 5 min.

Sinus barotrauma.   Sinus squeeze may occur when the ostia that vent the sinuses are obstructed. It may be experienced during descent, presenting as increasing pain in the sinus(es) involved. Since the pressure in affected sinuses decreases relative to ambient, oedema of the mucosa and haemorrhage into the sinus cavity may occur. If an ostium becomes blocked during a dive, which can occur as a result of breathing cold gas, barotrauma during descent, etc., sinus barotrauma may occur during the ascent phase of a dive. In such cases, the sinus pain is caused by a relatively increased pressure within the sinus and this may persist for some hours after the dive. Quite commonly, relief is accompanied by a squeaking sound, as gas, often accompanied by a discharge, escapes from the sinus.

External ear squeeze (reversed ears).   If the external auditory meatus is blocked by an obstruction, such as wax, a tight-fitting hood, ear plugs or otitis externa, the pressure in the outer ear can not equalise with the ambient pressure. During descent, a relative vacuum develops in both the outer and middle ear. When the ears are cleared, which returns the middle-ear pressure to ambient, the tympanic membrane balloons outwards, in the opposite direction to that which occurs in more conventional middle-ear barotrauma—hence 'reversed' ears. If this persists for more than a few minutes, injury to the epithelial lining of the external auditory meatus and the tympanum may occur; this consists of oedema and petechial haemorrhages. Occasionally haemorrhagic 'grape-like' blisters form and may burst to produce substantial haemorrhage into the ear canal.

Barotraumatic facial palsy.   In a small number of individuals the facial nerve is exposed to middle-ear pressure as it traverses the temporal bone. If the middle ear is pressurised during ascent, due to failure of the eustachian tube to vent, the vascular supply of the facial nerve may be compromised, resulting in an ischaemic neuropraxia. Generally, 10–30 min of overpressure are necessary for symptoms to appear. During this period there may be nausea and vertigo. The syndrome is characterised by a unilateral facial palsy of the lower motor neuron type. When the syndrome presents shortly after surfacing, it may be difficult to distinguish the condition from DCI. Once the middle ear vents, full facial function generally returns in between 10 min and 2 h.

Gastrointestinal barotrauma.   Gas within the intestine expands during decompression and may result in eructation, flatus or abdominal discomfort. Rarely, colicky abdominal pain, abdominal distension and 'tinkling' bowel sounds occur, which may resemble bowel obstruction. As a preventative measure, heavy meals and carbonated drinks should be avoided before a dive. Swallowing gas (aerophagia) when under pressure is dangerous because serious gastrointestinal barotrauma, possibly resulting in rupture of the bowel, may occur during ascent. Gastric rupture has been reported following very rapid ascents, as well as in individuals who have undergone fundoplication for repair of hiatus hernia. Individuals with para-oesophageal hiatus hernia should not dive, as any gas trapped in the gastric remnant within the chest will expand during ascent and may cause gastric rupture.

Pulmonary barotrauma. Pulmonary barotrauma is a serious and potentially life-threatening complication of diving that has already been discussed.

Conditions that require recompression therapy

Decompression Illness

Because bubbles can form in any tissue, or travel to any tissue in the case of arterial gas emboli, any part of the body can be affected. DCI is thus a multisystem disease that can manifest in a wide variety of forms. Furthermore, as, with time, more bubbles may come out of solution, or existing bubbles may grow in size, DCI is a dynamic process with changing symptoms and progression of symptoms.

Although DCI is a multisystem disease, there are certain systems that are affected more frequently than others. The British Hyperbaric Association's Diving Accident Database contains data on more than 1200 cases of DCI, over 75% of the cases presenting with neurological manifestations. These manifestations include muscle weakness, objective and subjective sensory changes, altered balance and coordination and, more rarely, visual and auditory disturbances and impairment of higher mental function. Although neurological dysfunction is the most common presentation of DCI, limb pain is present in approximately 50% of cases. This limb pain is a deep, aching, boring pain that is poorly localised to the area around a joint. The intensity of the pain is not affected by position or movement of the joint and the joint is not tender on palpation. In a small proportion of cases (5%) the diver will present complaining of a dull aching pain in the back, often radiating anteriorly in a girdle-like distribution. Such girdle pain is an ominous manifestation usually implying involvement of the spinal cord and frequently precedes the onset of objective motor and sensory loss.

Other manifestations of DCI include constitutional symptoms (general malaise, lethargy, fatigue, headache and nausea), pulmonary symptoms and cutaneous manifestations, which include itching and skin rashes (an erythematous rash which may progress to cyanotic mottling or marbling of the skin.) Although very rare, DCI may present with lymphatic obstruction. In most cases of DCI the diver will present with two, three or more manifestations.

MANAGEMENT OF DECOMPRESSION ILLNESS

The definitive treatment of DCI is recompression and administration of hyperbaric oxygen. However, the recompression chamber may be some distance from the dive site, and thus it may be necessary to support the diver for some hours while awaiting, and during, transport to the recompression facility. The initial treatment of the injured diver should not differ from that of any casualty but should, in addition, include administration of 100% oxygen and fluids. The theoretical justification for oxygen administration is that it both promotes the reabsorption of gas bubbles by providing a favourable tissue–bubble gas diffusion gradient, and, by increasing the tissue oxygen levels, the effect of tissue damage resulting from bubble formation is minimised.

Practical experience has revealed that oxygen administration does indeed slow the progression of DCI and may in some cases result in the complete resolution of symptoms. This should not be taken as an indication that recompression therapy is no longer required, as almost invariably symptoms recur when oxygen administration ceases. Oxygen should thus be administered from initial diagnosis of DCI to arrival at a recompression chamber.

Intravascular bubbles may result in activation of platelets, leucocytes and certain biochemical pathways (Francis and Gorman, 1993), the end-result of which will be an increase in vascular resistance and decreased tissue blood flow. This may be exacerbated by relative dehydration, common in divers, due to a combination of immersion and cold diuresis. Furthermore, some divers deliberately restrict their fluid intake before a dive as it is impracticable to urinate while wearing a diving dry suit. The conscious diver can be given any nonalcoholic fluid orally, aiming at about 1 litre in the first hour, while the unconscious diver should be given either normal saline or Hartmann's solution, once again aiming for 1 litre in the first hour. When administering such quantities of fluid it should be noted that urinary catheterisation may be required, as bladder dysfunction and urinary retention may be a symptom of decompression illness.

Although divers with limb pain or girdle pain may be in quite severe pain, it is essential that unless there is likely to be a long delay in transferring the diver to a recompression facility, analgesics are not given. Analgesics may cause diagnostic and management difficulties by masking certain DCI symptoms, such as pain and altered higher mental function. If it is necessary to administer an analgesic, the drug of choice is paracetamol. Under no circumstances should a 50:50 mixture of nitrous oxide and oxygen (Entonox) be administered to a diver, as not only will it mask symptoms but also, because of its solubility, the nitrous oxide may diffuse into existing bubbles, causing them to enlarge and thus exacerbate the diver's symptoms.

Recompression Therapy

Once the diagnosis of DCI has been made, the aim should be to transport the diver to a recompression chamber as rapidly as possible. The method of transport will depend upon what is available but the priority should always be to transfer the diver speedily and at as low an altitude as possible. Speed is essential as the shorter the time from onset of symptoms to commencement of recompression the better the prognosis (Moon and Gorman, 1993). If a helicopter is used to transport the diver, it should not exceed an altitude of 300 m, thereby avoiding a significant decrease in atmospheric pressure, which would result in the enlargement of any bubbles and exacerbation of symptoms.

Recompression therapy has three prime actions:

The reduction in volume (Boyle's law) of any gas bubbles.
The resorption of gas bubbles by providing a favourable tissue–bubble gas diffusion gradient.
The provision of oxygen to tissues damaged by bubble formation.

Recompression chambers come in a wide variety of shapes and sizes, ranging from small monoplace chambers, which only accommodate the injured diver, to large multiplace chambers in which a suitably qualified attendant accompanies the diver. Some multiplace chambers are capable of providing all the facilities to be found in an intensive care unit. This is essential in the management of the seriously injured diver or a patient receiving hyperbaric oxygen therapy for a nondiving-related clinical indication, such as carbon monoxide poisoning or necrotising fasciitis.

Once the diver has arrived at the recompression chamber, standard treatment protocols are followed and, depending upon the diver's presenting symptoms and response to recompression therapy, one of a range of different therapeutic recompression tables may be utilised. These tables range in duration from 135 min (Royal Navy Table 61/ US Navy Table 5), which is used for limb pain-only DCI rapidly resolving on recompression, to 4+ days for severe cases (Royal Navy Table 65/ US Navy 7). The therapeutic table most frequently used is the Royal Navy Table 62/US Navy Table 6 (Figure 16.2). This table is 285 min long, during which time the diver breathes 100% oxygen at both 18 m chamber depth (Pio_2 280 kPa) and also at 9 m chamber depth (Pio_2 190 kPa). The oxygen-breathing periods are interspersed by short breaks during which the diver breaths chamber air. These air-breaks reduce the probability of both pulmonary and CNS oxygen toxicity.

Following recompression therapy the diver must be admitted to a hospital for a period of at least 12 h, and preferably 24 h, for observation. The diver should be assessed regularly during this period of observation as, although uncommon, there may be a recurrence of signs and symptoms. In such cases it is essential that recognition is prompt and the diver is recompressed. Before being discharged, all patients should be briefed on what

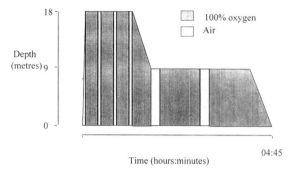

Figure 16.2　Royal Navy Table 62/US Navy Table 6 (standard oxygen recompression therapy)

action to take in the event of a recurrence of symptoms.

Outcome

Unfortunately, not all cases of DCI are cured by recompression therapy, only 55% of divers making a complete recovery after the initial recompression therapy. Fortunately this figure rises to 75% after retreatment but still leaves 25% of divers who do not fully recover. Although in most cases the residual symptoms are relatively minor, each year a small number of divers (1–2% of cases of DCI) are left with severe and disabling residual symptoms following recompression therapy and require extensive and long-term rehabilitation.

Flying after Recompression Therapy

Flying after therapeutic recompression therapy should be avoided for at least 7 days as it may precipitate a recurrence of symptoms. This is because, even following recompression therapy in which there has been complete symptomatic relief, small microbubbles may still remain in tissues; these may expand and produce symptoms in response to the reduction in cabin pressure. Symptoms may also be caused by damaged tissues, especially those of the central nervous system, becoming hypoxic when exposed to the reduced Po_2 of the aircraft cabin at altitude.

If it is impossible to delay flying for 7 days then arrangements should be made for oxygen to be available for the full duration of the flight. Even if oxygen is available, divers with limb pain or lymphatic or cutaneous DCI who have had complete resolution of all symptoms must not fly for 24 h after completing the therapeutic table. Patients with neurological, pulmonary or multisystem DCI who have had a complete resolution must not fly for a minimum of 48 h. Divers with residual symptoms should not fly for at least 72 h after completion of their final recompression table, and then only after consultation with a diving medicine specialist.

Drugs

Although recompression therapy is the definitive treatment of DCI, various drugs have been suggested as being of possible benefit as an adjuvant in treatment. The role of steroids is currently under review, while lignocaine, which presumably provides benefit by virtue of membrane stabilisation, is currently being assessed in a large trial in Australasia, from where preliminary results appear encouraging.

HEALTH ADVICE AND PROTECTIVE MEASURES

Perhaps the most important advice with regard to dive safety is to ensure that the diver receives adequate and appropriate training. Accidents are far more common with inexperienced divers, as shown by a study of 747 diving fatalities that occurred in the United States between 1989 and 1996 (Caruso et al., 1998). This study revealed that 8.1% of fatalities involved divers who had completed five or fewer dives, and 18.7% of fatalities involved divers who had completed between 6 and 20 dives. Within the UK and worldwide there are a number of recreational dive training organisations, all of which offer comprehensive training. The largest training organisations active within the UK are the British Sub-Aqua Club (BSAC) and the Professional Association of Diving Instructors (PADI) (see Additional Resources).

When travelling abroad to dive it is essential that travel insurance is purchased and that this insurance covers the costs associated with the treatment of diving accidents. Although, increasingly, travel policies do cover recreational diving, they often contain limits as to the maximum depth of dive or only apply when diving with a qualified instructor. Furthermore, some policies will only cover the cost of recompression therapy and not the cost of air evacuation, which may be many thousands of pounds, to the nearest recompression chamber.

REFERENCES

Benton PJ, Woodfine JD and Westwood PR (1996) Arterial gas embolism following a one metre ascent during helicopter escape training. *Aviation, Space and Environmental Medicine*, **67**, 63–64.

Caruso JL, Hobgood JA, Uguccioni DM et al. (1998) Inexperience kills: the relationship between lack of diving experience and fatal diving mishaps. *Undersea and Hyperbaric Medicine*, **25** (suppl), 32.

Denison DM and Francis TJRF (1999) Lung rupture, diving and submarine escape. In *The Lung at Depth* (eds CEG Lundgren, JN Miller), pp 295–374. Marcel Dekker, New York.

DMAC (1994) Guidance on assessing fitness to return to diving after decompression illness. DMAC 013. Diving Medical Advisory Committee, London.

DMAC (1998) Problems relating to the potential side effects from using mefloquine. DMAC information note 01. Diving Medical Advisory Committee, London.

Eggleston PA, Ward BH, Pierson WE et al. (1974) Radiographic abnormalities in acute asthma in children. *Pediatrics*, **54**, 442–449.

Elliott DH (1990) Residual effects and the return to diving. In *Diving Accident Management*, 41st Undersea and Hyperbaric Medical Workshop (eds PB Bennett and RE Moon), pp 235–243. Undersea Hyperbaric Medical Society, Bethesda MD.

Elliott DH (ed.) (1995) Pulmonary fitness. In *Medical Assessment of Fitness to Dive*, pp 109–153. Biomedical Seminars, Ewall.

Elliott DH and Moon RE (1993) Long term health effects of diving. In *The Physiology and Medicine of Diving* (eds PB Bennett and DH Elliott), 4th edn, pp 585–604. Baillière, Tindall and Cassell, London.

Francis TJR and Gorman DF (1993) Pathogenesis of the decompression disorders. In *The Physiology and Medicine of Diving* (eds PB Bennett and DH Elliott DH), pp 454–480. Baillière, Tindall and Cassell, London.

Light RW (1994) Pneumothorax. In *Textbook of Respiratory Medicine* (eds JF Murray and JA Nadel), 2nd edn, pp 2193–2210. WB Saunders, Philadelphia.

Lippert HL, Lund O, Blegvad S et al. (1991) Independent risk factors for cumulative recurrence rate after first spontaneous pneumothorax. *European Respiratory Journal*, **4**, 324–331.

Malhotra MS and Wright HC (1961) The effects of a raised intrapulmonary pressure on the lungs of fresh unchilled cadavers. *Journal of Pathology and Bacteriology*, **82**, 198–202.

Marsden CD (1988) Neurology. In *Oxford Textbook of Medicine* (eds DJ Weatherall, JGG Ledingham and DA Warrell), 2nd edn, p. 21.1. Oxford University Press, Oxford.

Moon RE and Gorman DF (1993) Treatment of the decompression disorders. In *The Physiology and Medicine of Diving* (eds PB Bennett and DH Elliott, pp 454–480. Baillière, Tindall and Cassell, London.

Palmer AC, Calder IM and Hughes JT (1987) Spinal cord degeneration in divers. *Lancet*, **ii**, 1365–1366.

Sutherland AFN, Veale AG and Gorman DF (1993) The neuropsychological problems prevalent in a population of recreational divers one year after treatment for decompression illness. *Journal of the South Pacific Undersea Medical Society*, **23**, 7–11.

Voge VM and Anthracite R (1986) Spontaneous pneumothorax in the USAF aircrew population: a retrospective study. *Aviation, Space and Environmental Medicine*, **57**, 939–949.

FURTHER READING

Bennett PB and Elliott DH (eds) (1993) *The Physiology and Medicine of Diving*, 4th edn. Baillière, Tindall and Cassell, London.

Bove AA and Davis JC (eds) (1997) *Diving Medicine*, 3rd edn. WB Saunders, Philadelphia.

Edmonds C, Lowry C and Pennefather J (1992) *Diving and Subaquatic Medicine*, 3rd edn. Butterworth-Heinemann, Oxford.

Elliott DH (ed.) (1995) *Medical Assessment of Fitness to Dive*. Proceedings of an International Conference at the Edinburgh Conference Centre 8–11 March 1994. Biomedical Seminars, Ewell.

ADDITIONAL RESOURCES

UK Training Organisations

British Sub-Aqua Club
BSAC headquarters
Telford's Quay
Ellesmere Port
South Wirral
Cheshire CH65 4FL, UK

Professional Association of Diving Instructors
PADI International
Unit 7, Albert Road
St Phillips Central
Bristol BS2 0PD, UK

Diving Emergency Helpline (24 hours)

Undersea Medicine Division, Institute of Naval Medicine
Tel (within the UK): 07831 151523
Tel (outside the UK): + 44 7831 151523

17

Travel Health at Sea: Cruise Ship Medicine

Robert E. Wheeler

Voyager Medical Seminars, Amherst, New Hampshire, USA

INTRODUCTION

The sea has drawn adventurers, explorers and settlers, as well as the recreational traveler, to its shores and beyond for centuries. This fascination with the sea continues into the present day, with tourists flocking not only to beaches and oceanfront resorts but also to fleets of cruise ships that sail worldwide.

Ten million people will travel in the year 2001 to a variety of destinations around the globe on the more than 250 cruise ships that make up the world's fleet. North American clients constitute approximately 75% of the world's cruise line passengers. Although there are currently only two large US-flagged ocean-going cruise ships (the SS *Independence* of American Hawaii Cruises and the MV *Patriot* of United States Line), 60% of the world fleet is based in North America to service this major market, with the Caribbean Sea as the primary destination for half of all cruises.

The availability of qualified medical personnel in a properly equipped medical facility aboard ship is a key element in providing for the appropriate medical care and safety of a cruise line's passengers and crew members. Cruise ship medicine is the practice of medicine designed to provide cruise line passengers and crew members with timely access to comprehensive medical services for minor to severe illness and injury. It is important, however, to view a ship's medical facility as an infirmary or sickbay and not a full-service hospital. Although most of the medical conditions that arise aboard ship can be treated as they would at a doctor's office or ambulatory care center at home, more severe problems may require emergency evacuation to a fully staffed and equipped shore-side hospital after the patient is stabilized in the ship's medical facility.

There is often a misconception, both by the general public and the medical profession, of what cruise ship medicine really entails. Many think that the maladies encountered aboard a cruise ship are limited to seasickness, sunburn and gastroenteritis, and that the doctors and nurses are merely on holiday. The reality of cruise ship medicine, however, is very different. On a weekly basis, the ship's medical staff will evaluate passengers and crew members with myriad complaints, similar to those that one would expect to see in a low-volume (though not necessarily low-acuity) emergency department, casualty clinic or ambulatory care center (Table 17.1).

Important elements of cruise ship medicine, as well as other sectors of travel medicine, are anticipation, preparation, improvisation, observation and transportation. The ship's medical staff must try to anticipate the medical needs of the passengers and crew members and prepare for the delivery of the proper care to meet these needs. At times it may be necessary to improvise medical services owing to limitations in the shipboard medical facility's equipment, formulary and staff. A victim of serious illness or injury may need to be observed in the shipboard facility until safe transportation to an appropriate shore-side medical facility becomes available.

On average, during a 1 week cruise to the Caribbean, a ship's medical staff will see 3–5% of the passengers and 10–15% of the crew members for some type of illness or injury. Typically, more than half of all visits to the infirmary are made by crew members; 80–90% of the visits to the infirmary will be for nonurgent medical problems, 10–15% for urgent problems, and 5–10% for serious illness or injury that may require temporary shipboard hospitalization and/or emergency medical evacuation to a full-service shore-side medical facility. Fortunately, less than 1% of shipboard patients require emergency transfer to a shore-side hospital.

PLANNING FOR A SAFE AND HEALTHY VOYAGE

Travel can be one of life's most exciting adventures. Whether by sea, land or air, it can provide countless opportunities to explore exotic places, experience novel activities and meet a variety of interesting people. Many travelers spend a significant amount of time planning

Principles and Practice of Travel Medicine. Edited by Jane N. Zuckerman.
© 2001 John Wiley & Sons Ltd.

Table 17.1 Comparison of the 10 principal diagnoses for passengers on board cruise ships versus US emergency departments (Dahl, 1999; Peake, 1999; McCraig, 2000)

Cruise ships		US emergency departments	
Organ system	%	Organ system	%
Respiratory	26–29	Injury-related and poisoning	30
Injury-related	12–18		
Nervous and sense organs	9	Respiratory	12.5
		Nervous and sense organs	5.7
Gastrointestinal	12–16		
Cardiovascular	3–7	Gastrointestinal	5.6
Genitourinary	3	Musculoskeletal and connective tissue	4.5
Musculoskeletal and connective tissue	3		
		Cardiovascular	4.2
Skin and subcutaneous tissue	3–13	Genitourinary	4.2
		Mental disorders	3.1
Endocrine and immune	0.8	Skin and subcutaneous tissue	2.8
Mental disorders	0.7	Endocrine and metabolic	1.4

their budget, itinerary, transportation and accommodations for a trip, but they often fail to consider contingencies for unexpected illness or injury that can occur at any time or place along their journey. Foresight and preparedness for possible medical mishaps during a trip can help to avert unnecessary inconvenience or even an unforeseen disaster.

Trip Readiness

The United States Coast Guard's motto, *Semper Paratus* (always prepared), is a useful concept for cruise travelers to bear in mind before the start of any voyage. This is especially important when the journey involves travel to developing countries or wilderness areas. Medical resources can be very limited or absent altogether in these areas and it may be up to the individual traveler to provide initial treatment for him- or herself or a companion should a medical mishap occur. A major benefit of traveling by cruise ship is the availability of shipboard medical services that often exceed those available shore side at exotic ports.

Research on the destinations along the route prior to departure can be very helpful. Cruise travelers should know if there are any unusual diseases that require special precautions, immunizations or medications. Such problems include infectious diarrhea, dengue fever, malaria, hepatitis, yellow fever and cholera. They should find out if the shore-side water is safe to drink and the food supply safe to eat without special preparation. Checking on the reliability of the area's transportation system and equipment can help to avoid motor vehicle incidents. Cruise

travelers should be aware of any societal and political unrest that could interfere with their shore-side exploration. They should also use common sense when considering new adventure activities in order to avoid unnecessary injuries. The cruise lines provide much of this information to the passengers before and during their cruise. Additional information can easily be obtained from travel agents, travel literature and Internet travel sites.

If planning to embark on an extensive or particularly rigorous trip, travelers should visit their health care provider to discuss any personal health issues that they may need to address. This is particularly important for people with chronic medical conditions, such as heart disease, lung disease, renal failure, diabetes, seizure disorders and immune disorders. They must consider the stress and physical exertion associated with long distance land, air and sea travel and the risks of travel outside their home territory, where medical services for their particular condition may be limited. To help minimize this stress and risk, some tour operators specialize in cruises for passengers with special medical needs, most commonly those requiring hemodialysis for chronic renal failure or oxygen for chronic lung disease. The operators provide the specialized equipment and supplies for the particular group, as well as their own medical staff of appropriate doctors, nurses and technicians to address the specific needs of the group.

It is essential that passengers with chronic medical conditions and special medical needs prepare carefully for their voyage. They should hand-carry sufficient quantities of their daily medications and medical supplies to avoid losing them in luggage misplaced during travel. Passengers can contact the cruise line passenger services or medical departments regarding any special medical needs or equipment that they may need during the cruise, such as oxygen (via portable tanks or oxygen concentrators), wheelchair, and needle and other biohazardous waste disposal containers. If not routinely available aboard ship, the cruise line can assist the passenger in obtaining the necessary equipment from reliable shore-side vendors. Special staterooms for passengers with disabilities are available on most large cruise ships built over the past 10 years. These cabins can provide wider entry doors without the usual raised threshold, wheelchair-accessible bathrooms, additional floor space, oxygen outlets, warning lights for the deaf and emergency call buttons.

For trips to exotic foreign destinations, travelers should also consider consulting a travel medicine specialist at least 6–8 weeks prior to their departure to determine if they need special immunizations or medications for the cruise. They can locate a travel medicine specialist through their own health care provider, local and state medical societies or other organizations, such as the American Society of Tropical Medicine and Hygiene, the International Association for Medical Assistance to Travellers and the International Society of Travel Medicine.

Travel Medical Insurance

A serious illness or injury while traveling can result in significant financial liability for the unfortunate tourist. Not only can out-of-pocket expenses be significant but emergency air medical evacuation can run into tens of thousands of dollars. Medical insurance for these events can be provided by a traditional health insurer or by one specializing in health insurance for the traveler. Many people with health insurance at home will be covered for medical services in another country; however, medical providers and facilities outside of the traveler's home country may not have the capacity to invoice the traveler's insurer for services rendered and may expect direct payment from them at the time of service. It is important for travelers to review their insurance policy regarding specific coverage for services outside their local area and reimbursement for direct payment for services. United States Medicare typically does not cover medical services outside US territories. A telephone call to the traveler's health insurer prior to leaving on the trip can provide additional information on health care benefits while traveling. It is important to discuss precisely what medical services are covered and whether emergency air evacuation is included in the policy. If the benefits from the primary health insurance are insufficient, the traveler should consider purchasing supplemental coverage, either from the same provider or from a travel insurance company. The medical illness and injury benefit should be at least $US20 000. The emergency medical evacuation portion of the policy (for North American cruise ship passengers) should provide up to $US15 000 of coverage for trips to Alaska, Bermuda, Canada, the Caribbean and Central America; $US60 000 for travel to Europe, South America and other readily accessible locations; and up to $US100 000 for trips to Africa, Antarctica, Asia, Australia and other remote or exotic areas. The traveler should also be sure that any pre-existing medical conditions are covered by the policy.

In addition to medical and evacuation policies, various other types of travel-related insurance are available. These include trip cancellation/delay/interruption, lost luggage, tour operator default/failure, accidental death/ repatriation of remains, and travel assistance coverage. Home and business insurance policies, credit card programs or transportation providers may offer limited coverage for some of these potential losses. These types of coverage are often bundled into a comprehensive insurance package along with the medical and evacuation insurance. The premium for a comprehensive insurance plan, good for the duration of the cruise or air/land tour, is typically 5–7% of the total cost of the travel package. If travelers need only supplemental medical and evacuation insurance, it can cost as little as $US50 per person for a year's coverage.

Traveler's First-aid Kit

Most illnesses and injuries incurred while traveling are

Table 17.2 Suggestions for a traveler's first-aid kit

A small flashlight is very handy if there is a power outage or if the kit is needed out of doors	Eyeglass repair kit
	Spare eyeglasses, contacts and sunglasses
Pen and notepad to keep track of supplies and make notations about important incidents	Antihistamine/decongestant medications for allergic symptoms and congestion.
Aspirin, acetaminophen or ibuprofen are effective for the treatment of pain and fever. Acetaminophen is the preferred medication for children with fever.	Eye drops
	Cough medicine and throat lozenges
	Lip balm, canker gel, dental floss
Oil of cloves for toothache	Hydrocortisone cream for insect bites and itch
A pair of round-tipped scissors is useful for cutting bandages and other items	Antifungal cream for athlete's foot and yeast infections
Tweezers, safety pins and a Swiss Army-type knife are all tools that have multiple uses	Antacid and heartburn relief tablets
Tape, bandages, cutton swabs and antibiotic ointment are used to treat scrapes, cuts and burns. Blister dressings	Laxative and antidiarrheal medication
	Sunscreen, factor 15 or greater
Elastic wraps and triangular bandages can help immobilize injured limbs	Sea/motion sickness tablets
Instant ice pack (or disposable freezer bag)	Insect repellent when traveling to insect-prone destinations
Rubber gloves protect your hands and reduce the risk of infection when treating open wounds	Personal medications and prescriptions
Thermometer with case	Personal medical information form

All medications should be stored out of reach of children; only products with child safety caps should be used.
First-aid kits should be in a carry-on bag, not in checked luggage.

not life threatening; however, if travelers are not prepared to treat them they can easily disrupt an otherwise enjoyable trip. A personal first-aid kit is an efficient way to prepare for these unexpected emergencies, both while traveling and at home. A standard kit can be purchased at most pharmacies and sporting goods stores or travelers may wish to design a specialized first-aid kit that meets their own particular needs (Table 17.2).

A small tote bag is a convenient way to store all of the supplies in the kit. It allows enough room for the essential items and it ensures easy portability for travel. Certain items should be included in any first-aid kit. A small flashlight is very handy if there is a power cut or if the kit is needed out of doors. A pen and notepad help to keep track of supplies and make notations about important incidents. A pair of rounded-tip scissors is useful for cutting bandages and other items. Tweezers, safety pins and a Swiss Army-type knife are all tools that have multiple uses. Tape, bandages, cotton swabs, antibiotic ointment and blister dressings are used to treat cuts, scrapes and blisters. Elastic wraps and triangular bandages can help immobilize injured limbs. Rubber gloves provide a protective barrier to reduce the risk of infection when treating open wounds. Acetaminophen, aspirin and ibuprofen are effective for the treatment of pain or fever. Nonprescription medications for colds, allergies, motion sickness, heartburn and diarrhea are commonly needed when traveling. Sunscreen and insect repellent are important for trips to sunny and insect-prone destinations. It is important for the cruise traveler to include an adequate supply of any prescription medications, including eyeglasses and/or contact lenses, to last the entire trip. They should also enclose a written list or copies of their medication and eyeglass prescriptions in the kit.

The final component of the first-aid kit should be a personal medical information form (Figure 17.1). This is a convenient way of ensuring that essential medical information will be available to traveling companions and medical personnel when needed. The form identifies the next of kin, doctors, hospital and insurance carrier. It lists any past and present illnesses, medications, allergies, blood type and immunization status. People with a history of heart disease may want to attach a copy of their most recent electrocardiogram. The form indicates who is to be notified in an emergency. That person should have a copy of the form outlining the traveler's entire medical history.

MEDICAL CARE AT SEA

Many people think of a cruise as the trip of a lifetime. For others it is the only way to travel. A modern cruise ship offers one of the most luxurious and safe ways of exploring international destinations. From the smaller ships of less than 100 m in length which carry fewer than 100 passengers, to the truly titanic 300 m vessels sailing with more than 3000 passengers and 1000 crew members, cruise ships provide their guests with amenities that rival, and even exceed, those experienced at renowned shore-side resorts. A beautiful vessel, luxurious accommodations, great food, the leisurely life at sea and exotic ports of call all add up to a fabulous holiday. But what if the unexpected happens and the cruise traveler suddenly becomes ill or injured? They are far away from home on the high seas and in need of prompt evaluation and treatment. It is comforting to both passengers and crew members to know that the ship's medical staff is just a few decks away.

Cruise Ship Medical Facility

Several factors influence the specific requirements for medical staff and equipment onboard a cruise ship. These include:

• the size of the ship.

• the total number of passengers and crew members.
• the average age of the passengers, their baseline health status, and their planned activities. Industry-wide, the average cruise line passenger is 45–50 years of age. Certain cruise lines attract a senior clientele, while others cater to the younger crowd. An older age group will tend to have more chronic medical problems, such as heart and lung disease, which may act up while they are traveling. A younger age group may have more injuries due to alcohol use and sports activities.
• The destination and length of the cruise. Longer periods away from the home port, especially days at sea, necessitate stocking up on more frequently used supplies. Common ailments, such as respiratory infections, may increase in frequency on longer cruises. Knowledge of the types and quality of medical facilities along the itinerary is important to determine whether passenters or crew members can be sent shore side for additional care or whether they need to be evacuated by air back to the home port.

A well-designed cruise ship medical department requires careful planning. Adequate space must be assigned in the architectural plans of the ship to allow for the delivery of necessary medical services for passengers and crew members. The medical facility must be equipped with essential diagnostic and therapeutic supplies and equipment. An efficient medical care delivery system is needed in order to meet the needs of passengers and crew members despite limitations in equipment and staff when compared with a shore-side hospital. There should be a contingency plan in place to provide emergency medical services in designated locations in the event of an on-board disaster and the primary medical facility becoming inaccessible due to fire, smoke or water damage. Most importantly, the medical department must be staffed by qualified doctors and nurses who are capable of working in an isolated environment. The final plan for any particular medical department will also be influenced by the ship's size and design, total number of passengers and crew members, guest demographics, expected number of medical facility patient visits, and the ship's itineraries.

Until recently, most cruise lines worked independently to address these shipboard medical facility issues. In 1990, however, the American College of Emergency Physicians (ACEP) Cruise Ship and Maritime Medicine Section was founded and created a forum for cruise ship medicine practitioners and others in the cruise industry to discuss these topics.

The Cruise Ship and Maritime Medicine Section was organized by members of the ACEP experienced in the practice of cruise ship medicine. The objectives of the Section are to:

1. Serve as a resource to the cruise industry, their medical departments, and physicians interested in cruise ship medicine.
2. Develop guidelines for quality and consistent medical care aboard cruise ships.

Personal Medical Information Form

Name:	Date of Birth:
Street:	
City:	Social Security Number:
State/Province:	Passport Number:
Postal/Zip Code:	
Country:	Telephone Number:

Health Insurance Plan **Supplemental / Travel Insurance Plan**

Provider:	Provider:
Member ID Number:	Member ID Number:
Street:	Street:
City:	City:
State/Province:	State/Province:
Postal/Zip Code:	Postal/Zip Code:
Telephone Number:	Telephone Number:

Doctor **Hospital**

Name:	Name:
Street:	Street:
City:	City:
State/Province:	State/Province:
Postal/Zip Code:	Postal/Zip Code:
Telephone Number:	Telephone Number:

Emergency Contact Person

Name:	Relationship:
Street:	
City:	Telephone Number:
State/Province:	
Postal/Zip Code:	

Present & Past Medical Conditions

Figure 17.1 An example of a personal medical information form

Allergies & Drug Sensitivities   **Blood Type**

Medications

Name (generic)	Dose	Schedule

Vaccines & Preventative Medications

Type	Yes	No	Date Last Received
Routine Immunizations:			
DTP, Td (diphtheria-**tetanus**-pertussis)			
Haemophilus influenza B (sepsis)			
Influenza			
MMR (measles-mumps-rubella)			
Pneumococcus (pneumonia)			
Polio			
Varicella (chicken pox)			
Other: (as determined by destination) *			

*Cholera, hepatitis A, hepatitis B, immune globulin, Japanese encephalitis, malaria prophylaxis, meningo-coccal meningitis, plague, rabies, tick-borne encephalitis, tuberculosis, typhoid fever, yellow fever

If you have a history of heart disease please attach a copy of a recent **EKG**.

Provide a copy of this form to family members and emergency contact designees.

Take this form with you when you seek medical attention.

Figure 17.1   (*cont.*)

3. Encourage research on cruise ship medicine.
4. Provide educational opportunities for cruise ship medical and administrative staff members.
5. Promote the importance and enhancement of on-board medical care.
6. Educate the medical establishment about the content and complexity of cruise ship medicine.

There are minimal international maritime regulations pertaining to medical services aboard cruise ships and these mainly address the needs of the crew members, not cruise ship passengers; for example, there is no international requirement to have a doctor aboard ship. Additional regulations may apply to cruise ships depending upon the country of registry, but many of these regulations are vague in nature and do not address specific recommendations for a cruise ship's medical facility or its medical staff.

One of the major accomplishments of the ACEP Cruise Ship and Maritime Medicine Section has been the development of the *Health Care Guidelines for Cruise Ship Medical Facilities*, first released in 1995 and then revised in 1997 (American College of Emergency Physicians, 1997) (see Additional Resources). The guidelines are the recommendations of several cruise line medical directors and experienced ship's physicians from within the industry and authorized to practice medicine in United States, British, Canadian, Norwegian and other land-based facilities. The guidelines provide invaluable assistance to cruise ship medicine practitioners in the development of shipboard medical departments, and to the cruise industry as a quality improvement tool for medical services at sea.

These guidelines are an adjunct to the international maritime safety regulations (International Safety Management Code (ISM), Safety Management System (SMS) and Safety of Life at Sea (SOLAS)) as established by the International Maritime Organization and International Labor Organization. The International Council of Cruise Lines (ICCL), a major cruise industry trade group based in the United States and representing 16 of the world's largest cruise lines, has adopted a modified version of the guidelines for its membership. The major cruise lines sailing to United States ports and many other cruise lines worldwide currently adhere to the ACEP and ICCL guidelines on a voluntary basis. The ICCL is working within the cruise industry to integrate the guidelines into the ISM code and the SMS as the standard for medical services aboard cruise ships.

The ACEP Cruise Ship and Maritime Medicine Section is currently reviewing the *Health Care Guidelines for Cruise Ship Medical Facilities* for another revision. Topics that are being considered for addition to the Policy Resource and Education Paper (PREP) include recommendations for a standardized formulary list, contingency plans for medical services in the event that the infirmary becomes inaccessible, expanded laboratory capabilities, travel insurance, emergency evacuation procedures and shore-side medical facility evaluation.

Cruise Ship Physician

The cruise ship physician's main responsibility is to provide medical services for all shipboard personnel and passengers. He or she is also involved in public health, hygiene and safety issues on board ship. In addition, the physician is a ship's senior officer who represents not only the medical department but also the ship and the cruise line. The ship's physician should never underestimate his or her responsibilities aboard ship, nor overestimate his or her authority. Cruise ships typically have a strict hierarchy of command and it is very important that the physician keep superiors informed of any health issues that could impact the ship's operations, such as an infectious disease outbreak or the need for an emergency medical evacuation.

As with the cruise industry in general, cruise ship medicine is made up of an international group of participants. North American physicians staff about 10% of the world's fleet. Physicians from various countries, such as the UK, Norway, Sweden, Denmark, Greece, Italy and South Africa, staff majority of the remainder. Tours of duty aboard ship run from a few weeks to several months, as determined by the respective cruise line's staffing policy. Depending upon the size of the ship and the number of passengers and crew members, the doctor may be the only medical staff member aboard ship or he or she may be part of a medical team consisting of an additional doctor and 3–5 nurses. Cruise ship nurses are typically well trained and experienced in emergency and critical care services. They play a pivotal role in providing quality medical care to the passengers and fellow crew members. They also often serve as triage officers for the ship's sickbay and office managers for the Medical Department.

SHIPBOARD MALADIES

Although the types of illness and injury encountered aboard a cruise ship are similar to those seen at shore-side outpatient clinics, there are certain medical problems that many people associate with ocean travel or that pose particular diagnostic and therapeutic dilemmas when they arise on board a ship. It is important for the ship's medical staff to be familiar with the common illnesses and injuries that that are seen aboard ship and be prepared to treat and stabilize patients with life-threatening conditions, who can also present to the ship's infirmary.

Sea Sickness

Sea sickness is a primary concern for many cruise travelers, but in reality it is seldom a significant problem. Most cruise itineraries are in calm seas and modern cruise ships have port and starboard stabilizers that help to minimize excessive motion in rougher waters. Unfortunately, some people are very sensitive to the motion not only of ships but also airplanes, automobiles, trains and amusement park rides. These cruise ship passengers are more likely to develop sea sickness even in smooth seas. As the churn of the sea increases, so does the incidence of sea sickness among both passengers and crew members. Nearly everyone will eventually exceed their threshold for sea sickness as ocean conditions worsen.

Humans sense their orientation in three-dimensional space via visual input from the eyes, proprioceptive input from muscles and joints, and vestibular (apparatus) input from the inner ear. Sea sickness, as well as motion sickness in general, is currently considered to be caused by visual, proprioceptive and vestibular sensory conflict, or neural mismatch, that results in the cholinergic stimulation of the brain's vomiting center and the parasympathetic nervous system. Hence, signs and symptoms of sea sickness can range from a vague feeling of being 'unwell' to headache, pallor, anxiety, warmth, cold sweats, fatigue, dizziness, vertigo, and finally nausea and vomiting (Gahlinger, 2000).

Several factors can influence one's susceptibility to sea sickness. An unfamiliar pattern of motion, such as that encountered aboard a boat or ship, is the main cause of symptoms. A ship's motion can be categorized as roll (rotation around the ship's longitudinal axis), pitch (rotation around the horizontal axis), yaw (rotation around the vertical axis) and heave (movement along the vertical axis). Although rhythmic motion around any one of these axes can precipitate sea sickness, it is typically a combination of these movements that one encounters at sea. A roll, pitch, yaw or heave periodicity of one cycle every 2–5 s (0.2–0.5 Hz) is most effective in causing symptoms when compared to other periodicity rates. Adaptation to the motion tends to occur over 2–3 days as cruise travelers get their 'sea legs' and symptoms then often abate. Infants under the age of 2 years are rarely affected, whereas children between the ages of 4 and 12 years are most likely to become ill from the adverse motion. Women tend to be more prone to sea sickness than men, especially when pregnant. Overzealous dietary intake or excessive alcohol consumption can aggravate the symptoms of sea sickness. In rough seas when many people become afflicted, a psychosomatic component may trigger sea sickness in travelers who otherwise could weather the storm.

The treatment of sea sickness can be approached using environmental alterations, pharmacological agents and nonpharmacological devices. Since the unfamiliar rhythmic motion encountered aboard ship is the major precipitant of sea sickness, actions to minimize the motion can be effective in preventing progression of symptoms. These include moving amidships near the vessel's center of gravity, where the motion should be less pronounced. Stepping out on deck for some cool fresh air and looking off to the horizon may help to diminish the conflicting visual sensory input. Stateroom location aboard ship has been considered to be a factor for the incidence of sea sickness, those closer to the center of the ship having less motion and their occupants suffering less sea sickness, but a recent small study disputes this (Gah-

linger, 1999). What may be more important is the actual position of the occupant. A supine position parallel to the axis of major motion helps to minimize the effects of the motion on the vestibular apparatus in the inner ear. Closing the eyes to inhibit visual stimulation and stabilizing the head with pillows to prevent side-to-side motion help to decrease contradictory visual and vestibular sensory input.

Mal de débarquement is another disorder that is associated with ocean travel. Following a few days at sea, with or without suffering from sea sickness, the cruise ship passenger may develop symptoms of motion sickness *after* returning to terra firma in port. This is felt to be a result of the traveler's habituation to the motion of the ship and the sudden exposure to the now unfamiliar absence of motion. Symptoms are usually mild and resolve within hours or a few days. More severe or protracted symptoms warrant consideration of other conditions such as benign paroxysmal positional vertigo and Meniere disease. Mal de débarquement syndrome (MDDS) is a chronic form of this disorder. What causes MDDS is unclear. Vestibular dysfunction, depression, hormonal imbalance and migraine variant have all been proposed as possible etiologies. Symptoms can be mild to severe and persist for many years. Treatment regimens may include the use of sedatives, antidepressants, female hormones and physical therapy (Hain *et al.*, 1999).

The pharmacological treatment of sea sickness involves the use of various antihistamine, anticholinergic and antiemetic agents (Table 17.3). The antihistamine medications dimenhydrinate, meclozine, cyclizine, buclizine, cinnarizine and diphenhydramine are the most widely used drugs for sea sickness. They can be very effective in preventing sea sickness if ingested 1–2 h prior to embarking on a voyage. When taken in the recommended doses, these drugs have minimal side-effects, mainly mild sedation and dry mouth.

Hyoscine (scopolamine) in the form of a transdermal patch is one of the most effective prophylactic medications for sea sickness. The 1.5 mg unit dose patch is placed behind the ear at least 4 h prior to sailing. The patch can be left in place for 3 days and then replaced if needed. Up to 60% of users develop a dry mouth but drowsiness is less common than with the antihistamine and antiemetic medications. Other potential side-effects include blurred vision, urinary retention (especially on older men), confusion and hallucinations. Due to the unit dosing, people with a smaller body mass may be more prone to side-effects. Hyoscine in tablet form, often taken with dexamfetamine or ephedrine to counteract drowsiness, is also very effective for the prevention and treatment of sea sickness.

Antiemetic medications are typically given parenterally or via rectal suppository to people who are vomiting or are having progressive symptoms despite taking the primary oral medications. Promethazine, prochlorperazine, metoclopramide and trimethobenzamide are all very effective in alleviating the nausea and vomiting of sea sickness. As with the antihistamines, their anticholinergic

Table 17.3 Medications commonly used for the prevention and treatment of sea sickness

Medication	Dose
Antihistamines	
Buclizine	50 mg p.o. 6–8 h
Cinnarizine	15–30 mg p.o. 6–8 h
Cyclizine	50 mg p.o. or i.m. 4–6 h
Dimenhydrinate	25–50 mg p.o. or i.m. 4–6 h
Diphenhydramine	25–50 mg p.o. or i.m. 4–6 h
Meclozine	25 mg p.o. 6–8 h
Anticholinergics	
Hyoscine	
(scopppolamine)	1.5 mg transdermal patch, 72 h
	0.3 mg p.o. 4–6 h (also taken in combination with dexamfetamine 5 mg or ephedrine 25 mg)
Antiemetics	
Metoclopramide	10 mg p.o., i.m. or i.v. 6–8 h
Prochlorperazine	10 mg p.o., i.m. or i.v. 6–8 h
	25 mg p.r. 12 h
Promethazine	25 mg p.r. or i.m. 4–6 h
	25 mg p.o. 4–6 h (also taken in combination with ephedrine 25 mg)
Trimethobenzamide	250 mg p.o. 6–8 h
	200 mg p.r. or i.m. 6–8 h
Other	
Ginger root	1 g p.o. 6–12 h

effects also decrease the efferent cholinergic impulses from the vestibular apparatus.

Ginger root is a popular alternative herbal treatment for sea sickness. It can be used either as a preventative or for the active treatment of symptoms. One gram is typically taken in tablet or capsule form prior to the start of the voyage. It may then be repeated every 6–12 h as needed. The most common side-effect associated with prolonged ginger root use is dyspepsia (Udani, 1998).

Nonpharmacological therapy for sea sickness is also available. Wrist bands that apply acupressure or electrical stimulation to the palmar surface of the wrists may be helpful in preventing sea sickness. The basis for their use is the stimulation of the P6 or Neiguan acupuncture point at the wrist. The acupressure wrist bands have been shown to decrease the morning sickness associated with pregnancy but studies evaluating the use of these and the electrical stimulation wrist bands for sea sickness have provided conflicting results (Bruce *et al.*, 1990; Hu, 1995).

Respiratory Illness

Respiratory ailments constitute the most common diagnosis in most ships' infirmaries. This is merely a manifestation of what one might term the traveler's respiratory syndrome. As they travel long distances over several hours or days in crowded trains, planes and cruise ships, travelers are often exposed to dry, recirculated air, a variety of unfamiliar viral and bacterial pathogens and new environmental allergens. All of these factors can contribute to inflammation and infection of the upper respiratory system in healthy individuals and aggravate respiratory conditions in others with chronic problems. Most of these cases are self-limited and the patients can be treated symptomatically with fluids, antipyretic, antitussive and antihistamine medications. Should a bacterial infection be suspected or diagnosed, appropriate antibiotics can be administered from the ship's pharmacy.

In recent years, outbreaks of influenza A have occurred aboard cruise ships worldwide, including outbreaks in New England, Alaska, the Mediterranean and Australia (CDC, 1998a, 1998b; Health Canada, 1998). In some cases the outbreak occurred outside the area's typical influenza season, with the virus being imported from another hemisphere with an active influenza season. Passengers unknowingly carried the virus to the various ships, infecting other guests and crew members. Although the cruise ships were not the actual source of the virus, they unfortunately became a reservoir for the virus on later cruises. The outbreaks were brought under control with antiviral medications and influenza vaccination for susceptible passengers and crew members. Annual influenza vaccination programs were then instituted for all crew members to prevent recurrent outbreaks during subsequent cruise seasons. In addition, active and passive influenza surveillance programs were instituted by several major cruise lines to assist in the early detection of any new outbreaks. In light of these outbreaks and others worldwide, and the ease of modern international travel from continent to continent and hemisphere to hemisphere, influenza is no longer considered to be a truly seasonal disease (CDC, 1999).

Food- and Water-Borne Illness

Isolated cases of gastrointestinal illness aboard cruise ships are common, comprising 5–10% of sickbay visits. Many of these cases are precipitated by changes in diet, overindulgence and food and water ingested off the ship in developing countries. Fortunately, outbreaks of food- and water-borne illness are rare. As with shore-side outbreaks, more than half are due to the Norwalk (or related) virus or an undetermined agent. The rest are due to a variety of bacterial agents, most notably enterotoxigenic *Escherichia coli*, salmonella, shigella, *Staphylococcus aureus*, *Clostridium perfringens* and campylobacter (CDC, 2000a, 2001).

The cruise industry is ever vigilant to ensure that the water and food stores aboard its ships are safe and reliable. An outbreak of food- or water-borne illness on a cruise ship can potentially afflict hundreds of passengers and crew members in a very short time. It can also quickly tarnish the reputation of even the most respected cruise line, as well as the cruise industry as a whole. A study by the United States Centers for Disease Control and Prevention (CDC) on the epidemiology of diarrheal disease outbreaks on cruise ships between 1986 and 1993 revealed that the incidence was only 2.3 outbreaks per 10 million passenger days (equivalent to a 1500 passenger ship sailing 50 weeks per year having a single outbreak once every 10 years). They noted that the incidence of outbreaks had decreased by nearly a third since the previous study period, 1980–1985. The CDC also suggested that a significant further decrease in future outbreaks could be accomplished merely by: (1) thoroughly cooking all meat, fish and poultry; (2) using pasteurized eggs for all pooled egg recipes; (3) not allowing food handlers to work with any gastrointestinal symptoms; and (4) not using onshore food vendors where quality control may be diminished (Koo, 1993).

The Vessel Sanitation Program (VSP), developed and administered by the CDC, has been instrumental in the steady decline of gastrointestinal outbreaks aboard cruise ships. The VSP was established in 1975 as a cooperative activity with the cruise industry to develop and implement comprehensive sanitation programs aimed at minimizing the risk of gastrointestinal diseases. Biannual, unannounced food safety and environmental sanitation inspections are performed on all vessels with a foreign itinerary calling on a United States port and carrying 13 or more passengers. The Vessel Sanitation Inspection Report, with a possible maximum score of 100, is completed during the inspection. A score of 86 or higher is considered to be satisfactory. Lower scores result in an unsatisfactory rating for the vessel and requires immediate corrective action. Inspection results are compiled in the VSP 'Green Sheet', which is made available to the public via mail and the CDC web site (CDC, 2000b).

In addition to the VSP, cruise lines utilize the Hazard Analysis Critical Control Point (HACCP) program to help prevent food-borne illness aboard ship. The HACCP program outlines procedures to ensure the proper storage, handling and preparation of food. It also addresses hygiene and sanitation regulations for food handlers and food preparation areas (US Department of Health and Human Services, 1999).

CRITICAL CARE AT SEA

A critically ill patient can be difficult to manage even in a full-service shore-side hospital. The critically ill passenger or crew member on board a cruise ship can provide a significant challenge for even the most seasoned cruise ship physician. With limited diagnostic equipment and medical staff available aboard ship, the physician's main resource for properly diagnosing and treating the patient may be his or her own clinical skills and experience. Admitting a patient from your hometown emergency department into the intensive care unit is relatively easy, but arranging for a costly emergency medical evacuation that requires diversion of the ship to another port, or air transport to an appropriate medical facility, must be coordinated with the ship's Master (Captain) and other superiors. The physician must take these logistical issues

into consideration when deciding whether to keep a critically ill patient aboard ship or disembarking them to an 'appropriate' shore-side medical facility that may be hundreds or even thousands of miles away via air transport.

A helicopter rescue at sea may be an exciting spectator sport for the ship's passengers, but it is used only as a last resort for patients that must get to a shore-side medical facility immediately, such as for severe gastrointestinal bleeding, cardiogenic shock, surgical abdomen, massive trauma or any other condition where time to definitive treatment is critical. A helicopter rescue is inherently dangerous because the helicopter must hover above the ship and the patient is raised in a basket. A crash of the helicopter on to the ship would undoubtedly result in extensive damage to the helicopter and ship and possibly multiple casualties on board both vessels. Therefore, most patients are stabilized aboard ship and then disembarked at the next available port.

The spectrum of serious illness and injury seen aboard cruise ships is very broad. Although incidents do occur that result in multiple trauma, most critical patients suffer from a variety of medical problems that include acute respiratory failure, stroke, gastrointestinal bleeding, acute abdomen, sepsis, ectopic pregnancy and abdominal aortic aneurysm. A particular concern is the patient with massive hemorrhage. Blood is not stored on board cruise ships. It is seldom needed, requires a special refrigeration unit and it has a short storage life of 35–40 days. However, when the need arises, it is most urgent that blood be made available. All efforts are made to obtain typed and screened O-negative blood from reliable shore-side sources in a timely fashion. If necessary it can be dropped from an aircraft to the ship. If banked blood is not available and the patient is at high risk of dying from the blood loss, then blood can be obtained from previously screened and low-risk crew members. Using simple diagnostic kits, the blood is typed, tested for HIV and then transfused to the patient. Such unconventional improvisation has proven to be life saving during these critical episodes.

The most common critical illness encountered is acute myocardial infarction. As in most industrialized countries, this is also the leading cause of death on cruise ships. Patients may initially present with sudden cardiac arrest, but more often they arrive at the infirmary to be evaluated for chest pain. As is done at shore-side medical facilities, they are promptly placed on a cardiac monitor and nasal oxygen and intravenous access is obtained. Evaluation of their chest pain includes a medical history, physical examination and electrocardiogram. If the ECG is consistent with acute myocardial infarction and there are no contraindications for its use, a fibrinolytic agent is given to abort the infarction, along with aspirin, heparin and a beta blocker, as per established advanced life support (ALS) guidelines. An initial nondiagnostic ECG will prompt blood tests for serial cardiac enzymes (using bedside diagnostic kits for myoglobin, CK-MB and troponin I) and serial ECGs. If a diagnosis of acute myocardial infarction can be made, fibrinolytic therapy is then reconsidered. If all tests are negative over a 6–8 h observation period and the patient is symptom-free, he or she can be released from the infirmary and advised to limit physical activity until re-evaluated the following day.

Cruise Ship Telemedicine

Although often viewed as a recent development, telemedicine has been used for decades to extend the reach of medical experts. The current state-of-the-art real-time videoconferencing is at one end of the telemedicine spectrum—very complex, very expensive. Near the other end are the less complex, less expensive applications. With respect to the maritime industry, these include the signal flag, the two-way radio, the satellite telephone/fax and more recently the Internet.

Telemedicine allows the often isolated cruise ship physician and nurse to consult with a specialist concerning a perplexing diagnosis or difficult case management. It also allows the ship's medical staff to provide consultation services to others in need. A few of the newer cruise ships have the capability for real-time videoconferencing but its utilization has been limited. Qualified cruise ship physicians can manage most cases that they are presented with, and most consultations can be done over a radio or satellite telephone. If graphical information (ECG, photographs) is requested by the consultant, it can be sent via fax or e-mail. A particularly useful shipboard telemedicine component is the digitized radiograph. The radiograph can be sent over the Internet via satellite to a radiologist anywhere in the world for either a primary diagnostic reading or as part of a quality management program. Regardless of what telemedicine modality is available on board a particular ship, it should be considered merely as a communications tool that can be used to enhance the medical services aboard ship. It must never be viewed as a substitute for a qualified and experienced cruise ship medical staff.

REFERENCES

American College of Emergency Physicians (1997) *Health Care Guidelines for Cruise Ship Medical Facilities.* ACEP, Washington DC.

Bruce D, Golding JF, Hockenhull N *et al.* (1990) Acupressure and motion sickness. *Aviation, Space and Environmental Medicine*, **61**, 361–365.

CDC (1998a) Outbreak of influenza A infection: Alaska and the Yukon Territory, June–July 1998. *Morbidity and Mortality Weekly Report*, **47**, 638.

CDC (1998b) Outbreak of influenza A infection: Alaska and the Yukon Territory, June–August 1998. *Morbidity and Mortality Weekly Report*, **47**, 685–688.

CDC (1999) *Preliminary Guidelines for the Prevention and Control of Influenza-Like Illness Among Passemgers and Crew Members on Cruise Ships.* Centers for Disease Control, Atlanta GA.

CDC (2008a) CDC Surveillance summaries, March 17, 2000. Surveillance for foodborne-disease outbreaks: United States, 1993–1997. *Morbidity and Mortality Weekly Report*, **49** (no. SS-1).

CDC (2000b) *Vessel Sanitation Program Operations Manual.* Centers for Disease Control, Atlanta, GA.

CDC (2001) Diagnosis and management of foodborne illnesses: a primer for physicians. *Morbidity and Mortality Weekly Report*, **50** (no. RR-2).

Dahl E (1999) Anatomy of a world cruise. *Journal of Travel Medicine*, **6**, 168–171.

Gahlinger P (1999) Motion Sickness, How to Help Your Patients Treat Travel Travail. *Postgraduate Medicine*, **106**, 177–184.

Gahlinger P (2000) Cabin location and the likelihood of motion sickness in cruise ship passengers. *Journal of Travel Medicine*, **7**, 120–124.

Hain TC, Hanna PA and Rheinberger MA (1999) Mal de debarquement. *Archives of Otolaryngology—Head and Neck Surgery*, **125**, 615–620.

Health Canada (1998) Influenza A outbreak on a cruise ship. *Canada Communicable Disease Report*, **24**, 9–11.

Hu S (1995) P6 acupressure reduces symptoms of vection-induced motion sickness. *Aviation, Space and Environmental Medicine*, **66**, 631–634.

Koo D (1993) Epidemiology of diarrheal disease outbreaks on cruise ships, 1986 through 1993. *Journal of the American Medical Association*, **275**, 545–547.

McCaig L (2000) National Hospital Medical Care Survey: 1998 Emergency Department Summary. Advance Data NCHS 313. National Center for Health Statistics, Hyattsville, MD.

Peake D (1999) Descriptive epidemiology of injury and illness among cruise ship passengers. *Annals of Emergency Medicine*, **33**, 67–72.

Udani J (1998) Ginger for motion sickness, hyperemesis gravidarum and anesthesia. *Alternative Medicine Alert*, **1**(12): 133–144.

US Department of Health and Human Services, Public Health Services, FDA (1999) *Food Code.* USDHHS, Washington DC.

ADDITIONAL RESOURCES

Useful Addresses

American College of Emergency Physicians
Section of Cruise Ship and Maritime Medicine
PO Box 619911
Dallas, TX 75261-9911, USA
+ 1 800 798 1822
www.acep.org

American Society of Tropical Medicine and Hygiene
60 Revere Drive, Suite 500
Northbrook, IL 60062, USA
+ 1 847 480 9592
www.astmh.org

Centers for Disease Control and Prevention
1600 Clifton Road
Atlanta, GA 30333, USA
+ 1 800 311 1345, 404 639 3534
Traveler's Hotline 877 394 8747
www.cdc.gov

Health Canada
AL 0904A
Ottawa, K1A 0K9, Canada
+ 1 613 957 2991
www.hc-sc.gc.ca

International Association for Medical Assistance to
Travellers
Regal Road
Guelph, Ontario N1K1B5, Canada
+ 1 519 836 0102
www.iamat@sentex.net

International Association for Medical Assistance to
Travellers (USA)
417 Center Street
Lewiston, NY 14092, USA
+ 1 716 754 4883

International Council of Cruise Lines
2111 Wilson Boulevard 8th Floor
Arlington, VA 22201, USA
+ 1 703 522 8463
www.iccl.org

International Maritime Health Association
Italielei 51
B-2000 Antwerp, Belgium
+ 32 3 229 07 76
www.semm.org/IMHA/IMHA.html

International Maritime Organization
4 Albert Embankment
London SE1 7SR, UK
+ 44 020 7735 7611
www.imo.org

International Society of Travel Medicine
PO Box 871089
Stone Mountain, GA 30087-0028, USA
+ 1 770 736 6732
www.istm.org

Pan American Health Organization
(WHO Regional Office)
525 23rd Street, NW
Washington, DC 20037, USA
+ 1 202 974 3000

US State Department Travel Warnings
+ 1 202 647 5225
http://travel.state.gov/travel_warnings.html

Wilderness Medical Society
3595 E. Fountain Blvd. Suite A1
Colorado Springs, CO 80910, USA
+ 1 719 572 9255
www.wms.org

World Health Organization
Avenue Appia 20
1211 Geneva 27, Switzerland
+ 41 22 791 21 11
www.who.ch

**Health Care Guidelines for Cruise Ship Medical
Facilities** (Reproduced by permission from
American College of Emergency Physicians, 1997)

The American College of Emergency Physicians believes
that appropriate emergency care and health care maintenance for passengers and crew members aboard ships
sailing in international waters are desirable. The cruise
ship industry and its medical departments should retain
medical personnel who can:

- Provide quality maritime medical care for passengers
  and crew members aboard cruise ships.
- Initiate appropriate stabilization, diagnostic and therapeutic maneuvers for the critically ill or medically unstable patient.
- Support, comfort and care for patients on board ship.
- Assist, in conjunction with the cruise line, the medical
  evacuation of patients in a timely fashion when appropriate.

Health Care Guidelines for Cruise Ship Medical Facilities: Policy Resource and Education Paper (PREP)

The specific medical needs of a cruise ship are dependent
on variables such as ship size, itinerary, patient (passenger
and crew) demographics, number of medical facility visits,
etc. These factors will modify the applicability of these
guidelines, especially with regards to staffing, medical
equipment and the ship's formulary.

Medical care on cruise ships would be enhanced by
ensuring that cruise ships have:

1. A ship medical center with medical staff (physicians
   and registered nurses) on call 24 h a day, examination
   and treatment areas, and an inpatient medical holding
   unit adequate for the size of the ship.
   A medical center with adequate space for diagnosis
   and treatment of passengers and crew members with
   360° patient accessibility around all beds/stretchers
   and adequate space for storage.
   - One examination/stabilization room per ship
   - One intensive care room per ship
   - Minimum number of inpatient beds: 1 bed per 1000
     passengers and crew
   - Isolation room or the capability to provide isolation
     of patients
   - Access by wheelchair and stretcher
   - Wheelchair-accessible toilet on all new builds de-
     livered after January 1, 1997
2. Physicians with:
   - Current medical licensure
   - 3 years of postmedical school clinical practice
   - Board certification in: emergency medicine, family
     practice, internal medicine, or general practice and
     emergency medicine experience
   - Competent skill level in advanced life support and
     cardiac care

- Minor surgical skill (i.e. suturing, incision and drainage of abscesses, etc.)
3. A medical staff:
   - Fluent in the official language of the cruise line
   - Fluent in English
   - Maintaining well-organized and legible standardized documentation of all medical care
4. Emergency medical equipment, medications and procedures:

   Equipment
   - Airway equipment: bag valve mask, pocket mask, endotracheal tubes, stylet, lubricant, vasoconstrictor, portable suction equipment
   - Cardiac monitor and back-up monitor (total of two)
   - Defibrillator (portable), total of two, one of which may be a semiautomatic defibrillator
   - External cardiac pacing capability
   - Electrocardiograph
   - Infusion pump
   - Pulse oximeter
   - Nebulizer
   - Automatic or manual respiratory support equipment
   - Oxygen (including portable oxygen)
   - Wheelchair
   - Stair chair and stretcher
   - Refrigerator/freezer
   - Long and short back boards, cervical spine immobilization equipment
   - Trauma cart supplies

   Medications
   - Emergency/code cart medications and supplies for management of common medical emergencies that include sufficient quantities of advanced life support medications for the management of two complex cardiac arrests

   Procedures
   - Medical operations manual as required by International Safety Management Code requirements
   - Medical staff orientation to the medical center
   - Maintenance for all medical equipment
   - Code team trained and updated regularly
   - Mock codes as recommended by the ship's physician
   - Emergency preparedness plan as required by the International Safety Management Code
5. Basic laboratory and X-ray capabilities:
   - Hemoglobin/hematocrit estimations, urinalysis, pregnancy test, blood glucose (all test procedures with a quality control program as recommended by the manufacturer).

     (*Modern cruise ships are now often equipped with a desktop laboratory and diagnostic kits that allow the medical staff to perform complete blood counts, blood chemistry testing, basic blood typing and cardiac enzyme evaluations.*)
   - X-ray machine for new builds delivered after January 1, 1997
6. A request for passengers to provide information regarding any personal medical conditions that may require attention aboard ship
7. A health, hygiene and safety program for medical personnel that includes an annual tuberculosis screening program.

Section V

Environmental Hazards of Travel

18

Travel-related Injury

Robert Grenfell

Grenfell Health Consulting Pty Ltd, Horsham, Australia

INTRODUCTION

Inherent in the desire to travel is the desire for new experience. The exposure to different surroundings and the excitement of the change itself yield the traveller to risks of unfamiliar proportion. All too often a journey ends prematurely as the result of injury. This chapter provides an overview of current knowledge concerning travel-related injury, and provides a broad framework that can be used to minimise actively the occurrence and impact of injury.

EPIDEMIOLOGY

To analyse the epidemiology of travel-related injury one looks at morbidity and mortality studies to define the overall population status.

In the formative study by Hargarten (Hargarten *et al.*, 1991) of the deaths of 2463 American travellers over a 10 year period, it was found that 24% were caused by injury. Of these, motor vehicle crashes were the most common (27%), followed by drowning (16%). In an analysis of cases transported back to the USA by emergency medical air transport over a 3 year period (Hargarten and Bouc, 1993), 44% were due to injury. Over half of these were the result of motor vehicle accidents. Studies from other countries echo these data. The deaths of Scottish citizens abroad from associated injury have been measured at 21% (Paixo *et al.*, 1991). The deaths of Australians overseas have been quantified (Prociv, 1995): 35% cardiovascular, 18% injury and 2% infection. The deaths due to injury were mainly the result of motor vehicle accidents. Within Australia, the deaths of visitors to the state of Victoria were found to be due to cardiovascular disease (47%) and injury (19%) (Grenfell *et al.*, 1997). The injuries were mainly motor vehicle accidents; other causes were drowning, suicide or multitraumatic. Of overseas visitors admitted to a hospital in the Australian state of Queensland over a 12 month period (Nicol *et al.*, 1996), the main reason for admission was for injury and poisoning (38%). The other reasons were cardiovascular (12%), gastrointestinal (10%) and genitourinary (9%).

These studies present a tantalising glimpse of the magnitude of travel-related injury, but unfortunately they are at best fragmented. There are many surveys of health service utilisation that indicate that injury is a common event while travelling (Bewes, 1993); however the information is of an uncontrolled nature, and as such only offers snapshot views of morbidity and mortality. We await the larger scale controlled studies that will take into account the various exposure indices, such as length of stay or activities undertaken, and individual indices, such as age or sex. These types of studies, when combined with available population statistics, will allow injury rate calculation and a more in-depth account of injury mechanism.

As a consequence of the diversity of exposure and accident types, the epidemiology is poorly defined. This is not too dissimilar to all other areas of injury research, and indeed many areas of public health. There are difficulties in the definitions of both cases and injury types. Surveillance is fragmented, or even absent. Interventional studies are rare indeed.

In order to attempt to analyse travel-related injury it is necessary to utilise a risk-based approach. This involves risk identification and risk management. Risk can be sourced from the environment that the travellers are in, through to the individuals themselves. An individual has many variables, such as age and sex, activities planned, behaviours adopted, precautions taken and, most importantly, what their particular perception of risk is. The environment poses an infinite array of risks.

CASE-BASED APPROACH

As with other areas of public health where the data are limited, it is desirable to review issues on a case study format. To illustrate the case-by-case nature of injury, let us consider the following actual cases:

Principles and Practice of Travel Medicine. Edited by Jane N. Zuckerman.
© 2001 John Wiley & Sons Ltd.

1. A tourist awaits her bag at the luggage carousel at an airport. The bag weighs in excess of 30 kg. The ergonomics of the situation are very poor: a moving heavy load at shin height, the tourist with a bent back and an outstretched arm. A wrenched shoulder and an acute lumbar disc prolapse result. Conservative management of the back injury fails and spinal surgery is required.

2. A group of travellers on an organised coach tour elect to participate in an optional excursion canyoning with a suggested local operator. All are complete novices to the sport, but the activity includes guides and equipment. While they are deep in a ravine, heavy rains upstream cause flash flooding, with resulting confusion and chaos; 18 young tourists drown.

3. On a quiet river in Africa, canoeing close to shore, a tourist is unseated when a hippopotamus overturns the craft. In the resulting confusion the hippopotamus attacks and bites the tourist, killing him.

4. A couple of experienced divers are diving while on holiday with a small group operator. The dive concludes, and the boat returns to port. It is noted that the two divers are missing. Extensive search and rescue only finds fragments of diving equipment; the divers are never found.

5. A middle-aged tourist on a self-drive tour stops to climb a look-out. While descending he loses his footing and falls some 15 m. This results in serious head injuries and multiple fractures. The rescue response takes over 2 h to extract him and transport him to the nearest hospital.

6. Honeymooners on a self-directed trip decide on a white water rafting day tour. All safety equipment and guides are included. While passing through some rapids, one of the pair falls from the craft. Tossed about in the water, she strikes her shoulder heavily against some rocks, fracturing the humerus. A quick extraction from the water by the vigilant guide prevents further mishap.

7. Resting outside the clubhouse of a golf club, a visitor is struck on the head by a misdirected golf ball. The resultant skull fracture and loss of consciousness requires him to spend a few days in hospital and shortens his holiday.

The lesson from these cases is that travel-related injury is heavily reliant on individual and activity-related factors. From each of these cases it can be seen that there are a multitude of factors involved. There are two ways to view an accident: that it is the individual who is at fault and that he or she should change behaviour, or that the accident occurred as a systematic error and not as a single point event. Injury prevention research is directing attention away from the individual to the organisational level. Let us consider the issues involved in the above case examples:

1. The tourist with the back injury could be blamed for packing such a heavy suitcase and for not lifting it correctly. But what of the design of the luggage carou-sel? It presents the suitcase at a height too low for correct lifting, and it is also moving. Even consider the design of the suitcase. Why are they made so big and cumbersome?

2. Of the 18 deaths following a canyoning adventure, it could be said that inexperience in the participants was a major factor, and that the activity was dangerous and they were taking a risk. Were they warned of this risk? Why was the activity allowed in such dangerous weather conditions? Were there warning systems in place to signal the guides of impending flooding? Was there a disaster plan? The legal issues around this case could indicate corporate negligence, involving both the overall tour organiser and the activity organiser.

3. Hippos are dangerous. Do all tourists know this? Why was an unsuspecting paddler allowed so close to one?

4. The diving case highlights the problem of lack of attention to procedures. When this case occurred the press suggested that the victims were part of a suicide pact. The inquest into the deaths found the dive operator negligent in not following correct occupational health and safety procedures.

5. Falls involving tourists are a frequent occurrence. Are we to blame the tourist for the fall because he was wearing inappropriate footwear, was fatigued or was unfit? What of the walkway itself: what type of surface was it, were the steps well placed, were the safety rails adequate? The rescue response was poor and required review.

6. White water rafting is often considered to be safe by tourists. How common are such events? Are tourists adequately warned of these? The rescue by the guide demonstrates a high level of competence.

7. There is a real danger around a golf course of being struck by an errant ball. Whose responsibility is it? The person struck, the hitter or the course management? Was any attempt made to minimise the occurrence of such an event, such as protective screens, or relocation of the rest area?

All these cases could be examined further. Examination can be systemised by the use of a framework: one that is particularly helpful is that illustrated in Figure 18.1. The terms used in the framework are easily explained.

• The context refers to the setting of the tourist activity, the environment and the individual.
• The identification of the risks requires a review of the available data, be that from morbidity and mortality data, case reports, service utilisation patterns or other available sources.
• To analyse the risks is to determine the mechanism of injury. What actually happened?
• An evaluation of the risk requires an appreciation of the frequency of that particular event, whether it has a high impact, and whether there is a simple solution.
• Treating the risk could involve a multitude of methods, from educational activities to engineering modifications.
• Most important is the continued monitoring and re-

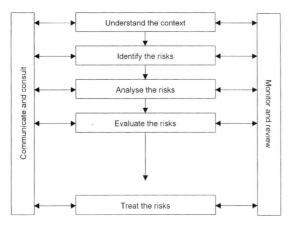

Figure 18.1 Australian/New Zealand standard framework for risk management. See text for explanation

view of the whole process, as with a disease surveillance system.
• Communication and consultation are also vital—with the individual, the tourist operator and any other relevant organisation.

The systematic analysis of each of the above cases would piece together what went wrong, identifying risks and areas that could be modified to reduce this risk.

Using the framework for case analysis starts with the analysis of existing morbidity and mortality data, from which is determined the pattern of injury. Injury mechanism is then determined, pertaining both to the individual and to the environment. From here, assumptions can be made on the causative factors for injury. A safety profile is then developed, so that reasonable action for risk reduction may be undertaken. To appreciate the process of developing strategies for specific problems relating to adverse health outcomes in the tourist setting, beach-related trauma and motor vehicle accidents will be considered in more detail.

Beach-related trauma

A visit to the beach is a common tourist activity. Consider this case study analysed using the risk management framework.

Risk Identification and Analysis

Two studies carried out on an Australian beach found the following (Grenfell and Ross, 1992; Grenfell, 1996): lacerations were very common, mostly to the feet but many to the head; drownings, near-drownings, ocean rescues, major limb fractures, joint dislocations, sunburn and various marine bites were occurring; the causes of injuries included rocks, litter and surfcraft; there were falls from walkways; and individuals were being caught in strong sea currents.

Utilising available beach usage data, a rate of injury was calculated at 100 per 100 000. This means that for every 1000 beach users, one person can expect to have to visit a doctor after the beach trip.

To add to the data from these studies, information related to various specific activities, such as drowning, ocean rescues, snorkelling and surfing, can be analysed. Drownings have been extensively studied (Manolios and Mackie, 1988) along the same region as the beach studies. This study found that the following features are common: male sex, consumption of alcohol and swimming alone outside patrolled beach areas. Ocean rescues occur more frequently outside patrolled areas, involve overseas visitors disproportionately, and occur more frequently in people who live more than 50 km from the coast (Short et al., 1991). A study of mortality reports of people who died while snorkelling (Edmonds and Walker, 1999) indicated a disproportionate number of overseas visitors, a lack of wearing of flippers and the absence of snorkelling with a 'buddy'. Surfing studies have indicated that collision with the rider's own board is a common source of laceration (Grenfell and Ross, 1992).

Risk Evaluation

High-impact risks ('nasty events') include those that result in death or hospitalisation. Frequent events are falls and cut feet. Simple preventative measures include using safety equipment that is already available, appropriate footwear, sunscreen and safety rails.

Treatment of Risk

This could include:

• Environmental factors—water currents, manmade structures such as walkways, natural hazards such as vegetation.
• Litter—control methods, collection, individual behaviours such as litter disposal and the wearing of footwear, fines for errant behaviour.
• Surfcraft—activity zones, board design, nose tips, helmets, education.
• Human factors—alcohol, overexertion, behavioural (attitude, bravado), lack of skills, education, protective apparel.
• Service provision—formal team approach, incorporation of beach safety into the planning phase of coastal developments, training, lifesavers, search and rescue, health infrastructure, first aid, emergency location systems, surveillance of service utilisation.
• Location—beach access, effective beach user traffic control, designation of water activity zones.
• Advertising—on a large scale by public education in

the press, at the airport, on the airline arrival video, in hotel brochures; or locally by the use of appropriate signs, delineating hazards.
• Education—of beach users, on hazard identification, beach behaviour and how to swim.

Communication and Consultation

In Australia, the bodies responsible for the management of the beach area include local management bodies (foreshore committee), regional authorities (Shire, State Government departments), national authorities (Federal Government), service providers (Surf Life Saving Association, medical colleges, ambulance service), regulatory bodies (consumer affairs). In response to a spate of beach drownings, a National Water Safety Council was formed and developed a national water safety strategy. Its success requires local action on the recommendations.

Monitoring and Review

If events and the circumstances of their occurrence are recorded, it is possible to determine trends in incidents and whether interventions have been effective. Sadly this is not occurring for beach-related injuries, nor is it on the agenda. It is essential for the refinement of beach injury control.

Motor Vehicle Accidents

Motor vehicle accidents emerge consistently as the most common cause of tourist death due to injury (Wilks, 1999). Let us consider an analysis of travel-related motor vehicle accidents in the context of the Australian state of Queensland, where a recent volume of research has been conducted.

Risk Identification

Using data from road crash investigations, hospital records and insurance claims, it was determined that over a 5 year period there were 39 fatalities and 397 hospitalisations of international drivers in Queensland (Wilks and Watson, 1998). Calculations of the social costs of road crashes determined that for the year 1997 these amounted to $A18 million. International visitors were more likely to be involved in head-on collisions.

Risk Analysis

The factors identified as contributing to motor vehicle accidents involving tourists were disorientation, fatigue, unfamiliarity with driving conditions and omitting to wear a seatbelt (Wilks and Watson, 1999a). Disorientation relates to the side of the road visitors drive on in their home country. Fatigue relates to the long distances travelled in Australia, compounded by jet lag and travel fatigue. The driving conditions vary: the road surface, the road signs, the presence of wildlife and other Australian nuances. Home country attitudes to alcohol use while driving and the wearing of seatbelts affect the tourist's compliance with Australian road laws. International literature confirms these factors as important sources of road accidents (Hargarten, 1991; Carey and Aitkin, 1996; Petridou et al., 1997, 1999).

Risk Evaluation

'Nasty events' need close attention; again, these are the events that lead to death or hospitalisation. Various strategies could be undertaken to minimise the risks. Increasing the use of seatbelts, minimising disorientation, tackling fatigue and increasing awareness of differences in road conditions could be included in national road safety initiatives for all road users, not just for tourists.

Treatment of Risk

This could include:

• Advice and driver education. Predeparture advice could consist of a discussion of the effects of medication, alcohol and jet lag on driving; the use of seatbelts; and the use of rest stops to counter fatigue. On collection of the hire vehicle there could be a screening of a video highlighting vehicle safety. A familiarisation programme of the vehicle to be hired could be conducted at the time of its collection.
• Placing stickers in the vehicle could be used to prompt the use of seatbelts. One initiative could involve engine immobilisers that cut the engine if the driver's seatbelt is not fastened.
• Hiring well-maintained vehicles with accepted safety features such as advanced braking systems and air bags. In-vehicle satellite navigation systems reduce driver distraction considerably.
• For off-road and remote driving, the supply of detailed manuals, first-aid kits and satellite locaters is sensible.
• Emergency services need to be maintained and well funded to assist in the rapid response to crashes.
• Tourists need to purchase insurance cover that will provide for medical assistance and rescue.

Communication and Consultation

In the Queensland case, a state government inquiry into the international road crash issue was held. This forum allowed medical specialists, accident researchers, tour operators, and representatives from the insurance industry and government departments of transport and tourism to discuss issues involving international visitors and road safety. Continued dialogue between these parties could lead to the development and implementation of many safety initiatives. A review was published after the forum (Wilks and Watson, 1999b).

Monitoring and Review

Ongoing monitoring of the situation can be conducted by accident research centres, analysing crash reports, coroners' reports, road mortality and morbidity data and insurance claims.

CONCLUDING REMARKS

Use of the management framework allows for an integrated approach to risk management. It relies on best-available evidence-based actions, allows input from the various stakeholders, from the tourist to the operator, and can be nationally coordinated with policy support. What it demonstrates is the multifaceted causation of injuries and how a systematic approach can lead to rational and evidence-based responses.

Areas of action that can be taken when considering travel-related injury are discussed below.

Travel Health Physician

The basic provision of structured injury prevention and risk minimisation advice is paramount; this includes the determination of the risks apparent from a detailed account of the traveller's proposed itinerary and any particular health conditions that he or she may have:

- Highlight the consequences of risk exposure.
- Strengthen the advice with brief, to the point, written material.
- Advise pertinent preventative actions: for example, travel with an organised tour group if undertaking adventure activities (with a reputable organisation, standards would be expected to be higher, and risks correspondingly reduced); hire a car and a driver; wear protective equipment; do not mix alcohol with physical activities; seek local safety information, e.g. fire escapes, safe areas to swim.
- Explain the value of travel insurance, as medical evacuations are expensive and access to high-quality health services is often limited, due to language, knowledge, distance from centres, and infrastructure deficiency.

Travel health physicians are in an ideal position to continue research into specific travel injury risks. Much information is needed on the incidence, rate and causation of travel-related injury, as is more information on effective proven strategies to reduce the injury caseload.

Tourism Industry

This includes all levels of the industry, from the individual operator to the regional authorities. Guidelines for the risk management of a tourist activity or a tourist site development should minimise risk at the planning stage. There must be an assessment of the impact of the development on safety. Safety plans need to be prepared, specifying safety resources to match predicted usage patterns, identifying problem areas and controlling the risks. Users and service providers need education about risks and preventative strategies. Litigious exposure should be minimised.

There is a requirement for the development of standards of operation that include safety mapping, entailing the audit of safety risks, management of these risks and maintenance of an injury register. This entails the development of a safety plan and direct action on it. All too often the best intentions still lead to inactivity. Incidents need investigating, which is certainly a process that occurs in many other industries, from which many important lessons can be learned for refinement of risk control. Management of legal risk is essential, and legal security is part of a complete risk management programme (Grenfell and Ranson, 1997) that is often referred to as loss control. Indeed, changes in insurance premiums can often produce changes in attitude and actions of errant operators: as the number of claims increase, so does the premium.

Insurance Industry

Travel insurance packages must provide broader cover. The 'small print' needs to be large, so that travellers know what is and is not covered, and can then make an informed decision about purchasing the appropriate policy.

Older travellers are increasing in number and, more than any other group, need insurance cover. The habit of not covering existing medical conditions is nonsensical. For example, an 80-year-old man with ischaemic heart disease is likely to experience a cardiac event, so he should be encouraged to cover such an event and should be able to obtain a reasonably priced policy to do so.

The adventure traveller needs specialised cover that includes the activities to be undertaken. It is all too easy to say 'rock climbing not included' but, when that is the purpose of the trip, the insurance broker must be able to provide an adjusted policy that does cover rock climbing. The exclusion of motor cycle riding (either in defined areas or as a blanket clause) by a number of policies may act as a deterrent for many travellers—that is, if they are aware of the exclusion. But what of the traveller who has no other option to a motorcycle as a means of transport? There should be a policy variation to cover this situation.

Governments

Many countries rely heavily on tourism for revenue; in

Australia, for example, tourism is a major industry employing over 6.9% of the workforce and generating over $A46.9 billion (Department of Industry, Science and Tourism, 1996). It would therefore seem obvious that it is very important to protect the industry by the provision of adequate health and safety management. This is not the case. It seems absurd that health and safety in tourism settings are not regarded with as much importance as they are in the mining industry. Government departments need to focus on health and safety management in tourism, with legislation providing a backbone for operation. This would include the enforcement of codes of conduct and the prosecution of unsafe practices. Planning is necessary for the designation of specified activity zones. With each new tourist area developed, consideration of the safety implications is required. Placing a resort in an isolated area next to a serious hazard, for example a beach that is unsafe for swimming, is a reason for concern, raising questions about adequate monitoring of water activities and how serious mishaps are to be managed. The service infrastructure is vital in such cases. Not only does this cover the provision of adequate transport but it should also provide for appropriate rescue services, evacuation services, primary treatment facilities, and so on.

SUMMARY

Injuries associated with travel are very common but the exact nature and incidence is not precisely known; however, in order to appreciate the risks of a specific activity, it is possible to analyse it with a generic framework. Injury prevention requires a systems approach, attempting to identify process errors, as there are usually a multitude of causative factors for each particular injury. It must be remembered that in cases of injury it is all too easy to blame the individual, when very often it is not the individual's fault.

REFERENCES

Bewes P (1993) Trauma and accidents: practical aspects of the prevention and management of trauma associated with travel. British Medical Bulletin, 49, 454–464.

Carey M and Aitken M (1996) Motorbike injuries in Bermuda: a risk for tourists. Annals of Emergency Medicine, 28, 424–429.

Department of Industry, Science and Tourism (1996) Impact: Tourism Facts. DIST, Canberra.

Edmonds C and Walker D (1999) Snorkelling deaths in Australia, 1987–1996. Medical Journal of Australia, 171, 591–594.

Grenfell R (1996) Beach related injuries. Medical Journal of Australia, 166, 390.

Grenfell RD and Ranson D (1997) Tourism and recreational injuries. Journal of Law and Medicine, 4.

Grenfell R and Ross K (1992) How dangerous is that visit to the beach? A pilot study of beach injuries. Australian Family Physician, 23, 1145–1148.

Grenfell R, Ranson D and Hargarten S (1997) Mortality of visitors to Victoria Australia. In Proceedings of an ISTM conference, Geneva.

Hargarten SW (1991) International travel and motor vehicle crash deaths: the problem, risks, and prevention. Travel Medicine International, 106–110.

Hargarten S and Bouc G (1993) Emergency air medical transport of US citizen tourists: 1988 to 1990. Air Medicine Journal, 12, 398–402.

Hargarten S, Baker T and Guptill K (1991) Overseas fatalities of United States citizen travellers: an analysis of deaths related to international travel. Annals of Emergency Medicine, 20, 622–626.

Manolios N and Mackie I (1988) Drowning and near-drowning on Australian beaches patrolled by life-savers: a 10 year study, 1973–83. Medical Journal of Australia, 148, 165–171.

Nicol J, Wilks J and Wood M (1996) Tourists as inpatients in queensland regional hospitals. Australian Health Review, 19(4), 55–72.

Paixao M, Dewar R, Cossar J et al. (1991) What do Scots die from abroad? Scottish Medical Journal, 36, 114–116.

Petridou E, Askitopoulou H, Vourvahakis D et al. (1997) Epidemiology of road traffic accidents during pleasure travelling: the evidence from the island of Crete. Accident Analysis and Prevention, 29, 687–693.

Petridou E, Dessypris N, Skalidou A et al. (1999) Are traffic injuries disproportionately more common among tourists in Greece? Struggling with incomplete data. Accident Analysis and Prevention, 31, 611–615.

Prociv P (1995) Deaths of Australian travellers overseas. Medical Journal of Australia, 163, 27–30.

Short A, May A and Hogan C (1991) A three year study into the circumstances behind surf based rescues. NSW Beach Safety Program Report 91. Sydney Coastal Studies Unit, University of Sydney.

Wilks J (1999) International tourists, motor vehicles and road safety. Journal of Travel Medicine, 6, 115–121.

Wilks J and Watson B (1998) Road safety and international visitors in Australia: looking beyond the tip of the iceberg. Travel Medicine International, 16, 194–198.

Wilks J and Watson B (1999a) International drivers in unfamiliar surroundings: the problem of disorientation. Travel Medicine International, 17.

Wilks J, Watson B and Hansen R (1999b) International Visitors and Road Safety in Australia: A Status Report. Australian Transport Safety Bureau, Canberra.

19

Aeromedical Repatriation

Alex T. Dewhurst and John C. Goldstone

Middlesex Hospital, London, UK

INTRODUCTION

The increase in foreign travel, the rise in holidays to exotic locations and the enthusiasm for adventure holidays has led to an increase in the requirements for medical repatriation services in the last decade. An ageing population with increased disposable income is expected to lead to a rise in the number of air ambulance transfers each year. People who fall ill or have an accident abroad can be repatriated to the UK by a number of methods:

- They may organise their own transport, either alone or with an escort.
- They may travel on a scheduled flight with a doctor or nurse escort.
- They may require an air ambulance on a scheduled flight or chartered aircraft.

In the region of 3000 patients a year are repatriated on scheduled airline services with a nurse escort and there are approximately 900–1000 air ambulance transfers into the UK per annum (Morton *et al.*, 1997). In Europe, the German Air Rescue service has shown a steady increase in the number of flights, from 322 in 1976, 704 in 1983 to 1468 in 1993 (Kramer *et al.*, 1996). This chapter will focus on the logistics and problems associated with air ambulance transfers.

MEDICAL TRANSFERS

The medical transfer of a patient can be designated as primary or secondary: primary transfer is from the scene of injury or illness to the initial treating hospital; secondary transfer is the movement of a patient from one hospital to another for medical or social reasons. All cases of medical repatriation should be deemed secondary transfers, although some may be undertaken with a degree of urgency and without definitive treatment having been performed. In the majority of cases, patients will have been treated in countries in which the health care facilities are of a good standard. In these situations transfer usually occurs once the patient has been fully stabilised and all urgent therapy initiated. However, these patients may still require a high degree of supportive therapy, including intensive care. In countries where the health care resources are felt to be inadequate, the patient may be transferred back to the UK at an earlier stage of the illness. In some cases the air ambulance team may need to institute resuscitative and supportive procedures before the patient is deemed fit to fly. In the rare situation where medical care is completely inadequate or unavailable, a primary rescue flight may need to be undertaken. Occasionally the patient may be transferred locally to a region or country that can provide the required resources. If communications are difficult and the clinical situation is not clear, a doctor may be flown out to assess the patient and decide if transfer is required.

All transfers place the patient at some risk, and poorly conducted transfers have been shown to be detrimental to outcome (Waddell, 1975; Gentleman and Jennett, 1981; Bion *et al.*, 1988). The risk of transfer should be balanced against the risk of deterioration in a suboptimal environment. For an escorted scheduled flight, the patient's condition should be unlikely to deteriorate, not contagious, not disturbing to other passengers, require minimum nursing or medical care and the patient should be able to travel seated. If the patient requires high-dependency or intensive care or needs to be transported on a stretcher, an air ambulance transfer should be performed either via a scheduled carrier or in a chartered jet. The use of a scheduled flight or chartered aircraft will depend on the clinical condition, the distance to travel, the availability of flights and the conditions stipulated by the carrier. Approximately 90% of stretcher cases are transported on small chartered aircraft (Kramer *et al.*, 1996).

Organisation of Repatriation Services

Air ambulance flights are expensive. Prices quoted vary from £5000 to £19 000 to return from Mediterranean countries, £35 000 to £50 000 from Africa and £60 000

Table 19.1 Factors involved in making the decision to repatriate

- Health care facilities at the treating unit
- Patients condition and progress
- Expected duration of treatment and level of expertise available
- Potential detrimental effects of transport
- Potential risk to the patient if not transferred
- Availability of aircraft
- Availability of beds within UK, particularly intensive care beds

Table 19.2 People involved in making the decision to repatriate

- Referring doctor
- Assistance company doctor
- Receiving doctor
- Air ambulance company
- Air ambulance escorting doctor and nurse
- General practitioner in the UK
- Relatives, next of kin or legal guardian

from the USA. However, these prices should be balanced against the cost of health care itself, particularly the cost abroad of major procedures and intensive care therapy. Fortunately, most people carry health insurance while travelling. On each insurance document is a telephone number to contact in case of a problem. This is the number of an assistance company, the first point of contact the patient or relative makes with the repatriation services. There are approximately 20 major assistance companies within the UK. They provide a 24 h telephone service and aid in organising logistical support for anyone with a problem abroad. In the event of an air ambulance being required, a quarter of the assistance companies provide their own in-house service; the remainder will subcontract to a company that supplies repatriation services. There are four major repatriation service providers within the UK, and numerous smaller operators. There are also European air ambulance companies available, some of which are subsidised by governmental ambulance systems.

Deciding When to Repatriate a Patient

The decision to repatriate depends on medical, social and political factors (Table 19.1). The assistance company will have a medical director—either a consultant or general practitioner with experience in repatriation. It is the duty of the medical director, or the deputy, to liaise with the treating and the receiving hospital medical staff. If an air ambulance company is involved, they will have their own medical staff in the communication loop (Figure 19.1), with separate responsibility for care of the patient during transport. In an ideal world there would be a complete assessment and discussion of the case between all medical parties involved and the final decision to repatriate would be made at consultant level or the equivalent (Table 19.2). However, in reality many problems are encountered. There are difficulties in communication and language, and in some cases disagreement on patient management. Social factors also come into play. There is a question of finance: will the insurance cover the cost of transport or will the repatriation be undertaken privately? If privately, financial securities are required before initiation of an air ambulance and this causes delays. The patient's expectations of being repatriated may not agree with the insurance company's views. Social reasons for repatriation can be an expectation of a long period of therapy, a language barrier, lack of nursing care, problems with diet and climate. Most patients prefer to be in a familiar environment where their family and friends are close and can provide emotional support. It is likely that the rate of recovery and the incidence of complications such as in-

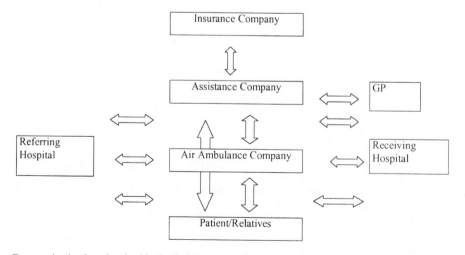

Figure 19.1 Communication loop involved in the decision to transfer a patient

Table 19.3 Physical changes associated with increasing altitude

Altitude (feet)	Pressure (kPa)	Gas volume (litres)	P_AO_2 breathing air (kPa)
0	101	1	14
5 000 (1 500)	84	1.2	10
8 000 (2 400)	75	1.35	8.5
10 000 (3 000)	70	1.44	8.4
20 000 (6 000)	46	2	5
38 000 (11 600)	21	5	NA

Values in parentheses are metres.
NA = not applicable.

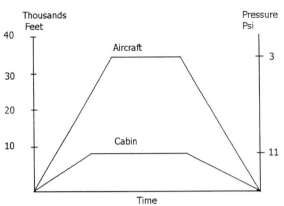

Figure 19.2 Cabin versus aircraft altitude

tensive care psychosis may be affected by factors that reduce communication between patient and medical staff. It is hard to motivate a patient who cannot understand what you are saying!

PHYSICS AND PHYSIOLOGY OF AIR TRAVEL

The density of the atmosphere decreases exponentially with altitude. With increasing altitude there is a drop in the molecular concentration of gas particles, expansion of gas volume and a reduction in pressure (Table 19.3). These physical changes can lead to alterations in the physiological status of patients during aeromedical repatriations (Ernsting *et al.*, 1999).

Pressure Changes

Air ambulance flights are carried out in turboprop or subsonic jet aircraft that fly at altitudes of between 25 000 and 40 000 feet. To allow the occupants to breath air and move freely within the cabin, the aircraft is pressurised. There are a variety of terms used to describe aircraft cabin pressure. The absolute cabin pressure is the internal pressure within the cabin itself. Atmospheric pressure is the outside atmospheric pressure at the altitude at which the aircraft is flying. The cabin differential pressure is the difference between the external and internal pressures:

Cabin differential pressure = cabin pressure − atmospheric pressure

During ascent the pressure within the cabin falls until it reaches a predetermined minimum absolute cabin pressure, usually described in terms of equivalent cabin altitude (Figure 19.2). As the aircraft climbs further, the cabin altitude is maintained and a cabin differential pressure results between the internal cabin pressure and the external atmospheric pressure. The cabin differential pressure reaches a maximum at the operational ceiling of the

aircraft. The aircrew can adjust the cabin differential pressure during flight. If the aircraft is flying below its operational ceiling, increasing the cabin differential to its maximum will maintain a low cabin altitude and will minimise the effects of altitude-related environmental changes. Air ambulance cabin altitudes range from 6000 to 8000 feet (1800–2400 m); the absolute cabin pressure therefore ranges between 81 kPa (609 mmHg, 11.8 p.s.i.) to 72 kPa (543 mmHg, 10.5 p.s.i.).

The most important features of this pressure change that affect patient physiology during ascent are:

1. The rate of change in cabin pressure. This determines the rate of volume change within gas-filled cavities. It is described in terms of rate of climb or descent. Ascent is usually better tolerated than descent and in commercial aircraft the rate of descent of cabin altitude is kept below 300 feet (90 m) per minute, which is less that the actual rate of descent of the aircraft.
2. The end cabin altitude [maximum 8000 feet (2400 m)], which determines total volume of gas expansion and the drop in partial pressure of oxygen.
3. The final aircraft altitude, which determines the degree to which cabin pressure must fall and also the effects of accidental loss of cabin pressure (see below).

Hypobaric Hypoxia

During ascent through the atmosphere there is a fall in density of air and a reduction in the molecular concentration of oxygen. This in turn leads to a fall in the partial pressure of oxygen within the lung, and hence the blood. At 8000 feet (2400 m), atmospheric pressure is reduced by 25%, from 101 kPa to 75 kPa. The alveolar partial pressure of oxygen (P_AO_2) drops from 14 kPa to 8.5 kPa. There is minimal effect on the physiology of fit individuals, other than some minor reversible deterioration in mental performance for novel tasks, detected on psychometric tests. The patient's susceptibility to hypoxia depends on the underlying cardiopulmonary function, intercurrent disease, physical activity and metabolic rate. The drop in partial pressure of oxygen at cabin altitudes of 8000 feet (2400 m) is sufficient to cause tissue hypoxia and the development of symptoms in patients with reduced cardiopulmonary reserve. The physiological response to this hypoxia is to increase ventilation, which leads to a reduction in alveolar carbon dioxide and a rise in alveolar oxygen tension. This is explained by the simplified alveolar gas equation:

$$P_AO_2 = P_IO_2 - P_ACO_2/RQ$$

where P_AO_2 is the alveolar oxygen tension, P_IO_2 is the tracheal oxygen tension, P_ACO_2 is the alveolar carbon dioxide tension and RQ is the respiratory quotient. In extreme cases, the degree of hyperventilation and hypocapnia can itself induce a separate group of symptoms.

Gas Expansion

Boyle's law states that the volume of a gas is inversely proportional to its absolute pressure; therefore, as atmospheric pressure falls with ascent, gas expands (Table 19.3). In the pressurised aircraft, cabin ascent to an altitude of 8000 feet (2400 m) leads to gas volume increasing by 35%. This gas expansion can affect the gas-filled body cavities, depending on the degree with which they communicate with the external environment. The lungs, middle ear, paranasal sinuses and the gastrointestinal tract are all potential problem areas. In a fit individual there are few problems with this degree of gas expansion, other than mild middle-ear discomfort. However, certain conditions may become significantly worse and even life threatening with this change in volume. Patients with pneumothoracies, pneumocephalus, severe bowel distension or obstructed middle ears should be taken to altitude with caution.

Acceleration/Deceleration

During take off and landing, patients laying flat maybe exposed to forces of acceleration in the longitudinal (G_z) plane of the body. Acceleration describes the rate of change of velocity of an object and can be positive $(+ G_z)$ or negative, sometimes described as deceleration $(- G_z)$. In aviation, acceleration is expressed as multiples of the force of acceleration exerted on a body by gravity (g) which is equal to $9.8\,m\,s^{-2}$:

$$G = applied\ acceleration/g$$

The effects of G on the body depend on duration and direction. Short or intermediate duration forces are those associated with an abrupt deceleration, such as vehicle crashes. Long duration accelerations of more than 2 s occur mainly in military aircraft. In commercial aircraft, linear acceleration seldom reach magnitudes of any sig-

nificance, especially in the seated patient. The horizontal patient is unlikely to experience forces greater than 1–2 $+ G_z$ on take off in a small subsonic jet. In the fit volunteer, a force of 4–6 $+ G_z$ is required to experience grey-out (loss of peripheral vision), black-out (total loss of vision) and G-LOC (G-related loss of consciousness). These are manifestations of reduced perfusion of the retina and brain as a result of the effects of hydrostatic forces on the cardiovascular system. There is also a progressive fall in mean arterial pressure at the level of the heart over 6–12 s, due to a decrease in peripheral vascular resistance and reduction cardiac return. A compensatory reflex tachycardia and vasoconstriction then occurs in response to reduced pressure in the carotid sinus.

The critically ill patient may be volume depleted, vasodilated, possess a poor myocardium and have a depressed sympathetic response due to drugs or pathology. In such cases even the relatively small acceleration forces experienced combined with the 45° head-up tilt of take off may be enough to cause a deterioration in cardiovascular function. This is easily prevented by adequate monitoring and volume loading before take off.

Deceleration forces may cause increased blood flow to the head and neck, leading to carotid sinus distension. Reflex bradycardias and other arrhythmias have been reported in experimental situations with high G forces. Once again, it is unlikely that the forces experienced in commercial aircraft are great enough to cause these problems.

Cabin Decompression

Cabin decompression is a rare event that can occur rapidly or slowly. A rapid decompression can be explosive in nature when a major defect occurs in the aircraft frame. It results in a near normal environment being quickly converted to an extreme environment, with lack of oxygen, cold and the effects of gas expansion putting the lives of patient and crew at risk. The effects of gas expansion depend on the cabin differential pressure, the altitude of the aircraft and the size of the defect in the aircraft frame in relation to the cabin volume. The medical risks from decompression are: rapid loss of consciousness from hypoxia, barotrauma to the middle ear or sinuses, inducement of a pneumothorax and altitude decompression sickness. In the event of a cabin decompression, oxygen masks are automatically released and the aircraft is brought to a lower altitude. Aircrew are advised to place their own oxygen mask on before helping others because of the risk of becoming incapacitated by hypoxia.

DETRIMENTAL EFFECTS OF TRANSPORT

The majority of medical transfers are simple escorted cases that pass off with the minimum of problems. Transporting critically ill patients is more difficult, requiring continuation of organ support and invasive monitoring.

Table 19.4 Defining a detrimental effect of transportation

- Deterioration in vital signs
  Change in vital signs by more than 20% from baseline
  Change outside 'normal' range for patient
- Mechanical, equipment or human error leading to an adverse effect on patient
  Airway, ventilator problems
  Handling, loading problems
  Loss of I.V. access, failure of infusion system
  Power failure
  Failure of oxygen supply
  Aircraft incidents

It has been shown that critical incidents, which have a detrimental effect on outcome, occur while moving these patients (Venkataraman and Orr, 1992). The environmental factors of flight mentioned in the previous section, factors associated with road transport and the logistics involved in moving the intensive care patient can all lead to adverse effects. These can be divided into major, requiring immediate intervention, and minor, leading to little disturbance to the patient. The causes can be defined as changes in physiology in response to transfer, leading to disturbed organ function and mechanical or equipment-related errors. It is difficult to stipulate when a change to physiology becomes detrimental and even harder to show a difference in outcome as a result of such a change. However, commonly used definitions of significant change are either movement from baseline vital signs by 20% or readings that fall outside the 'normal' range for the patient (Table 19.4).

SPECIFIC HAZARDS AND THEIR MANAGEMENT DURING TRANSPORT

Respiratory

- The reduced oxygen tension at altitude may lead to symptoms of hypobaric hypoxia. Arterial oxygen saturation should be monitored and supplementary oxygen administrated if indicated. If gas exchange is critical, the aircraft may have to fly at a lower altitude to maintain a sea-level cabin pressure.
- The dry atmosphere of the cabin may lead to thickening of bronchial secretion and paralysis of respiratory cilia. This can cause a deterioration in respiratory function, especially in patients whose natural humidification processes are bypassed by an artificial airway. The end-result maybe a spontaneously ventilating patient requiring mechanical ventilation (Armitage et al., 1990). Efforts should be made to humidify inspired gases using heat moisture exchange filters and nebulisers. Patients should receive regular chest physiotherapy, manual bagging and suction to clear secretions during transport.

- Gas expansion will increase the volume of pneumothoracies, which may lead to respiratory compromise. All pneumothoracies, or even suspected pneumothoracies, should be drained via an intercostal drain before ascent to altitude or the aircraft should maintain a sea-level cabin pressure. In trauma patients with fractured ribs there should be a low threshold for placing an intercostal drain. The use of a Heimlich valve rather than an underwater seal makes transfer simpler.
- Patients who are stable on mechanical ventilation are safe to transfer. However, caution is required if the inspired oxygen concentration is greater than 60%, lung inflation pressures are higher than 35 cmH$_2$O, or more than 10 cmH$_2$O of positive end-expiratory pressure (PEEP) is in use. In some cases a more sophisticated ventilator than the standard transport ventilator may be required. Consideration should be made to sedating and formally ventilating patients who are on a weaning mode of ventilation. Transferring a patient is thought to set weaning back by 1 day.
- Gas-filled endotracheal cuffs increase in volume with altitude and may cause tracheal mucosal ischaemia. They should be filled with saline or their pressures monitored regularly.
- Drugs and equipment should be available for treating respiratory emergencies.

Cardiovascular

- Cardiovascular events are the leading cause of death during air travel (Gong, 1992).
- Any movement and stimulation of critically ill patients may cause hypertensive or hypotensive episodes (Waddell, 1975). There are haemodynamic changes associated with air ambulance transport, possibly due to the effects of gravitational forces and hypoxia (Malagon et al., 1996). The force of acceleration on take off may cause a reduction in cardiac output, especially in patients who are volume depleted, vasodilated and have poor myocardial function. Adequate monitoring, including invasive arterial and central venous pressures, with institution of therapy to maintain haemodynamic stability may reduce such complications.
- Reduced inspired oxygen concentration may precipitate angina or heart failure. Oxygen should be administrated to these patients during flight.
- Despite the risks, unstable angina patients have been transferred over long distances by air. However they require intensive therapy unit level care, adequate monitoring and sedation (Castillo and Lyons, 1999).
- Any collections of mediastinal air will enlarge, potentially causing cardiovascular compromise.
- Patients on inotropic infusions are at risk of inadvertent changes in the rate of infusions. Pumps with alarms and short, stiff infusion lines should be used. Lines should be labelled and not used for boluses.

- Noninvasive blood pressure readings have been shown to underread systolic and overread diastolic pressures during transport. Direct methods of blood pressure readings should be used in critically ill patients (Runcie et al., 1990). The pressure transducer should be re-zeroed at altitude.
- There is an increased risk of thromboembolic events during flight because of dehydration and immobility (Cruickshank et al., 1988). Support stockings may be considered and heparin prophylaxis administrated unless contraindicated.

Gastrointestinal

- Motion sickness can be treated with prophylactic anti-emetics. Escorting staff should not suffer unduly from motion sickness.
- In the normal subject, gas expansion within the bowel causes little problem unless ascent is to altitudes greater than 25 000–28 000 feet (7600–8500 m). However, in patients with cardiorespiratory compromise and intestinal distension, even ascent up to moderate altitudes of 8000 feet (2400 m) can cause distress. Consideration should be given to restricting cabin altitude to less than 6000 feet (1800 m) in those patients with severe abdominal distension.
- Gastric distension and intestinal obstruction lead to an increased risk of aspiration of gastric contents. During transport, restricted access to the patient means that in the event of vomiting the oropharynx cannot be easily cleared. A nasogastric tube should be placed, aspirated and left on free drainage. Patients who have reduced airway protective reflexes should be considered for intubation.
- Gas expansion in the small and large bowel increases the risk of perforation in cases of severe bowel distension. There is a theoretical risk to surgical anastomoses.
- Air in the peritoneal cavity may expand and it is recommended that 10 days be allowed between abdominal surgery and transport in an aircraft not pressured to sea level.
- Ileus may be prolonged.
- Patients with abdominal or chest trauma should have no evidence of continuing intra-abdominal haemorrhage before transfer.
- Limited cleaning facilities make severe diarrhoea a major problem. Laxatives and suppositories should be avoided before travel.

Renal

- Patients receiving renal support should be dialysis 24 h before flight, aiming to have a normal electrolyte and fluid balance. Care must be taken to ensure normovolaemia.

- All critically ill patients need to be catheterised to allow monitoring of their urine output.

Neurological

- Head-injured patients should be managed to maintain cerebral perfusion pressures within a safe range: the ultimate aim being to prevent secondary brain injury. Standard guidelines for the management of head-injured patients during transport are followed (Gentleman et al., 1993).
- Patients with air in the skull or fractures through sinus cavities are at risk of gas expansion. This may lead to a tension pneumocephalus or the risk of bacterial meningitis. Following neurosurgery, flying other than at sea level should be delayed until CT shows no evidence of intracranial air.
- Patients with recent subarachnoid haemorrhages should preferably have had definitive surgery if the cause of bleeding is amenable to operative intervention and if expertise is available. If surgery has not been performed, the blood pressure must be adequately monitored and controlled. Infusions of nimodipine need to be continued. If an extraventricular drain is in situ it should be closely monitored during flight and turned off while the patient is moved.
- Patients with a spinal cord injury must be treated as if the injury is unstable, unless cleared by an orthopaedic or neurosurgeon. They are at increased risk of requiring ventilatory assistance and need to be transferred by a doctor able to institute mechanical ventilation (Armitage et al., 1990). Spinal shock and autonomic hyperreflexia should have been adequately treated.

TRANSFERRING PATIENTS WITH SPECIAL NEEDS

Paediatric/Neonatal Patients

Neonatal, infant and paediatric transfers require special consideration. These transfers are complicated by the smaller size of the patient, different physiology and pathology. Specialist equipment such as a transport incubator and neonatal ventilator are required. Personnel should be skilled in neonatal and paediatric intensive care. The medical crew should include at least one doctor, either a neonatal paediatrician or paediatric anaesthetist, and a nurse with neonatal experience. Many neonates are transferred to specialist units for management of congenital disorders; specific protocols for management are available.

Obstetric Patients

Scheduled airlines restrict the carriage of pregnant

women to those under 32–36 weeks of pregnancy, depending on the airline and the distance to be travelled. Obstetric patients may require an air ambulance transfer for standard medical or surgical reasons. Obstetric indications for air ambulance transfer are: complicated pregnancies in countries with poor health care facilities; and premature labour at gestation ages where neonates would be expected to survive if the neonatal facilities were adequate. Transfers maybe done before or after delivery.

These are complicated transfers involving two patients, incubator, neonatal staff and staff to care for the mother. If the mother is undelivered, precautions in these cases include supplementary oxygen at altitude, left lateral tilt to prevent aortocaval compression and antacid therapy. There is also the increased risk of thromboembolic events at all stages and prophylaxis should be given unless contraindicated.

Psychiatric Patients

Psychiatric patients are observed before flight long enough to assess their suitability for transfer. They can be categorised as patients who are cooperative and can travel as seated passengers, those who are not grossly disturbed but may react badly to travel, and those who are frankly disturbed. Patients in the last two groups may require sedation and adequate monitoring. They may even need to be moved as a stretcher cases, with heavy sedation and the additional escort of a registered psychiatric nurse.

OTHER PROBLEMS

Despite the environmental challenges faced by the patient during transfer, the majority of problems arising are due to logistic reasons rather a deterioration in the patient's condition, provided that the patient has been adequately assessed and prepared for the journey. In an unpublished audit of air ambulance transfers the most common problems encountered were untoward, and causes included:

- Human error
- Equipment failure, power failure
- Delay in ambulance or aircraft
- Problem with medical liaison and transfer of care of patient to transporting team
- Customs clearance for drugs and equipment
- Injury to medical staff, particularly in loading and unloading
- Aircraft problems, such as oil leaks, cabin decompression and other mechanical failures, some requiring emergency landing.

EQUIPMENT

All equipment taken should be robust, lightweight and battery powered. The minimal monitoring required for a ventilated critically ill patient is ECG, pulse oximetry, blood pressure and end-tidal carbon dioxide. All alarms should be visual and auditory. Two mechanical ventilators should be carried, together with a self-inflating bag for manual ventilation. The ventilators should have adjustable inspired oxygen concentration, variable tidal volumes and frequency. There should be a disconnection alarm, the ability to supply PEEP and to alter the inspiratory/expiratory ratio. The amount of oxygen carried should cover ventilation with an inspired oxygen concentration of 100% for the duration of the journey and with 1–2 h spare. In most countries, transporting road ambulances will carry oxygen.

Equipment and drugs need to be regularly checked and labelled ready for use. They should be comprehensive and packed in easy-access bags (Figure 19.3). For the average air ambulance a total of 12 bags or items are taken, together with 3–4 oxygen cylinders and the personal kit of the medical staff (Table 19.5).

AIRCRAFT

The ideal aircraft should have good access, fitted medical equipment, methods for loading and unloading, be comfortable and have reasonable speed and range (Figure 19.4). The type of aircraft used depends on availability, distance to travel and cost. Aircraft vary from twin prop Beechcraft King Air to small business jets such as the Lear 35 and HS125. In the UK most operators charter aircraft that are normally used for business purposes. They have little fitted medical equipment other than a stretcher, oxygen supply, suction and drip stand. Some air ambulance companies, particularly the European operators, have their own designated aircraft with fitted medical equipment, while others just have a fitted stretcher, with all other medical equipment carried as separate items. The Civil Aviation Authority (CAA) defines a dedicated air ambulance aircraft as one in which medical equipment has been installed permanently and has been approved by their inspectors. Other noninstalled equipment and supplies carried should comply with regulations and be securely stored during flight. The flight commander is in overall charge of the stowage and the decision to use medical equipment.

STAGES OF A STANDARD AIR AMBULANCE TRANSFER

Initial Information

Once contact has been established between the patient and assistance company, regular updates on the patient's condition are made. A decision is made on the optimal time for transfer and the air ambulance company contacted.

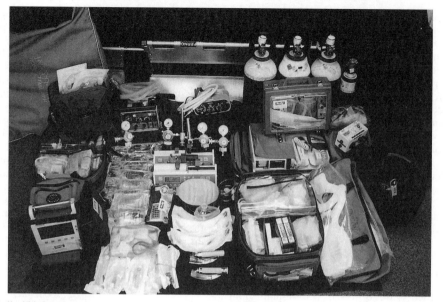

Figure 19.3 Medical kit for air ambulance transfer

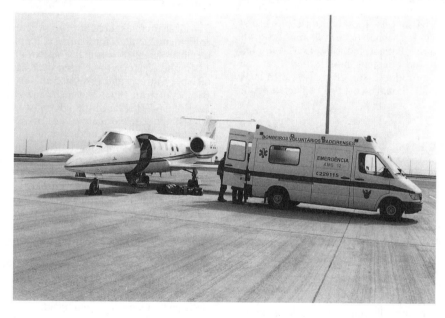

Figure 19.4 Example of an aircraft used for air ambulance transfer

Information received by the air ambulance company on the patient's condition varies widely in content and accuracy, depending on the referring hospital and number of parties involved in the communication chain. Standard information requested is the history of the presenting illness, past medical history, progress of disease and results of investigations or tests. Often very little is received other than a diagnosis and statement that the patient is felt to be fit for transfer. In this situation the air ambulance team must assume the worst case scenario and prepare for all eventualities. The most important information the retrieval team require is whether the patient is cardiovascularly stable, on inotropes, what the ventilator parameters are and what the patient's gas exchange is like. With this information it is usually possible to establish with some accuracy whether it is safe to transfer the patient. It is useful to have a form that can be faxed to the referring hospital requesting this information (Figure

Table 19.5 Equipment and drugs taken on air ambulance

Defibrillator
Portable suction
Monitor (Propaq)
Two ventilators
Bedding/vacuum matress/scoop
Oxygen cylinders
Infusion pumps
Battery

Respiratory bag
Intubation pack—kit for intubation
Laedal bag, mask, reservoir
Guedel airways
Oxygen pack—masks, nebulisers, tubing
Intercostal drain set
Ipratropium bromide
Salbutamol
Diazepam
Etomidate
Midazolam
Propofol
Thiopental
Suxamethonium
Vecuronium

Invasive monitoring bag
Heparinised saline 1 litre
Pressure transducers and cables
CVP line, drum catheter, A-lines

Miscellaneous
Variety of syringes, needles, swabs, gloves
Portable blood gas analyser
BNF
Sharps bin
Nurse's bag
Sthethescope
BM stix

Drug bag
Intravenous
Adrenaline (epinephrine)
Amiodarone
Dobutamine
Dopamine
Furosemide (frusemide)
Glyceryl trinitrate
Isoprenaline

Magnesium sulphate
Midazolam
Noradrenaline (norepinephrine)
Propofol
Vecuronium

Others
Aminophylline
Doxapram
Buscopan
Chlorphenamine (chlorpheniramine)
Dexamethasone
Hydrocortisone
Haloperidol
Naloxone
Phenytoin

Minijets
Adrenaline (epinephrine)
Atropine
Calcium chloride
Lidocaine (lignocaine)
Sodium bicarbonate
5% Glucose

Cardiac drugs
Adenosine
Atropine
Digoxin
Hydralazine
Labetolol

Oral
Aspirin
Co-dydramol
Diazepam
Furosemide (frusemide)
Metoclopramide
Nifedipine
Paracetamol
GTN spray/patch
Volterol

Fluids bag
Elohaes 1 litre
Saline 1 litre
5% Glucose 1 litre
Dextrose saline 1 litre
Mannitol p.r.n.
Blood p.r.n.

19.5). This should be simple and easy to understand, using internationally recognised terms and translated to the relevant language.

Planning Prior to Repatriation

This involves planning the transfer, briefing crew, checking equipment and organising aircraft. The duration of ground transfer and flight time should be estimated. Any extra drugs, equipment, fluids or blood products not normally carried should be ordered.

Arrival at Hospital

It is important to establish a rapport with the referring medical team caring for the patient. They must be given time adequately to hand over the patient, and undue criticism should not be made of any perceived deficiencies

Name.............................   DoB..................

Sex   M/F   Weight..............   Height................

Diagnosis...

Past medical history...

Allergies....................   Temp..................

Cardiovascular:

HR/Rhythm................   BP............. CVP.........Inotropes Y/N

Respiratory:

FiO_2.......... Sats.......... PaO_2.......... $PaCO_2$...........BE..........

Mode of ventilation.....................   PEEP.......... I:E..........

Tidal volume (Vt)...........   Rate (f)...........   PAP...........

Vascular access:

Peripheral line   Y/N   CVP   Y/N   Arterial line   Y/N

Renal/GIT/Neuro:

Urinary catheter   Y/N   Urine output.................

Nasogastric tube   Y/N   Diarrhoea   Y/N   Abdo surgery Y/N

GCS..........   Focal signs   Y/N   Cervical spine stable   Y/N

Results: **Drugs and infusions:**

Na..........   Hb..............   ....

K..........   WBC.............   ....

Urea......... Platelets.......... ....

Creat......Glucose......Clotting...... ....

Table 19.6 Checklist for pretransfer assessment

Before transfer
Staff prepared-fully briefed
ICU bed available
Drugs and equipment checked
Any extra equipment needed

Patient safe to transfer

Respiratory
Airway secure, is intubation required?
Ventilation adequate $Pao_2 > 13\,kPa$
$\qquad\qquad\qquad Spo_2 > 95\%$
$\qquad\qquad\qquad Paco_2\ 4–5\,kPa$
Chest drain needed?

Cardiovascular
Heart rate/blood pressure controlled and stable
Circulating volume adequate
Intravenous access established and secure
Inotrope infusions moderate and stable

Renal
Catheterised
Adequate urine output

Neurological
Glasgow coma scale stable
No air in skull
Spine stabilised

Abdominal
Nasogastric tube free drainage
Major intra-abdominal haemorrhage excluded
Any further investigations or treatment required?
Established and stable on monitors and transport ventilator

in treatment. Once care of the patient has been transferred to the transporting team a full examination and assessment of bedside results can be made. It is now time to make the final decision on whether the patient is fit for transfer. The patient's relatives need to be located and be given a summary of the patient's condition and an explanation of the proposed plan for transfer and the associated risks.

Preparing the Patient for Transfer

The patient should be optimised for transfer (Table 19.6). The following areas are assessed:

- Cardiac output
- Oxygenation
- Ventilation
- Volume status
- Intravenous access
- Analgesia/sedation
- Monitoring
- Gas-filled spaces
- Thromboembolic prophylaxis.

In patients who are unstable and require resuscitation and ventilation the following order of optimisation is

suggested:

1. Administer oxygen and establish monitoring
2. Secure intravenous access and infuse intravenous fluids
3. Insert arterial line under local anaesthesia
4. Rapid sequence induction, intubation and ventilation
5. Central access
6. Inotropes if necessary
7. Urinary catheter
8. Review patient, check arterial blood gases, chest X-ray if possible
9. Transfer if stable.

If invasive procedures are to be performed, this should be explained to the referring medical staff as being necessary for a safe transfer. Cases have been reported of the transferring medical staff being forcibly removed from the patient's side by hospital security staff after having initiated an invasive procedure without clear communication to referring medical staff. It may become necessary to delay the transfer to stabilise and review the patient.

During transfer the patient will be moved four times from various beds, trolleys and stretchers. To simplify these movements the patient is placed on a vacuum mattress, which is then secured to a scoop stretcher (Figure 19.6). The scoop stretcher can now be used to lift the patient and can also be secured to the ambulance and aircraft stretchers.

Ground Transfer to Aircraft

Ground transport is usually undertaken in a local ambulance. Most are of good standard with trained crew and adequate equipment. Often the ambulance will pick up the medical crew and equipment from the airfield. This allows the medical crew to assess the quality of the ambulance and possibly leave some of the medical kit on the aircraft. They should always check for the availability of a functioning defibrillator, suction and oxygen before leaving their equipment with the aircraft. Sufficient oxygen should be taken for the duration of the journey and a spare method of ventilating the patient should be carried. Most European ambulances do not have the correct connections for UK portable ventilators; therefore if the ambulance oxygen is to be used during transfer the patient must be hand ventilated. Adequate time should be allowed for traffic congestion and customs controls, which can be lengthy in some countries despite the presence of a ventilated patient.

Arrival at the Aircraft

Once the ambulance is clear of customs and on the airfield the aircraft is readied for loading. During this period the patient should be kept in the ambulance, accompanied by one of the medical staff at all times. Once the aircraft is prepared for loading the air and ground crew

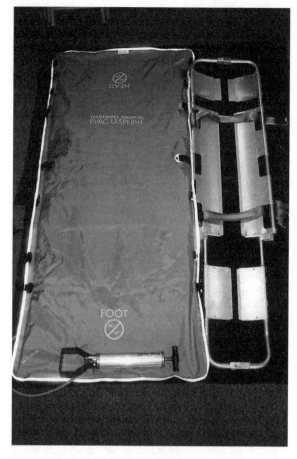

Figure 19.6   Vacuum mattress and scoop stretcher

can be briefed on the plans for loading. The assistance of keen but untrained non-English-speaking ground handlers can cause problems, with intravenous lines being pulled out and potential accidental extubations. In most chartered aircraft, manual loading is required and this involves lifting the patient on a scoop stretcher. Considerable difficulty may be encountered with very tall or morbidly obese patients. Some aircraft have specifically designed loading mechanisms, such as ramps and other crane mechanisms. Once loaded, the patient is reassessed. The monitors and ventilator are checked to make sure that no accidental disconnection or changes to settings have occurred. The medical kit must be stowed securely, with certain essential items being easily available.

Take Off and Ascent

During take off the medical staff monitor the patient carefully for signs of any problems associated with acceleration or gas expansion. At altitude the monitors are adjusted and rezeroed if necessary. Basic care and monitoring should continue and any indicated therapy

instituted. Light aircraft experience greater effects from turbulence and care should be taken that equipment is secured. In the event of severe turbulence crew should remain seated and use their safety belts.

Descent, Landing and Second Ground Transfer

On arrival at the destination airport the medical staff maybe fatigued and it is often cold, dark and raining. The ambulance staff should be briefed on the patient's condition and the unloading technique. Transfer to the receiving hospital is carried out at a normal speed; there is very rarely an indication for a 'blue light' transfer. On arrival at the receiving hospital a full medical handover, including details of the transfer, should be made to both nursing and medical staff.

GUIDELINES

There are a variety of bodies involved in producing guidelines. The recommended standards for UK fixed wing transfers were published in the *Journal of the Royal Society of Medicine* (Bristow *et al.*, 1992). The Intensive Care Society and the Association of Anaesthetists have both produced guidelines for the transfer of critically ill patients with in the UK and these should be taken as the gold standard when transferring critically ill patients. The major points are summarised as follows:

- The decision to transfer should be made by consultant medical staff after discussion between appropriate medical staff. Transfer should be initiated for patient benefit.
- Fixed wing aircraft should be used for distances over 150 miles (240 km).
- Specialised air ambulance providers should be used
- A minimum of two escorts are required: (1) an experienced medical practitioner with training in intensive care and transport medicine, at least 2 years experience in anaesthesia, intensive care or other equivalent speciality, and competent in resuscitation, airway support, ventilation and organ support; (2) another experienced assistant, either nurse, operating department assistant, or paramedic.

SUMMARY

There are an increasing number of medical repatriations into the UK. The majority of cases are stable patients requiring the minimum of intervention. These usually return on a scheduled flight with a nurse escort. Air ambulance transfers of critically ill patients involve a specialist team of anaesthetists and intensive care trained nurses with previous experience in flight medicine. Most patients can be safely transferred providing they are adequately prepared, optimised and monitored. However, there are risks to transporting any patient. The decision to transfer should involve careful discussion between all the parties concerned, the ultimate aim being a safe transfer with overall benefit to the patient.

REFERENCES

Armitage J, Pyne A, Williams S *et al.* (1990) Respiratory problems of air travel in patients with spinal cord injuries. *British Medical Journal*, **300**, 1498–1499.

Bion J, Wilson I and Taylor P (1988) Transporting critically ill patients by ambulance: audit by sickness scoring. *British Medical Journal*, **296**, 170.

Bristow A, Toff N, Baskett P *et al.* (1992) A report: recommended standards for UK fixed wing medical air transport systems and for patient management during transfer by fixed wing aircraft. *Journal of the Royal Society of Medicine*, **85**, 767–771.

Castillo C and Lyons T (1999) The transoceanic air evacuation of unstable angina patients. *Aviation, Space and Environmental Medicine*, **70**, 103–106.

Cruickshank J, Gorlin R and Jennet B (1988) Air travel and thrombotic episodes: the economy class syndrome. *Lancet*, **ii**, 497–498.

Ernsting J, Nicholson A and Rainford D (1999) *Aviation Medicine*. Butterworth-Heinemann, Oxford.

Gentleman D and Jennett B (1981) Hazards of inter-hospital transfer of comatose head-injured patients. *Lancet*, **ii**, 853–855.

Gentleman D, Dearden M, Midgley S *et al.* (1993) Guidelines for resuscitation and transfer of patients with serious head injury. *British Medical Journal*, **307**, 547–552.

Gong H (1992) Air travel and oxygen therapy in cardiopulmonary patients. *Chest*, **101**, 1104–1113.

Kramer W, Domres B, Durner, P *et al.* (1996) Evaluation of repatriation parameters: an analysis of patient data of the German Air Rescue. *Aviation, Space and Environmental Medicine*, **67**, 885–889.

Malagon I, Grounds R and Bennett E (1996) Changes in cardiac output during air ambulance repatriation. *Intensive Care Medicine*, **22**, 1396–1399.

Morton N, Pollack M and Wallace P (1997) *Stabilisation and Transport of the Critically Ill*. Churchill Livingstone, London.

Runcie C, Reeve W, Reidy J *et al.* (1990) Blood pressure measurement during transport. A comparison of direct and oscillotonometric readings in critically ill patients. *Anaesthesia*, **45**, 659–665.

Venkataraman S and Orr R (1992) Intrahospital transport of critically ill patients. *Critical Care Clinics*, **8**, 525–531.

Waddell G (1975) Movement of critically ill patients within hospital. *British Medical Journal*, **2**, 417–419.

20

Poisons and Travel

Virginia Murray

Medical Toxicology Unit, London, UK

INTRODUCTION

Travel medicine has not included many issues relating to medical toxicology as part of the routine information required by travellers; however, in the experience of the Medical Toxicology Unit, many such enquiries are received and these have often presented difficult medical problems to manage.

The chemically related health problems reported by travellers have included:

- Use of local pharmaceutical products
- Use of local household and domestic products
- Exposure to local traditional remedies when abroad
- Concern about toxic plants, snakes and insect envenomations
- Exposure to chemically contaminated air, water, soil and food products.

Some of these exposures have occurred abroad but others have also been reported on the traveller's return to the country of origin. Other exposures have occurred during travelling. This chapter provides some examples of the types of chemically related health problems identified, together with sources of advice within the UK and elsewhere.

THE MEDICAL TOXICOLOGY UNIT

The Medical Toxicology Unit (MTU) was formed in 1967 when the laboratory was established alongside the information service, which had been in existence since 1963. The MTU is a National Health Service (NHS) unit with regional and national roles, part of the Guy's and St Thomas' Trust, one of London's leading university hospitals. The MTU is also part of the King's College School of Health and Life Sciences and a member of the Interdisciplinary Research Group, the GKT Institute of Toxicology (IOT). International activities have been developed chiefly through the MTU's role as a participating institution in the WHO-based International Programme on Chemical Safety (IPCS—World Health Organisation/International Labour Organisation/United Nations Environment Programme, Geneva).

The MTU has developed in four key areas, providing information, clinical services, laboratory services and chemical incident response. These services respond to demands from the full range of health service functions, including hospitals, primary care and public health. The services are only available to medical professionals. It includes:

- National Poisons Information Service (NPIS), London
- Chemical Incident Response Service (CIRS)
- Analytical toxicology laboratory
- Medical toxicology clinical services.

Medical toxicology encompasses all aspects of human toxicology: drug poisoning; poisoning from chemicals encountered in domestic and industrial settings; and poisoning from natural toxins. Exposure may be acute or chronic, deliberate or unintentional, in circumstances varying from domestic or industrial to environmental. The main aims of the MTU are to strive to improve its services to the medical profession and emergency services and to make a key contribution to the NHS national priorities for health care, including:

- Providing prompt and effective emergency care
- Ensuring continuing and effective protection of the public's health with regard to the health effects of environmental and chemical hazards
- Providing information for health
- Developing and expanding the training and outreach programme to contribute to the national NHS initiative on training, education and staff development
- Developing a strategy to deliver high-quality research, working with the Trust and GKT Medical School.

National Poisons Information Service, London

The National Poisons Information Service (NPIS), London, is one of six UK-based national poisons information

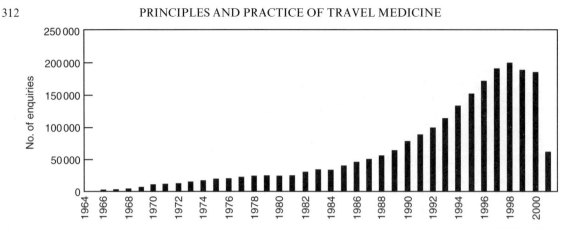

Figure 20.1   Number of emergency case enquiries received by the National Poisons Information Service (London), 1964–2000

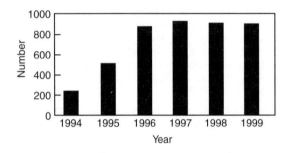

Figure 20.2   Number of chemical incidents reported to the Chemical Incident Response Service, 1994–1999

services. It provides information and advice to medical professionals and emergency services only on the identification, investigation and management of poisoned or potentially poisoned patients. Figure 20.1 shows the numbers of emergency case enquiries received by the service since 1963.

Chemical Incident Response Service

The Chemical Incident Response Service (CIRS) is one of five newly evolved chemical incident provider units developed at the request of the Department of Health. CIRS was formed in 1995 as a specialised department as a result of increasing reports of 'chemical incidents' to NPIS laboratory and clinical services. Figure 20.2 shows the number of incidents reported between 1994 and 1999. CIRS has contracts with 73 health authorities, serving a population of approximately 38 million across England. The service provides 24 h consultant lead response.

The principal functions of the CIRS are to:

- Assist in identifying the chemical hazard and determine the toxic risk
- Provide the relevant medical toxicological information and advice

- Advise on decontamination, treatment, laboratory sampling and follow-up
- Advise and assist with epidemiology, incident documentation and surveillance
- Provide environmental toxicology information
- Carry out site visits where appropriate
- Provide training and materials to public health and health care professionals.

Figure 20.3 provides a breakdown of the types of incidents reported, although some incidents such as fires may cause air contamination from the plume, water contamination from the fire water run off and soil and food contamination as an a longer term outcome.

Medical Toxicology Laboratory

Clinical assessment of travellers where a differential diagnosis includes a toxidrome, together with early collection of biochemical and physiological data obtained from local laboratories, can sometimes point to the type of chemical involved, but proper confirmation can come only from analytical work (Murray and Widdop, 1999). Environmental samples (air, soil, water, etc.) are the easiest to deal with, but if these are not available biological materials are the other alternative. Samples of blood and urine should be taken immediately and it is vital to guard against contamination and to ensure that the correct containers are used. For a 'blind screen' in adults, 10 ml of lithium heparinised blood, 4 ml of EDTA blood and 50 ml of unpreserved urine suffice. The samples must be transported to the laboratory as quickly as possible to avoid losses of chemicals during storage.

Techniques available in the Medical Toxicology Laboratory, such as gas–liquid chromatography (GLC) and high-performance liquid chromatography (HPLC) cover a wide range of chemicals. Ideally, these should be linked to a mass spectrometer which provides unequivocal analytical evidence. Mass spectrometers are equipped with vast libraries of spectra that can be matched to those of

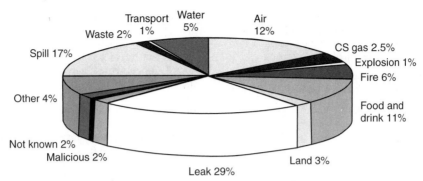

Figure 20.3 Chemical incidents reported to the Chemical Incident Response Service, by type, 1999

the unknown chemical within minutes. Groups of compounds that can be detected include volatile solvents, alcohols, glycol ethers, pesticides and drugs. For toxic metals, inductively coupled plasma mass spectrometry (IPC-MS) is the best technique and can screen for elevated levels of over 30 elements in less than an hour.

No amount of investment in these expensive analytical instruments will bear fruit without having a team of fully trained and experienced analytical toxicologists available to undertake the assays. By using the experience gained from the work of the two services, the following data are provided on poisons and travel.

From the NPIS, London database:

- Traditional and alternative remedies
- Exposure to potentially harmful plants
- Use of domestic products
- Individual risks from toxicity to the traveller.

Several cases reported to NPIS, London are not presented but are mentioned for completeness only. These include cases or health concerns occurring after exposure to imported venomous and nonvenomous animals into the UK (usually found in personal luggage) and use of pharmaceuticals purchased overseas.

From the CIRS database:

- Food-related issues
- Water contamination
- Air contamination
- Pesticide exposure
- Travelling incidents.

Where appropriate, additional information from incident reports is included to give a view of the complexity of drawing together data from sources to show risks to travellers from poisoning.

NPIS, LONDON DATABASE

Traditional and Alternative Remedies

NPIS, London and the MTU has received a series of case reports about the use of traditional and alternative reme-

dies resulting in adverse health effects. Some of these remedies are potentially harmful if used inappropriately without adequate medical supervision. The following case report by Seng and Anderson (1999) documents the concern raised about a recent case.

Case History

Recently a 48-year-old woman resident of Harrow with multiple sclerosis was investigated following complaints of fatigue, loss of appetite, constipation and myalgia. She was found to have severe anaemia caused by lead poisoning. For several weeks she had been taking various 'remedies' given to her by an Ayurvedic practitioner who had visited her at home. These remedies were analysed at the MTU laboratory, Guy's and St Thomas' Hospital Trust and two were found to have very high levels of lead and arsenic. These were Guggul (lead 29 000 p.p.m.) and Pulsineuron (lead 12 000 p.p.m. and arsenic 46 000 p.p.m.).

Comment. The Department of Health and the Medicines Control Agency (MCA) were notified immediately. The MCA found that the remedies had been unofficially introduced into the country from India by a relative of the practitioner. The extent of the distribution of these two medicines is unknown. The authors found that there was no protocol for rapid dissemination of information for such incidents:

- For *contaminated food* there is health hazard system in the UK which can be triggered rapidly. Within hours of the issue of a warning, the environmental health departments can be alerted and the suspected products removed from the shelves.
- A similar mechanism exists for *licensed drugs*. Health Authorities are sent urgent messages via a dedicated electronic network (EPINET). The hospitals and general practitioners of that district are then sent the message by fax or, to those without fax, by first-class mail.
- It is worrying that with the increasing use of *alternative*

medicines in the UK, there is no established national mechanism for ensuring the safety of these medicines and also no rapid system of warning the public against taking those remedies identified as dangerous.

Concern must exist as to mechanisms of alert in other countries, although some, such as Australia, are developing sophisticated networks.

Lead

Lead is also toxic by ingestion of contaminated water from lead pipes, lead-lined tanks and cooking utensils; it is also present in a few Asian cosmetics and as a constituent or contaminant of traditional medicines from other developing countries.

Lead and lead salts (Bates, 2000a) are ubiquitous in our environment. Acute clinical effects include commonly gastrointestinal colic with nausea, vomiting, anorexia and abdominal pain, leading to malaise, convulsions, coma, encephalopathy, hepatic and renal damage, anaemia, hypertension and bradycardia may occur (Khan *et al.*, 1983; Carton *et al.*, 1987; Parras *et al.*, 1989).

Chronic clinical effects from exposure to inorganic lead are summarised as follows: clinical effects from chronic exposures include severe gastrointestinal disturbances with constipation, abdominal pain tenderness. Other effects include anaemia, weakness, pallor, anorexia, insomnia, renal hypertension and mental fatigue. Rarely there may be a bluish 'lead line' on the gums. Lead may also be drawn to areas of the skeleton that grow most rapidly and in some cases hypermineralisation of the radius, tibia and femur can be seen on X-ray with the development of metaphyseal lines (Davies, 1984). Neuromuscular dysfunction may result in signs of motor weakness and paralysis of the extensor muscles of the wrist and ankles. Encephalopathy can occur in patients with previously mild symptoms. Effects include vomiting, confusion, ataxia, apathy, bizarre behaviour and coma and convulsions due to cerebral oedema. Nephropathy may occur and is characterised by albuminuria, glycosuria and renal tubular acidosis. Gout has also been reported.

Early diagnosis and management are essential to minimise harm, with removal from exposure and institution of control of source. Children are particularly at risk. Information and advice are available from local Poisons Information Centres.

Exposure to Potentially Harmful Plants

Many plants are potentially harmful to humans and our knowledge of those found abroad can be limited. Much work has been undertaken on this aspect of the toxicology at the MTU and the NPIS, London. This work has been undertaken in collaboration with the Royal Botanic Gardens, Kew. As a result of the current work programme the CD-Rom *Poisonous Plants and Fungi in Brit-*

ain and Ireland (Dauncey, 2000) and its sister publication in German, covering the flora of northern Europe, were published in September 2000.

An example of one of the frequently found and frequently documented harmful plant is the *Brugmansia* species. A detailed report by Bates (2000b) on this plant has been prepared and can be found on the CD-Rom. The *Brugmansia* species, also known as angels' trumpets, brugmansia or tree datura, is known for its dramatic, fragrant hanging flower heads, often up to 10–15 cm long. In summary, poisoning from *Brugmansia* species causes anticholinergic effects, with dry mouth, blurred vision and dilated pupils, tachycardia, warm and dry skin, reduced bowel sounds, urinary retention and hallucinations. Its main toxins are the tropane alkaloids, hyoscyamine (L-atropine), atropine (DL-hyoscyamine) and scopolamine (hyoscine). Deaths have occurred from abuse of *Brugmansia* (Mendelson, 1976a, 1976b, 1976c; McHenry and Hall, 1978), but are rare. Fatalities may be due to the toxic effects of the alkaloids or from inappropriate behaviour secondary to altered mental state, e.g. from drowning (Hall *et al.*, 1977) or exposure. Abuse of *Brugmansia* appears to occur in periodic epidemics and is particularly prevalent among adolescents and young adults.

Two examples of case reports are given to show the toxicity of the plant.

Case History : *Accidental Ingestion*
A 76-year-old male made 'moon flower' wine from *Brugmansia suaveolens* and ingested 5 ml to test the final product. Some days later he drank 15–20 ml over a 1 h period. Shortly afterwards, he experienced loss of coordination of his hands and feet, followed by sensory loss. Ninety minutes later he was rushed to hospital with respiratory difficulty, partial body paralysis and muscle weakness. He was fully conscious on arrival but unable to communicate. He left hospital several hours later after refusing to stay. Analysis of his wine revealed a scopolamine concentration of 29 mg ml^{-1}. No atropine was detected. This patient had ingested 435–580 mg of scopolamine (Smith *et al.*, 1991).

Case History : *Intentional Abuse*
Two 15-year-old boys were found by police wandering naked and delirious in a field. One of them was holding a flower later identified as *Brugmansia suaveolens*. Within 5 min of admission one of them developed profound muscular weakness and suffered a convulsion which was treated with diazepam. He had tachycardia, tachypnoeia, pyrexia, dry flushed skin, dry mouth, fixed dilated pupils and a positive Babinski sign. Muscular weakness was so marked that he was unable to stand. He was confused, disorientated in time, place and person

---

and had terrifying visual hallucinations. He was given physostigmine and improved but continued to complain of intermittent hallucinations for 4 days after treatment and had persistently dilated pupils. He had recent memory loss and diminished ability to imprint new short-term memories for 1 week. Analysis of his urine revealed a mixture of alkaloids, with scopolamine predominating. Both boys had eaten *Brugmansia* flowers before becoming delirious. The other boy, who was only mildly intoxicated, having eaten less of the flowers, reported that his friend had eaten 5 or 6 flowers (Hall *et al.*, 1977; McHenry and Hall, 1978).

Overseas Domestic Products

Case reports exist of toxicity arising from use of overseas products designed for dealing with domestic issues. Some relate to the overuse of pesticides and others to inappropriate use of similarly named products containing a different ingredient to a UK brand. All such exposures present risks; however, some of the potentially more concerning exposures can occur with the use of chemicals that are not available for domestic purposes in the British Isles. An example of such a chemical is hydrofluoric acid. Products containing this chemical are reported to be available for over-the-counter purchase as a cleaning preparation in countries such as the United States. Local case reports (Eddelman, 1992, personal communication) demonstrate severe adverse health effects from contact when inadequate precautions are taken.

Hydrofluoric Acid

Hydrofluoric acid is a colourless to green fuming liquid, which is extremely corrosive and has a strong irritating odour. Hydrofluoric acid is extremely toxic and all exposures should be regarded seriously. It readily penetrates intact skin, getting under nails and into deep tissue layers, causing liquefactive necrosis of soft tissues and decalcification and corrosion of bone; this may be extremely painful and prolonged for days. Systemic toxicity can occur from all routes of exposure, especially oral and dermal.

The classic acute clinical effects from dermal contact include the following:

* Skin irritation, rash and burning sensation may occur
* Erythema, central blanching with peripheral erythema, pain, which may be severe, swelling and vesiculation can occur from minimal exposure
* In severe cases there may also be ulceration, a blue-grey discoloration of the skin and necrosis and bone decalcification
* Tendonitis and tenosynovitis may result.

With high or continuing exposure, systemic effects have been reported. These include hypocalaemia and hypomagnesaemia, which may lead to cardiac arrhythmias, and metabolic acidosis (Hathaway *et al.*, 1996). Although chronic effects are reported, these are less likely to be of concern to families living abroad.

Early management is the removal of any contaminated clothing, placing it in double, sealed, clear bags, labelling it and storing it in a secure area away from patients and staff. The affected area should be irrigated immediately with copious amounts of water. Specific treatment with calcium gluconate gel massaged into the affected area for a minimum of 30 min or injected, as appropriate, is required. Information and advice are available from local Poisons Information Centres.

Individual Risks from Toxicity to the Traveller

In order to assess whether there is a risk to a traveller from exposure to pesticides used to prevent the carriage of insects, the NPIS, London emergency case enquiries database was searched (Murray *et al.*, 2000). It collects information primarily on cases with acute exposures presenting to hospitals and is a representative but not a complete coverage of exposures in the southeast of England. The total number of enquiries between 1995 and 2000 was 1 006 550. In order to identify the number of aircraft-related enquiries, additional searches of the database showed:

* 6472 insecticide-related case enquiries
* 2445 pyrethroid-related case enquiries
* 59 transport-related emergency cases enquiries.

Two cases of pyrethroid pesticide exposure were identified and are summarised below. As far as the MTU can ascertain, in the light of the toxicological reviews, neither person was likely to have developed long-term health effects as a result of the exposure in the cabin environment.

Case History
A 41-year-old woman was concerned about exposure to insecticides during several intercontinental flights and that she had thus developed a chronic eye condition, which was diagnosed in 1992. On attendance at the medical toxicology clinic, she reported that she was exposed to aircraft disinfectant treatment with pesticides in 1990 and 1991. It was apparent that she had developed mild eye irritation and lachrymation of the eyes approximately 48 h after arrival at her destinations on these occasions and that this had been self-limiting. The active ingredient of the products to which she was concerned that she had been exposed was pyrethroid.

Case History

An adult woman reported being exposed to aircraft disinfectant treatment with pesticides on a flight in November 1995. She was reported as developing acute ocular symptoms at the time of the flight; these were thought to be self-limiting. In addition, she reported continuing harm leading to injury to sight, teeth or facial bones. She required various operations to correct her sight and teeth. She was reported to have become legally blind. As a non-UK resident she was not seen in the MTU clinic and details of her illness could not be verified. The active ingredient of the products to which she was concerned that she had been exposed was also pyrethroid.

Pyrethroids and Pyrethrins

Pyrethroids and pyrethrins have been reviewed by Schofield (2000). Pyrethrins are brown, viscous liquids or solids with the characteristic odour of the carrier vehicle. The name pyrethrins (or pyrethrum) refers to the six naturally occurring insecticidal components of *Pyrethrum* chrysanthemums. Pyrethroids are synthetic substances similar to pyrethrins, modified to improve stability.

In all acute exposures the toxicity of the carrier, usually a hydrocarbon or a talc-based powder, must be considered. By inhalation, many preparations will cause local irritation to the upper respiratory tract, leading to coughing, wheezing and rhinitis. By contact with the skin, most pyrethroids will cause local irritation and drying, and may sensitise. By ocular exposure, the fumes or splash contact may cause a burning sensation or itching, and irritation with the carrier ingredients, e.g. solvents, shampoo, may be responsible for other effects. In summary, the chronic clinical effects that have been reported show that sensitisation may occur, resulting in dermatitis upon re-exposure, particularly with pyrethrins. In sensitised patients re-exposure may lead to asthmatic attacks; this is particularly noted with pyrethrins.

For those exposed, provide reassurance and symptomatic and supportive care. Information and advice are available from local Poisons Information Centres.

CIRS DATABASE

Since 1996, over 60 overseas incidents have been referred to CIRS for information and advice. These incidents can be divided into the following main groups of concern:

- Food-related issues
- Water contamination
- Air contamination
- Malicious events
- Travel-related incidents.

Food-related Issues

These incidents can be divided into two main groups: those that occur in the UK from ingestion of imported products, and those occurring abroad. Three examples of the incidents that have been reported as a result of purchases made abroad and the product being brought back and consumed in the UK, leading to adverse health effects, are given:

- Botulinum-contaminated bottled fungi from Italy
- Ground glass found in curry sauce
- Frozen broccoli purchased in Europe—noted to be looking 'blue'. On analysis the presence of hydroxycoumarin, a rodenticide, was detected.

The following are examples of events where exposure has occurred abroad:

- Botulinum-contaminated mascarpone cheese in Italy
- Concern over mercury levels in water at a dairy farm, leading to contamination of dairy products
- Concern over the use of cyanide to kill fish
- Lead battery factories contaminating irrigation water with lead; water going to salad and crop vegetables
- Ingestion of illicit alcohol containing methanol
- Ingestion of contaminated beer, brewed in Europe
- Soft-drink contamination
- Concern over apparent Coca-Cola contamination in Belgium.

A review of the Belgian Coca-Cola incident was published by Nemery *et al.* (1999). Although many cases of real and apparent illness were reported, it was considered by the authors that the cause was likely to have been a mass sociogenic illness. The incident was thought to have occurred as two separate events:

- Returnable glass bottles from a plant in Antwerp with carbon dioxide in the head space of the drink had a 'musty' smell
- Cans from a plant in Dunkirk with a chlorinated phenol compound on the outside of the can resulted in a smell on the cans but did not lead to direct contamination of the drink (Murray, 1999a).

Water Contamination

Some of these incidents have been listed under food-related incidents, above. Water contamination incidents can be divided into raw and drinking water contamination. An overturned lorry carrying a tanker load of chemicals, including cyanide, which spilled its contents into a land-locked lake provides an example or raw water contamination. Drinking water supply contamination with chemicals such as ammonia and antifouling paint cause considerable concern. Sometimes the adverse health effects reported have come from exposure in swimming pools. Chronic issues related to water contamination have occurred as a result of lead from lead solder seeping into the pipes of housing development water systems in Europe.

Air Contamination

Enquiries about adverse health effects arising from acute and chronic air pollution can prove difficult to manage unless detailed information is available.

Classic examples of acute exposure include concern about products of combustion from industrial fires. An example relates to a transformer fire in Belgium in 1999, when questions about polychlorinated biphenyls and dioxin exposure were raised. With the help of the Meteorological Office's NAME model (Maryon, 1994), it was possible to see that the risk was towards Europe and away from the UK. Fortunately the fire was rapidly extinguished and little harm was reported.

Exposure to chronic air pollution from fires of longer duration are complex issues to manage. For example, smoke from forest fires in Indonesia was reported in May 1997 and affected Indonesia, Malaysia, Singapore, Thailand, Brunei, Philippines and Hong Kong. The haze resulted in poor visibility until October 1997 and led, for example, to the closure of some airports and several airplane and ship collisions and other accidents. Adverse effects reported included increased incidence of upper respiratory tract infections, sore eyes, exacerbation of asthma and bronchitis. In one retrospective study by a medical centre in Singapore between October 1997 and April 1998, of 500 soldiers aged 18–24 years, the authors found lower airways disease and conjunctivitis with significant correlation to their pollution standard index ($p = 0.037$ and $p = 0.02$) and concluded that under such conditions strenuous exercise requires precautionary measures (Murray, 1999b).

Other sources of chronic air pollution referred to CIRS have included concerns about a scrap metal foundry in a village on a Mediterranean island, which is thought to be possibly responsible for a cluster of cancers in the villagers.

More domestic, but frequently potentially highly toxic, are exposures to family members, particularly children. These include exposure to carbon monoxide from faulty boilers, sometimes causing fatalities and severe chronic adverse health effects. Other domestic exposures include inhalation of lead dust and fumes from sanding lead paint inside the house.

Carbon Monoxide

Carbon monoxide (Scott, 2000) is a colourless, odourless gas. Acute inhalation effects are summarised below:

- Mild to moderate exposures cause headache, weakness, fatigue, nausea, vomiting, irritability, dizziness, drowsiness, disorientation, incoordination, visual disturbances, hypotension, tachycardia and hyperventilation

- Severe exposures can rapidly cause coma, convulsions, severe hypotension, respiratory depression, cardiovascular collapse, cerebral oedema, death
- Low-level exposure to carbon monoxide causes non-specific symptoms that are often mistaken for other illnesses, e.g. viral illness or food poisoning
- Permanent neurological sequelae following recovery from acute symptoms of poisoning include dementia, amnestic syndromes, psychosis, paralysis, apraxias and agnosias.

Chronic inhalation effects from carbon monoxide include problems associated with repeated exposure to low levels of carbon monoxide, which can cause nausea, diarrhoea, abdominal pain, headache, fatigue, dizziness, paraesthesiae, chest pain and palpitations (Meredith and Vale, 1988). The symptoms are protean in nature and can be mistakenly attributed to other illnesses, e.g. food poisoning or viral illness. Signs that may indicate chronic carbon monoxide poisoning as a possible cause for unexplained illness include the fact that symptoms tend to occur in bad weather (due to heating systems being switched on), recurrent episodes are common, several people are affected simultaneously (e.g. a whole family) and spontaneous recovery occurs when the patient is outside the home (Crawford et al., 1990).

Early diagnosis and management are essential to minimise harm, with removal from exposure and institution of control of source. Information and advice are available from local Poisons Information Centres.

Travel-related Chemical Incidents

The CIRS database is structured to capture information about circumstances to allow specific incident types to be identified and retrieved. The total number of chemical incidents recorded between 1994 and 2000 in the CIRS database is 5243. The CIRS database was searched for:

- 39 transport-related incidents
- 20 airport-related incidents.

The following three incidents provide examples of the types of travelling events documented by CIRS and in the literature.

Incident 1: A Travelling Incident

At 04.00 h on 9 April 1997 a courier company's plane with two pilots and an engineer landed at West Midlands airport. The hold contained, among other goods, two 25 kg drums of rose oxide. While unloading, the engineer noticed an unusual smell in the hold and requested help from a local company to clean up the plane. The plane then flew on to Scotland where the engineer reported feeling unwell and, along with both pilots, was sent to the local accident and emergency department for assessment and treatment.

Meanwhile the drums were transferred to the courier's Derby warehouse. At 13.59 h an enquiry was received by NPIS, London, seeking information about rose oxide, as six staff of the warehouse had arrived at a Derby Royal Infirmary accident and emergency department complaining of light headedness, headache, dry mouth and throat and chest pain. Following the recommended clinical assessment they were discharged well later that afternoon.

The drums were meanwhile sent on by van to the Maidstone warehouse. An employee discovered that one of the drums was leaking. Ninety minutes later he developed dizziness, headache and ataxia, which progressed to a dry mouth and throat with chest tightness and shortness of breath. He was taken to the local accident and emergency department where on examination no abnormality was noted, other than that his peak flow changed from $520 l min^{-1}$ at 18.40 to $580 l min^{-1}$ at 21.10, when he was discharged. By the next day his peak flow had improved to $620 l min^{-1}$.

On contacting the company, one of the senior managers reported that other goods that had been near the drums had also been contaminated and that these had been taken to warehouses in Manchester, Liverpool and London. All had been concerned by the smell and in Manchester advice was sought from the local Fire Brigade, who advised evacuation of the warehouse.

Concerned that further enquiries might arise from this, CIRS notified several health authorities in Trent and South Thames Regions.

Toxicological commentary on rose oxide. Rose oxide is tetrahydro-2-(2-methyl-1-propenyl)-4-methylpyran, a naturally occurring substance that is used as a scenting agent in some household products. It is normally considered to be of low toxicity with an oral-rat LD_{50} of $4300 mg kg^{-1}$. It has been reported as causing skin irritation.

Commentary on incident. Previous experience at CIRS of 'travelling' chemical incidents has caused concern, and on some occasions more casualties than in this incident. Many companies use courier services to transport raw materials and products rapidly. Couriers usually have little knowledge of the toxicological consequences of exposure to accidental spills or leaks. Vigilance and better alerting mechanisms are therefore required when transporting any chemicals, in order to identify damaged containers and minimise health and safety issues.

Incident 2: The Fireman's Tale (Millership, 2000)

Background. A fireman visited his general practitioner—very concerned about an exposure to radiation, as he was planning to start a family. His story was as follows.

On a cold wet night in December 1999, 3 weeks earlier, a cargo plane crashed into woods shortly after take off. He was a member of the first two fire crews on the scene. The plane was burning fiercely with a large plume of smoke and it took 2.5 h to bring it under control. The fireman was wearing his ordinary protective clothing (helmet, suit and boots), which he would have worn for any fire. After about 3 h he was advised to wear a dust mask, but no explanation was given for this advice. The fireman was on the site for about 5 h. The aircraft and parts of the surrounding woods were still smouldering the next morning. He returned to assist and, in all, spent about 17 h in the area.

The only casualties were the four crew members, who all died. No one else was injured. As far as the members of the fire crews were concerned the incident was over; however, in early January press reports of uranium in the plane began to circulate. The fireman remembered sitting with a group of colleagues when he was told about this by his union representative. He was very worried, especially as he felt no one seemed to know anything about the health hazards. He went to see his general practitioner for advice about the possible dangers to the children he might have.

The Public health problem. The local hospital accident department was cleared for a major incident but was stood down within 30 min as there were no survivors. The local health authority public health department had an agreement with the ambulance service to notify chemical and radiation incidents, but there was no requirement to do so for other major incidents. Although the public health department was aware of the crash within 30 min via press and other reports, few details were available at the time. The full extent of the fire was not recognised until the following day, when several public health concerns emerged:

- There were press reports of benzene in the atmosphere as a consequence of spilled fuel.
- The contents of the cargo were unknown except that there were 13 litres of a 'hazardous substance', thought to have been completely destroyed in the fire, and press reports of detonator fuses on board. Neither police nor fire service would confirm the contents of the cargo manifest.
- No mention was made that the tail section of the plane had broken up, distributing its ballast of 24 depleted uranium ingots in the woods and nearby lake.

Public health investigation. Benzene is well known to act as a carcinogen on prolonged exposure; however, it is likely that any present in the fuel was destroyed during the fire.

The Air Accident Investigation branch of the Department of the Environment, Transport and the Regions (DETR) supplied the cargo manifest, which is a public document. There were 125 consignment notes, with between 1 and 20 separate items listed on each. These were principally clothing, machine parts and office equipment but included seven named chemicals or products, none more than 15 litres in volume, and, in addition, diagnostic kits with 'limited quantities of radioactive material' were also present. The Air Accident Branch confirmed that these were medical kits with 25 cl vials for immunoassay purposes. All the above, except the diagnostic kits, were likely to have been destroyed in the fire.

The Environment Agency monitored the crash site for radioactivity to locate the uranium ingots. So far 20 of the 24 rods have been recovered, of which one was in two pieces and the rest were intact. The ingots are depleted uranium (DU), which has a lower proportion of the more radioactive constituents of natural uranium. Typically DU is 0.2% ^{235}U. The alpha emissions can be stopped by intact skin, beta emissions by a few millimetres of plastic or metal, and there is no significant external hazard from gamma radiation. The ingots were encased in metal, and therefore not a health hazard unless broken or burnt, with the production of dust. Once in a soluble form, uranium is a highly toxic heavy metal as well as being a radiation hazard if ingested. There was no evidence that any ingot burnt; this requires a temperature of 700 °C for 4 h. Only one ingot was broken into two pieces, which fitted together. The remaining missing ingots are believed to be at the bottom of a lake near the crash site.

Extensive monitoring failed to show any other signs of radioactivity elsewhere, apart from the radioactive material in the medical kits.

Discussion. The press identified two issues regarded as public health concerns: benzene in the fuel, and uranium in the tail section of the aircraft. Further enquiry revealed a list of chemicals and the presence of radioactive material in the cargo. Fortunately, further investigation showed that health fears were groundless (M.J. Clark, 2000, personal communication). The author was able to reassure the fireman and local doctors without undertaking health surveillance.

Commentary on incident. Experience at CIRS reinforces the need for early incident identification, investigation and management. Only with all the data about an event available is it possible to assess the risk to travellers effectively.

Incident 3: Underground Spread and Petroleum-related Incidents

Numerous petroleum product-related incidents have occurred around the world. These incidents present particular difficulties in their management, as they have potential to present explosive or fire hazards, contamination of land, water and indoor air and major coastal problems from tanker spills.

Contamination of drains with petrol is potentially very dangerous because it can lead to widespread explosive and fire damage (Murray, 2000). The quantity of contaminant does not need to be large, as demonstrated in the incident described above. Possibly one of the worst and unfortunately most memorable incidents of this nature in the last 10 years occurred at Guadalajara in Mexico. There was extensive television reporting of the event at the time, however recent searches revealed no report in the scientific literature relating to this incident. All details provided below are therefore obtained from information gathered for reports to insurance underwriters.

On 22 April 1992, a series of explosions ripped through Guadalajara, killing possibly as many as 252 people, injuring approximately 1440, with more than 15 000 left homeless. The explosions started at 10.00 h and continued well into the night, with a total of 17 blasts being recorded within 12 h. A strong smell of gas was reported at the site of the first explosion.

Initially conflicting evidence as to the cause was reported. However, it seemed likely that the explosions were triggered by an undetermined quantity of petrol escaping from a ruptured petrol pipeline. This pipeline came from a major fuel depot near the city. Petroleos Mexicanos, responsible for the depot, later reported a loss of approximately 1000 barrels of gasoline, which presumably had filtered into the subsoil and from this into the central drainage and sewage system of the city. As a result of this incident and the reported rupture of the pipeline, Petroleos Mexicanos extracted 900 barrels of gasoline from the subsoil by 3 May 1992.

Reports suggested that the approximate estimated damage was between 300 million and 1 billion US dollars: 2.6 square miles (6.7 km^2) with 8 km of streets were destroyed or damaged; about 600 vehicles were destroyed and buried; at least one vehicle was found on the roof of a house; damage to 1124 houses and 450 businesses was reported. Residents were reluctant to return because of continuing concern about further explosions.

CONCLUSION

Travellers are at risk of poisoning while abroad, travelling or at home from the products they may bring with them. It is essential that the adverse health effects reported by travellers should include a toxicological differential diagnosis and relevant information and advice, and, if necessary, analytical investigation of the patients biological samples or suspect material should be sought if appropriate.

REFERENCES

Bates N (2000a) Lead and lead salts information sheet. In *Chemical Incident Management Handbook* (eds C Farrow *et al.*). Stationery Office, London.

Bates N (2000b) Brugmansia. In *Poisonous Plants and Fungi in Britain and Ireland: Interactive Identification Systems on CD-Rom* (ed. E Dauncey). Royal Botanic Gardens, Kew.

Carton JA, Maradona JA and Arribas JM (1987) Acute-subacute lead poisoning. *Archives of Internal Medicine*, **147**, 697–703.

Crawford R, Campbell DGD and Ross J (1990) Carbon monoxide poisoning in the home: recognition and treatment. *British Journal of Medicine*, **301**, 977–979.

Dauncey E (ed.) (2000) *Poisonous Plants and Fungi in Britain and Ireland: Interactive Identification Systems on CD-Rom*. Royal Botanic Gardens, Kew.

Davies JM (1984) Lung cancer mortality among workers making lead chromate and zinc chromate pigments at three English factories. *British Journal of Industrial Medicine*, **41**, 158–169.

Hathaway GJ, Proctor NH and Hughes JP (1996) *Proctor and Hughes' Chemical Hazards of the Workplace*, 4th edn. Van Nostrand Reinhold, New York.

Hall RCW, Popkin MK and McHenry LE (1977) Angel's trumpet psychosis: a central nervous system anticholinergic syndrome. *American Journal of Psychiatry*, **134**, 312–314.

Khan AJ, Patel U, Rafecq M *et al.* (1983) Reversible acute renal failure in lead poisoning. *Clinical Laboratory Observations*, **102**, 147–149.

Maryon RH (1994) Modelling the long range transport of radionuclides following a nuclear accident. *Nuclear Energy*, **33**, 119–128.

McHenry LE and Hall RCW (1978) Angel's trumpet. Lethal and psychogenic aspects. *Journal of the Florida Medical Association*, **65**, 192–196.

Mendelson G (1976a) Poisoning due to *Datura fastuosa* (letter). *Journal of Tropical Medicine and Hygiene*, **79**, 163.

Mendelson G (1976b) Reversal by physostigmine of delirium induced by ingestion of the flowers of the plant *Datura stramonium* (letter). *Anesthesia and Analgesia (Cleve)*, **55**, 260.

Mendelson G (1976c) Treatment of hallucinogenic-plant toxicity (letter). *Annals of Internal Medicine*, **85**, 126.

Meredith T and Vale A (1988) Carbon monoxide poisoning. *British Journal of Medicine*, **296**, 77–79.

Millership S (2000) The fireman's tale. *Chemical Incident Report*, January.

Murray V (1999a) Food and drink related incidents. *Chemical Incident Report*, July, 14–16.

Murray V (1999b) Conference Report: 11th World Congress on Disaster and Emergency Medicine: World Association of Disaster and Emergency Medicine, Osaka, Japan, May 10–13 1999. *Chemical Incident Report*, July, 17–18.

Murray V (2000) Petroleum related incidents. *Chemical Incident Report*, January, 14–17.

Murray V, Cullen G, Kamanyire R *et al.* (2000) Call for evidence on the aircraft cabin environment. Evidence from the Medical Toxicology Unit, Science and Technology Committee, House of Lords, May.

Murray V and Widdop B (1999) Detection and identification of unknown poisonous substances from patients material: the experience of the Chemical Incident Response Service, London. *Chemical Incident Report*, July, 16.

Nemery B, Fischler B, Boogaerts M *et al.* (1999) Dioxins, Coca-Cola and mass sociogenic illness in Belgium. *Lancet*, **354**, 77.

Parras F, Patier JL and Ezpeleta C (1989) Lead contaminated heroin as a source of inorganic lead intoxication. *New England Journal of Medicine*, **316**, 755.

Schofield N (2000) Pyrethrins and pyrethroids information sheet. In *Chemical Incident Management Handbook* (eds C Farrow *et al.*). Stationery Office, London.

Scott N (2000) Carbon monoxide information sheet. In *Chemical Incident Management Handbook* (eds C Farrow *et al.*). Stationery Office, London.

Seng C and Anderson S (1999) Ensuring the protection of the public against dangerous, unlicensed, alternative medicines— whose responsibility? *Chemical Incident Report*, April, 14.

Smith EA, Meloan CE, Pickell JA *et al.* (1991) Scopolamine poisoning from homemade 'moon flower' wine. *Journal of Analytical Toxicology*, **15**, 216–219.

ADDITIONAL RESOURCES

Guadalajara Incident Sources of Information

Lloyds Weekly Casualty Report 1.5.1992
Lloyds Weekly Casualty Report 8.5.1992
Lloyds Weekly Casualty Report 15.5.1992

21

Venomous Bites and Stings

R. David G. Theakston and David G. Lalloo

Liverpool School of Tropical Medicine, Liverpool, UK

INTRODUCTION

Travel throughout the world is becoming easier and easier every year with air travel enabling any individual with even limited means to visit almost any region of the world. Thus contact with venomous animals, which has in the past been mainly confined to the inhabitants of tropical or subtropical zones, is rapidly becoming a danger worthy of consideration by the world traveller. It is therefore important that the traveller should be aware of the hazards relating to bites and stings by venomous animals and of the safest, simplest and most appropriate methods for dealing with accidents.

Venomous creatures produce venom in a gland or in specialised cells, and can deliver it during a bite or sting. All venoms contain a complex mixture of toxins, which can be experimentally fractionated into enzymes and polypeptides with widely varying biological, pharmacological and autopharmacological properties.

Toxic effects depend both on the type and amount of venom injected. Although death can result from venomous bites or stings, more commonly, little or no envenoming occurs as a result of bites or stings by a venomous animal because little or no venom is injected; for example, following bites by venomous snakes only 50–70% of victims show signs of envenoming.

SNAKE BITES

Venomous Snakes

The majority of venomous snakes have fangs at the front of their mouths which enable them to inject venom. This is produced by the venom glands, of which there are two, one on each side of the head behind the eye. Each gland is surrounded by muscle, which, on contraction, forces the venom out of the lumen of the gland, along the venom duct, which is positioned on either side of the upper jaw, and then down the canal or groove in the fang. Venomous snakes are divided into three major groups: elapids (fam-ily Elapidae), sea snakes (family Hydrophiidae) and vipers (family Viperidae). There is also a small group of venomous colubrids (back-fanged snakes) which include the boomslang (*Dispholidus typus*) found in southern Africa and the red-neck keel-back snake (*Rhabdophis subminiatus*) in Southeast Asia. Elapids are landsnakes with short fixed fangs covered by a gum-fold, the vagina dentis. Sea snakes have very short fixed fangs and characteristic flattened tails; they are most common in Asian coastal waters. The Viperidae is divided into the true vipers (Viperinae) and the pit vipers (Crotalinae). These snakes have long, erectile fangs and triangular heads (Figure 21.1); their bodies are usually shorter and fatter than those of most elapids. The pit vipers possess a thermosensitive (loreal) pit between the eye and the nostril which is used for detecting warm-blooded prey in the dark; most snakes have diurnal hunting habits. The true vipers do not possess these loreal pits.

Viper bites are much more common than elapid bites, except in the Pacific Australasian area where vipers do not naturally occur. Sea snake bites used to be common among fishing folk of Asian and western Pacific coastal areas but, because of recent modernisation of fishing methods, they have become much rarer. In South and Central America, snakes of medical importance include *Bothrops atrox* (the Barba amarilla, often miscalled ferde-lance, which probably causes more deaths in South and Central America than any other snake) and the tropical rattlesnake (*Crotalus durissus*). In Africa, the puff adder (*Bitis arietans*), cobras (mostly *Naja* species), mambas (four species of *Dendroaspis*) and the carpet or saw-scaled viper (*Echis* species) are common. Members of the genus *Echis* almost certainly cause more snakebite deaths than any other snake in the world, particularly in farmers. In parts of Asia, Russell's viper (*Daboia russelii*), the Malayan pit viper (*Calloselasma rhodostoma*), the saw-scaled viper (*Echis carinatus*), the sharp-nosed pit viper (*Agkistrodon acutus*), the Mamushi pit viper (*A. halys*), the Habu viper (*Trimeresurus flavoviridis*), cobras (mainly *Naja* species) and kraits (*Bungarus caeruleus* and *B. multicinctus*) are important. In Australasia, which has some of

Principles and Practice of Travel Medicine. Edited by Jane N. Zuckerman.

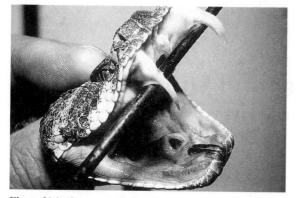

Figure 21.1   Long erectile fangs of a viperine snake. (Reproduced with permission from Dr J White)

the most venomous land snakes in the world, there are no vipers. One of the most important species in this region is probably the Papuan taipan (*Oxyuranus scutellatus canni*) which is the main cause of death due to snake bite in Papua New Guinea and probably also in Irian Jaya.

Epidemiology

Snake bite is mainly a rural and occupational hazard and therefore affects men more than women; farmers, plantation workers, herdsmen and hunter gatherers are at greatest risk. Children also are frequently bitten due to their inquisitive nature; for example, they may play with snakes or put their hands down old rat holes or behind piles of stones or sticks where snakes may be lurking. Travellers and foreign visitors are entering rural areas of the tropics more frequently and this is resulting in more accidents. Most bites occur in the daytime and involve the foot, toe or lower leg as a result of accidentally disturbing a snake; however, some species of snake (e.g. kraits) may bite sleeping victims at night. Bites by sea snakes, although rare, may occur in holiday makers who swim in the sea or in rivers to which sea snakes have access.

Snake bite statistics based on hospital figures are misleading because in the rural tropics, where snake bite is common, victims rarely go to hospital, preferring treatment from traditional healers. In Bangladesh, for example, snake bite victims will visit the ohzas, in Sri Lanka the ayurvedic healers and in Ecuador the local shamans. In Nigeria, one such healer treats several hundred snake bite patients each year, his house being just a mile from one of the largest university teaching hospitals in Africa, which records only about five cases annually. It is unclear whether traditional therapy has benefits; most local healers do not wish to give away their secrets. The main problem when patients visit such healers is that the admission of patients to the hospital is delayed. This delay, in cases of severe envenoming, can result in a fatal outcome. Some years ago when sea snake bite was a

problem in Asian coastal areas, less than 15% of those bitten sought treatment from the government medical services.

Enzyme-linked immunosorbent assay (ELISA) has been used, combined with information obtained from survey questionnaires, to reliably identify specific venom antibodies in the blood of individuals envenomed by snakes in the past (Theakston *et al.*, 1977; Theakston, 1991). Such detailed rural survey procedures have revealed a higher incidence of snake bite, and a higher mortality from this cause, than previously suspected. This reinforces the fact that hospital figures grossly underestimate the real extent of the problem. On the basis of such findings in northern Nigeria, it is estimated that snake bite causes many thousands of deaths per annum in the West African savannah, mainly due to the carpet viper, *Echis ocellatus* (Pugh and Theakston, 1980). Likewise, in Amazonian Ecuador and Brazil, the incidence and mortality due to snake bite in the indigenous Indian populations, such as the Waorani in Ecuador and the Kaxinawa in northwest Brazil, is simply not recorded in the snake bite statistics of the country. It is estimated that almost 5% of Waorani Indians in northeastern Ecuador die annually from snake bite. A group of anthropologists reported that 45% of the population had experienced at least one snake bite and 95% of all adult males have been bitten once (Larrick *et al.*, 1978). These risks also apply to travellers, especially in remote areas such as this which are now readily accessible by small aeroplane or by road following the opening up of many regions in the Amazon and other remote areas by oil and timber companies.

The incidence of snake bite in Sri Lanka, a popular holiday location, is currently one of the highest in the world, with 400 bites and six deaths per 100 000 population per year. Here the most important species from the medical point of view is Russell's viper (*D. russelii*), which is common in the paddy fields during sowing and harvesting of rice (Phillips *et al.*, 1988). At these times of the year, there is a massive increase in the incidence of snake bite corresponding to the period when the farmers are in the paddies. A similar problem exists in Burma (Myanmar) where bites by Russell's viper are reckoned to be the fifth most common cause of death. In areas of Thailand, bites by the Thai cobra (*N. kaouthia*) represent a major problem in many rice-growing and fish-farming regions (Virivan *et al.*, 1986). Further south, in the rubber plantations of Thailand and Malaysia, bites by the Malayan pit viper (*Calloselasma rhodostoma*) are a major cause of morbidity with some associated mortality (Warrell *et al.*, 1986).

Reliable observations suggest that more than half of all those sustaining bites escape with minor or no poisoning because little or no venom is injected. On the other hand, mortality can be high when adequate medical treatment is not given for serious envenoming. It can be as high as 50% following envenoming by sea snakes (which occurs in 20% of all sea snake bites) and 10–15% in cases of *E. ocellatus* envenoming in West Africa. Snake bite in its early stages is very unpredictable and all victims should

Table 21.1   Precautions that should be taken to avoid snake bites

---

- Cut the grass short around houses or camp sites
- Wear proper shoes or boots, and ideally long trousers, when walking in the dark or in undergrowth where snakes are known to occur
- Make a noise when walking in areas where snakes are common
- Use a torch when walking at night
- Avoid sleeping on the ground: snakes are attracted to the warmth of the human body
- Take care after heavy rain: flooding may force snakes into the open in a confined area
- Avoid snakes as far as possible. Do not attack or corner a snake
- Do not handle snakes, even if you think that they are nonvenomous
- Never put your hand down holes/burrows or behind wood piles without looking
- Pay attention to warnings by members of the local community
- Take care swimming in waters where sea snakes are known to be active

---

be observed closely for at least 24 h to assess the severity of poisoning and to ensure rational treatment.

Avoiding Snake Bite

For the traveller, there are several measures that are invaluable for avoiding snake bite and these should be strictly adhered to in areas where venomous snakes are found. They are summarised in Table 21.1.

Pathophysiology of Snake Envenoming

The major important clinical effects of venom may be classified as follows:

1. Local effects: increased vascular permeability and/or direct cytolytic action leading to pain, swelling and/or tissue necrosis.
2. Systemic effects:
   (a) Shock
   (b) Bleeding
   (c) Coagulopathy
   (d) Neurotoxicity
   (e) Myotoxicity, cardiotoxicity and nephrotoxicity (less common).

Local effects.   Many different venoms contain components such as proteases, haemorrhagins, hyaluronidase, cytotoxins and phospholipases. These act to increase vascular permeability, damage vascular endothelium and destroy skin and subcutaneous tissue, leading to swelling,

bruising and necrosis of a bitten limb.

Shock or hypotension is a prominent feature of envenoming by some species, particularly vipers. Syncope is sometimes reported soon after the bite; this may be an autopharmacological effect in which venoms contain substances that cause release of endogenous kinins or histamines. Later or prolonged hypotension is usually due to loss of fluid from the circulation because of changes in vascular permeability or because of haemorrhage. Some venoms may also cause direct myocardial toxicity or lead to vasodilatation.

Bleeding.   The rapid development of intense local haemorrhage and systemic bleeding is a feature of envenoming by a number of species. These effects are caused by venom haemorrhagic factors (haemorrhagins), potent zinc metalloproteinases which degrade proteins of the extracellular endothelial matrix (with resulting haemorrhage) and which can also affect platelet function by inhibiting aggregation. Haemorrhagins are responsible for the frequently observed gingival haemorrhage, or bleeding from old wounds/sores, etc. In combination with a coagulopathy, they can lead to life-threatening bleeding into tissues such as the brain and the gut.

Coagulopathy.   The venoms of many vipers and some elapids contain substances capable of activating clotting factors. These may act on the clotting cascade at a number of sites, activating prothrombin and/or factors X and V or converting fibrinogen directly to fibrin (thrombin-like enzyme). In small animals, the effect of such actions is to cause total intravascular coagulation of the whole circulation. In humans, envenomed patients often develop a consumption coagulopathy or a disseminated intravascular coagulation (DIC)-like state, with low fibrinogen levels, prolonged prothrombin and activated partial thromboplastin times and elevated levels of fibrin(ogen) degradation products. Although some venoms contain substances that act as anticoagulants *in vitro*, these are rarely clinically significant. Thrombocytopenia may occur because of consumption of platelets, but may also be due to a direct effect of venoms on platelet numbers and function.

Neurotoxicity.   This is a prominent and life-threatening effect of envenoming by many elapids. A vast number of individual neurotoxins have been described and isolated; venom from one species often contains a mixture of different neurotoxins. They can be divided broadly by their major site of action: presynaptic or postsynaptic. Presynaptic neurotoxins are predominately phospholipases A_2, which tend to bind with poor reversibility to the motor endplate and damage the nerve terminal, preventing transmitter release. Recovery is by regrowth and resprouting of axons. Postsynaptic neurotoxins tend to bind reversibly to postsynaptic receptors, and hence are more amenable to treatment.

Renal failure.   Acute tubular necrosis occurs following

Table 21.2 Main clinical features of snake bite

Snake	No poisoning (%)	Effects of poisoning		Natural mortality (approximate) (%)	Average death (time)
		Local	Systemic		
Elapids	50	Slow swelling, then necrosis by Asian cobras, African spitting cobras Usually no local effects with other elapids	Neurotoxic effects: ptosis, bulbar palsy Respiratory paralysis	10	5–20 h
Sea snakes	80	None	Myotoxic effects: Myalgia on moving Paresis Myoglobinuria Hyperkalaemia	10	15 h
Vipers	30	Rapid swelling Necrosis in 5–10% (some vipers only)	Haemorrhagic effects and abnormal bleeding Nonclotting blood (some vipers only) Shock	1–15	2 days

bites by a number of species. In some cases, it may simply be due to the effects of prolonged hypovolaemia. However, direct venom nephrotoxicity, DIC and rhabdomyolysis and myoglobinuria are all important mechanisms following bites by certain species. Renal ischaemia and renal cortical necrosis may also occur.

Cardiotoxicity. ECG changes have been reported following envenoming by a large number of different species, although clinically significant cardiotoxicity is much less common. These changes are caused by a number of different mechanisms, including a direct effect of venom components on myocardial or conducting tissue function, myocardial damage due to myotoxins or myocardial haemorrhage, or alterations in coronary blood flow due to coronary vasospasm, coronary thrombi or hypotension.

Myotoxicity. The venoms of sea snakes, certain rattlesnakes and some Russell's vipers contain phospholipases A_2, which act directly to break down skeletal muscle cells, causing rhabdomyolysis, myoglobinaemia and myoglobinuria. Renal failure is a common accompaniment of this syndrome in untreated patients.

Clinical Features

These are summarised in Table 21.2. Fright and anxiety often causes signs and symptoms that may mimic systemic envenoming.

Local Envenoming

Early Features

Local swelling starts within a few minutes of a viper bite if venom is injected (Figure 21.2). It is a valuable clinical sign because, if swelling is absent and it is known that the biting snake was a viper, then envenoming may be quickly excluded. Local swelling is also a feature of envenoming in bites by Asian cobras and the African spitting cobra, *N. nigricollis*, although it may not appear for 1–2 h. Bites by other elapids (nonspitting African cobras, mambas, kraits, coral snakes) and sea snakes do not usually cause swelling.

Local pain and fang marks are extremely variable and of no help in diagnosis. In bites by some snakes, usually vipers, early blackening at the bite site may be a sign of impending local necrosis or may be due to the local bleeding caused by the local action of venom haemorrhagins.

Later Features

Local swelling caused by viperine envenoming can extend to the trunk after 2–3 days and can become extensive. Provided necrosis does not develop, it resolves completely in 2–4 weeks, often with discoloration similar to the stages of a bruise. Swelling of a snake-bitten limb may suggest increased intracompartmental pressure in the anterior tibial compartment or the digital pulp spaces. However, compartmental syndromes are relatively rare and tend to be overdiagnosed in snake bites, particularly by surgeons.

Blisters extending up the limb suggest that local necrosis will follow. Local necrosis is common in Asian and

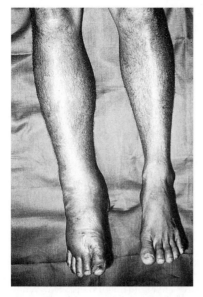

Figure 21.2 Swelling following the bite of a Malayan pit viper. The bite occurred on the dorsum of the right foot

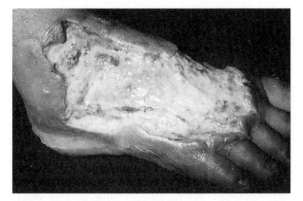

Figure 21.3 Debrided wound following local necrosis after a bite by an Asian common cobra. Similar necrosis occurs in bites by the African spitting cobra, *Naja nigricollis*

African spitting cobra bites, and in 5–10% of some viper bites (such as those caused by the African puff adder). Necrosis becomes evident a few days after the bite by a darkening of the skin, together with an offensive 'putrid' smell, which is particularly marked in cobra bite necrosis. Necrosis can be extensive (Figure 21.3) but it is usually superficial; involvement of tendons, muscle and bones is exceptional. Bacterial infection may follow necrosis and may spread to deep tissues. In the absence of necrosis or harmful local 'treatment' measures, such as incisions, fasciotomy or application of dirty dressings, bacterial infection is rare in snake bite.

Systemic Envenoming

Nonspecific Early Signs

There are three important nonspecific early signs of systemic envenoming:

1. Vomiting (sometimes of emotional origin but more often denotes systemic envenoming)
2. Hypotension (elapid and viper bites, but not sea snake bites)
3. Polymorph leucocytosis (varies according to species).

In envenoming by some species of snake, painful enlargement of the draining local lymph nodes (most commonly in the femoral region) is an extremely useful sign that significant amounts of venom have been absorbed into the lymphatic system.

Specific Signs

Specific early signs of systemic envenoming may develop within 15 min of the bite but their onset may be delayed up to 18 h after an elapid bite. Thus, it is important to observe carefully all patients after a snake bite. These specific signs depend upon the biting species and can be broadly divided into three groups. *Viper bites* may result in abnormal bleeding from gums and old wounds, incoagulable blood and shock. In *elapid bites* the most common feature is neurotoxicity, and in *sea snake bites* there is usually generalised myalgia, myoglobinuria and paresis.

Shock. Hypotension often associated with fluid loss into a limb.

Coagulopathy and haemorrhage. Bleeding may occur from the bite site, injection sites, the gums (Figure 21.4) or old wounds. Blood may be found in the sputum, vomit or stool. Discoid ecchymoses may be observed. Spontaneous capillary haemorrhage may occur into vital organs, especially the brain. This may be delayed from 3 days to a week after a viper bite if effective antivenom is not given, and is often, although not inevitably, fatal.

Neurotoxicity. Ptosis is the commonest early sign of neurotoxicity. This may progress to cause ophthalmoplegia and bulbar paralysis: patients are unable to speak, cough, swallow or protrude their tongue (Figure 21.5). Paralysis of the limbs occurs and ultimately ventilatory failure may occur due to paralysis of the intercostal muscles and the diaphragm. Respiratory paralysis may be preceded by shallow breathing, rise in pulse, respiration rate and blood pressure, increased sweating, cyanosis, confusion and stupor. Coma, nonreactive dilated pupils, twitchings, and convulsions presage death.

Myotoxicity. Severe myalgia and tenderness may be followed by myoglobinuria. Peripheral paresis may occur

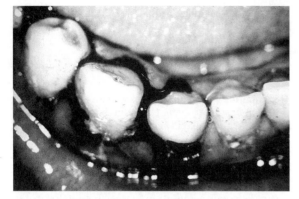

Figure 21.4   Bleeding from the gums following a bite by *Echis ocellatus*, the carpet viper. (Reproduced with permission from Professor D.A. Warrell)

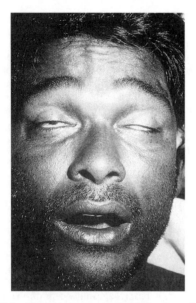

Figure 21.5   Neurotoxic envenoming following a bite by the Indian krait, *Bungarus caeruleus*. (Reproduced with permission from Professor D.A. Warrell)

after some hours, tendon reflexes become depressed, then absent. Respiratory failure from muscle weakness may supervene within a few hours or as long as 60 h after the bite. Some patients succumb from hyperkalaemic cardiac arrest or (later) from acute renal failure.

Renal failure.   There may be oliguria, abnormal electrolytes and raised urea and creatinine on presentation, but these often develop during the course of envenoming in hospital.

Severe systemic envenoming is indicated by the following:

• *Viperine envenoming.* Shock, swelling extending above elbow or knee, haemorrhagic signs and/or incoagulable blood within 30 min of the bite. T wave inversion and ST depression on ECG.

• *Elapid envenoming.* Neurotoxic signs usually within an hour of the bite, with rapid progression. Shock may also occur. T wave inversion and ST depression on ECG.

• *Sea snake envenoming.* Myoglobinuria within 1–2 h and/or signs of respiratory failure. Tall, peaked T waves in chest leads of ECG give warning of impending death due to hyperkalaemia or renal failure.

There are rare exceptions to the rule of haemorrhage and coagulopathy occurring in vipers and neurotoxicity in elapids. Venoms of some Australasian elapids such as the taipan, *O. scutellatus*, cause incoagulable blood and systemic bleeding in addition to causing characteristic neurotoxicity (Lalloo *et al.*, 1995). Venoms of some viperine snakes such as *C. durissus terrificus*, the South American tropical rattlesnake, and the South African Berg adder, *Bitis caudalis*, also cause neurotoxic signs in systemically envenomed humans. The venom of some viperine snakes (e.g. *C. d. terrificus* and *D. russelii*) may also be myotoxic, causing rhabdomyolysis and myoglobinuria in a similar fashion to sea snake bites.

Diagnosis

The diagnostic importance of local swelling in viperine poisoning has already been stressed. For some viper bites, nonclotting blood may be the earliest and only sign of envenoming. This should be looked for by a simple and very sensitive bedside test of systemic envenoming (Table 21.3). This test is extremely useful for the diagnosis of systemic envenoming, especially in areas where laboratory facilities do not exist. Along with careful clinical observation, it may also be useful in helping to diagnose the biting species. For example, in parts of West Africa and Southeast Asia, an abnormal clotting test is diagnostic of viper bite and eliminates bites by elapids. Nonclotting blood can also differentiate envenoming by one type of viper from that of another; for example, in Africa *E. ocellatus* envenoming causes nonclotting blood, whereas envenoming by *B. arietans* does not. Recognition of the dangerous local species and their clinical pattern of envenoming is extremely useful in making subsequent treatment decisions.

Definitive diagnosis of the envenoming species can only be made if the snake is reliably identified; however, victims seldom bring the snake with them and species identification by the victim or associates at the time of the bite is notoriously unreliable. Many victims claim to have been bitten by a 'big black snake' when the snake responsible is in fact a small brown snake! Although a dead snake is useful, victims or the local population should be dissuaded from attempting to kill the snake responsible for the bite as this may result in a second bite. Even when the snake is brought to the hospital, medical and nursing

Table 21.3 Twenty minute whole blood clotting test

- Place a few millilitres of freshly sampled blood in a new, clean, dry glass tube or bottle
- Leave undisturbed for 20 min at ambient temperature
- Tip the vessel once
- If the blood is still liquid (unclotted) and runs out, the patient has hypofibrinogenaemia ('incoagulable blood') as a result of venom-induced consumption coagulopathy

Table 21.4 Summary of emergency management procedures for snake bite

- Reassure the patient
- Avoid manoeuvres that may do harm (incision, suction etc.)
- Immobilise the bitten limb
- Transfer the patient to hospital as rapidly as possible
- A pressure immobilisation bandage may be appropriate if the bite of the snake is unlikely to cause tissue necrosis
- Maintain an airway
- Avoid oral fluids or drugs (especially aspirin or sedatives)
- Take the snake to hospital if it has been killed (care!)

personnel often misidentify the species; local knowledge is not always reliable.

ELISA can provide a more objective, although usually retrospective, means of reliable identification of the species causing the envenoming (Theakston, 1991). It can be used to detect specific venom at the bite site or in an aspirate taken from a venom-induced blister or wound aspirate and to quantify the amount of venom present in body fluids such as serum and urine. Rapid ELISA tests, which can provide an accurate diagnosis within 30 min, have been developed in Australia and may be useful for the traveller in that country. They permit the use of the correct monospecific antivenom for treatment; however, the costs of such tests have precluded their development and use in most developing countries. It is important to emphasise that the detection of specific venom on the skin at the bite site does not necessarily mean that envenoming has occurred; other signs of envenoming must be looked for.

First Aid and Prehospital Treatment

The aims of first aid for bites and stings by snakes and other venomous animals should be to treat or delay life-threatening effects which may develop before the patient reaches medical care, to hasten the safe transfer of the patients to a hospital, clinic or dispensary and to avoid harmful measures (Table 21.4):

1. Panic is a common response to snake bite. The patient should be reassured that not all bites result in envenoming, that most snakes are nonvenomous and that modern hospital treatment is effective.
2. Harmful measures should be avoided at all costs. Wound incision is of no benefit, will aggravate bleeding in victims who have a venom-induced coagulopathy, may damage nerves and tendons and may introduce infection. There is no evidence that application of suction is effective in removing venom from the wound. It may introduce secondary infection and may aggravate the problems of venom-induced local necrosis. Tourniquets or constriction bands should be avoided. Electric shock therapy, application or injection of chemicals locally to the site of the injury, local application of ice packs, and excessive and potentially dangerous traditional methods (e.g. black snake stone, forcible inhalation of oil) should be avoided.

3. The patient should be transferred as quickly as possible to the nearest place where medical attention is available. Minimising movement of the bitten limb will reduce the spread of venom from the bite site through the lymphatic system into the circulation. Splinting is a useful way of immobilising the limb.
4. If evacuation time to a hospital or clinic with antivenom facilities is likely to exceed 30 min, application of a pressure bandage may be useful. Although there is no formal clinical trial evidence for its efficacy, animal experiments and anecdotal reports from Australia suggest that it may be effective in delaying absorption of venom via the lymphatics. A compressive crepe bandage should be applied firmly, as for a sprain, over the bite and up the entire limb (White, 1987) (Figure 21.6). Strips of torn clothing can be used as a substitute. This bandage, or alternative, should not be released during transit. This procedure is only appropriate for bites by snakes whose venom does *not* cause local necrosis and swelling (e.g. Australasian elapids, kraits, coral snakes, sea snakes). If used for snakes with necrosis-inducing venoms, this treatment may concentrate the venom at the bite site, thus worsening the local cytolytic effect.
5. Oral intake of food, alcohol, drugs (especially aspirin or sedatives) or drinks should be avoided unless necessary to avoid dehydration.
6. A clear airway should be maintained by lying the patient head-down on the side. This will prevent aspiration of vomitus or oral secretions. If a patient stops breathing, expired air ventilation with or without external cardiac massage should be commenced. In patients with severe neurotoxicity, artificial ventilation can be successfully maintained for a number of hours until the patient reaches medical care.
7. If the snake has been killed, it should be taken to the hospital with the victim. Careful handling is necessary: the biting reflexes of a recently dead snake may cause a second bite.
8. Introduction of venom into the eye by the African and Asian spitting cobras should be treated by liberal irrigation with water or other available bland fluids (e.g. milk or even urine).

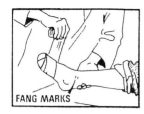

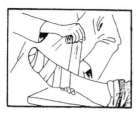

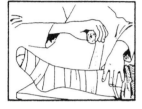

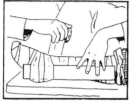

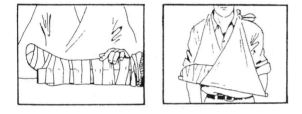

Figure 21.6 Crepe bandage technique for limb immobilisation following snake bite. (Reproduced with permission from Dr B. Currie)

Table 21.5   Initial clinical assessment of the envenomed patient

- Whole blood clotting test. This should be repeated at 6-hourly intervals if envenoming by a viper whose venom causes fibrinogen consumption is suspected
- Careful examination of gums, injection sites and old wounds for signs of bleeding
- Examination for ptosis, limb weakness or difficulties in breathing, talking or swallowing
- Regular recording of pulse, respiration, blood pressure and urine output
- Examination for muscle tenderness and myoglobinuria in sea snake bites
- Measurement of limb swelling (comparing the circumference at different levels with unbitten limb)
- Recording of local necrosis (skin colour, blisters, putrid smell)
- Electrocardiograph

Table 21.6   Useful laboratory tests in envenoming

White blood cell count
Haemoglobin level
Platelet count
Prothrombin time, APTT and fibrinogen levels if available
Serum urea and creatinine
Creatine phosphokinase (CPK) (reflecting skeletal muscle damage)

Early Management

Initial Assessment

It is very important that staff neither panic nor dismiss a case of snake bite as trivial, without proper observation. Except for cases in which envenoming can be *reliably* excluded, the patient should be carefully observed for at least 24 h; fatalities have occurred in patients discharged from hospital with presumed minor envenoming only. Initial observations which should be performed are shown in Table 21.5 and useful laboratory tests in Table 21.6.

Local Site

On admission to hospital, the compression bandage, or any tourniquet which was applied earlier, should be released. There are case reports of sudden systemic envenoming following removal of tourniquets; patients should be carefully observed over this period. After cleansing if necessary, the site of the bite should be left alone. Local dressings should not be applied as they increase the risk of secondary bacterial infection. It is now recommended that blisters should be aspirated using a sterile syringe. They may contain large amounts of free venom which could theoretically gain later entry to the circulation and exacerbate the clinical situation.

Although bacteria are found commonly in the oral cavities of snakes (Theakston *et al.*, 1990), infection at the site of the wound is relatively uncommon unless skin necrosis is present. Routine antibiotic prophylaxis is therefore not recommended unless necrosis is present. The commonest organisms found from infected clinical specimens are Gram-negative, but Gram-positive aerobic cocci and anaerobes also cause problems. From the few limited clinical studies, chloramphenicol or a combination of penicillin and an aminoglycocide would be suitable initial therapy until sensitivities become available. Although reports of tetanus following snake bite are extremely rare, tetanus toxoid should be given to all patients with a snake bite.

Antivenoms

Indications for Use

Antivenom is the most important factor in the treatment of serious systemic envenoming. It can reverse systemic effects of the venom when given hours or even days after the bite. The major indication for the administration of antivenom is systemic envenoming (usually neurotoxicity, incoagulable blood and bleeding or hypotension and shock).

The indications for the use of antivenom in local envenoming are less clear; further research is needed to assess indications and efficacy in this situation. However, antivenom treatment should be considered in patients presenting within hours of a bite by a known or suspected necrotising snake, such as Asian cobras, African spitting cobras and puff adders, who have swelling extending to cover more than half the length of the bitten limb (e.g. a bite on the hand or foot with swelling extending to the elbow or knee).

Antivenom remains effective for treating a coagulopathy for a number of days after a bite; however, in most cases when a patient presents with neurotoxicity more than 24 h after a bite, antivenom is only indicated if life-threatening neurotoxicity is present or develops subsequently. Antivenom should not be given routinely in all cases of snake bite because of adverse anaphylactic-type reactions in about 1–80% (Cardoso *et al.*, 1993) of individuals, depending on the antivenom. It is also expensive and often in short supply in many developing countries; it should therefore not be used unnecessarily.

Choice of Antivenom

Antivenoms are produced by immunising large animals (usually horses) with gradually increasing amounts of venom. Once hyperimmunised, the animal is bled and the plasma or serum harvested. Pools of individual venoms obtained from a large number of snakes of the same species are used; this eliminates venom variation, which can be extensive even within single species from the same geographical area. If a venom pool from a single species is used for immunisation, the serum is termed monospecific or monovalent; if venom from more than one species is used, it is termed polyspecific or polyvalent.

Monospecific antivenoms are theoretically more effective and less likely to cause reactions than polyspecific antivenoms; their neutralising activity for a particular venom is greater and therefore less foreign protein is required for treatment. Polyspecific antivenoms, which are usually prepared by immunising the animal against 4 or 5 venoms from snakes within a geographical area, contain more foreign protein, with a consequent higher rate of early, potentially life-threatening reactions. Monospecific antivenoms are useful when the snake can be definitively identified or when there is one predominant venomous species in a particular area. Use of monospecific antivenoms may be facilitated by venom detection kits, as described previously in Australia. Polyspecific antivenoms are useful when the species of the biting species is not known and usually will cover most of the important venomous species for a particular area.

Although whole purified or crude IgG has been used in the past, most commercial antivenoms currently produced use pepsin to remove the Fc fragment, leaving an antivenom composed of F(ab')$_2$ fragments (Figure 21.7). Providing that the Fc fragment has been effectively removed during the purification procedure, F(ab')$_2$ antivenoms do not bind complement or macrophages, eliminating a common source of antivenom reactions.

Recently, antivenoms have been produced which consist of smaller, Fab fragments prepared from the whole IgG molecule by papain digestion (Theakston and Smith, 1995). This has theoretical advantages. Fab antivenoms only have one antigen binding site and do not form immune complexes of sufficient size to cause type III hypersensitivity reactions. Due to their smaller size, Fab fragments have greater volumes of distribution and more rapid kinetics than either IgG or F(ab')$_2$ (Meyer *et al.*, 1997). This means that, potentially, they may penetrate tissue spaces better, which may be of particular importance at the neuromuscular junction. However, it also means that they are rapidly cleared from the circulation via the kidney; about five times more rapidly than the clearance of F(ab')$_2$ fragment antivenoms. Frequent redosing of Fab antivenoms may therefore be needed in order to neutralise venom antigen which is redistributed from tissues to blood or absorbed from a venom depot at the bite site. Currently, most antivenoms are of the F(ab')$_2$ fragment type; it is felt that the disadvantages of an Fab antivenom outweigh the potential advantages.

Dose and Administration

The dose of antivenom is primarily dependent on its neutralising efficacy, which varies considerably between different manufacturers. In most cases, local advice should be sought, which may be more reliable than the manufacturer's instructions. Recommended initial doses of antivenom may vary according to the severity of envenoming. *Doses of antivenom for children are the same as those for adults* because the amount of venom introduced by the snake bears no relationship to the age or to the size of the victim.

Ideally, antivenom should be diluted two- to three-fold in saline and be given by intravenous infusion. Dextrose saline can be used in children to avoid a large sodium load. The infusion should be started off slowly and the rate progressively increased so that it is completed within an hour. In the absence of infusion apparatus, antivenom can be given by slow direct push injection over 10–15 min. Before use, antivenom should be checked for any opacities, which precede loss of potency. Clear antivenom is fully effective and, in areas where it is in short supply, expired antivenom which retains its clarity should not be discarded.

The administration of further doses of antivenom is dependent upon careful observation of the patient's clinical response to antivenom. Correction of a venom-induced coagulopathy is a good marker of the efficacy of antivenom in patients envenomed by viperine snakes

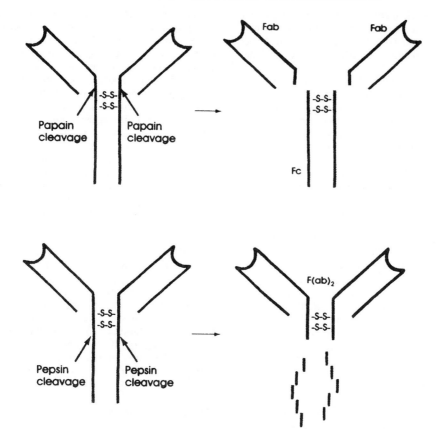

Figure 21.7   Schematic representation of the IgG molecule highlighting both F(ab′)$_2$, Fab and Fc regions

whose venom causes fibrinogen consumption. On admission to hospital such patients often have incoagulable blood, measured by the 20 min whole blood clotting test (20WBCT; Sano-Martins *et al.*, 1994). Six hours after antivenom, the 20WBCT should be repeated. Resolution of coagulation is evidence that the antivenom is effective; if the blood is still nonclotting, then a further dose of antivenom is indicated. As incoagulable blood can reoccur after apparent successful treatment with antivenom, the whole blood clotting test should be repeated at 6-hourly intervals for the first 2 days.

It is generally more difficult to judge the need for further antivenom when the predominant problem is neurotoxicity. In envenoming by some species (e.g. the Australasian death adder or the Philippine cobra) an effective antivenom will reverse neurotoxic signs such as ptosis, external ophthalmoplegia and respiratory paralysis. For these species, if there is no improvement in neuromuscular function, then further doses of antivenom should be given; however, for other species of elapid, especially those with neurotoxins that bind presynaptically, neurotoxic signs are more difficult to reverse even with adequate doses of antivenom. This appears to be because toxin binding is poorly reversible. In such cases,

the clinical response does not help in deciding whether further antivenom is needed.

Enzyme immunoassay can be used as a research tool to look at the rate of permanent venom clearance. Circulating venom and antivenom levels can be assessed quantitatively on retrospective samples and may help to determine the optimum dose of a particular antivenom (Figure 21.8). The time taken by the antivenom to clear venom permanently from the circulation correlates well with correction of venom-induced systemic effects, such as the restoration of blood coagulability.

Antivenom Reactions

Prediction and Prevention

All patients given antivenom treatment should be regarded as likely to have a reaction, although the incidence of reaction varies widely between different antivenoms (1–80%; Cardoso *et al.*, 1993). Skin sensitivity tests have no predictive value for reactions (Warrell, 1983). They should not be used; they delay treatment and can themselves be sensitising. A history of a significant allergic

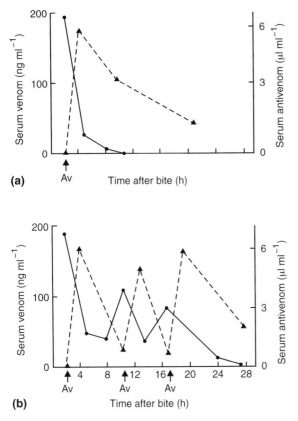

Figure 21.8 Venom and antivenom (AV) levels in a patient treated with (a) an effective antivenom and (b) a relatively ineffective antivenom. Venom levels (•) are shown by unbroken lines and antivenom levels (▲) by broken lines

adrenaline (epinephrine), especially in patients with co-agulopathies. While the efficacy of prophylaxis with adrenaline (epinephrine) appears promising, there are not yet adequate safety data to routinely recommend adrenaline (epinephrine) prophylaxis, especially as life-threatening reactions are rare. The benefit : harm ratio of adrenaline (epinephrine) will depend considerably upon the incidence of severe antivenom reactions for a particular antivenom.

Early Reactions

The majority of early antivenom reactions appear to be due to complement activation, often by the presence of $F(ab')_2$, or Fab, aggregates in the antivenom. The incidence of antivenom reactions is closely related to the quality of purification of antivenoms. Both immediate (potentially life-threatening) and delayed serum reactions may be more common with polyspecific antivenoms than with monospecific antivenoms because of the larger volumes of antivenom required. Although intravenous infusion is advocated, it has been shown that there are no significant differences in the incidence of early reactions when antivenom is administered by slow intravenous push injection or by slow intravenous infusion (Malasit et al., 1986).

In routine antivenom therapy, adrenaline (epinephrine) should be drawn up for use before the infusion is started. The initial drip rate should be slow and at the first sign of any anaphylactoid reaction (e.g. a few spots of urticaria, start of itching, tachycardia or restlessness) antivenom infusion should be temporarily stopped. Adrenaline (epinephrine) [0.5 mg; 0.5 ml of 1 : 1000 adrenaline (epinephrine)] should be injected intramuscularly into the deltoid muscle. In the case of children, the recommended dose is $0.01 \, mg \, kg^{-1}$ body weight intramuscularly. This is usually quickly effective. After minor reactions, the antivenom infusion can then be cautiously restarted, along with antihistamine treatment (e.g. H1-blockers such as chlorpheniramine maleate: adults 10 mg, children $0.2 \, mg \, kg^{-1}$ by intravenous injection over a few minutes).

Pyrogenic Reactions

Some antivenoms contain impurities (endotoxins) due to inadequate purification; these can cause pyrogenic reactions. Such reactions are treated by cooling the patient physically, giving antipyretics, such as paracetamol, by mouth and intravenous fluids to correct hypovolaemia.

Late Serum Sickness Reactions

These usually occur 7–10 days after antivenom. Clinical features include fever, itching, recurrent urticaria, arthralgia, lymphadenopathy, periarticular swellings, mononeuritis multiplex, proteinuria with immune complex

reaction to antivenom is a relative contraindication to its use unless the risk of death from envenoming is high. In that rare event, small amounts of adrenaline (epinephrine), (0.2–0.5 ml of 1 : 1000 adrenaline (epinephrine) solution) should be given subcutaneously before antivenom administration and should be repeated if a reaction occurs.

Routine prophylaxis against antivenom reactions is controversial. Adrenaline (epinephrine), antihistamines and steroids have all been used in various regions of the world. There is no rationale for the use of steroids in early reactions and their role will not be considered further. There is no evidence that routine prophylaxis with antihistamines is effective; one small Brazilian clinical trial demonstrated no reduction in either early or late antivenom reactions (Fan et al., 1999). A recent trial in Sri Lanka suggested that routine use of adrenaline (epinephrine) prophylaxis reduced the incidence of early antivenom reactions from 43% to 11%. (Premawardhena et al., 1999). The trial excluded certain categories of patients in view of concerns about the possible adverse effects of nephritis and rarely encephalopathy. These reactions may be treated with an oral antihistamine combined with a steroid such as prednisolone (15–20 mg day^{-1}).

Venom-induced Anaphylaxis

Individuals who have been exposed to venom previously or who have worked with venomous snakes and/or venoms are at risk from IgE-mediated anaphylactic shock. People sensitised in this way may well suffer severe and life-threatening reactions in the event of a snake bite.

The Traveller and Antivenom

In general, it is not recommended that the overseas traveller purchases antivenom to take with him or her when visiting areas in which snake bite is a problem. The reasons for this are:

- Hospitals in areas where bites are a problem would normally be expected to stock appropriate antivenoms.
- Antivenom can cause severe and potentially life-threatening reactions. Medically qualified individuals trained in its delivery must therefore administer it in a hospital environment (preferably under intensive care conditions).
- Antivenom must be given by the intravenous route, requiring qualified personnel. It is a waste of time to give antivenom locally or by any other route.
- Antivenoms should ideally be stored at 4 °C.

However, there may be exceptions to this rule; for example, the traveller may be visiting areas where snake bite is a major problem and where no antivenoms are available locally. Under these conditions there would be a case for purchasing the antivenom in advance, after taking expert advice as to the optimum type and source of the antivenom. In this situation, a polyspecific antivenom would be the most appropriate.

It cannot be stressed strongly enough that antivenom *should not be administered by a lay or inexperienced person* for the reasons already given. In the unlikely event of a bite, the antivenom should be taken to the hospital with the victim. In most circumstances, even in remote areas when incidents happen, arrangements can be made to get the bitten individual to hospital in plenty of time. Intramuscular administration of most snake antivenoms is not effective.

Supportive Therapy

Although antivenom is of prime importance in treating snake bite, supportive therapy of the patient may be crucial in minimising both mortality and morbidity.

Neurotoxicity

As antivenom is not always effective in reversing neurotoxicity, maintenance and protection of the airway and assisting ventilation are life-saving interventions. Patients with early signs of neurotoxicity need careful observation. The inability of a patient to swallow saliva, leading to pooling and dribbling of secretions, is an important sign that a patient is unable to guard the airway. They should be nursed head-down, on the side and endotracheal (ET) intubation should be performed, if possible, to protect the airway.

If further progression of neurotoxicity occurs, assisted ventilation should be performed via an ET tube or tracheostomy. In the absence of mechanical ventilators, patients have been successfully ventilated by hand for a number of days, sometimes utilising relays of relatives. Ventilation may need to be continued for up to 5 days before recovery of neuromuscular function occurs. Patients should be lightly sedated, as although they may appear unconscious and unable to react to stimuli, this is a function of profound neuromuscular paralysis; few venoms affect the central nervous system.

One extremely useful adjunct for the treatment of neurotoxicity is the use of anticholinesterases. These appear to be particularly effective in bites by species which have neurotoxins that act primarily postsynaptically (e.g. many cobras or Australasian death adders). Initially, one should evaluate the effectiveness of anticholinesterases by performing a 'Tensilon test'. A short-acting anticholinesterase drug such as edrophonium chloride (2 mg initially, then 8 mg) should be injected intravenously along with atropine sulphate to avoid undesirable side-effects. The patient should be observed over 10–20 min. If neurotoxic signs such as ptosis disappear or the ventilatory capacity improves, then a longer-acting anticholinesterase such as neostigmine can be given combined with atropine. In some patients, the response to anticholinesterases can be dramatic and may obviate the need for antivenom. Unfortunately, these drugs are not effective for venoms that cause presynaptic neuromuscular blockade.

Coagulopathy and Bleeding

Strenuous efforts should be made to prevent complications from bleeding in a patient with a coagulopathy. Intramuscular injections and invasive procedures should be avoided; patients should avoid activities that may lead to trauma. After adequate treatment with antivenom, the restoration of normal clotting is dependent upon the hepatic synthesis of clotting factors, which takes several hours. There is no role for clotting factors, fresh frozen plasma or fresh blood unless there are signs of significant active bleeding. Even then, they should not be used until sufficient antivenom has been given to neutralise venom procoagulant components; giving blood products before this point may lead theoretically to a worsening of a coagulopathy and to clot deposition in small vessels.

Shock

Fluid replacement or blood transfusion may occasionally be indicated for victims of viper bites who are in shock, but specific antivenom is usually dramatically successful in viperine shock if given in adequate dosage. Central venous pressure lines may be helpful in determining fluid requirements, especially if there is concomitant renal impairment. Very rarely, inotropic drugs such as adrenaline (epinephrine) may be needed. Arrythmias are rare, but occasionally, atropine is needed for bradycardias.

Renal Impairment

This occurs due to a number of mechanisms, including direct nephrotoxicity of the venom. In many cases, careful fluid balance is all that is required. Peritoneal dialysis can be set up in quite primitive conditions and has been used very effectively in areas such as Burma, where renal failure following Russell's viper bite is common. Renal impairment in association with rhabdomyolysis and myoglobinuria (as in sea snake bites) may be avoided by the early use of alkaline diuresis and mannitol.

Late Management of Local Wounds

As soon as local necrosis is obvious, sloughs should be excised. There have been good results with the use of early skin grafting, even if infection is still evident. As previously discussed, the considerable swelling following bites by some species may lead to clinical suspicion of compartmental syndromes. Fasciotomy should not be considered unless the intracompartmental pressure exceeds 45 mmHg (less in children). This can be simply measured by the introduction of a cannula into the compartment, which is connected to a transducer (or simple fluid manometer). Special care may needed with the management of bites affecting the pulp space of the fingers. It is vital that haemostatic disorders are corrected before surgery; many patients have bled to death from unnecessary fasciotomies.

Eye Injuries

Some cobra species in Africa and Asia are able to 'spit' from fang tips whose venom duct exits are directed forwards instead of downwards. These cobras can eject venom up to 2 m and venom may enter the eyes of the victims. If this occurs, the eyes should be thoroughly irrigated with liberal amounts of water or other available bland liquid. If the eyes are promptly bathed with water, only mild inflammation results. Instillation of 0.5% adrenaline (epinephrine) drops is reported to relieve the pain and inflammation. Because of the slight risk of corneal abrasion, examination by fluorescein staining or slit lamp is advisable. Otherwise, topical antimicrobials such as tetracycline or chloramphenicol should be applied.

If Antivenom is Not Available

Unfortunately, in many areas of the world, appropriate antivenoms are sometimes unavailable. If neurotoxicity occurs, supportive therapy as indicated above (airway management and artificial ventilation) can prevent death. Recovery from neurotoxicity will eventually occur, although this may take a number of days. Coagulopathies may also spontaneously recover; avoidance of trauma and prevention of bleeding become the major priorities. Fresh frozen plasma, clotting factors, cryoprecipitates or fresh whole blood can be transfused to prevent serious bleeding, but this procedure runs the theoretical risk of making things worse.

SCORPION STINGS

In many areas of the world, scorpion stings are medically much more important than snake bites. Such areas include Mexico, Trinidad, parts of Brazil, North Africa, the Middle East, and India. A 1979 survey in Libya revealed an estimated yearly total of over 6500 scorpion stings in a population of 3 million people, with at least 50 deaths, most of which were in children under 2 years old. In Mexico there are an estimated 300 000 cases a year, with about 1000 deaths (WHO, 1981). The extent of the problem in some areas is also increasing; for example, in Minas Gerais State in Brazil, scorpions such as *Tityus serrulatus* are rapidly colonising urban areas.

Scorpions have four pairs of legs, a pair of claws, a body with a broader front part and a six-jointed tail-like abdomen. The terminal segment of the 'tail' is called the telson (Figure 21.9) and contains two venom glands connecting with the curved, needle-sharp sting which is used either in defence or in obtaining food. The tail with its sting is always brought forward in front of the scorpion. Scorpions never sting backwards and this feature enables safe handling of scorpions (provided one is familiar with their habits). The length of adult scorpions varies from under 2 cm up to about 25 cm, but the length of the scorpion does not relate to its danger to humans.

Most scorpions are nocturnal, and feed on spiders and insects. During the daytime, they hide under stones, in cracks, among debris or in clothing; desert species often burrow, sometimes to a depth of as much as 2.5 m. Scorpions are divided into six families and all the dangerous ones are in the Buthidae family. Probably the five species most dangerous to humans are *Centruroides* (southern United States, Central America), *Tityus* (South America), *Androctonus* (Africa), *Leiurus* (Africa and Middle East), and *Buthus* (Africa, Middle East, Asia).

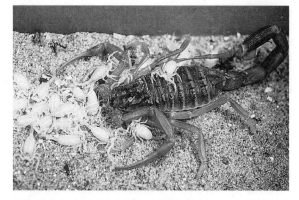

Figure 21.9 Scorpion, with young, showing the terminal segment or telson, which contains two venom glands. The sting is always brought forward over the abdomen

Avoiding Scorpion Sting

The traveller in areas where scorpions are common can take certain simple precautions to avoid being stung:

- Shoes should be worn when walking in the dark.
- Clothes, socks and footwear should be checked carefully for scorpions by shaking them in the morning before dressing.
- A torch should be used when searching in dark areas such as cupboards.
- Storing domestic rubbish near the house should be avoided.
- Travellers, especially children, should be actively discouraged from handling scorpions.

Clinical Features

These are partly dependent on the amount of venom injected relative to the weight of the victim. Pain around the bite site is the commonest feature; this can be severe and last for several hours, even 1–2 days. Local erythema and swelling are unusual, but itching and paraesthesia may be prominent and last for many days. Only a small proportion of victims develop systemic envenoming; this is more common in children and may occur within several minutes of the bite in severe cases. Symptoms and signs are caused primarily by activation of the autonomic nervous system by venom components, leading to an 'autonomic storm' (Table 21.7).

In severe envenoming, the cardiovascular manifestations of severe hypertension, acute pulmonary oedema and myocardial failure are particularly prominent. Respiratory failure may also occur, due to pulmonary oedema, bronchial hypersecretion and paralysis of respiratory muscles. Both tachycardias and bradycardias are common. Acute pancreatitis has been reported to occur in *Tityus* stings and, in India, necropsy evidence of intravascular coagulation has been reported in *Buthus* stings.

Table 21.7 Major signs and symptoms of scorpion envenoming

Tachypnoea
Excessive salivation
Nausea and vomiting
Lacrimation
Sweating
Abdominal pain
Muscle twitches and spasms
Hypertension
Pulmonary oedema
Cardiac arrhythmias
Hypotension
Respiratory failure

Treatment

First aid consists of reassuring the victim, immobilising the limb and getting the victim to hospital. If local pain is severe, the area should be infiltrated through the puncture wound with 2–5 ml 1% lidocaine (lignocaine) hydrochloride. Alternatively, opiates may be used, but care must be taken not to cause respiratory depression. Local injection of emetine hydrochloride has been used to control pain, but is not generally recommended because it sometimes causes local necrosis. Specific scorpion antivenom is available in many parts of the tropics, although supplies are variable. It is indicated, especially in children, for systemic envenoming (ideally, by intravenous infusion as in snake bite, but intramuscular administration may be effective). When antivenom is not available, supportive treatment is indicated. Prazosin appears to be effective in treating hypertension and cardiac failure; it may block the action of scorpion venom peripherally. Nifedipine has also been used to manage hypertension; opinion is divided on its efficacy and it should probably only be used in combination with prazosin. Pulmonary oedema should be treated by conventional means; intravenous vasodilators, such as sodium nitroprusside, may be needed in severe cases. Subcutaneous atropine and intravenous calcium gluconate have been advocated to alleviate systemic symptoms, but evidence of their efficacy is lacking and they could theoretically be harmful.

SPIDER BITES

As with scorpions and many snakes, the harmfulness of a spider cannot be judged from its appearance: many of the large brown fearsome tarantula-like spiders are harmless to humans. Perhaps the most dangerous are the black widow spiders of the genus *Latrodectus*, which are found in most tropical and subtropical countries including North America, Argentina, the Mediterranean region, Middle East, southern Russia, Arabia, Ethiopia, southern and eastern Africa, Madagascar, south and Southeast Asia and New Zealand. The bodies of these spiders

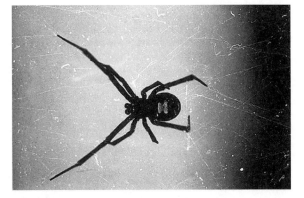

Figure 21.10 The black widow spider, *Latrodectus*, showing the typical abdominal red marking

Table 21.8 Symptoms and signs of latrodectism

Sweating
Hypersalivation
Rhinitis and lacrimation
Nausea and vomiting
Intense cramp-like muscle pain
Generalised weakness
Tachycardia or badycardia
Hypertension
Breathing difficulties
Insomnia and mental agitation
Restlessness and feeling of impending doom
Generalised rash (late)

measure only 1 cm in length (Figure 21.10).

Another biting genus, *Loxosceles*, distributed throughout the American continent, the Mediterranean region and the Middle East, is brown and about the same size as *Latrodectus*. In the United States of America about 3000 bites, primarily by species of these genera, are reported each year, and in Australia, bites by the funnel-web spider (*Atrax robustus*) are fairly common. The highly aggressive Brazilian wolf spider, *Phoneutria nigriventer*, is distributed from southern Brazil to Central America and causes frequent bites; it is responsible for the majority of accidents involving spider bite in Brazil, although very few deaths have been recorded. Spider bite may be difficult to diagnose: the spider responsible is often not found. With a few exceptions, the female spider is usually responsible for envenoming; it is larger than the male and therefore can inject more venom.

Avoiding Spider Bite

It is difficult to avoid bites because the medically important spiders are usually small and, having bitten, are almost impossible to find. It is sensible to wear gloves when working in areas where venomous species are common, and keeping houses/huts free of insects likely to attract spiders may also help. In the unusual event of the spider responsible for the bite being killed, it is a good idea to take the dead animal to the local hospital for possible identification. As mentioned above, all spiders are venomous and many can cause a painful bite; however, fortunately only very few species can cause severe problems.

Clinical Features

Latrodectus spp are not usually aggressive and bite always in self-defence. *L. mactans* is considered to be the most dangerous species. The predominant symptom is pain at the bite site, which usually occurs within an hour

of the bite and may become severe. Bite site reactions are often slight or, at most, demonstrate slight blanching, erythema or urticaria. The majority of patients do not develop systemic signs or symptoms.

In patients who do develop systemic envenoming, the pain may spread from the site to local lymph nodes and become either generalised or affect parts of the body close to the bitten limb. This may take a number of hours to occur. Abdominal pain is common in lower limb bites, and may mimic an acute abdomen. Other features of systemic envenoming are mainly due to transmitter release from skeletal and autonomic nerve endings (Table 21.8).

Some authors describe a characteristic appearance of an envenomed patient, especially in bites in Europe, 'facies lactrodectismica'. Patients have a flushed and sweating face, swollen eyelids, blepharoconjunctivitis and a painful grimace. Hypertension is also a characteristic feature of systemic lactrodectism and may be severe. Electrocardiographic abnormalities have been observed but, overall, death appears to be relatively rare. Recovery is usually complete within 24 h but can take up to a week. Weakness, fatigue, pains, headaches, drowsiness and impotence may persist for several months.

The clinical picture following *Loxosceles* bites is quite different. Although the initial bite may be painless, local pain subsequently develops over a number of hours; patients may present 12–48 h after the bite. A slowly evolving white ischaemic area may be seen at the site of the bite, surrounded by redness and extravasated blood. The white area later turns violaceous, then black and dry by 3–7 days (Figure 21.11). The eschar separates, leaving a deep ulcer. Healing is slow, taking from 3 weeks to 5 months, and sometimes may cause severe scarring. In the rare severely affected patient, systemic manifestations of haemolysis, haemoglobinuria, DIC and ultimately acute renal failure may occur.

The Sydney funnel-web spider, *Atrax robustus*, is medically the most important species of the genus *Atrax* but, in the majority of bites, systemic envenoming does not occur. However, the large fangs and aggressive attack of this spider may result in intense local pain of short duration. Systemic envenoming may develop rapidly, initially causing numbness around the mouth and spasm of

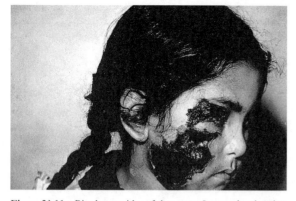

Figure 21.11 Bite by a spider of the genus *Loxosceles* showing the black eschar

the tongue. Nausea and vomiting, abdominal pain, profuse sweating, and excessive salivation and lacrimation may develop. Muscle fasciculation and spasms occur and changes in mental state leading to coma may be observed. Severe hypertension and arrhythmias may occur in the first few hours and acute pulmonary oedema is particularly problematic in children. In some untreated patients, symptoms appear to settle before progressive hypotension occurs, which may culminate in irreversible cardiac arrest.

Systemic envenoming does not occur in the majority of *Phoneutria* bites. Local burning pains at the site of the bite usually radiate to the entire limb and even to the trunk within 10–20 min of the bite. When it occurs, systemic envenoming may develop rapidly, initially causing tachycardia, hypertension, vertigo, fever and sweating (mainly in the neck region). Loss of sight, nausea, vomiting, abdominal pain and priapism, particularly in children, may occur. Confusion, bradycardia, hypotension, pulmonary oedema and shock may occur in severe cases.

Treatment

The pressure immobilisation first aid method is advocated for bites by *Atrax* species, but there are no other specific methods for bites by other species. Antivenoms against spider venoms are produced for treating systemic *Latrodectus* envenoming in Australia, South Africa and Croatia; antivenoms are produced against *Loxosceles* and *Phoneutria* venoms in Brazil. They should be administered in the same way and using the same precautions as for treating snake bite.

There has been considerable debate about the indications for antivenom in *Latrodectus* envenoming. If available, it is indicated for systemic envenoming and many would advocate its use for any significant symptoms. Many other therapies have been used, either as adjuncts to or instead of antivenom. These include intravenous calcium gluconate, muscle relaxants including diazepam,

opiates, atropine, and chlorpromazine. Although calcium gluconate is used extensively in the USA, there is little clinical evidence for its efficacy. One observational study has demonstrated faster resolution of symptoms, predominantly pain, with antivenom. It also suggested that opiates and diazepam together were far more effective for symptomatic relief than calcium gluconate.

The evidence that antivenom is efficacious for bites by *Loxosceles* species is disappointing; many patients present late after the bite when necrosis is already established. Therapy with dapsone is often used in the USA, although there is no proven benefit. Steroids have received both favourable and unfavourable comment, but small trials show no benefit. The role of surgery is also controversial; many surgeons now believe that surgery should not be performed until clear demarcation of the necrotic lesion has occurred, and skin grafting only appears to be necessary in around 3–5% of patients. Hyperbaric oxygen has been suggested as therapy; experimental animal studies conflict in their conclusions about its efficacy.

Antivenom for funnel-web spider bites has significantly improved the prognosis following bites by this species and is indicated for any patient with systemic envenoming. Intensive care support my be required to control pulmonary oedema and circulatory failure. Although excessive autonomic nerve activity appears to be involved in the pathogenesis of severe envenoming, pharmacological intervention is not usually required.

BEE, WASP AND HORNET STINGS

Until recently, the main medical problem posed by bee and other hymenopteran stings has been the development of hypersensitivity with the risk of fatal anaphylaxis. However, multiple stings by honey bees and other hymenoptera can cause fatal envenoming. For example, in adults up to 500 bee stings and in children 30–50 stings are enough to cause death by direct toxicity. Following the introduction of the aggressive Africanised honey bee (*Apis mellifera scutellata* or *A.m.adamsonii*) into South America in 1957, mass attacks in humans have become more common. A recent study shows that three out of five victims died after mass attack in São Paulo state, Brazil (França *et al.*, 1994). Deaths have been reported after only 30–60 honey bee stings but usually 400–600 stings are necessary to kill an adult, and survival has been reported after as many as 2243 stings. It is estimated that there were 700–1000 such deaths in Latin America between 1957 and 1985.

Clinical Features

Local pain is the most common clinical feature; however, in victims with multiple stings, clinical features include rhabdomyolysis (myoglobinuria and myoglobinaemia), intravascular haemolysis, hepatic dysfunction, hypertension and myocardial damage, possibly due to the release of endogenous catecholamines by venom phospholipase A_2 and mellitin. Sick patients may develop respiratory distress with ARDS, shock, coma, acute renal failure and bleeding. Laboratory findings include a severe neutrophil leucocytosis in addition to evidence of rhabdomyolysis and impaired renal and hepatic function.

Another serious, and much more common, aspect of wasp, bee and hornet stings is an allergic reaction. If highly sensitised, symptoms may start within a few seconds, with tingling of the scalp, vasodilatation, hypotension, and death within 1–2 min. In most patients, the reaction begins after 1–2 min with generalised urticaria, followed over the next hour by oedema of the glottis, bronchoconstriction, hypotension, and coma. Subsequent reactions to further stings starts progressively sooner and may be more severe. Delayed allergic reactions may also occur 1–7 days after the sting, with fever, urticaria, enlarged lymph nodes, joint pains, and leucocytosis. These episodes usually last between 1 and 2 weeks.

Treatment

The sting, a tiny black shaft with the white poison sac attached to its free end, should be carefully removed. It should not be grasped with forceps or fingers as this can express more venom from the sac into the skin, but should be scraped from the flesh with the fingernail or the blade of a knife. Local antiseptic should be applied and pethidine given for pain if necessary. Meat tenderiser is claimed to relieve all pain in seconds, when rubbed into the skin in a dilute solution (1:4 ratio of tenderiser to water). Papaya extracts in the tenderiser provide papain, which may break down venom and kinins at the site of the sting.

No antivenoms are currently available commercially to treat multiple stings. A prototype antivenom has been produced in Brazil, by the Instituto Butantan, which is highly effective in an experimental animal model; clinical trials are currently underway in humans. In a patient with multiple envenoming, the first priority is to remove as many stings as possible using the methods outlined above; this will limit the amount of venom injected. Serious complications, such as intravascular haemolysis and the consequences of rhabdomyolysis, should be anticipated. Renal failure may be avoided by the early use of mannitol and bicarbonate. The empirical use of large doses of antihistamines and corticosteroids may be helpful in treating the massive release of histamine; drugs such as prazosin and nifedipine have been advocated to control the clinical manifestations of catecholamine release.

Adrenaline (epinephrine) is indicated for anaphylactic reactions, and is given by injection or inhalation. Inhalation of an adrenaline (epinephrine) aerosol (Medihaler, EPI, Riker), similar to the type used by asthma sufferers, works more rapidly than injection (Epipen). Children known to be allergic to bee or wasp stings should always carry such an inhaler. Alternatively, a tablet of sublingual isoprenaline (Aleudrin) may be carried, wrapped up in foil. Desensitisation is possible but is usually temporary unless maintenance desensitising injections are continued indefinitely every 1–4 months.

FISH STINGS

Fish stings represent a real risk to holiday makers who are relaxing in the sea, or even in freshwater where the fresh water sting ray can cause problems. Venomous fish generally have bony spines covered by venom-secreting tissues and most individuals are stung when they tread on or touch a fish that possesses a venom apparatus (Warrell, 1983). There are a number of families of venomous species found worldwide in tropical waters. Stingrays have a flat, triangular-shaped body varying in width from a few centimetres to over 5 m. When trodden on they whip their tail forward, which possesses a retroserrate sting. Catfish are mostly riverine, sometimes coastal, fish with serrated spines and whiskery mouthparts. Scorpionfish (Scorpaenidae) are widely distributed in tropical seas, especially around coral reefs. They have multiple dorsal spines and include *Trachinus* species (weeverfish), *Pterois* species (zebrafish, lionfish, tigerfish, etc.) and *Synanceja* (stonefish) species. Venom is injected by mechanical pressure of the victim's tissue upon the venom gland around a spine.

Avoiding Fish Stings

If swimming or bathing in areas where such fish are known to be present, it is sensible to wear some sort of protective footwear (e.g. 'flip-flops' or plastic lightweight sandals). Care should be exercised when swimming near or touching items on sandy bottoms.

Clinical Features

The main effect of stings by these fish is an intense and often agonising local pain. This is often stated to be the worst pain ever experienced by the victim and may lead to extreme distress and incoherence. Stingray injuries may cause significant lacerations and even deep puncture wounds. Systemic symptoms are generally rare in envenoming by fish, although there are reports of deaths from some areas of the world following stonefish, zebrafish and weeverfish stings. Most species cause rapid swelling and a bluish discoloration around the sting; stonefish do not cause local necrosis, but this may be a prominent feature in weeverfish and catfish stings. Spines may becomes detached and remain embedded, leading to a chronic infection and discharge.

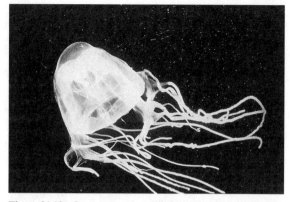

Figure 21.12 Sea wasp or box jellyfish, *Chironex fleckeri*, the jellyfish most dangerous to humans. In its natural waters it is translucent and very difficult to see. (Photograph courtesy of J. Gillet)

Treatment

The most effective treatment for the local pain of venomous fish stings is hot water, as many marine toxins are heat labile. The part stung is immersed in water as hot as the patient can bear; care must be taken to avoid burning and blistering as the severe pain may alter the sensation of the affected limb. The clinician should check that he or she can bear the water temperature without pain and asking the patient to check the temperature with the other limb is sometimes useful. The pain may be relieved rapidly, but continued immersion and maintenance of the temperature is necessary; this may be achieved by continually adding boiling water to the immersing water to keep it as *constantly hot* as the patient can bear (with repeated checking by the clinician). Regional nerve block may be helpful and, if the part stung is unsuitable for immersion in hot water (for example, the face or trunk), the area should be infiltrated through the puncture wound with 2–5 ml of 1% lidocaine (lignocaine) hydrochloride. Stonefish antivenom is available in Australia (only for intramuscular use) and appears to be very effective in relieving the pain. Stingray injuries may require surgical exploration and debridement.

JELLYFISH STINGS

Jellyfish have myriads of microscopic stinging capsules called nematocysts on their tentacles. When touched, these capsules rapidly fire a sting, which can inject venom; however, only a small number of jellyfish have stings that can penetrate intact human skin. The most dangerous jellyfish, the cubomedusan or box jellyfish, sometimes called sea-wasp, *Chironex fleckeri*, is confined to tropical waters, mainly off the eastern coast of Australia in the region of the Great Barrier Reef and around the coasts of Papua New Guinea and Irian Jaya (Figure 21.12). It has a

cuboidal body or float, up to 200 mm in diameter, and a leash of several tentacles growing from each of the four body corners. It is translucent and difficult to see in the water. Sea-wasps of the family Chirodropidae have been found in tropical waters of all continents of the world. *Physalia* spp. ('Portuguese man-o'-war' in Atlantic waters, 'bluebottle' in Pacific waters) has a coloured float from which numerous minor tentacles hang, together with a single main tentacle that can be up to 10 m in length. A smaller cubomedusan, *Carukia barnesi*, occurring in Indo-Pacific waters causes the 'Irukandji syndrome', so-named after an Australian aboriginal tribe.

Avoiding of Jellyfish Sting

If jellyfish are common on a beach, it is obviously sensible to keep out of the water; local knowledge about safe beaches and seasons may help. In Australia, there are frequently warning signs on the beaches and special jellyfish-free areas may be cordoned off for swimmers. Protective clothing ('stinger suits') may offer some protection but cannot be relied on to prevent venomous jellyfish stings.

Clinical Features

Stings by most jellyfish only cause local wheals with tingling and discomfort, usually lasting a few hours; however, a few species cause systemic syndromes, which may be life-threatening. *Physalia* species have an evil reputation, but severe envenoming is relatively rare by either Atlantic or Pacific species; fatal stings are extremely rare. Long linear wheals are usually associated with severe pain which passes off without treatment. In the Irukandji syndrome, local symptoms are minimal and the jellyfish is never seen. However, after 10–20 min, violent generalised muscle pains ensue, with restlessness, vomiting, sweating, and prostration. Symptoms appear to be produced by the release of large amounts of catecholamines; severe hypertension and, rarely, cardiac decompensation can occur. Symptoms may continue for 2 days, but the sting is rarely fatal.

In contrast, a number of deaths have been recorded following stings by the box jellyfish, *C. fleckeri* (Figure 21.12) in Australian waters. Wheals on the skin are normally multiple and 'cross-hatched'. Death can follow rapid collapse within a few minutes of the sting, probably due to myocardial toxicity, although respiratory arrest has also been recorded. Abnormal autonomic nerve activity has been observed. In nonfatal envenoming, swelling and subsequently local skin damage and necrosis can occur.

Treatment

In most jellyfish stings, only a small proportion (about

10–20%) of the nematocysts discharge their stings and venom. This has important implications for the first aid and treatment of jellyfish envenoming. For all species, care should be taken to avoid triggering undischarged nematocysts. The stung area should not be rubbed with wet hands or a wet cloth. Vinegar has clearly been shown to be effective in preventing the discharge of nematocysts following *Chironex* stings and is also advocated for the Irukandji syndrome. It should be poured liberally over the affected area. However, as there is some evidence that vinegar may cause firing of nematocysts from some *Physalia* species, these stings should be washed with sea water and adherent tentacles gently removed. In stings that are not life-threatening, pain relief is an important part of management. This may be achieved by the use of ice, but this is not effective for all species.

Although not proven to be effective, Australian authorities advocate the use of the compression–immobilisation bandaging method, described previously, for severe *Chironex* stings. In severe *Chironex* envenoming, artificial resuscitation on the shore may be needed; patients may develop extremely rapid envenoming after stings by this species. A potent *Chironex* antivenom is available from CSL Ltd, Australia and administration intramuscularly by first-aid teams on the beach has resulted in dramatic recovery from severe envenoming by *C. fleckeri*. Patients may require considerable intensive care support and repeated doses of antivenom in hospital (Fenner, 1998). Although no antivenom is available for the treatment of the Irukandji syndrome, analgesia with opiates and use of alpha blockers such as phentolamine may be necessary in severe cases.

ECHINODERM STING

Stings by the spiny varieties of sea urchins are very common in travellers who may be bathing off generally rocky or stony beaches. They can be extremely painful, but are resolved by using the hot water treatment described above for treating fish stings. Again, the venom is heat labile and responds well to this type of therapy. Small spines, which normally break off in the victim's foot, can be left and will be absorbed after a few weeks or months. Larger spines may need to be removed to prevent infection and granuloma formation.

CONE SHELLS

These are marine snails which have evolved venoms and an elaborate harpoon-like venom apparatus. They are found particularly in Indo-Pacific waters. Their shells are particularly attractive, leading to human envenoming when they are picked up; in some regions the snails are eaten. Those cone snails that normally hunt fish may be particularly dangerous; the venom contains a mixture of neurotoxins that cause severe local pain and the rapid

(within 30–60 min) onset of profound neurotoxicity, leading to respiratory paralysis and death. Management hinges upon preventing absorption of the toxin by immobilisation and possibly pressure bandages and getting the victim to medical care. Antivenom is not available but supportive treatment with intubation and ventilation may be life saving. As some of the neurotoxins act postsynaptically, a trial of anticholinesterases is worthwhile, although there is no clear evidence of benefit.

REFERENCES

Cardoso JLC, Fan HW, França FOS *et al.* (1993) Randomized comparative trial of three antivenoms in the treatment of envenoming by lance-headed vipers (*Bothrops jararaca*) in São Paulo, Brazil. *Quarterly Journal of Medicine*, **86**, 315–325.

Fan HW, Marcopito LF, Cardoso JLC *et al.* (1999) A randomised double-blind trial of promethazine prophylaxis against early anaphylactic reactions to antivenom in patients bitten by Bothrops snakes in São Paulo, Brazil. *BMJ*, **318**, 1451–1453.

Fenner PJ (1998) Dangers in the ocean: the traveler and marine envenomation. I. Jellyfish. *Journal of Travel Medicine*, **5**, 135–141.

França FOS, Benvenuti LA, Fan HW *et al.* (1994) Severe and fatal attacks by 'killer' bees (Africanized honey bees—*Apis mellifera scutellata*) in Brazil: clinicopathological studies with measurement of serum venom concentrations. *Quarterly Journal of Medicine*, **87**, 269–282.

Lalloo DG., Trevett AJ, Korinhona A *et al.* (1995) Snakebites by the Papuan Taipan (*Oxyuranus scutellatus canni*): paralysis, haemostatic and electrocardiographic abnormalities and effects of antivenom. *American Journal of Tropical Medicine and Hygiene*, **52**, 525–531.

Larrick JW, Yost JA and Kaplan J (1978) Snake bite among the Waorani Indians of eastern Ecuador. *Transactions of the Royal Society of Tropical Medicine and Hygiene*, **72**, 542–543.

Malasit P, Warrell DA, Chanthavanich P *et al.* (1986) Prediction, prevention and mechanism of early (anaphylactic) antivenom reactions in victims of snake bites. *BMJ*, **292**, 17–20.

Meyer WP, Habib HG, Onayade AA *et al.* (1997) First clinical experiences with a new ovine Fab *Echis ocellatus* snakebite antivenom in Nigeria: randomised comparative trial with Institute Pasteur serum (Ipser) Africa antivenom. *American Journal of Tropical Medicine and Hygiene*, **56**, 291–300.

Phillips RE, Theakston RDG, Warrell DA *et al.* (1988) Paralysis, rhabdomyolysis and haemolysis caused by bites of Russell's viper (*Vipera russelli pulchella*) in Sri Lanka: failure of Indian (Haffkine) antivenom. *Quarterly Journal of Medicine*, **68**, 691–716.

Premawardhena AP, de Silva CE, Fonseka MM *et al.* (1999) Low dose subcutaneous adrenaline to prevent acute adverse reactions to antivenom serum in people bitten by snakes: randomised, placebo controlled trial. *BMJ*, **318**, 1041–1043.

Pugh RNH and Theakston RDG (1980) The incidence and mortality of snake bite in savanna Nigeria. *Lancet*, **ii**, 1181–1183.

Sano-Martins IS, Fan HW, Castro SCB *et al.* (1994) Reliability of the simple 20 minute whole blood clotting test (WBCT20) as an indicator of low plasma fibrinogen concentration in patients envenomed by *Bothrops* snakes. *Toxicon*, **32**, 1045–1050.

Theakston RDG (1991) Immunological aspects of snake venom research. In *Handbook of Natural Toxins*, vol. 5 *Reptile and*

Amphibian Venoms (ed. AT Tu), pp 495–527. Marcel Dekker, New York.

Theakston RDG and Smith DC (1995) Therapeutic antibodies to snake venoms. In *Therapeutic Antibodies* (eds J Landon and T Chard), pp 109–133. Springer-Verlag, New York.

Theakston RDG and Warrell DA (1991) Antivenoms: a list of hyperimmune sera currently available for the treatment of envenoming by bites and stings. *Toxicon*, **29**, 1419–1470.

Theakston RDG, Lloyd-Jones MJ and Reid HA (1977). Micro-ELISA for detecting and assaying snake venom and venom antibody. *Lancet*, **ii**, 639–641.

Theakston RDG, Phillips RE, Looareesuwan S *et al.* (1990) Bacteriological studies of the venom and mouth cavities of wild Malayan pit vipers (*Calloselasma rhodostoma*) in southern Thailand. *Transactions of the Royal Society of Tropical Medicine and Hygiene*, **84**, 875–879.

Virivan C, Veeravat U, Warrell MJ *et al.* (1986) ELISA confirmation of acute and past envenoming by the monocellate Thai cobra (*Naja kaouthia*). *American Journal of Tropical Medicine and Hygiene*, **35**, 173–181.

Warrell DA (1983) Injuries, envenoming, poisoning, and allergic reactions caused by animals. In *Oxford Textbook of Medicine*, vol. 1 *Chemical and Physical Injuries, Climatic and Occupational Diseases* (eds DJ Weatherall, JGG Ledingham and DA Warrell), pp 6.35–6.47. Oxford University Press, Oxford.

Warrell DA, Looareesuwan S, Theakston RDG *et al.* (1986) Randomized comparative trial of three monospecific antivenoms for bites by the Malayan pit viper (*Calloselasma rhodostoma*) in southern Thailand: clinical and laboratory correlations. *American Journal of Tropical Medicine and Hygiene*, **35**, 1235–1247.

White J (1987) Elapid snakes: management of bites. In *Toxic Plants and Animals. A Guide for Australia* (eds J Covacevich, P Davie and J Pearn), pp 431–457. Queensland Museum, Brisbane.

WHO (1981) *Progress in the Characterization of Venoms and Standardization of Antivenoms*, WHO Offset Publication No.58, World Health Organization, Geneva.

FURTHER READING

Fenner PJ (1998) Dangers in the ocean: the traveler and marine envenomation. II. Marine vertebrates. *Journal of Medicine*, **5**, 213–216.

Meier J and White J (1995) *Handbook of Clinical Toxicology of Animal Venoms and Poisons*. CRC Press, New York.

ADDITIONAL RESOURCES

Some Institutes Making Antivenom

For a more complete list see Theakston and Warrell (1991).

1. *Algeria.* Institut Pasteur d'Algeria, Rue Docteur Laveran, Algiers.
2. *Argentina.* Instituto Nacional de Microbiologia, Av. Velez Sarsfield 563, Buenos Aires.
3. *Australia.* CSL Ltd, 45 Poplar Road, Parkville, Victoria 3052.
4. *Brazil.* (a) Instituto Butantan, Caixa Postal 65, Sao Paulo.
5. (b) Fundacao Ezequiel Dias, Rua Conde Pereira Carneiro 80, Belo Horizonte.
6. *Burma* (Myanmar). Industrie & Pharmaceutical Co., Rangoon (Yangon).
7. *China.* Shanghai Vaccine and Serum Institute, 1262 Yang An Road (W), Shanghai.
8. *Colombia.* Instituto Nacional de Salud, Av. Eldorado con Carrera, Zona G, Bogota.
9. *Costa Rica.* Instituto Clodomiro Picado, San Jose.
10. *Croatia.* Institute of Immunology, Rockerfellerova 2, Zagreb.
11. *Czech Republic.* Institute of Sera and Vaccines, W. Piecka Str. 108, 10 103 Prague 10.
12. *Ecuador.* Instituto Nacional de Higiene y Medicina Tropical, Casilla Postal 3961, Guayaquil.
13. *Egypt.* Al Algousa Sharea, Alvezara, Cairo.
14. *France.* Pasteur-Merieux Serum et Vaccins SA, Av. Leclerc, BP7046,Leon.
15. *Germany.* Knoll Pharmaceuticals, Postfach 21 08 05, Ludwigshafen.
16. *India.* (a) Central Research Institute, Kasauli, R.I., Punjab.
17. (b) Haffkine Bio-Pharmaceutical Corporation, Parel, Bombay 12.
18. (c) Serum Institute of India, 212/2 Hadaspar, Pune-411 028.
19. *Indonesia.* Perusahaan Negara Bio Farma, 9 Djalan Pasteur, Bandung.
20. *Iran.* Institut d'Etat des Serums et Vaccins Razi, Boite Postale 656, Tehran.
21. *Israel.* Ministry of Health, POB 6115, Jerusalem 91060.
22. *Italy.* Instituto Sieroterapico Vaccinogeno, Via Fiorentina 1, 53100 Siena.
23. *Japan.* Takeda Chemical Industries Ltd, Osaka.
24. *Morocco.* Institut Pasteur, Place Charles-Nicolle, Casablanca.
25. *Pakistan.* National Institute of Health, Islamabad.
26. *Peru.* Instituto Nacional de Salud, Calle Capac Yupanqui 1400, Lima.
27. *Philippines.* Serum and Vaccine Laboratories, Alabang Multinlupa, Rizal.
28. *Russia.* Ministry of Public Health, 101 431, GSP 4, Moscow K-51.
29. *South Africa.* South African Institute for Medical Research, PO Box 1038, Johannesburg 2000.
30. *Sri Lanka.* Protherics UK Ltd, 14–15 Newbury Street, London EC1A 7HU, UK.
31. *Switzerland.* Institut Serotherapique et Vaccinal Suisse, CP 2707, 3001 Berne.
32. *Taiwan.* National Institute of Preventive Medicine, 161 Kun Yang St., Taipei.
33. *Thailand.* Queen Saovabha Memorial Institute, Bangkok.
34. *Tunisia.* Institut Pasteur, 13 Place Pasteur, Tunis.
35. *United States.* (a) Wyeth-Ayerst Laboratories, Box 8299, Philadelphia, 1, PA.
36. (b) Arizona State University, Temp, Arizona 85287-2701.
37. (c) Protherics UK Ltd., 14–15 Newbury St., London EC1A 7HU, UK.
38. (d) Merck, Sharp and Dohme Int., POB 2000, Rahway, NJ 07065.
39. *West Africa.* Protherics UK Ltd., 14–15 Newbury Street, London EC1A 7HU, UK.

Scorpion antivenoms are made at institutes 1, 4, 10, 15, 16, 20, 24, 29 and 34; spider antivenoms at institutes 3, 4, 20, 26, 29 and 38; jellyfish (sea-wasp) at institute 3 and fish antivenoms at institutes 3 and 10.

Doctors who need supplies of antivenom for use in various geographical areas may find the following most useful.

Americas: polyvalent viper antivenom from 2, 4, 5, 8, 9, 12, 26 or 35; coral snake antivenom from 2, 4, 5, 9, 26 or 35.

North Africa: viper antivenom from 1, 13, 14, 20, 21, 24, 29 or 34.

Mid-Africa: polyvalent antivenom from 14 or 29.

South Africa: polyvalent antivenom from 29.

Middle East: viper–cobra antivenom from 14 or 20.

Asia: (sea snake bite) sea snake or tiger snake antivenom from 3.

India and Pakistan: cobra–krait–viper antivenom from 16, 17, 18 or 25.

Burma (Myanmar): cobra–viper antivenom from 6.

Cambodia, Laos, Malaysia, Vietnam, Thailand: viper and cobra antivenoms from 33.

Indonesia: cobra–krait–viper antivenom from 19.

Japan: viper antivenom from 23.

Philippines and Taiwan: cobra–krait–viper antivenom from 32.

22

Ophthalmic Conditions in Travellers

Theresa Richardson and Clare Davey

Royal Free Hampstead NHS Trust, London, UK

SUNLIGHT EXPOSURE

The eye is the only organ, apart from the skin, that is directly exposed to radiation from the sun. Biologically, the most damaging wavelengths encountered are ultraviolet B (UVB) and, to a lesser extent, ultraviolet A (UVA) and blue light (Figure 22.1).

Ten per cent of all light energy reaching the earth's surface is ultraviolet light. Ninety per cent of this is UVA (320–400 nm). Most of the rest is the longer wavelengths of UVB (320–280 nm). Ultraviolet C (UVC) light is filtered by the ozone layer and the upper atmosphere. The shorter the wavelength the greater the energy content (Planck's equation). The ozone layer is 2–3 mm in thickness and produced in the stratosphere as a photochemical reaction fuelled by UVC and possibly by lightning. This ozone layer filters out most of the shorter ultraviolet wavelengths from the solar emission. There has been a 3–6% per decade decrease in the ozone layer, producing holes over the Antarctic and Arctic regions and thinning all over. The loss of the ozone layer is believed to be due to chlorine from pollutants, particularly chlorofluorocarbon gas in aerosols and refrigerators. For every 1% reduction in ozone, there is an approximate 1% increase in ultraviolet light reaching the earth's surface.

VULNERABILITY TO ULTRAVIOLET LIGHT DAMAGE

Youth

With increasing age there is protection from sunlight by overhanging eyelid skin, bushier eyebrows, relative corneal opacification, smaller pupils and increasing absorption of shorter wavelengths by the lens, which causes increased protection of the retina from ultraviolet light. Additionally, young people today tend to spend more time out of doors than elderly people and youth is a relative risk factor for ultraviolet light damage.

Pigmentation

Lightly pigmented individuals are more at risk from sunburn, basal cell carcinoma of the eyelids and age-related macular degeneration. Cataract and pterygium susceptibility also appears to be greater in lightly pigmented individuals.

Occupation

Clearly the amount of ultraviolet light reaching the eyes is related closely to occupation and to wearing of wide-brimmed hats or sunglasses while out of doors. The Maryland waterman study showed a 20-fold difference of exposure to ultraviolet light between men who worked on deck to those who worked inside the boats.

Eyelid Damage

Sunburn

Acute sunburn of the eyelids is uncommon in people walking about. Sunbathing, lying flat on the back, can result in unpleasant, but not dangerous, sunburn to the eyelids. Clouds do not filter out ultraviolet light very well and there may also be reflection by sand and water; thus, there may be only limited protection from beach umbrellas and hats and therefore sunbathers should be careful about exposure under these circumstances and wear sunglasses.

Chronic Lid Exposure

Superficial punctate keratosis, age spots, comedones and sebaceous hyperplasia, as well as premalignant and malignant lesions, are all induced by chronic exposure to ultraviolet light.

Principles and Practice of Travel Medicine. Edited by Jane N. Zuckerman.
© 2001 John Wiley & Sons Ltd.

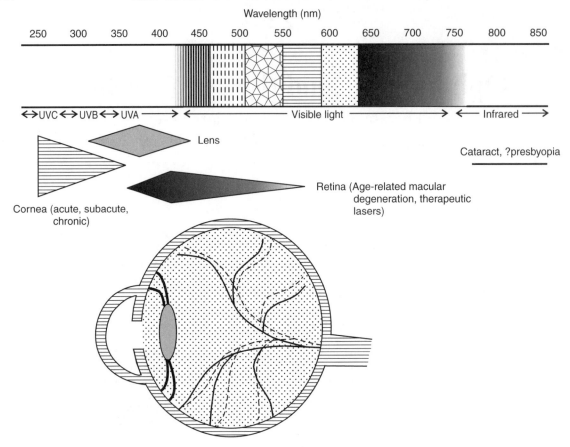

Figure 22.1 Ocular damage by ultraviolet, visible and infrared light

Malignant Tumours

Actinic keratosis is a premalignant squamous change seen in the eyelids. Squamous cell carcinoma is rarer than basal cell carcinoma. Malignant melanoma of the lids is very rare and constitutes well under 1% of all malignant lesions of the eyelids. All these conditions are related to ultraviolet light exposure.

Basal cell carcinomas (Figure 22.2) are extremely common in Caucasians living in sunny countries such as Australia and South Africa. Both these countries have vigorous education campaigns, such as the 'No hat, no play' rule for school children.

Cornea

Damage to the cornea by ultraviolet light is both intensity- and wavelength-dependent.

Acute Keratitis

UVC and very short wavelength ultraviolet light of 260–290 nm are maximally absorbed by the corneal proteins, such that only a very brief exposure can cause an acute keratitis (inflammation of the cornea). Most of these short wavelengths are filtered out by the ozone layer. Acute keratitis, in practice, is mostly seen as an effect of a welder's flash (approximately 320 nm), the victim feels no abnormality until 4–10 h after the exposure and then suffers severe painful, photophobic, red, watery eyes. The main effects last for 12 h, with some residual discomfort for 2–4 days. The main treatment is time and reassurance. It is reasonable to instil local anaesthetic drops to help the patient sleep, but these should not be instilled more than twice as there is a risk of delayed healing and of unnoticed trauma. Antibiotics are not needed.

Snow blindness occurs as a result of longer exposure to UVB (320–400 nm) reflected off the snow; those who forget or lose their sunglasses or goggles are particularly at risk. It should be remembered that freshly fallen snow reflects 80% of the ultraviolet light.

Sunbeds can be a risk, but those mainly of an older variety emit UVB as well as UVA, which does not cause acute keratitis but is implicated in pterygia and cataract.

Appropriate ocular protection is the mainstay in

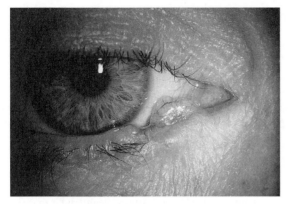

Figure 22.2 Basal cell carcinoma of lower lid

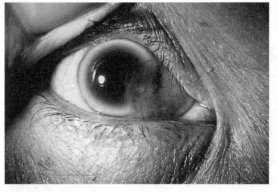

Figure 22.3 Pterygium

preventing acute and subacute keratitis. Travellers, who are often unused to seeing welding in their own country, may be tempted to watch welders in action at the roadside, but should not do so because of the risk of acute keratitis and of ocular foreign bodies. Skiers and mountain climbers must wear adequate UV protection. Those who lose their sunglasses (typically down a crevasse while crossing a glacier) should wrap a scarf around the head, leaving only a small horizontal slit to see through in much the same way as the Inuit do in the Arctic.

Chronic Keratitis

Climatic droplet keratopathy and Labrador keratitis are names for chronic exposure to ultraviolet radiation that results in yellow or golden subepithelial droplets in the cornea, which are initially clear but later become opaque, spreading from the periphery of the cornea to the centre. It is seen predominantely in the Inuit in Northern Canada and in Arab desert dwellers. Males are typically affected much more than females.

Pingueculum

This is an elastotic degeneration of the conjunctiva and is frequently seen in elderly people; it is thought to be the result of cumulative damage to the conjunctiva by ultraviolet light.

Pterygium

Pterygium (Figure 22.3) is the growth of a membrane, consisting of blood vessels and degenerative fibres, that extends across the cornea. The nasal side of the cornea is affected more frequently than the temporal. It is more common with exposure to sunlight and proximity to the equator. It is also more common in windy countries, suggesting that mechanical abrasion is a factor in devel-

opment. It is therefore seen particularly in coastal areas and in desert people. Pterygia seem to develop many years after exposure to sunny, windy conditions: this is particulary evident, for instance in the UK, where West Indians immigrating in early adulthood do not develop their pterygia until years later, living in less than sunny Britain.

Pterygia are unlikely to be sight threatening in travellers and are likely only to cause chronic mild discomfort and to be cosmetically disfiguring. Surgery for pterygia is usually done for cosmetic reasons. Unfortunately, it is complicated by frequent recurrences. The currently favoured surgical technique to avoid recurrence is to remove the pterygium and then place a free conjunctival graft between the conjunctiva and the cornea. Beta irradiation and cytotoxic agents are no longer used because of later side-effects.

Cataract

A cataract is an opacity in the lens of the eye (Figure 22.4). The prevalence of cataract increases with age in all societies. There are, however, very great differences in prevalence between countries. Population surveys are often difficult to compare because of different definitions used to define cataract. Notwithstanding, there is definitely a greater incidence and prevalence in Asia compared with Britain, of between four- and tenfold in most age groups. In the last 20 years many useful surveys have attempted to elucidate the reasons for these differences.

Risk Factors

Sunlight exposure, diabetes, diarrhoea, alcohol and cigarette smoking are all strongly associated with cataracts.

Sunlight exposure. The lens absorbs both UVB and UVA light, and with increasing age the lens absorbs more short wave visible spectrum light, i.e. blue light. Experimentally, short bursts of UVB cause cataract but UVA

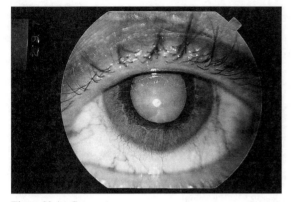

Figure 22.4 Cataract

and blue light do not. Human lenses are exposed to chronic low levels of UVA and visible light. Epidemiolocal studies have shown a greater instance of cataracts with increasing levels of ultraviolet and visible light. Calculating an individual's exposure to light, however, is complicated and depends on factors such as how much time is spent indoors and whether a hat is worn, etc. The Maryland waterman study took these factors into consideration and compared ambient ocular exposure between different fishermen and found as much as a 20-fold increase of exposure to ultraviolet and visible light in some fishermen compared with others. Increased occurrence of some types of cataract was found in those exposed to most visible light and ultraviolet light.

This study and others have definitely linked exposure to sunshine to cataracts. This has enormous significance both for personal behaviour and for economics worldwide. Much concern has been raised over the depletion of the ozone layer and increasing levels of UVB radiation and the likely increase of cataracts in future years. A recent study of people living in Chile under the hole in the ozone layer did not demonstrate changes, but these would not necessarily be expected as increased levels of cataract would take many years to develop.

Protection from sunlight exposure. It is recommended that young people and children, in particular, wear hats and sunglasses during long periods of time in the sunshine, especially at the beach and when engaged in water sports.

Dark glasses. On a bright sunny day, the high light levels saturate the retina and reduce overall visual performance, particularly distinguishing between fine levels of contrast in objects of similar colour and shade. Most sunglasses will absorb 70–80% of incident light of all wavelengths and will improve visual function.

Polaroid sunglasses reduce glare from reflective light from the road or water. Wide sunglasses that curve around the eyes reduce glare from the side.

Photochromic lenses darken when exposed to short wavelength light; they may be made of glass or plastic. In

the case of glass there is a chemical reaction of conversion of silver ion to elemental silver. The reaction is reversible when the glass is returned to the dark. At its most dark, about 80% of the light is absorbed, and at its most light about 20% of light is absorbed. It takes longer for the glass to lighten than it does for it to darken.

Plastic photochromic lenses depend for their property on a chemical coating that lightens and darkens with exposure to short wavelength light. The chemical coating is more easily damaged than that of the glass lenses.

Almost all dark glasses absorb most ultraviolet light. Even toy sunglasses can absorb over 90%; however, there is no guarantee. Children should wear British Standard approved ('kite' marked) sunglasses. Blue lenses are much less effective at absorbing short wavelength light than are lenses of other colours and should not be used. Dark sunglasses should be worn; blue tints should be avoided.

AIRCRAFT TRAVEL AND THE EYE

The atmosphere of an aircraft is drier and is under lower pressure than normal. In addition there are often blowers above seats that cause increased evaporation of tears. Travellers often cannot sleep on long haul flights and will attempt to while away time by reading, using their computers and watching triple movie screenings. When people are overtired their rate of blinking also decreases. These conditions can aggravate existing eye problems as well as giving rise to symptoms in people who do not ordinarily suffer from dry eyes.

The Dry Eye

People who have never experienced dry eyes may get symptoms. Likely sufferers are people with thyroid disease, pregnant women, perimenopausal women, and rheumatoid arthritis sufferers.

Blepharitis is a very common condition caused by alterations of tear film. These people suffer already from gritty and sensitive red eyes, which may be aggravated by air travel. It is advisable for susceptible travellers to take artificial tears with them, which can easily be bought over the counter at most good pharmacies. A range of products is available: before travelling they can try different preparations to see which suits them best. Drops should be instilled throughout the flight.

Management

When on the aircraft, if eyes become red or gritty it will help if the blowers above the seats are turned off. Artificial teardrops should be instilled when the eyes feel gritty—up to as often as every 15 min. Those with severe dry eye or who are sensitive to preservatives can use preservative-free drops (also available 'over the counter').

Corneal Abrasion and Recurrences

Many people who have had previous corneal scratches or abrasion may experience a recurrence. This presents with a sudden onset of pain, watering and photophobia, usually on waking or after minor trauma. Treatment is the same as for a corneal abrasion with chloramphenicol ointment. To prevent the pain recurring, patients are advised to use ocular lubricants and simple eye ointment before sleeping.

Contact Lens Wear

The special problems of contact lens wearers is discussed in a later section.

Following Eye Operations

It is generally safe to travel by air following most eye operations, including for squints, cataracts, glaucoma, corneal grafts and after laser treatment for diabetic eye disease.

Patients who have had surgery less than 6 weeks previously are often advised by doctors not to do too much heavy lifting of luggage. This is because it is possible that straining can increase the pressure in the eye and could lead to rupture of the fine sutures holding the cornea. Nowadays most cataract surgery is carried out using small incision without sutures and therefore this precaution is probably unnecessary. Most patients who have cataract surgery are elderly and are therefore unlikely to be carrying large suitcases unaided but common sense should prevail.

Accidental eye damage is more likely and a more common scenario when a patient has had cataract surgery and vision is still not clear. These patients are more susceptible to bumping their face and operated eye when travelling, especially when attempting to load the overhead luggage rack. It may be better in the first 6 postoperative weeks to wear an eye shield for the transit periods. These can be of clear acrylic material for those with only one good eye.

Accidental Injury to the Operated Eye

If a bump to the eye is sustained on board the aircraft an attendant can usually tell if something serious has happened by asking the patient if there is a change of vision. Next, look at the pupil of the eye and see if it is round. If it is of a teardrop shape then there may be a rupture of the corneal wound. There may even be a blood level in the anterior chamber. Ask the patient if he or she remembers the pupil being irregularly shaped just after surgery: sometimes this predates the operation.

If a rupture of the wound is suspected, do not panic, because most injuries can wait for 24 h for repair. Cover the eye with a clean eye pad and plastic shield if available, to avoid pressure on the eye. (If a shield is not available then fashion one out of a polystyrene coffee cup, just cutting an oval in it and taping it over the eye, without exerting any undue pressure.) Do not instil antibiotic creams and drops as the intraocular contents need preservative-free drops and some antibiotics, e.g. gentamicin, are retinotoxic; however, oral ciprofloxacin should be given and this has good ocular penetration. If patients have a blood level, hyphaema, in the eye then it is probably best to keep them sitting upright in the aircraft seat to assist resolution, but the position adopted is not very important.

Retinal Detachment Surgery

Following retinal detachment surgery the surgeon will advise whether or not it is safe to fly. It depends on whether and which substances were used to tamponade the detachment. This could be either gases such as air, SF6 (sulphur hexafluoride) or C3F8, or silicone oil. Gases injected into the eye during surgery will expand because of the lower cabin pressure and cause a dangerous rise in intraocular pressure (Figure 22.5). Patients who have had C3F8, a heavy gas, have to wait about 6 weeks to allow absorption of the gas. In the case of air 2–3 days is usually sufficient, and with SF6 2–3 weeks.

Ocular Pain after Aircraft Travel

Air travel can precipitate sinusitis. People with a tendency to sinus problems often experience pain around the eye on descent of the aircraft. This is due to a relative vacuum in the sinuses. Air is unable to enter due to mucosal swelling acting as a valve. Tenderness is present over the affected sinus. Nose blowing and nasal decongestants are helpful. Pain is usually described as a dull ache behind the eye. Ask the patient if the pain shifts on sleeping or tilting the head to one side: this will indicate the presence of fluid in the sinuses.

Recently, people have been choosing holidays to the Far East to take advantage of the cheaper dental treatment. Root canal work with a dental abscess can result in pain referred to the eye. Treat with oral amoxicillin and refer to a dentist for further evaluation.

Sinus problems can develop into orbital cellulitis.

Diabetic Retinopathy

Patients who need treatment for diabetic eye disease should finish the course of treatment prior to travel. There is no evidence that vitreous haemorrhages are more likely during aircraft travel. However, trauma should be avoided. Diabetics need to continue good control of the diabetes despite the variation in diet and daily

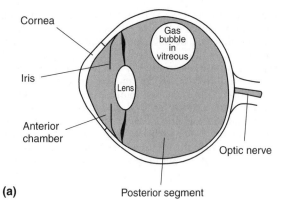

(a)

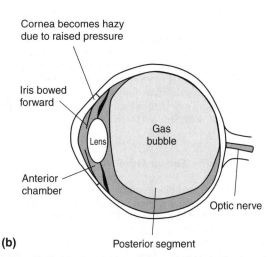

(b)

Figure 22.5 (a) The position of the gas bubble in the posterior segment following retinal detachment surgery. (b) As the air cabin pressure falls, the air bubble expands within the eye, pushing the lens forward and compressing the anterior chamber

routine, as well as jet lag. Blurring of vision can occur during hypoglycaemic attacks.

OCULAR CHANGES AT ALTITUDE

Examination of the retinas of people climbing on Everest expeditions have shown the common occurrence of small, flame-shaped haemorrhages in the retina. These are not sight threatening. Most visual problems at altitude are related to exposure of the corneas to wind, cold and ultraviolet light. Wind and cold cause mechanical abrasions and drying of the cornea. Ultraviolet light damage causes snow blindness. Extreme precautions against exposure to ultraviolet light and wind damage must be taken, with dark goggles that protect from the side as well.

Hyperbaric Oxygen

Hyperbaric oxygen used to treat frost bitten limbs often causes temporary loss of vision due to constriction of retinal arterioles. This is reversible.

THE RED EYE

The major problems facing a traveller are whether and how to obtain treatment for a red eye and deciding what is a serious red eye problem, needing repatriation and what can be treated with simple measures. Nonophthalmologists often shy away from even thinking about how to resolve red eye problems, but in fact a systematic approach, a torch, a Snellen chart (or even simpler means of checking vision) and fluorescein strips will sort out most problems and indicate what needs urgent attention.

Symptoms

Some symptoms are helpful as they point their way to the diagnosis; others need clarification to understand precisely what the patient means:

- *Blurred vision.* This may be the result of a reduction of visual acuity or diplopia or simply a need for a change in glasses, or even a bit of mucous that intermittently smears across the vision and clears on blinking.
- *Double vision.* This may indicate diplopia, in which case try to work out if it is present in one eye only or in both eyes. Often patients will refer to double vision, meaning that their vision is blurred or that there is ghosting of objects around the edges.
- *Haloes.* These may refer to glare or dazzle seen in cataracts. Coloured or rainbow haloes suggest corneal oedema, which is seen in acute angle closure glaucoma, in which case it will be associated with pain and the patient should be referred urgently.
- *Photophobia.* This may be due to corneal disease or uveitis, or the patient may be referring to the glare of cataract, or to migraine or meningism.
- *Pain.* This, as opposed to discomfort, suggests a serious cause, e.g. corneal disease, uveitis or acute glaucoma. Urgent referral should be considered.
- *Grittiness.* This is usually the result of dry eyes and occasionally blepharitis.
- *Foreign body sensation.* This may be caused by the presence of an actual foreign body, or by a corneal abrasion, or dry eyes.
- *Sticky discharge.* This usually occurs as a result of bacterial infection -conjunctivitis, or occasionally blepharitis and sometimes accompanies an acute allergic reaction.

- *Itchy eyes.* These are usually due to allergy, but are sometimes due to blepharitis.

Examination

Visual Acuity

A Snellen chart may or may not be available. It is important to get some estimation of vision. The eyes must be tested separately and using the patient's distance glasses. If there is no reasonable distance acuity measure, simply reading the newspaper (with reading glasses, if needed of course!) testing each eye separately, will give an approximate vision of N8 (roughly corresponds to 6/18 Snellen chart), which is the type size that most newspapers use.

If the eye has a reduced visual acuity and it is painful and red, a serious cause should be sought for the problem.

Eyelids

Look at the eye and eyelids generally with a torch, looking for lid swelling, red rims and redness of the eyes and for the presence of pus.

Light Reflection from the Eye

Shine a torch into the eye and look at the reflection from the cornea. If the reflection is cloudy or hazy in the presence of a painful eye, look for a serious cause such as corneal ulcer or acute glaucoma.

Redness

Redness all over the conjunctiva associated with severe pain may be due to acute glaucoma. Redness associated with mild pain or discomfort may be due to conjunctivitis. Redness around the cornea only may be the result of corneal disease or uveitis. A patch of redness may be episcleritis, scleritis or subconjunctival haemorrhage.

Fluorescein Staining

Moisten a strip of fluorescein paper with saline, retract the lower lid and place it on the inside so that the fluorescein is blinked across the eye. Examination should preferably be performed with a blue light, but even a bright white light will suffice. If green staining is seen, and does not move on blinking, this suggests an epithelial defect in the cornea; if it due to anything other than a small traumatic abrasion the patient should be referred urgently.

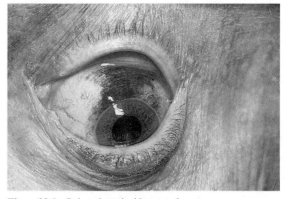

Figure 22.6   Subconjunctival haemorrhage

SPECIFIC OCULAR CONDITIONS

Conjunctiva

Subconjunctival Haemorrhage

Spontaneous subconjunctival haemorrhage (Figure 22.6) involves an isolated patch of redness, no discomfort and normal vision.

Treatment.   Reassure the patient that it will go away in a week or two.

Acute Bacterial Conjunctivitis

Acute bacterial conjunctivitis involves an uncomfortable but not painful sticky discharge, especially in the morning, with redness all over the conjunctiva and a normal visual acuity. It is usually bilateral.

Treatment.   Clean the lids three times a day and use drops of chloramphenicol 2-hourly for the first day, then four times a day for 4 days. If it does not respond to chloramphenicol consider another diagnosis, as it is unlikely to be bacterial conjunctivitis. Other useful antibiotics are fucidic acid, ofloxacin and gentamicin.

Chlamydial Conjunctivitis

Chlamydial conjunctivitis may be sexually transmitted or may be trachoma. Most travellers will not pick up trachoma, but it is a diagnosis worth considering in those who have been staying in poor areas, with poor sanitation. Symptoms are of a chronic red, sticky eye.

Treatment.   Referral should be made for confirmation of the diagnosis and treatment with topical and systemic tetracycline. The patient and contacts may need to be referred to the sexually transmitted diseases clinic.

Viral Conjunctivitis

This condition produces an uncomfortable red eye which may be painful. It is usually bilateral, with a watery discharge and sensitivity to light. There is usually a tender lymph node in front of the ear.

Treatment.   There is no effective treatment; refer if it is painful.

Episcleritis

Episcleritis causes discomfort but no pain; there is an isolated patch of redness and normal vision. It may be associated with inflammatory bowel disease or gout.

Treatment.   Refer if uncertain; otherwise reassure the patient that it will subside by itself. Recurrent episcleritis may be treated with topical steroid drops for a short reducing course of no more than 1 month.

Scleritis

Scleritis is rare. It produces a severely painful and photophobic eye, usually unilateral and usually with a history of rheumatoid arthritis or other autoimmune condition.

Examination.   There should be a characteristic patch of redness and swelling about 6 mm behind the cornea, with possible reduced vision.

Treatment.   Refer urgently.

Dry Eye

Dry eye (Figure 22.7) is a chronic problem usually affecting middle-aged women more than men. Symptoms are of a gritty sensation and a mild discharge; there may be a history of rheumatoid arthritis or sarcoidosis.

Examination.   The eye may appear white. Vision is usually normal and there may be spotty staining with fluorescein in the area of the eye exposed to air.

Treatment.   Regular, from 6-hourly to 1-hourly, instillation of artificial teardrops, e.g. hypromellose, as required, depending on the severity of the symptoms. Other useful drops are Liquifilm Tears, Viscotears and simple eye ointment.

Pterygium

Pterygia are usually seen in people brought up in sunny countries or who have spent a long time in sunny countries. They may produce a gritty, uncomfortable sensa-

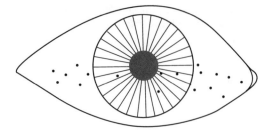

Figure 22.7   Dry eye

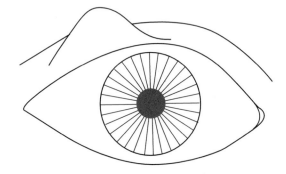

Figure 22.8   Chalazion

tion. It is rare for travellers to grow a pterygium that extends across the visual axis.

Treatment.   Surgery is undertaken for cosmetic reasons. There is a high recurrence rate. The currently favoured surgical technique involves a free conjunctival graft.

Management.   Refer routinely.

Eyelids and Orbit

Chalazion

Chalazion (meibomian cyst; Figure 22.8) is a chronic isolated lid swelling, either minimally tender or not tender at all.

Treatment.   Hot compresses applied with a flannel for 5 min twice a day sometimes help. If there is no resolution within 1 week refer routinely.

Stye

A stye (Figure 22.9) is a tender small swelling on the lid margin (infections of the eyelash follicle).

Treatment.   Hot compresses (as for chalazion). They usually resolve within 48 h.

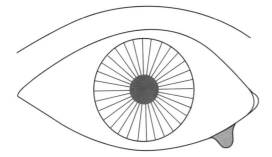

Figure 22.9 Stye

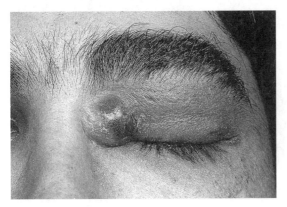

Figure 22.10 Preseptal cellulitis

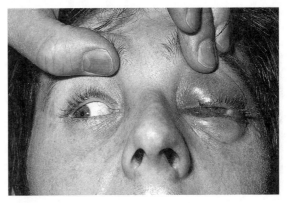

Figure 22.11 Left orbital cellulitis

Table 22.1 Signs and symptoms of preseptal and orbital cellulitis

Preseptal cellulitis	Orbital cellulitis
White globe	Red globe
No diplopia, normal ocular movements	Diplopia if severe, with reduction in ocular motility
No reduction in acuity	Reduction in acuity
Normal pupil reactions	Relative afferent defect if severe
No red desaturation	Red desaturation
No proptosis	Proptosed

Preseptal Cellulitis

Preseptal cellulitis (Figure 22.10) is a tense swelling of the eyelid with no proptosis of the eye.

Treatment. Oral ampicillin and flucloxacillin. If there is no resolution within 2 days refer urgently.

Orbital Cellulitis

Orbital cellulitis (Figure 22.11) is a tense swelling of the orbit with proptosis of the eye (Table 22.1). Eye movements and vision may be impaired. The patient is usually febrile. Refer to a centre urgently. See Table 22.1.

Blepharitis

Blepharitis (Figure 22.12) is a chronic problem involving itchy redness of the eyelids. Crusts may be seen on the lashes.

Treatment. Clean eyelids carefully with cotton wool dipped in warm, weak, baby shampoo solution twice a day and continue indefinitely. Rub ointment of chloramphenicol into the eyelids for courses of no longer than 10 days at a time, once or twice a day. Symptoms may improve with a steroid cream, but if this is used for a long time there is a risk of inducing glaucoma or herpes simplex keratitis.

Advise patients that while it is an irritating and recurrent problem it is at least benign and not sight threatening.

Cornea

Herpes Simplex (Dendritic Ulcer)

This condition produces a painful watery eye which is photophobic. It is unilateral and has a possible history of cold sores in the mouth.

Examination. There is circumcorneal redness, fine branch-like staining of the cornea with fluorescein. Figures 22.13 and 22.14 illustrate the importance of using fluorescein to demonstrate the ulcer. Vision may or may not be affected.

Treatment. Refer urgently. Do not use topical steroids.

Herpes Zoster Ophthalmicus

When the forehead skin is affected the eye will be affected

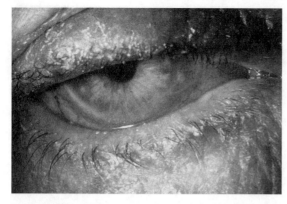

Figure 22.12 Blepharitis

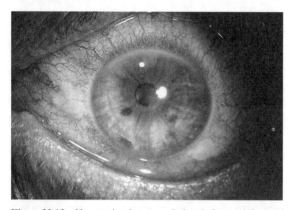

Figure 22.13 Herpes simplex corneal ulcer before staining with fluorescein

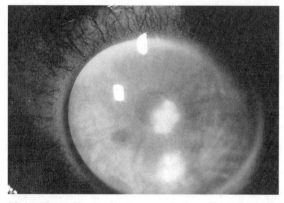

Figure 22.14 Herpes simplex corneal ulcer after staining with fluorescein

in 50% of cases. If the side of the nose is affected, then the eye is usually affected because both are supplied by the nasocillary branch of the ophthalmic division. If the eye is red, it is affected. There may be blepharitis, conjunctivitis, corneal ulcer, corneal anaesthesia, uveitis and other rarer manifestations. Refer urgently if the eye is affected or the patient is concerned.

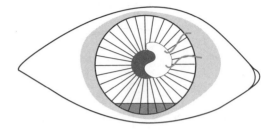

Figure 22.15 Corneal ulcer with hypopyon

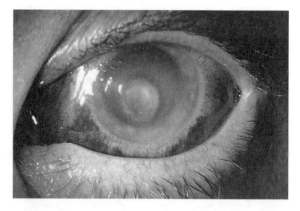

Figure 22.16 Bacterial corneal ulcer

Treatment. Aciclovir tablets 800 mg five times a day for 1 week orally, and chloramphenicol ointment three times a day to the eye to prevent secondary infection.

Bacterial Corneal Ulcer

Bacterial corneal ulcer (Figures 22.15 and 22.16) produces a painful eye, usually with a sticky discharge. It is unilateral, with a possible history of soft contact lens wear (see below), dry eye or previous herpes zoster infection.

Examination. Visual acuity is reduced. There is hazy reflection from the cornea and an area of whiteness can be seen in the cornea. There may be hypopyon (white cells accumulating in the anterior chamber).

Treatment. Refer urgently; if there is likely to be any appreciable delay start ofloxacin (preferably), gentamicin or chloramphenicol drops hourly.

Anterior Uveitis (acute iritis)

Anterior uveitis (Figure 22.17) involves (usually) unilateral redness, pain, photophobia, watering and a possible history of ankylosing spondylitis, sarcoidosis, the Reiter syndrome, inflammatory bowel disease and previous attacks of uveitis.

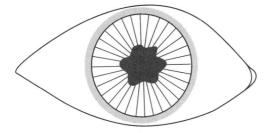

Figure 22.17 Acure iritis

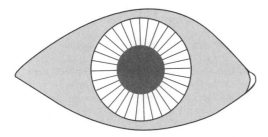

Figure 22.18 Acute glaucoma

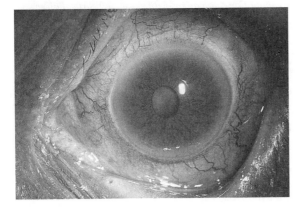

Figure 22.19 Acute glaucoma

Examination. Visual acuity may be reduced or normal. There will be circumcorneal redness, no staining, and there may be a small irregular pupil.

Treatment. Refer urgently. If the patient is known to have recurrent uveitis and is sure that this is the diagnosis, it may reasonable to start with topical dexamethasone drops hourly, until a proper examination of the eye can be made.

Acute Angle Closure Glaucoma

Acute glaucoma (Figures 22.18 and 22.19) affects middle-aged and elderly people. It occurs in hypermetropic (long-sighted) people and symptoms are of severe pain, redness and reduced vision. Coloured haloes may be seen, or have

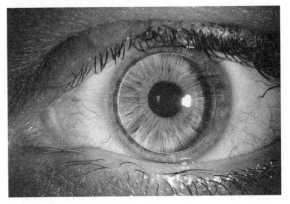

Figure 22.20 Normal hard contact lens

been seen in the previous weeks. Onset is usually in the evening.

Examination. There is reduced visual acuity, a hazy corneal reflection and a mid-dilated, vertically oval pupil.

Treatment. Refer urgently. The patient may need to be repatriated. If there is likely to be any delay start acetazolamide (Diamox) 250 mg four times a day.

Contact Lens Care and Complications

The wearing of contact lenses is hazardous alone, without adding the extra factor of travelling (Figure 22.20). The contact lens can sequester bacteria on its surface, forming a unique biofilm. This must be removed daily to prevent infection taking hold, which can happen when the corneal epithelium is breached. Poor hygiene and overwear may lead to corneal epithelial breakdown, resulting in bacterial corneal ulcer. In the aircraft all these factors could come together. Long flights and a dry atmosphere combine to increase the risk of corneal ulcers. Travelling breaks the daily routine of contact lens care, which involves hand washing before touching the lens, cleaning, sterilising and deproteinising of the actual lens, and adequate storage. Facilities for hand washing may be suboptimal, for example during a flight, camping in the bush, trekking, etc., so the normal routine is skimped. Inadvertent corneal abrasions with fingernails can occur, due to overwear, to attempts at removal without using a mirror (in the inexperienced) or, in cases where the atmosphere is drier, to the lens sticking fast to the cornea.

Contact lenses are small transparent objects that are easily lost either in the eye or in the aircraft; in either case the attempts to find them are more amusing to the onlooker than the person who has lost them.

There are two basic types of contact lens: hard and soft:

1. *Hard lenses.* These are rigid, and are either made of polymethylmethacrylate or of a gas-permeable ma-

terial. They are less likely than soft lenses to lead to ulcers because they do not sequester bacteria.

2. *Soft contact lenses.* These can be further divided into:

(a) Extended wear. These are rarely prescribed routinely but may be used in patients with other ocular problems. Wearers are more likely to suffer infection owing to poor oxygen penetration to the cornea.

(b) Disposables. These are the most common type of lens and can be 6-monthly, monthly or daily disposables.

(c) Daily wear. These are usually changed every year.

The monthly disposable lens is associated with the greatest risk of corneal ulcer; this is probably due to its inferior quality and because some wearers do not actually dispose of the lens when it is out of date and do not sterilise it properly. Wearers may often be tempted to extend the life of the lens for over a month, due to expense or convenience, especially young adolescent travellers.

Travellers should consider changing to daily disposable lenses, although they are more expensive. This will obviate the need to carry the necessary sterilising solutions and prevent devastating corneal infection. Alternatively, those using daily wear or monthly disposable lenses should check that the sterilising solution contains hydrogen peroxide, which is the only way of eradicating acanthamoeba cysts. A neutralising solution is needed to deactivate it. Patients should carry all contact lens solutions with them, because identical products are often unobtainable, even in European countries.

Lenses are stored in special plastic cases during travel. The traveller should always take a spare in case of loss. If going away for more than a month it is advisable to take a new case for each month to prevent build-up of acanthamoeba.

Daily disposables come in blister packs for ease of transport. Make sure that these are intact before use to ensure sterility.

Spare bottles of the solutions should be taken and a new bottle used each month, as open bottles in hot climates could soon become contaminated. In every case up-to-date glasses should always be carried as a back-up in case lenses are lost. Some opticians run an insurance scheme that will guarantee next day delivery of replacement lenses or glasses to most parts of the world. Make sure that all these necessary solutions, cases and spare glasses are carried in hand luggage, in case baggage is lost in the hold.

Common Contact Lens Problems and Some Rarer More Serious Complications

Contact lens loss in the eye. Unfortunately this is common, especially in dry climates where the lens sticks to the cornea and tears as it is removed. The advice is not to panic. If the wearer says he or she can feel the lens then it is probably there even if you cannot see it. Look careful-

ly for the lens, everting the upper lid if needed, and remove with a clean finger. If it cannot be found, leave it overnight. Advise the wearer to take a bath: the humidity improves lubrication, the contact lens miraculously appears and can be removed easily.

Special problem: acanthamoebae. These are unicellular organisms that proliferate in still water, even that which is supposedly clean. They can cause a devastating corneal infection in contact lens wearers who use tap water to clean their lenses. Acanthamoeba corneal infections are less common in the USA, where water comes straight from the mains and not from a tank.

Bacterial corneal infections. Most common corneal ulcers are seen in soft contact lens wearers, but can occur following mild ocular trauma if with a soiled object. This is more likely in hot humid climates such as in the Far East and Africa. It cannot be overemphasised that any patient who you suspect as having conjunctivitis must be asked about contact lens wear. It is then mandatory to exclude corneal ulcer.

Examination of a patient with suspected corneal ulcer.

• Testing visual acuity is a good way to diagnose a serious problem. If acuity is preserved there is less to worry about.

• Ask about a sticky discharge: pus usually suggests a bacterial infection. Using a good strong torch compare one eye with the other. If the shining normal reflex of the cornea is dull, then worry: if there are obvious white patches these may well be ulcers.

• Use fluorescein dye to show epithelial defects in the cornea, which show up as bright yellow with a blue light.

• Look at the anterior chamber of the eye. If there is a white collection of pus forming an obvious level, this is a hypopyon.

Management. The patient should be referred immediately to a specialist unit. If the patient is abroad and there is no access to adequate specialist facilities for 24 h or more, start a broad-spectrum topical antibiotic such as ofloxacin hourly. Ofloxacin covers the rapidly blinding infection with *Pseudomonas* that can melt and destroy a cornea overnight. If ofloxacin is not available, antibiotic drugs should be made up using intravenous preparations such as gentamicin or cefuroxime; however, chloramphenicol is better than nothing at all and if help is not at hand for more than 12 h. Unfortunately, some contact lens ulcers can lead to severe loss of vision if not attended urgently.

TRAUMA

Ocular injury when travelling can pose difficulties for patient and doctor, as there may not be adequate access

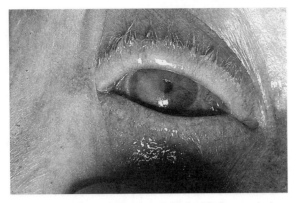

Figure 22.21 Corneal abrasion stained with fluorescein in a child

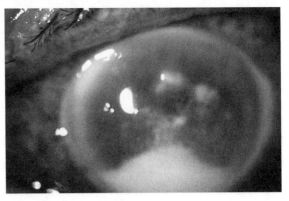

Figure 22.22 Fungal corneal ulcer

to diagnostic facilities. A decision may need to be made as to whether the patient should be transferred to a centre for assessment and surgical treatment. This section provides guidance on what to do in these circumstances.

Severe trauma to the eye can occur in road traffic accidents, with facial fracture and penetrating injury from metal or glass. Unfortunately, road traffic accidents are far more likely to occur when visiting countries abroad. Many factors contribute to this. The roads are unfamiliar, driving is often on the opposite side from that at home, road rules may be also be dramatically different, e.g. in Italy flashing lights means that a driver is going to take an action rather than give way. Car hire also contributes to the dangers: unfamiliar controls and poorly serviced vehicles lead to increased risk of accident. In the United Kingdom, following the introduction of the seat-belt law in 1981, the incidence of driving-related severe eye injuries was reduced to one-third. When travelling abroad the holiday maker is likely to relax and forget about wearing seat belts.

Minor Trauma

Fingernail or twig injuries usually cause corneal abrasions. Always take a history of the injury. Check and record visual acuity. Abrasions (Figure 22.21) can be diagnosed by the use of fluorescein stain and a pen torch. It is useful if the torch has a blue filter as this will show up any corneal epithelial deficit as a yellow area if fluorescein is instilled; however, even without a filter, it is possible to still see epithelial deficits. Check for any pupil distortion or corneal foreign body with a pen torch: it is possible to see them.

If experiencing difficulty examining a patient, instillation of a topical anaesthetic drop, such as benoxinate or proxymetacaine, will help. Everting an eyelid to remove subtarsal foreign bodies can be done with a cotton bud.

Treatment of Corneal Abrasions

Topical chloramphenicol ointment should be used 4 times a day for a minimum of 5 days. Chloramphenicol is cheap, is broad-spectrum and has the advantage of remaining relatively stable in heat. For pain relief some patients prefer a firm pad, others do not. Cyclopentolate 1% twice a day may help reduce pain by reducing ciliary spasm. Topical diclofenac (Voltarol) or ketorolac (Acular) may also be helpful. Oral paracetamol or nonsteroidal anti-inflammatory agents can be used. The regular use of topical anaesthetics should be avoided, as they slow the healing process.

Follow-up and Sequelae

If symptoms worsen or the eye becomes more painful after 3–4 days, referral to an ophthalmologist is essential. The corneal epithelium usually heals within 24–48 h. If the abrasion was caused by a dirty object, especially in the context of a rural or farming setting or in humid climates, there could be a risk of fungal infection (Figure 22.22). However, antifungals should not be used as a first-line treatment; if fungal infection is suspected, refer to ophthalmologist.

Recurrence of a corneal abrasion can occur at any time. Usually the patient awakes from sleep in the early hours of the morning in intense pain, perhaps on an aircraft where the dry atmosphere can predispose to recurrence. This is because the epithelium has failed to adhere properly and formed cystic spaces, which are weak. The theory is that during rapid eye movement sleep the epithelium can be easily reabraded. Treat in exactly the same way as the initial abrasion. If the symptoms persist, prescribe simple eye ointment at night for 3 months as prevention.

Treatment of Corneal Foreign Body

A superficial foreign body may be removed with a 'green'

needle using topical anaesthetic: the cornea is tough and is reasonably difficult to perforate! More deeply embedded foreign bodies should be removed by a specialist at a slit lamp. Leaving a rust ring can lead to a grumbling uncomfortable eye.

Major Trauma

Penetrating Injuries

History and examination. Any object that hits the eye at speed can enter it and leave very little evidence of its entry, particularly if it is thin and sharp. Ask if the patient has any disturbances of vision such as floaters or shadows and test the visual acuity; examine the eye carefully with a torch. Subconjunctival haemorrhages may hide an underlying scleral laceration. This would be unlikely if the vision is preserved and the conjunctiva intact.

If vision is affected, look carefully at the pupil for irregularity. When the cornea is perforated, the iris is sucked into the wound site, thus preventing further collapse of the eye; this shows as a teardrop-shaped pupil. You may need to be very careful to prevent further prolapse of ocular contents. Gently separate lids to examine the eye. If there is gross swelling, cotton buds used gently can facilitate the examination.

Management. If a perforating injury is suspected, tetanus status should be sought and prophylaxis given as necessary. Then pad the eye lightly with gauze and a shield to prevent pressure on the eye. Do not instil antibiotics which may be retinotoxic, especially aminoglycosides. Oral antibiotics such as ciprofloxacin should be initiated, as well as analgesia. Transfer to hospital is then necessary for an X-ray to detect any retained intraocular foreign body and for repair. Whether the patient is repatriated for surgery depends on local access to expertise. Liaison with the International Centre for Eye Health in London is a good idea. Delays in repair of 24 h or more are better than a poor repair locally. In general, a high-quality ophthalmic service can be found in most large cities in the Far East and India, all of Europe, the USA and Russia. Regrettably there are a few good units in Africa.

Retention of Intraocular Foreign Body

Retention of an intraocular foreign body (Figure 22.23) occurs with high-velocity missiles, such as in drilling, hammering, etc. Metal foreign bodies are toxic if retained in the eye, quickly setting up a severe inflammation, even if sterile. It is important to have a high index of suspicion as they can be easily missed. It is worthwhile to X-ray for intraocular foreign bodies, but this will not always detect them. Glass does not always show up on X-ray. The best way of ruling out a foreign body is by history taking, always recording Snellen visual acuity and conducting a

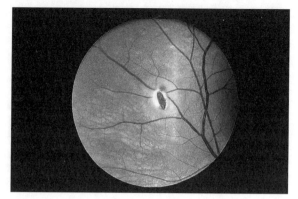

Figure 22.23 Intraocular foreign body

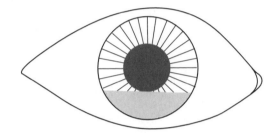

Figure 22.24 Traumatic hyphaema

careful examination with a dilated pupil. Never ignore the patient who tells you there is something floating in his or her vision following an ocular accident. Small thin shards of metal or glass can penetrate the clear cornea and lens or zonule with hardly a trace. Refer to an ophthalmologist if unsure. These foreign bodies will need to be removed by special vitrectomy procedures.

Blunt Injury

Blunt injury can result in hyphaema, dislocated lens, retinal detachment and retinal oedema (commotio retinae), vitreous detachment and haemorrhage. Trauma can also result in orbital wall fractures.

Hyphaema

Hyphaema (Figure 22.24) is a bleed into the anterior chamber of the eye. Sometimes in a severe bleed all of the anterior chamber fills with blood. This will soon settle down if the patient is kept in an upright position, and a blood level will form.

The blood originates usually from a tear in the iris or iris root. The hyphaema usually settles quickly in 48–72 h. The problems associated with hyphaema are those of a short-term rise in ocular pressure and long-term risk of glaucoma, due to damage to the drainage mechanism of the eye if the injury was at the iris root. There is an increased risk of development of cataract in those who have had hyphaema.

Management. If the patient remains in a head-up position the vision will be clearer than lying flat; however, it is doubtful that the position influences the rate of clearing of the hyphaema. Raised ocular pressure does not usually develop immediately and it is more common in rebleeds. If the patient is on aspirin it may be better to stop it until the bleeding settles. If the pain is severe, check for an associated corneal abrasion. The use of cyclopentolate 1% is controversial: dilating the pupil can lead to a rebleed. However, it may provide some pain relief. Topical steroids, may reduce intraocular inflammation, e.g. dexamethasone 0.1% q.d.s. If there is corneal haziness the intraocular pressure may be high; a tablet of acetazolamide (Diamox) 250–500 mg will reduce the pressure and relieve pain.

As soon as possible, arrange follow-up with an ophthalmologist to check whether any other injury, such as retinal detachment, has occurred and whether the drainage angle has any damage. If there is greater than 50% damage to the angle there is a risk of development of glaucoma in the future and annual clinic or optometrist review is needed. Raised intraocular pressure following hyphaema can develop as late as 20 years after the event.

Flashes and Floaters Following Blunt Injury: retinal detachment or not?

Patients who have experienced a blow to the eye may not at first have any symptoms: in a younger patient the vitreous in the eye is well attached. After a few days, if a patient experiences flashing lights or floating objects in the vision then he or she could be developing a posterior vitreous detachment (Figure 22.25). This does not always mean there is a retinal detachment or retinal hole, but a dilated examination of the retina is necesssary (use tropicamide and phenylephrine for a very wide pupil to look for retinal detachment). Ask the patient if there is a shadow in the field of vision that does not float around, and is constant, indicating a retinal detachment (Figure 22.26). A good central vision does not mean that there is no detachment.

Management. Cases that need immediate repair are superior retinal detachments with good vision, as they do the best if operated on promptly. Those who have poor vision, that is 6/60 or less, probably have foveal involvement. The urgency for repair is less and delays of up to 72 h are acceptable. In this situation the prognosis for full visual recovery is poor, but without surgery the eye will become blind and possibly painful.

If access to a modern vitreoretinal service is not available, repatriation is best. If the diagnosis of a superior retinal detachment is made, it is probably better that the patient be transported in a prone position to prevent further peeling of the neurosensory retina. This is because

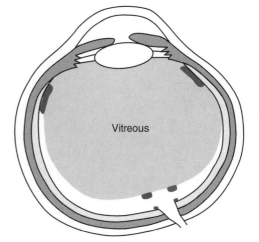

Figure 22.25 Posterior vitreous detachment causing floaters

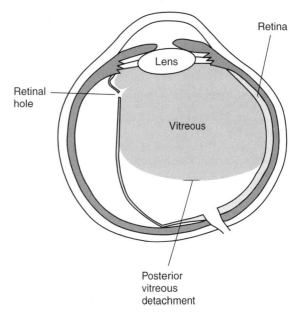

Figure 22.26 Retinal detachment due to a hole, with pre-existing posterior vitreous detachment

fluid can enter the tear in the detachment and, by gravity, increase the detachment. A prone position is achieved by lying on the tummy face down or in the sitting position, e.g. on an aircraft face down with the head resting on a pillow on the lap or the table in front.

Orbital Fracture

Fracture to the walls of the orbit commonly occurs from missiles such as a golf, tennis and squash balls. They also occur in fights between drunk and disorderly travellers!

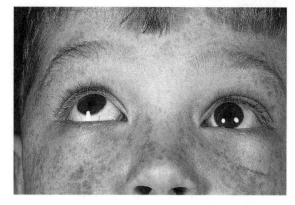

Figure 22.27 Limited left upgaze in blow-out fracture

The signs and symptoms will vary according to the wall that is fractured. The fracture that is often missed is the orbital floor fracture or blow-out fracture, sustained by direct impact on the globe, from a ball or fist for example. The force is transmitted from globe to delicate bone of the orbital floor, leading to prolapse of the orbital contents and entrapment of the tissues around the inferior rectus and consequent vertical diplopia (Figure 22.27).

Signs and symptoms of blow-out fractures. A blow-out fracture is diagnosed on history and examination; X-rays do not always easily show it. Patients who have vertical diplopia following injury almost invariably have a blow-out fracture. Paraesthesia of the cheek below the eye suggests damage to the infraorbital part of the maxillary nerve as it travels through the floor of the orbit. Check eye movements using a torch. Watch the excursions of the eye in the vertical plane. You will notice that there is reduction in upgaze in the affected eye due to tethering of the tissues around the inferior rectus.

Ask for an X-ray to show the floor of the orbit and maxillary sinuses. Usually blood can be seen in the antrum as a level. But this is not always the case, sometimes there is just entrapment of muscle; this is recognised by the teardrop sign.

If the patient blows the nose, surgical emphysema occurs due to air from the nose entering the space beneath the conjunctiva or lid (Figure 22.28). This is benign but broad-spectrum systemic antibiotics are advised.

Management of blow-out fracture. Broad-spectrum antibiotics are given to prevent spread of infection from sinuses to orbit. Pain relief is not usually necessary. Referral for further assessment of fracture is to both an ophthalmologist and a maxillary facial unit (or in some units ENT). The best time and type of repair depends on the nature of the injury. Delays result in fibrosis, and outcome can be compromised. Again, repatriation is best, ensuring that the patient knows that delays beyond 10 days are best avoided.

Other orbital fractures. Fractures of the rim of the orbit

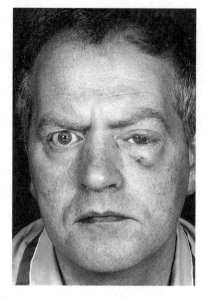

Figure 22.28 Surgical emphysema in fracture of ethmoid bone after blowing nose

and undisplaced fractures of the zygoma are stable and can be treated conservatively. Fractures of the roof of the orbit are more complex and must be referred to a neurosurgical unit. There is the risk of meningitis due to leak of cerebrospinal fluid, for which broad-spectrum antibiotics are necessary. If a patient complains of a runny nose, check the fluid for glucose using urinalysis sticks. The presence of glucose indicates that the fluid is cerebrospinal.

Damage to the Adnexal Tissues: Eyelids, Muscles and Canalicular Structures

Road traffic accidents, sports injuries and dog bites are the commonest causes of ocular adnexal tissue injury. Lid lacerations cause cosmetic and functional problems.

Assessment. When obvious damage has occurred to these areas, be aware that there may be globe perforation. (Check vision and look for iris prolapse.) If these can be ruled out, then proceed to assess the degree of damage. Full-thickness lacerations through the lid should be referred to an ophthalmologist for repair. Minor skin lacerations could be closed with sterile strips. Look for damage to the medial side of the lower lid to see if canalicular damage has occurred, as this may result in a watery eye (Figure 22.29). Check ocular movement for assessment of muscle damage, asking for symptoms of diplopia.

Management. Full-thickness lid lacerations should be repaired by an experienced ophthalmologist. Poor surgery can result in ectropion, entropion, ptosis and

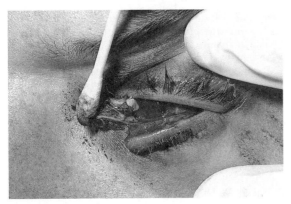

Figure 22.29 Lid laceration through lower canaliculus—risk of watering eye

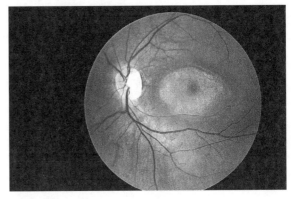

Figure 22.30   Chloroquine maculopathy

misalignment. If travelling abroad, surgery can be delayed for up to 24 h if adequate facilities cannot be reached. The wounds should be covered with sterile moistened dressings and the patient given a tetanus booster and broad-spectrum antibiotic. Reapposition of full-thickness lid lacerations should be accurate and performed in layers with appropriate fine suture such as 6-0 Prolene or silk to the skin and 5-0 absorbable to the tarsal plate and muscle layers. Care should be taken to realign the lashes. Damage to the levator aponeurosis, which attaches to the levator muscle of the lid, will cause a ptosis. Repair of this is very specialised, but it can be done as a secondary procedure with reasonable success.

Assessment of trauma around the eye requires examination of the lacrimal system. Tears drain from the conjunctival sac via the lacrimal puncta into the canaliculus. If there is damage to this area then there is a 50% chance of a chronic watery eye. Repair, even in the best hands, is difficult.

DRUGS AND TOXINS

Ocular Preparations

Stability at Extremes of Temperature

There is surprisingly little information about the stability of different ocular preparations at extremes of temperature; however, the following general statements can be made:

- Eye drops should ideally be stored between 2 and 6 °C. Almost all preparations are stable up to 25 °C.
- The more simple the preparation, the more likely it is to be stable at higher temperatures. For example, simple antibiotics such as chloramphenicol or gentamicin are more likely to be stable than those with a complex viscous carrier.
- Ointments are more likely than drops to be stable at a higher temperature.

- If given the choice, it is better to keep the preparations at too cold rather than too hot a temperature, as the active ingredient is likely to remain stable, even if the carrier becomes denatured. On return to normal temperature the bottle should be shaken thoroughly, particularly if the preparation is in a suspension, such as dexamethasone.
- All ocular preparations should be discarded 1 month after opening because the preservative becomes unstable. At higher temperatures the preservatives may become unstable earlier than 1 month and consideration should be given to discarding the preparation after 2 weeks.
- Drops can be made up from intravenous preparations of the drug, given suitable dilutions mixed with normal saline. These preparations, of course, are not preserved, but if kept refrigerated can safely be used for a few days.

Ocular Toxicity from Systemic Medication

Chloroquine/Hydroxychloroquine

Retinal toxicity from chloroquine (Figure 22.30) used for malarial prophylaxis at the recommended dosage does not occur, even in those people such as pilots on routes to malaria-infested areas who are on continuous prophylaxis. Massive overmedication with chloroquine by self-administration, when patients are feeling unwell and thinking they have a recurrence of malaria, has resulted in visual loss due to retinal toxicity. Hydroxychloroquine is less toxic than chloroquine and is usually used for treatment of rheumatoid arthritis and skin diseases. Treatment is at a much higher dosage than for malaria prophylaxis.

Screening of patients.   Patients taking chloroquine for malaria prophylaxis must be advised not to take more than the prescribed amount and to seek expert attention if a malaria attack is suspected. Those taking high levels of hydroxychloroquine for rheumatoid arthritis or associated conditions will be on a screening regimen for retinal toxicity. Only those taking over $6 \, mg \, kg^{-1} \, day^{-1}$ are considered to be at risk (usually 400 mg: two tablets a day or more in a person weighing 70 kg).

The current recommendations of the Royal College of Ophthalmologists are that the prescriber should check the visual acuity and central field with an Amsler chart if the patient is taking under the at-risk dose. An ophthalmologist should check those taking more than $6 \, mg \, kg^{-1} \, day^{-1}$, by central fields, visual acuity and retinal examination every 6 months.

Ethambutol

Ethambutol is used to treat drug-resistant tuberculosis, in combination with rifampicin and isoniazid. Some travellers returning from abroad having contracted TB may be on ethambutol. The ocular side-effects of optic neuropathy leading to irreversible loss of vision occur in a small number of patients. The effects are idiosyncratic and dose-related, 1% of patients on $15 \, mg \, kg^{-1}$ develop optic neuropathy, and this is more likely if there is poor renal function.

There are reports that Ethambutol toxicity is more common in alcoholics and diabetics.

Screening of Patients. Patients need examination for baseline visual acuity, colour vision, check of pupil reactions (for relative afferent defects) and ophthalmoscopy. Sometimes baseline visual fields to a red target are performed. These need to be documented in notes so that if side-effects are experienced by a patient the ophthalmologist can be sure that the effects are due to treatment and not due to pre-existing pathology. The most important part of the consultation is for the prescribing doctor to make the patient aware of the potential ocular effect of the drug and when to stop the drug and seek advice. Follow-up by the ophthalmologist should be every 3 months if the patient remains on ethambutol.

Acute Closed Angle Glaucoma Induced by Drugs Likely to be Used by a Traveller

Any drug that causes the pupil to dilate could result in the development of acute glaucoma (see Figure 22.18), but usually only in susceptible people. Patients who are longsighted (hypermetropic) and elderly are at greater risk of angle closure. Most preparations carry warnings about the use of a drug if the patient suffers from glaucoma. These refer to acute closed angle glaucoma rather than primary open angle glaucoma.

Most patients who know they are at risk will have had laser iridotomies which prevent an attack; such patients are therefore no longer at risk. The warnings are useless to those who do not know they are at risk because the condition is asymptomatic until the first attack. Acute glaucoma is characterised by pain and hazy vision and is

a result of a closing of the drainage angle in the eye. On examination the pupil will be nonreactive to light and oval-shaped and the cornea hazy. Chronic glaucoma is symptomless. If in doubt check with an ophthalmologist.

Common drugs that induce angle closure are antihistamines (used in travel sickness), anticholinergics, tricyclic antidepressants and illegal drugs such as cocaine.

Most people under the age of 60 are unlikely to develop angle closure unless very hypermetropic. The risk increases with age. Angle closure glaucoma is more common in Orientals (particularly people from Mongolia) and other Asians.

Acute glaucoma is an emergency and needs treatment to be instituted within hours. It is a diagnosis that should not be missed.

Eye Medications: Side-effects

Many patients forget to mention to their physician that topical eye medications are being used. The following drugs prescribed by ophthalmologists could have potentially serious side-effects or exacerbate existing health conditions.

Beta blockers, e.g. timolol, carteolol, betaxolol. These drugs may exacerbate asthma and chronic obstructive airways disease and cause heart block. Some are supposed to be cardioselective, but can still cause problems. If in doubt stop all drops. There is always a substitute possible and glaucoma is a slow process. It should not harm the patient to stop the drops for 2–3 weeks until an ophthalmologist can be seen.

Pilocarpine. Pilocarpine is a treatment for glaucoma. It may result in headaches and blurred vision. The pupils are constricted, which may cause problems in the assessment of head injury.

Chloramphenicol. Chloramphenicol is associated with the rare idosyncratic side-effect of bone marrow suppression, resulting in acute agranulocytosis. It is, however, an excellent antibiotic with good stability and a broad spectrum of activity and good ocular penetration.

Acetazolamide. Acetazolamide is a treatment for glaucoma. Patients are rarely on this treatment for long periods of time, as it has quite severe side-effects. The worst of these is Stevens–Johnson syndrome. Tingling of fingers, tiredness and depression are common. Renal stones and renal failure can also occur. Patients dehydrate as acetazolamide is a diuretic. It is useful in treatment of altitude sickness.

Alcohol Poisoning and Reduction in Vision

Travellers may be induced to imbibe some unusual alcoholic drinks when on their journeys. This should be avoided unless the contents and ingredients of these drinks can be ascertained. Travellers should avoid home-brewed alcoholic beverages, which could contain potentially toxic substances, particularly methanol. Methanol is toxic to the optic nerve.

Alcoholics develop vitamin B_{12} deficiency due to poor diet; and smoking of high-tar cigarettes and pipe tobacco can result in optic neuropathy (tobacco–alcohol amblyopia). This is a slow process and reversible in the early stages with hydroxocobalamin injections and a change of habit.

Snake Venom

The venom from spitting cobras can cause acute ophthalmic symptoms. They are found in Africa and Asia (Sumatran spitting cobra). Those snakes that are found in hotel lobby displays will be devenomised. The spitting cobra possesses great accuracy and can place venom in a victim's eye at up to 3 m. Fortunately, systemic toxicity does not occur; however, the venom binds to the cornea and causes corneal opacity, severe uveitis and blindness if not treated promptly.

The management is to irrigate immediately and copiously with any fluid that is to hand, preferably normal saline but any bland fluid, including milk, will do. To irrigate, get somebody to hold open the eyelids and pour fluid directly on to the cornea. If this is not possible due to severe blepharospasm, plunge the patient's head into bucket of water, to reduce the concentration of venom, and then retry. Use as much fluid as is possible, preferably 2–3 litres. Sedate the patient if you are having difficulty. Enlist the help of an ophthalmologist as soon as possible. The eye will look oedematous and inflamed with a whitish discharge. It will take some time for this to settle and the extent of damage to the be evaluated.

If a patient has been bitten, this is much more serious: be prepared for cardiovascular and neurological collapse.

Bee Stings

Bee stings around the ocular tissue are common but rarely serious. Incidents of multiple stings from African bees have been reported. Stings on the cornea have also been reported.

Management.   Reassure the patient. The eye and lid may be grossly swollen and look alarming. This will resolve. Remove the sting and give antihistamines if there is a large amount of swelling. A cold compress may also help. If corneal sting has occurred, a whitish opacity will be seen on the normally clear cornea associated with chemosis and congestion. Refer to an ophthalmologist for treatment with steroid drops. Cellulitis due to infection can follow a bee sting.

SPECIFIC INFECTIONS AFFECTING THE EYES IN TRAVELLERS

Ocular symptoms following travel are often a cause for great concern for both traveller and clinician alike. Some of the more esoteric and visually devastating ocular disease may well have been seen by travellers when visiting far-off countries such as India and Africa and South America. Travellers may then become anxious about whether they could have caught these diseases.

River Blindness or Onchocerciasis

Life Cycle of the Onchocerciasis Vector

This disease is endemic in equatorial Africa and certain areas of Central and South America. Its prevalence is related to the presence of the blackfly. The blackfly is the insect vector that spreads the parasitic microfilarial infection between humans. Blackflies breed in fast-flowing rivers, hence the name river blindness; this explains why the infected populations are focused along river locations. The parasite is spread when an infected human host is bitten by the female blackfly. The microfilaria becomes a larva in the fly. These then are passed on to another human host by biting. The larvae migrate through subcutaneous tissues and eventually develop into adults after 12 months, producing characteristic nodules, typically around the pelvis or head (onchocercomas). The adult worms mate and produce millions of microfilariae, which migrate through the tissues and into the eye and skin.

The infection risk from one bite of a blackfly is about 1 in 10 and many repeated bites over a period of time are probably needed to establish infestation. The actual bite of a blackfly is usually unnoticed, although a painful wheal often develops, subsiding in a few days. Ocular disease, although eventually blinding, is delayed in onset and needs repeated reinfections to establish.

Symptoms and Signs

Skin infestation always accompanies eye disease, with pruritus, hyperkeratosis, depigmentation or hyperpigmentation, as well as nodules. Skin snips are used commonly to make the diagnosis.

Early stages of the ocular infection may not be observed without a slit lamp to see the microfilariae swimming in the anterior chamber or in the cornea. The patient is asked to bend over to increase the load of microfilariae in the anterior chamber. When the microfilariae die they become more obvious due to inflammatory reactions. The cornea can take on the appearance of cracked ice, or have snowflake opacities. The retina and optic nerve can also be affected, with mottling of the retina and fibrosis. Optic nerve inflammation causes swelling and, in the later course of the disease, atrophy.

Reducing Risk

The traveller need not worry unnecessarily about contracting the disease unless going to endemic regions for a period of some years. Obviously it would be wise always to avoid being bitten by insects in areas of the world where insect vectors are common; this can be achieved by the use of insect repellent, covering bare skin and sleeping under nets.

Treatment should be managed by experienced clinicians because violent reaction to drug treatments is common, as millions of parasites are killed simultaneously, often leading to more damage, such as optic atrophy.

Trachoma

Trachomal conjunctivitis is seen in populations where there are close-knit living conditions, poverty and poor hygiene. It used to exist in the British Isles only a few decades ago in crowded living conditions, for example in Glasgow and Dublin. It is encountered now in the Middle East, Africa, Indonesia and Central and South America. Trachoma has been largely eradicated from India as a result of effective public health measures.

Chlamydia trachomatis has several strains, which cause different forms of conjunctivitis. The more common strain in the UK and USA is the milder form, which causes inclusion conjunctivitis. This form is more likely to be contracted by the less careful traveller, as it is sexually transmitted and can be easily transferred from genitalia to conjunctiva by fingers. Serotypes A, B and C of *C. trachomatis* cause classical trachoma.

Signs and Symptoms

Trachoma is usually a chronic disease with repeated reinfection; initial symptoms are usually of an irritable red eye with mucopurulent discharge. Symptoms may be mild and ignored, but after 2–3 weeks characteristic changes occur. These take the form of follicles, easily seen by naked eye when everting the lid. Without treatment, symptoms are seen to resolve after 8–12 weeks, or at least abate, but continuing reinfection in susceptible patients leads to blinding complications. Blinding occurs because of extensive corneal scarring; as a consequence of conjunctival scarring, which leads to distortion of the eyelid margin, entropion and trichiasis, and inward-growing lashes, the cornea suffers from repeated abrading from lashes and poor lubrication. None of these long-term complications would be seen if a patient who contracted trachoma were adequately treated and reinfection did not occur.

Trachoma Infection Reduction

Trachoma has been eradicated in Europe due to in-creased hygienic living conditions and disposal of waste. In the developing world it is usually spread by eye-seeking flies that feed off the ocular discharge. It is a sad fact that the blinding disease is entirely preventable by simple hygiene measures, yet is still affecting millions. The infection rate could easily be reduced by educating mothers to keep eyes and hands clean, and the frequent removal of waste from around living quarters, which could reduce the number of flies that also carry the infection to the faces of small children. Regular treatment of infection as it occurs, with a tube of cheap antibiotic such as tetracycline, could reduce reinfection and therefore prevent future long-term damage.

Diagnosis and Management of Chlamydial Infection in Travellers

The correct diagnosis involves a conjunctival scrape sent in special chlamydia transport medium (which should be available from a sexual health clinic or gynaecology department). The scrape must include conjunctival cells so it must be done quite firmly with a spatula. A smear can also be made from the scrape on to a glass slide, which will give a quick diagnosis, although serotyping will be necessary. If the sample is taken inadequately or in the wrong medium, the condition will go undiagnosed. The use of chloramphenicol before sampling reduces the rate of pick-up.

The patient can be treated with either oral or topical tetracycline or erythromycin. If the genitourinary form of chlamydia is suspected, it may be best to refer the patient to an appropriate clinic so that partners are also treated.

Those with chronic disease who have developed trichiasis and dry eye need specialist help. Entropion surgery, electryolysis and tear film supplements will help ease symptoms and prevent corneal scarring.

Loa loa

Infection with this filarial worm is not that uncommon in peoples from the equatorial rainforest of Central and West Africa. A biting fly of the genus *Chrysops* transmits the microfilariae. They develop into adult worms in the human host. The thought that a patient may have this infestation usually strikes revulsion in the westerner, but the people who live in this area are well used to its occurrence.

Symptoms

The symptoms are usually initially ignored by clinicians who are not familiar with the disease. These symptoms include itching, oedema and the patient reporting the feeling of something moving around the eye. Usually another member of the family has had a look in the eye and seen the translucent adult worm, which moves freely under the conjunctiva and subcutaneous tissues.

L. loa can survive for many years, evading capture. When they eventually die, they lead to a more severe reaction in the eye, with sudden severe swelling and itching. This gradually subsides and the tissues recover. (This swelling is sometimes called a Calabar, as it is common in the Calabar region of Nigeria.) The presence of *L. loa* is not associated with any visual loss.

The treatment is either physical removal or oral diethyl carbamazine. Physical removal is easier said than done. It involves the patient waiting in a darkened room until they feel the worm moving around the eye. At that point the clinician instils topical anaesthetic, preferably cocaine, and then makes a grasp for the worm with artery forceps. Then an incision is made in the conjunctiva to remove the worm. This usually involves some degree of skill and experience.

Leprosy

Leprosy is found in Africa, Asia and South America. The highest incidence is in Central and West Africa, but it is also seen in the Indian subcontinent among poorer communities. A quarter of a million leprosy patients are blind. There still remains uncertainty about how leprosy is contracted but it seems that close contact with an open case is necessary. Leprosy has not been seen in western Europe since the end of the 1800s. This is probably due to increased levels of hygiene. The organism prefers a cooler temperature and in the eye it is found in the lids, cornea, sclera and iris. Symptoms take 2–7 years to develop because the bacilli take 2 weeks to double in number. Clinical symptoms depend on the immunity of the patient. There is therefore a spectrum of disease, with two extremes called tuberculoid and lepromatous leprosy.

Ocular Involvement

Some of the systemic early signs that are seen include a seventh nerve palsy, erythema nodusum and joint pain. Leprosy does not always involve the eyes but it can be seen early on in the disease, so it is important to recognise this. There is madarosis or loss of eyebrows and eyelashes. Facial skin becomes thickened and nodular, especially the eyelids. Facial nerve palsy is often bilateral and therefore less obvious. The face loses its expression (lepromatous stare). Discrete characteristic changes in the cornea and anterior chamber can be seen. There is thickening of corneal nerves and corneal anaesthesia with secondary corneal ulceration. Iritis is common in advanced cases, with iris pearls and granulomatous change.

Treatment

Treatment is with dapsone, introduced in the 1940s, rifampicin and clofazimine. There are now problems with resistance, just as occurs in tuberculosis. Multiple drug regimens are usually used. BCG affords some protection against leprosy and a vaccine is being developed. Ocular involvement requires specialist referral usually to a corneal or uveitis clinic for specific treatments.

The likelihood of a traveller catching leprosy is small, in view of high levels of immunity and hygiene, and should not really be a concern.

Lyme Disease

The ocular manifestations of this tick-borne disease are unusual. Lyme disease is caused by the spirochaete *Borrelia burgdorferi*, which is spread by ixodid ticks and also by biting flies, carried on the white-tailed deer. This disease is endemic in parts of the USA, especially Connecticut, but also in Australia and Asia. In Britain it is seen in the New Forest. Ten per cent of patients have an early follicular conjunctivitis; a keratitis can follow months later, resembling adonoviral infection. Episcleritis, uveitis, vasculitis and ocular myositis can occur in later stages. A dramatic presentation is a seventh nerve palsy, but other cranial nerve palsies, including optic neuropathy, can also occur. In endemic regions, 25% of new cases of Bell palsy is due to Lyme disease.

Treatment

Doxycycline 100 mg b.d. or amoxicillin for children is effective in early stages. Later stages may need high dose penicillin or cephalosporin.

Toxoplasmosis

This organism is an obligate intracellular parasite. Humans become infected when eating undercooked meat, such as pork, beef or lamb, and possibly unpasteurised milk products; and if hands are contaminated with cysts following handling of cat litter trays. Infection at this stage is often not recognised. Symptoms like those of a mild 'flu are experienced. It is only when a pregnant woman is infected for the first time that serious consequences arise. Women who have positive antibodies to toxoplasmosis cannot transmit the disease. The parasite is spread transplacentally, to the fetus, with varying outcomes, depending on the gestational age of the fetus. In early pregnancy, stillbirth can occur. In the first trimester, neurological involvement can result in convuslions and mental handicap. In severe cases, ocular involvement results in scarring at the macula of the retina, but most milder cases can go unrecognised (Figure 22.31), until later in childhood or adult life when there could be a reactivation of old healed chorioretinitis, when dormant cysts rupture. Although infection is more likely later in a pregnancy, due to increased placental blood flow, the

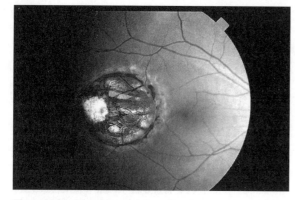

Figure 22.31   Toxoplasmosis scar

consequences of infection in early pregnancy are more serious.

Pregnant women should not eat undercooked meat in the UK or abroad, to avoid vertical transmission. In France, steak tartare should be avoided. Barbecued meats should be well grilled or avoided.

BLINDNESS: A GLOBAL PROBLEM

Travelling in the developing world, people from Britain are likely to be shocked by the number of people with poor vision they encounter—not only elderly people, although most causes of blindness are age-related, but also those of working age and children. Travellers must inevitably wonder why so many people have poor vision and what can be done to prevent or cure blindness.

Seventy-five per cent of those who are blind live in developing countries. As the populations of these countries are both ageing and increasing, the present level of blindness, at 45 million blind globally, is set to increase to 75 million in the next 20 years, given present levels of eye care provision. Eighty per cent of blindness is either preventable or treatable: the challenge is therefore to increase the provision of eye care globally. In the light of this, the World Health Organization, the International Agency for the Prevention of Blindness and nongovernmental development organisations held meetings to develop a strategy for action to control avoidable blindness. As a result of these meetings, the programme 'Vision 2020: the right to sight', was announced, with the mission statement: 'To eliminate the main causes of blindness in order to give all people of the world, particularly the millions of needlessly blind, the right to sight.' The strategies put forward include widespread use of paramedical workers, a community approach with mobile health workers, and prioritisation and cost analysis. In the first 5 years of a 25 year programme the focus will be on cataract surgery, trachoma, onchoceriasis, childhood blindness and refractive error.

Cataract

Cataract accounts for around 50% of global blindness. In 2000 about 10 million cataract operation were performed throughout the world. It is estimated that this will need to increase to 32 million a year by 2020 to address blindness from cataract.

Trachoma

Blindness from trachoma occurs in poor communities. It is estimated that 146 million people, mainly children, carry active infection and 5.9 million, mainly adults, are blind from trachoma. Treatment and control is based around facial cleanness, regular instillation of antibiotics in children, lid surgery to those with lid scarring and environmental cleanliness.

Onchoceriasis

It is estimated that 18 million people are infected and 300 000 are blind from onchoceriasis, mainly in Central Africa and Central America. Control programmes are centred on the larvicidal spraying of blackfly breeding sites and the distribution of ivermectin annually. The resulting decrease in infection is dramatic.

Childhood Blindness

The causes of childhood blindness vary from country to country. The major causes include vitamin A deficiency, often associated with measles, ophthalmia neonatorum and infections from the use of traditional eye medicines. Good hygiene and adequate nutrition are important to prevent blindness in this group. Some countries that are becoming industrialised, particularly in Latin America, have high levels of retinopathy of prematurity.

Refractive Errors

The provision of spectacles at an affordable price is one of the simplest ways of improving quality of life and income.

Vision 2020

The goals of the global initiative are achievable by simple and cost-effective means. Good eyesight makes an enormous personal and economic difference to whole families and communities, as well as to the individual involved. Prevention and treatment of blindness is one of the most important health issues of the twenty-first century.

Section VI

Practical Issues for Travellers

23

Traveling with Children

Philip R. Fischer

Mayo Clinic, Rochester, Minnesota, USA

INTRODUCTION

The principles guiding the practice of travel medicine are fairly constant regardless of the age of the traveler. The application of these principles, however, varies markedly between children and adults. Children are not merely 'little adults'. Children are unique in regard to size, development, behavioral risks, immune maturity, and tolerance of medications. Reviewing available data, this chapter gives practical guidance for medical practitioners providing care to children traveling internationally.

Millions of children cross international borders each year, and lives are frequently enriched from foreign experiences. Clearly, each specific trip carries its own individualized benefits and risks. Every traveling child faces issues of comfort, safety, exposure to germs, and readaptation. Pretravel guidance can help families maximize the benefits of international travel for their children while minimizing the health risks. Following travel, personally tailored evaluation and care can also facilitate a healthy entry or re-entry to the ongoing living situation.

In recent years, there has been increased interest in the particular needs of traveling children. Several review articles cover the broad area of pediatric travel medicine (Neumann, 1995; Fischer, 1998a; Hostetter, 1999; Knirsch, 1999).

MALARIA AND OTHER INSECT-BORNE DISEASES

Geographical considerations regarding the need for protection from malaria and other insect-borne diseases are similar for children and adults. Within endemic areas, however, the need for protection for children is a critical concern. Children can become very ill very quickly, and they do not always show easily localized signs of infection. Many different illnesses present with fever in children, and even where medical care is good, delayed diagnosis of malaria is common (Emanuel *et al.*, 1993;

Viani and Bromberg, 1999). Children carry the greatest burden of malaria's morbidity and mortality, so careful prevention is necessary for any child spending time in a malaria-endemic area.

No single intervention is 100% protective, and a multifaceted approach to the prevention of insect-borne diseases is needed. Vaccination and chemoprophylaxis are not available for many diseases transmitted by insects; thus, the avoidance of bites by mosquitoes and other insects should be a primary focus.

Personal Protective Measures

Adults traveling with children should be advised particularly to dress children comfortably with clothes exposing minimal amounts of skin and to keep the children in 'mosquito-free zones' during the evening and night hours. Rooms with closed doors and screened windows can keep many of the biting insects away from vulnerable young travelers. Expatriates and others spending prolonged periods in malaria-endemic areas should be advised to avoid leaving stagnant water (a breeding site for mosquitoes) around their dwellings.

Bednets are available commercially in forms that can fit over a variety of cribs and beds where children might be spending nights. Impregnating bednets or even curtains with insecticides can also help protect individuals and has even been shown to decrease morbidity in communities (D'Alessandro *et al.*, 1995; Habluetzel *et al.*, 1999). Permethrin-impregnated clothes and bednets are safe for use by children and can offer weeks to months of protection after a single impregnation.

N,N-diethyl-*meta*-toluamide (DEET) is the 'gold standard' for efficacy as an insect repellent and has been used in hundreds of millions of people of all ages over the past four decades. Newer repellents such as those containing citronella seem to be much less effective (Fradin, 1998). Nonetheless, there has been controversy over the safety of DEET-containing insect repellents in children.

Principles and Practice of Travel Medicine. Edited by Jane N. Zuckerman.

Table 23.1   Malaria chemoprophylaxis in children

Medication	Administration	Dose	Comments
Mefloquine	Weekly	$5\,mg\,kg^{-1}$	Suitable at any age
Doxycycline	Daily	$2\,mg\,kg^{-1}$	Not if < 8 years of age
Chloroquine	Weekly	$5\,mg\,kg^{-1}$	
+ proguanil	Daily	$4\,mg\,kg^{-1}$	
Atovaquone	Daily	$\frac{1}{4}$ pill per $10\,kg$	$250\,mg$ atovaquone +
+ proguanil		max. at $40\,kg$	$100\,mg$ proguanil per pill
Primaquine	Daily	$? \, 0.5\,mg\,kg^{-1} \, ?$	Only if no G6PD deficiency

Is DEET safe for use in young children? Millions of children use DEET each year, and there have been just 13 reports of adverse outcomes in children who were using DEET (Fischer and Christenson, 1998). One 6-year-old child with previously undiagnosed ornithine carbamoyl transferase deficiency had a fatal Reye-like syndrome (Heick *et al.*, 1980). Just before becoming encephalopathic, she had used 15% DEET on at least 10 occasions over extensive areas of skin. An 8-year-old girl had seizures and encephalopathy after using 'copious' amounts of DEET (unspecified concentration) and recovered after supportive care (Roland *et al.*, 1985). Similarly, a 5-year-old boy with underlying developmental delay seized after a total body application of 95% DEET followed by a repeat application of another DEET-containing formulation (Lipscomb *et al.*, 1992). In another case, an 18-month-old girl used 20% DEET daily for 3 months and was often noted to lick her skin following application of the DEET; she then developed ataxia (Edwards and Johnson, 1987). In a report of two children from Africa, a 5-year-old girl developed fatal encephalopathy and seizures after using 10% DEET nightly for 3 months, and an 18-month-old girl developed encephalopathy a day after incidentally using an unknown amount of DEET (Zadikoff, 1979). Details of exposure to DEET are less clear in the other reported cases (Osimitz and Murphy, 1997).

Studies of the percutaneous absorption of DEET have not been undertaken in children. Nonetheless, studies with similar compounds suggest that absorption is increased during the first few weeks of life but that children otherwise do not have greater absorption than adults (Osimitz and Murphy, 1997).

Clearly, DEET has been associated very rarely with tragic outcomes, but there is no clear evidence of causality. In cases where details were available, the exposure seemed to be either oral or over extensive skin surfaces in frequent applications. How should travel medicine practitioners interpret these data? Clearly, DEET is effective and is safely used in millions of children each year. It spares the inconvenience of insect bites and the risk of insect-borne disease. The use of DEET should be encouraged, but it should be used prudently. It should only be applied on exposed skin, and most of the skin should be covered with clothes. DEET, travel medicine practitioners should remind parents, should not be ingested orally. Thus, special attention should be placed on young children who lick their hands and arms. The concentration of DEET relates to the duration of effective protection but not to the risk of toxicity. Thus, DEET use by children can be encouraged with attention paid to using it only on the few areas of skin that are exposed to insects.

Personal protective measures are critically important, but they are not universally practiced or completely protective. Thus, chemoprophylaxis should be advised for travelers to areas where malaria is endemic. Protective immunity to malaria develops slowly over 2–5 years in children, so prophylactic medications can be necessary for years despite ongoing exposure to malaria parasites.

Malaria Chemoprophylaxis and Treatment

The geography of medication resistance by *Plasmodium* parasites is not age-dependent. Nonetheless, the delivery of medication to children differs from that to adults. Dosing details are noted in Table 23.1.

Mefloquine seems fully effective and safe in children. Despite hesitation during the earlier part of the past decade to use mefloquine in children, no significant toxic effects were reported. Its use is now accepted for children of any age. As in adults, mefloquine would not be given routinely to a child with a history of cardiac dysrhythmia or with a known psychiatric disorder. Attention deficit disorder and other behavioral problems have not been associated with mefloquine-induced toxicity. Children with active seizure disorders, however, should not take mefloquine. Since some children with simple febrile seizures go on to develop recurrent epileptiform seizures, it is probably best to be judicious about mefloquine use in children less than 6 years old with a history of a previous febrile convulsion. However, since mefloquine is by far the best prophylactic agent available for some areas, individualized decisions should be made, weighing the known risk of severe malaria with the unknown but probably small risk of mefloquine toxicity in a particular child.

Mefloquine, however, does not taste good, and it is not yet available in a liquid form. Weekly doses can be weighed and placed by a pharmacist into capsules; capsules can then be opened each week to give the appropriate dose of powdered mefloquine to the child. Alternatively, pills can be cut in quarters with doses rounded off to the nearest quarter pill to be given weekly. Anecdotal reports suggest that the taste of mefloquine is better tolerated when mixed with chocolate or cola-containing soft drinks.

Doxycycline is associated with discoloration of developing teeth and might adversely affect the growth of long bones. It is, thus, generally not used in children less than 8 years of age.

Chloroquine is completely safe in children and is effective against most of the malaria present in a few parts of the world. Even with long-term weekly use, toxicity has not been noted. Nonetheless, ocular damage has been reported with large doses of chloroquine used over shorter periods of time. Thus, chloroquine use in a child for more than 5 consecutive years should be undertaken only in careful consultation with an ophthalmologist who is following the condition of the child's retinas. As in adults, other rare but reversible adverse effects are possible. As with mefloquine, most children do not enjoy the taste of chloroquine, but attempts to 'hide' the taste may help.

The combination of weekly chloroquine with daily proguanil is also safe for children. Compliance is always an issue with children, so careful attention to regular daily administration is important.

The combination of atovaquone and proguanil has also been studied in children. This has recently been recommended for use and its seems safe and effective for children (Lell *et al.*, 1998).

The combination of sulfadoxine and pyrimethamine, like other sulfa-containing products, carries about a 1 in 5000 risk of life-threatening Stevens–Johnson syndrome. Thus, this combination is not routinely used in children.

The artemesinin derivatives are short-acting antimalarials developed from a plant originally used in China. Even for malaria treatment, they are effective only as short-term agents so are not used alone. Similarly, they are not effective as prophylactic agents.

There is increasing interest in using primaquine as an agent of causal prophylaxis. As in adults, this product should not be used in children until glucose-6-phosphate dehydrogenase (G6PD) deficiency is ruled out. Careful studies of the best dosing for long-term prophylaxis have not yet been completed.

Presumptive treatment is sometimes recommended for adults traveling beyond the reach of accessible medical care. This sort of prediagnosis use of malaria treatment is not generally advised for traveling children due to the risk of overtreatment of nonmalarial fevers as well as the risk of staying away from medical care when a child has malaria and could deteriorate rapidly.

When malaria treatment is needed in a traveler, the medication selection is the same as in adults. Chloroquine is used orally with a total cure of $25\,mg\,kg^{-1}$ ($10\,mg\,kg^{-1}$ once, $5\,mg\,kg^{-1}$ 8 h later, $5\,mg\,kg^{-1}$ 24 and 48 h after the initial dose). Parenteral chloroquine has a narrow therapeutic window and is only used with intensive care unit levels of monitoring. Quinine may be used in a dose of $10\,mg\,kg^{-1}$ three times daily for 7 days. The associated use of tetracyclines for 1 week in treating life-threatening infections is acceptable despite the slight risk of rapid tooth staining. Mefloquine is used either in a $15\,mg\,kg^{-1}$

single treatment dose or in two doses ($15\,mg\,kg^{-1}$ first, then $10\,mg\,kg^{-1}$) separated by 6 h. Artemesin derivatives would always be used in combination with a longer-acting antimalarial.

Malaria Vaccines

The initial optimism for the usefulness of a South American malaria vaccine has waned, as studies in other populations showed very limited efficacy in children. New DNA vaccines offering a combination of antigens in a prime-boost technique now hold great promise. Vaccines could be ready for clinical trials in children during the first few years of the twenty-first century.

DIARRHEA

Travelers' diarrhea occurs in children as in adults. Treatment, however, varies according to the age of the traveler.

Incidence

A retrospective survey done in the late 1980s provided age-specific epidemiology of travelers' diarrhea (Pitzinger *et al.*, 1991). The survey involved 363 children who had recently traveled to tropical developing areas of the world after receiving pretravel advice from an established Swiss travel clinic. Diarrhea occurred in 40% of travelers aged zero to 2 years, in 9% of children from 3 to 6 years, in 22% of children 7–14 years of age, and in 36% of travelers 15–20 years old. While the numbers of children included in each age group were not large, it seems clear that the incidence of travelers' diarrhea is similar in children and adults (Steffen *et al.*, 1999) but that the youngest children carry the highest risk. In addition, infants seem to have more severe diarrheal illness and had diarrhea for longer than the other travelers (Pitzinger *et al.*, 1991).

Etiology

There is no evidence that the microbiological causes of travelers' diarrhea differ between adults and children. Thus, the most common germ causing diarrhea in travelers is enterotoxigenic *Escherichia coli*. With varying rates in differing regions of the world, *Shigella*, *Salmonella*, and *Campylobacter* are also important pathogens for travelers (Paredes *et al.*, 2000). Other bacterial causes occur less frequently, as do parasites and viruses. In about a third of cases of traveler's diarrhea, no pathogenic agent is identified (Peltola and Gorbach, 1997).

Prevention

The microbes causing travelers' diarrhea typically follow

oral contamination. This is usually blamed on contaminated food and water. The higher incidence of diarrhea in young children (Pitzinger *et al.*, 1991), however, suggests that hand-to-mouth contamination is a likely source of microbes. For children, preventive efforts should include not only food and water hygiene but also handwashing, promotion of clean living spaces, and the avoidance of manual contact with germ-laden materials. Pacifiers and bottles should be handled only with clean hands as they are prepared for children. Special attention to handwashing around diaper changes is also important.

Primum non nocere (First, do no harm) is a fundamental principle guiding medical care. While it would be nice to prevent travelers' diarrhea in children, potential preventive medications carry significant risks for adverse effects. Bismuth subsalicylate is usually avoided in asymptomatic children due to the association of salicylates with Reye syndrome. Similarly, sulfa-containing antibiotics have been linked occasionally to Stevens–Johnson syndrome, and tetracyclines can stain teeth. Fluoroquinolone antibiotics carry a theoretical risk of damaging growing joints. Although readily used for ill children, these antibiotics are usually avoided in asymptomatic traveling children.

Prevention of traveler's diarrhea in children is thus based on careful food, water, and hand hygiene. Cleanliness is particularly important in young children who put their hands and other objects frequently in their mouths.

Treatment

Travelers' diarrhea is usually a self-limited illness, but it does seem to be more severe and more prolonged in young children (Pitzinger *et al.*, 1991). Thus, careful attention to prompt treatment is vital.

The mainstay of treatment of diarrhea in children is oral hydration (American Academy of Pediatrics, 1996). Indeed, oral hydration is considered by some to have been the greatest medical advance of the twentieth century. Fluids should be given generously to replace all excessive losses as soon as a child begins to have diarrhea. Even when dehydration is identified, oral fluids (with appropriate salt and sugar concentrations) are effective (American Academy of Pediatrics, 1996).

There is controversy over the use of antiperistaltic agents in children. While recent evidence suggests that one such agent is as effective as oral hydration in traveling young adults (Caerio *et al.*, 1999), there is no evidence that slowing peristalsis actually decreases fluid losses in young children. In a South African study, an antimotility agent did not change the course of dehydrated children with diarrhea (Bowie *et al.*, 1995). Some antimotility medications contain opioids which, when absorbed, cause sleepiness and altered mental status; they thus make the primary treatment, oral hydration, more difficult. Loperamide is minimally absorbed but is still not generally recommended for or used in young children (Gattuso and Kamm, 1994). Loperamide is probably both safe

and effective when used for the treatment of travelers' diarrhea in teenagers.

In adult travelers, the decision to initiate presumptive antibiotic therapy is made, in part, based on the social impact of diarrhea on the traveler's schedule and plans. Children usually have less time-sensitive itineraries, and therapy is often limited to oral hydration for simple (non-dysenteric) travelers' diarrhea.

When judged necessary, however, traveling children may carry antibiotics to use presumptively in the event of severe travelers' diarrhea. Of course, diarrheal illness with bloody stool or with fever should prompt the family to seek medical attention. In the United States, ciprofloxacin ($10\,\mathrm{mg\,kg^{-1}}$ twice daily) is not generally used for children due to concerns about musculoskeletal toxicity. In fact, this medication seems safe in children (Schaad *et al.*, 1995; Jick, 1997), but both the benefit and the potential risk would need to be considered in making individual decisions for prepubertal children. Co-trimoxazole (dose calculated based on 5 mg of the trimethoprim component per kilogram of body weight twice daily for 5 days) is safe in children and may readily be used for travelers' diarrhea; in many areas of the world, however, the microorganisms causing diarrhea are increasingly resistant to this product. Azithromycin has shown good efficacy against some of the etiologic agents of travelers' diarrhea (Khan *et al.*, 1997) and may be used orally in a dose of $10\,\mathrm{mg\,kg^{-1}}$ once followed by $5\,\mathrm{mg\,kg^{-1}}$ on each of 4 successive days. Though not studied in children with traveler's diarrhea, shorter courses of antibiotic therapy are likely to be equally effective.

VACCINATION

While prevention with behavioral changes and therapeutic medication use are often challenging in children, vaccines are well accepted and provide effective pretravel intervention that can decrease greatly the risk of many diseases. Attention should be paid to the timing of 'routine' childhood vaccines (Table 23.2) as well as to the use of special travel-related immunizations (Table 23.3). New vaccines are being developed, and expert recommendations change rapidly. Health care providers taking care of traveling children should consult up-to-date sources (such as www.cdc.gov) for current recommendations.

'Routine' Vaccinations

Diphtheria (D), tetanus (T), and pertussis (P) vaccines are commonly used in most countries of the world. Diphtheria is an unusual illness in many areas but became more common in Europe and Asia following the restructuring of the former Soviet Union; cases in adult travelers were reported. Tetanus is common around the world, and pertussis continues to cause significant morbidity and mortality in infants. The pertussis vaccine has been

Table 23.2 'Routine' vaccinations

Illness/vaccine	'Routine' administration	Acceptable 'early' administration
Hepatitis B	Ages 0–2, 2–4, 6–18 months	2nd and 3rd doses 1 and 4 months after 1st
Diphtheria	Ages 2, 4, 6 , 15, 60 months	Ages 6, 10 and 14 weeks, 1 and 5 years
Tetanus	Ages 2, 4, 6 , 15, 60 months, repeat each 10 years	Ages 6, 10 and 14 weeks, 1 and 5 years
Pertussis	Ages 2, 4, 6 , 15, 60 months	Ages 6, 10 and 14 weeks, 1 and 5 years
Haemophilus	Ages 2, 4, 6, 12 months. Only one dose after 12 months	Ages 6, 10, 14, 52 weeks
Polio	Ages 2, 4, 6–18, 60 months	Additional dose at birth
Measles	Age 12 and 60 months	'Extra' dose at 6–9 months. 2nd dose 1 month after 1st
Mumps	Prepuberty	Age 12 months
Rubella	Prepuberty	Age 12 months
Varicella	Age 12–18 months	Age 12 months
BCG	Controversial	1st days of life

Table 23.3 Travel-related vaccinations

Illness/vaccine	Usual age	Comments
Hepatitis A	> 2 years	? Any age if mother seronegative
Typhoid, Ty21a, oral	2–6 years	
Typhoid, Vi, intramuscular	2 years	
Yellow fever	9 months	Encephalitis risk < 4 months of age
Cholera	? 1 year ?	Limited infant data
E. coli	? Infancy ?	Limited pediatric data
Meningococcal	2 years	A component suitable for 3-month-old infants C component suitable for 2-year-old children
Japanese encephalitis	> 1 year	12–36-month-old children: $\frac{1}{2}$ adult dose
Rabies	> 1 year	Underused
Malaria		Pending

plagued by popular concern over side-effects, but the acellular vaccines (aP) are effective without as many adverse reactions. The initial series of injections is usually at 2, 4, and 6 months of age in industrialized countries, but it may be given as early as 6, 10, and 14 weeks of age. Traveling infants should be as completely protected as possible before departure. An additional immunization (DTaP) is given after the first birthday to complete the primary series. A booster of DTaP is given at 4–6 years of age. Older children have waning immunity to pertussis and can serve as reservoirs to pass the microorganisms to younger, at-risk individuals, but revaccination against pertussis is not widely recommended for children beyond 6 years of age. Tetanus vaccine booster doses, incorporating diphtheria vaccine as well, are given subsequently every 10 years.

Hepatitis B is common in Africa and Asia, and expatriates even without known body fluid exposure are at risk of this infection (Lange and Frame, 1990). To prevent both acute illness and the risks of later chronic hepatitis and of hepatocellular carcinoma, travelers should consider the full three-dose hepatitis B vaccination course. Administration may begin in the neonatal period, and subsequent doses are given 1–2 months later and then again 6–18 months after the first dose. Accelerated schedules have been proposed, sometimes with a later fourth dose, but have not been studied fully.

Poliomyelitis has been eradicated from the western hemisphere, but cases still occur in Africa and Asia. Travelers to areas that are still endemic should be vaccinated. The oral vaccine is effective but does carry a slight risk of causing vaccine-associated paralytic poliomyelitis. Each dose of either the injectable or the oral vaccine provides some protection, but three doses are usually needed to confer adequate protection against each of the three polio strains. If possible, pediatric travelers should have at least the three initial doses before traveling; doses may be given at 2, 4, and 6 months of age. Younger travelers may receive doses at 6, 10, and 14 weeks of age. A dose at birth is less immunogenic but may be given to children who would not otherwise receive all three initial doses before traveling.

Haemophilus influenzae type b is a major cause of meningitis, pneumonia, and other invasive diseases in children around the world. Several good vaccines are available; timing of doses varies with the different products, so package inserts should be consulted. Traveling children under 1 year of age should usually be given three doses of vaccine (usually at 2, 4, and 6 months of age; acceptable at 6, 10, and 14 weeks of age). A single vaccine dose is adequate to provide protection to children over 12 months of age. H. influenzae type b disease is very unusual after 5 years of age, so healthy older children do not need this vaccine before traveling if they have not received it previously.

Measles, mumps, and rubella are viral illnesses seen around the world. 'Routine' vaccination schedules vary between countries. Passively acquired maternal antibody can impair the effectiveness of these vaccines in young children, but such antibody influences rarely persist beyond the first birthday. Thus, measles vaccine (with or without accompanying mumps and rubella vaccine) may be given after 12 months of age. A second dose is recommended at least 1 month after the first dose to try to provide protection for the small percentage of children who fail to respond to the first dose. Children traveling between 6 and 12 months of age should have an additional dose of measles vaccine before traveling to provide protection in the event that their maternal antibody titers had already waned. Mumps and rubella are particularly problematic illnesses after puberty; unvaccinated traveling children who are nearing puberty should be vaccinated against these illnesses as well.

Varicella vaccine has become available in recent years and is affordable in many areas of the world. Although varicella illness is less common in some developing countries than in some industrialized regions, varicella vaccine could be given routinely to any immunocompetent pediatric traveler over 1 year of age who has not already had chickenpox. To ensure an adequate immune response, two doses of varicella vaccine are recommended for children 13 years of age and older; they may be given 4–8 weeks apart.

Rotavirus vaccine could also be considered for international travelers at risk of exposure to contaminated food and water. This oral vaccine is effective but has been associated with a slightly increased risk of intussusception (CDC, 1999a). Due to this risk, it is not available commercially in some areas.

The tuberculosis vaccine, BCG, is used routinely in many countries. This vaccine is of limited and variable efficacy but does seem to prevent some extrapulmonary tuberculosis. The vaccine may be given at any age. Later, if there is concern about possible tuberculous disease, the history of past BCG vaccination should not affect the interpretation Mantoux (PPD) skin testing.

Travel-related Vaccines

Hepatitis A is usually asymptomatic in young children and is only rarely associated with life-threatening complications. Nonetheless, children can serve as a reservoir to transmit disease to their older traveling companions or to contacts at home after they return from travel. Hepatitis A vaccines are safe and immunogenic. There does not seem to be any reason not to vaccinate pediatric travelers. Limited studies suggest that the vaccine is immunogenic in young children who did not receive hepatitis A antibody passively from their mothers (Troisi et al., 1997; Piazza et al., 1999). Thus, even though the vaccine is not usually given before 1 or 2 years of age, the offspring of seronegative women can probably receive the vaccine safely and effectively at any age. By 12–15 months of age, titres of passively acquired antibody have usually waned sufficiently to allow adequate vaccine immunogenicity. While recommendations often include administration of this vaccine 2 weeks prior to travel, to give time for the development of a protective immune response, the vaccine seems effective even when given after exposure (Sagliocca et al., 1999). Thus, vaccine may still be given with confidence up to the time of departure.

Typhoid vaccines have been developed recently and offer better immune protection and fewer side-effects than older vaccines. The Vi capsular vaccine is effective in providing some protection for 2 years when given intramuscularly to children 2 years of age and older. The current Ty21a oral vaccine must be swallowed in capsular form but has documented effectiveness in children. Dosing recommendations vary from a three (World Health Organization) to four (American licensing authorities) doses in the initial series, and the lowest age at which the vaccine is used also varies (2 years by WHO guidelines, 6 years in North America).

Yellow fever vaccine is required for entry into some countries and is recommended for travelers to some other endemic areas. There have been a few cases of vaccine-associated encephalitis, mostly in children under 4 months of age. The vaccine is, therefore, not advised for routine use in children under 9 months of age. Children between 4 and 9 months of age who are at particular risk of exposure to yellow fever might be considered candidates for vaccine use. As always, mosquito avoidance measures should also be integrated into the travel plans.

Newer, oral cholera vaccines have shown good efficacy in some parts of the world (Trach et al., 1997). While cholera is not a high-frequency problem in traveling children, the cholera vaccines do show good efficacy (Thompson, 1999). As these vaccines become increasingly available on the commercial market, it is expected that they will be useful in children as young as 1 year of age.

Vaccines against enterotoxigenic E. coli (ETEC) are being studied, some in association with cholera vaccine. A preliminary report suggests that there is some protective effect of an oral ETEC B-subunit-inactivated whole cell vaccine in traveling adults and children (Wiedermann et al., 2000). Further clinical studies are in progress.

Meningococcal vaccine has limited immunogenicity in young children. The group A vaccine component provides some protection to children as young as 3 months, but the group C component does not induce immune responses reliably before the age of 2 years (American Academy of Pediatrics, 1997). The vaccine is usually given to children 2 years of age and older, but full protective efficacy is not present until after 4 years of age. With ongoing exposure, revaccination would be considered annually until age 4 and then every 5 years if the previous dose was given after the fourth birthday. A newer conjugate vaccine active against groups A and C is immunogenic for both groups as early as 10 weeks of age (Campagne et al., 2000).

Japanese encephalitis virus vaccine indications are the same in adults and children. This vaccine may be used in children 1 year of age and older, but a half-sized dose is used for children 12–36 months of age.

Rabies is still common in much of the world. By their size and location near the ground and by their friendly curiosity with animals, children are particularly at risk. Even long-term expatriates in developing countries, however, often neglect rabies vaccination (Arguin et al., 2000). When needed, rabies vaccine may be given after the first year of age. As in adults, pre-exposure vaccination does not negate the need for some further care following a subsequent potentially rabid bite. Concurrent use of chloroquine (and, possibly, mefloquine) seems to impede the immune response to rabies vaccine, especially when it is given intradermally. Consequently, rabies vaccination should be completed before prophylactic chloroquine therapy is initiated (American Academy of Pediatrics, 1997).

Effective malaria vaccines hold the promise of saving the lives of a million children each year in Africa alone. Travelers, too, could be greatly aided by malaria vaccination. DNA vaccines using multiple genetic 'antigens' and unique immunologic boosting techniques are being developed and should be ready for field testing during the first decade of the twenty-first century.

COMFORT

The success and enjoyment of a family's travel often depends on how comfortable their children are. Pediatric travelers are most comfortable when parents view planning and scheduling at least partly from the child's perspective. Travel health practitioners can provide practical suggestions to help families traveling with children.

Long trips can be broken up into smaller segments. Periods of vigorous activity (whether exercise or games) can be mixed with sedate times of transit. Activities can be planned so that the child's mind and body can be occupied. Long waits leading only to 'boring' adult activities can be discouraging to children. Transit nights in hotels with some other activities can help break up trips between several continents.

Age appropriate activity packs can increase a young child's tolerance of long road and air trips. New snacks, games, or books may be opened and used either after a specified duration of travel or when crossing a particular landmark. In this manner, children not only get special new pleasures, but they also mark their advancing progress through the trip.

In airplanes, advanced seat selection can help minimize some of the stress of traveling with children. On intercontinental flights, infants can use fold-out cots attached to walls in front of the bulkhead (front row) seats. Without impeding parental leg room, children can thus stretch out for restful sleep. Families with toddlers should have aisle access for 'walks' around the cabin during long trips. Older children can select air seats with care to obtain a good view of the video screen.

Some families choose to medicate their children to help the child tolerate long periods of inactivity. Sedatives have not been subject to efficacy studies in pediatric travelers. Diphenhydramine (1 mg kg^{-1} per dose) is a commonly used antihistamine drug that provides a few hours of sedation for many children. If a family is going to use it, they should try a test dose before the trip; some children have a reaction of excitability that can clearly disrupt the trip. Chloral hydrate ($50–75 \text{ mg kg}^{-1}$ per dose) can provide sedation for medical procedures but is not generally recommended for behavioral control when a child is to be in a confined travel situation. Clearly, parents responsible for supervising traveling children should not personally be under the influence of sedative medications or alcohol.

Typically, the discomfort associated with jet lag seems to increase with age. Nonetheless, children who wake during the night while adjusting to new time zones can disrupt the entire family. Melatonin seems to be safe in neurologically healthy children, but detailed studies of melatonin for pediatric jet lag have not been done. As noted, sedatives may be given; most experts, however, do not advise traveling children to take sedatives. Families should plan their schedules and their accommodations in such a way that the disruption of awakening children will be minimized.

Changing cabin pressures in commercial aircraft with ascent and descent have been associated with eustachian tube obstruction and resulting earache in children. This is a particular concern during descent, when 10–15% of young children experience middle-ear discomfort (Buchanan et al., 1999). Recommendations for preflight use of antihistamines and decongestants have been published, but scientific studies do not demonstrate effectiveness of these products in traveling children. Pseudo-ephedrine has documented effectiveness in preventing earache in adults (Csortan et al., 1994) but it had no positive effect in a study of young children making commercial air flights (Buchanan et al., 1999).

Comfort is also a concern during road trips. Vehicles and car seats should be selected with the child's comfort in mind. The parents' seating location should also be planned to allow supervision and assistance to children without compromising safety.

Motion sickness is a problem for some children. A gentle flow of fresh air and a seat near the front of the vehicle can often help. Dimenhydrinate ($1–1.5 \text{ mg kg}^{-1}$ per dose) is often effective preventive treatment.

SAFETY

Accidents and injuries cause more deaths among travelers than do exotic diseases, and injuries are often preventable (Reid and Keystone, 1997). Safety should be a major priority of families traveling either domestically or internationally with children.

There is controversy about the seating of infants in aircraft. In general, air travel is safer than road travel, but turbulence and rare crashes do pose risks for incompletely restrained infants in airplanes. Car seats are designed both to restrain general movement and to protect children in accidents where there is a sudden cessation of forward motion. The physical forces caused by air turbulence and plane crashes are much less predictable than the movements of automobile accidents. There is, therefore, no ideally designed infant aircraft restraint seat. Use of car seats in airplanes would possibly prevent some injuries and rare deaths. On the other hand, the increased cost of a full airfare for infants using their own restraining seats would prompt some families to use alternative modes of transportation; these other means of transport are actually more likely to be associated with accidents and fatalities. Replacing expensive air trips by long road trips would probably actually increase the risks of infant injury and death. When feasible, families of infants traveling by air might consider using 'car seats' in airplanes to decrease further the already low risk of turbulence and crash-related injury.

Vehicular safety is paramount. Age-appropriate restraints should be available and correctly used for all travelers. Rear-facing car seats are best for children under 12 months of age, and forward-facing restraint seats can be used for children aged 1–5 years. Seat belts should be used by all travelers in cars, and back seats are safer than front seats during accidents. Advance planning is often required to ensure that vehicles of adequate size, with seat belts and car seats, will be available at a particular international destination. Parents of young children are advised to carry their own car seats. Allowing children to move freely about a car endangers the lives of all passengers.

Water-related accidents continue to account for injury and death in children and adolescents. Alcohol should not been consumed during boating. Swimming should always be well supervised with ready help available. Particular attention to boating and propeller safety is necessary (Fischer, 1998b).

In their homes, most parents are aware of 'child-proofing' and the need to ensure a safe living environment for children. While traveling, care should be paid to electrical outlets, cords, and water temperature. Doors, stairs, and balconies should be in good repair; a quick inspection at each new lodging site is advisable.

During travel, medicines, cleaning products, and chemicals (such as insect repellents) are often exposed and within reach of children. Parents should be especially careful to control a child's environment to decrease the risk of accidental ingestion during trips.

Some injuries occur when young children do not exercise adequate precautions about strangers. Avoiding clothes with visible personal identifiers can help decrease the risk that naive children will allow malintentioned adults to identify and 'befriend' them.

Skin safety is also important. Sunscreen is not generally advised for children under 6 months of age, and the infant should be either shaded or have covering clothes to prevent sunburn. Older children should use sunscreen with a sun protection factor (SPF) of 15–30; this provides a 93–96% reduction in exposure to ultraviolet B light (Kim et al., 1997). Blistering sunburn during childhood is a major risk factor for malignant skin problems later in life.

Travel medicine practitioners should discuss appropriate clothing during pretravel consultations. Children should wear closed shoes to decrease the risk of helmin-thic diseases in areas where parasite worms and larvae have contaminated the soil. Clothes and diapers/nappies should be ironed before use if they were dried on the ground in an area of tumbu fly infestation.

Despite good parental intentions and efforts, injuries happen and health problems occur. Families should consider traveling with a medical kit to allow prompt response to health problems incurred during their trip. A medical kit could include important health information about the child (name, birth date, weight, medical allergies, immunization history, doses of current medications, and blood type) as well as medicines and supplies. Routine first-aid supplies (bandages, tape, gauze, splints, disinfecting solutions) could be part of a traveling medical kit. Usual medications would be carried, often with two separate supplies in case the traveler is separated from part of the luggage during the trip. Antibacterial skin ointment, steroid creams, antihistamines, analgesics, and antipyretics could also be useful. Families should know the size-appropriate dosing for common medications (acetaminophen/paracetamol $10–15 \, mg \, kg^{-1}$ per dose every 4 h, ibuprofen $10 \, mg \, kg^{-1}$ per dose every 6 h as needed). Ipecac could be carried to use to help empty the stomach of a child who ingests potentially toxic material (but not hydrocarbons). Medications for travelers' diarrhea and malaria, when appropriate, could also be included. A family could put oral rehydration fluid packets, sunscreen, and insect repellents in their medical kit as well.

ALTITUDE CONCERNS

The Bible teaches that God created humans and placed them in a garden (Genesis 2:8), probably not far above sea level. There were problems, however, and the original couple were sent traveling (Genesis 3:23–24). Generations later, as the Bible records history, God sent Noah and his family on a high-altitude excursion. Noah's itinerary called for slow ascent en route to a high, mountainous elevation (Genesis 7:17). Travelers since that time have ascended to high altitude more quickly, and acclimatization challenges are well known.

Children, like adults, are at risk of high-altitude sickness. With the relative immaturity of their cardiovascular systems, however, there are questions about the best management of young children undergoing rapid elevation changes and the resultant exposure to widely varying pressure and oxygen conditions.

Air Travel and Infants

Anecdotally, there have been sudden, unexplained deaths in infants following long trips in commercial aircraft (Parkins et al., 1998). This should not be surprising because sudden infant death syndrome (SIDS) is both sudden and idiopathic. Tragically, infants might suddenly die after any coincidental activity, be it air travel, vaccination, or kissing. The anecdotal association of a few cases does not prove causality. To date, there is no documented evidence that air travel in pressurized craft increases the risk of sudden death for children. If air travel does increase the risk of SIDS, it is likely to be a less important factor than either prone sleep positioning or passive smoke exposure.

Air travel probably does, however, have physiologic effects on children. Aircraft are pressurized to simulate the atmosphere at an altitude of about 8000 feet (2500 m). Under laboratory conditions, some infants had either unusual degrees of hypoxia or increased episodes of abnormal respiratory patterns when subjected to hypoxic ambient air (Parkins et al., 1998). The clinical implications of these findings, if any, are not known. The data indicate that children respond to conditions simulating high altitude or aircraft exposures, but it is not clear that the responses are either pathologic or dangerous.

There is also a published recommendation that children under 6 weeks of age 'should not fly because their alveoli are not completely functional' (CDC, 1999b). In fact, this recommendation represents the conjecture of an established expert, but there are no reported data to suggest that this precaution is necessary.

In the face of incomplete data, therefore, what should travel medicine practitioners recommend for families who are considering air travel with infants? First, families should be aware that many babies fly commercially without known adverse outcome. Second, families should be told that medical knowledge on this subject is incomplete and that there could be previously undescribed risks. Third, extreme caution should be exercised for babies with a history of lung disease, who would presumably tolerate decreased oxygen tension less well. Finally, families can balance their own perceived benefits of the trip with the unknown and possibly nonexistent risk of travel with infants.

Chronic Altitude Exposure in Infancy

Infants undergo physiologic adaptation when exposed chronically to high altitudes. They initially show decreased oxygen saturations. Over time, they have enhanced oxygen uptake (compared with infants at sea level) with increased ventilation, increased lung compliance, and increased pulmonary diffusion. They also have elevations in pulmonary artery pressure and raised blood viscosity (DeMeer et al., 1995). These changes seem useful in providing adequate tissue oxygenation.

In some infants, however, chronic exposure to high altitude has negative effects. Pulmonary hypertension can lead to cardiac decompensation and death (Khoury and Hawes, 1963; Sui et al., 1988).

In Tibet, an autopsy study of 15 infants showed pathologic changes suggestive of response to hypoxia (Sui et al., 1988). While complete population data were not reported, it was notable that most of the involved infants

had been of non-Tibetan origin and had moved to high altitude within a few months of the fatal episode. This suggests that either genetic factors are important or that travelers to high altitude are at greater risk than those who are born at and then stay at altitude.

In Peru, children living at 14 000 feet (4500 m) elevation were studied. Pulmonary hypertension was common, but this seemed to be less common in older than in younger children (Sime et al., 1963). Similarly, a report from Colorado in the United States included 11 children with pulmonary hypertension (Khoury and Hawes, 1963). The nine survivors did well with treatment, relocation to a lower altitude, and time.

Putting these reports together, one can conclude that poor outcomes are possible in children developing pulmonary hypertension at high altitude. The exact risk is not quantified, but it appears that immigrants might be at greater risk than those born at altitude. Pending the availability of further data, families should be cautioned about unnecessarily exposing infants to high altitude, and they should be advised to seek medical attention at the earliest sign of any cardiorespiratory symptoms that might develop.

Besides sharing medical risk information, travel health practitioners can help guide the thought processes of parents wondering about taking their children to high altitudes. Clearly, a pleasure trip should not warrant placing the child at much risk at all. A family relocation for humanitarian service or for other less self-gratifying reasons, however, might prompt parents to accept carefully some risk but also to institute contingency plans to respond quickly to any problems that occur.

Altitude Sickness

Available information suggests that altitude sickness (be it acute mountain sickness, high-altitude pulmonary edema, or high-altitude cerebral edema) is essentially the same in children and adults. The communication of symptoms will differ with age, but the conditions are similar.

In North America's Rocky Mountains, 22% of 3–36-month-old children had symptoms compatible with acute mountain sickness (Yaron et al., 1998). This is similar to the incidence of acute mountain sickness in adults in that area. Previously, a study had noted that 28% of school-aged children had signs of acute mountain sickness during a vacation at 2835 m (Thies et al., 1993). Interestingly, however, 21% of a 'control' group vacationing at sea level in that study had similar symptoms. Clearly, other features of travel can mimic acute mountain sickness.

A retrospective review of cases of high-altitude pulmonary edema suggested that children, but not adults, were more likely to have had an antecedent viral upper respiratory infection when they developed their altitude-related illness (Durmowicz et al., 1997). Details of the pathophysiology of this relationship are not known, but families of children with colds might need to be particularly prudent about adjusting high-altitude itineraries and about promptly seeking medical attention (and descending!) if tachypnea develops.

Acetazolamide has not been studied systematically in children. Physiologically, one would expect it to be as effective as in adults, and anecdotal reports suggest nothing to the contrary.

In summary, acute complications of ascent to high altitude are similar in children and adults. Minor respiratory symptoms might predispose children to more severe pulmonary complications at altitude, but the preventive and therapeutic options are probably independent of age.

BODY FLUID EXPOSURES

Adolescents, like adults, may be at risk of sexually transmitted diseases. Through sexual exposure, body piercings, tatooings, and nonsterile medical procedures, even children can be exposed to *Hepatitis B virus* and *Human immunodeficiency virus* (HIV). For families traveling together, pretravel consultation should include reminders of these risks as well as suggestions regarding risk avoidance. For adolescents traveling with or without their families, confidential discussion of these issues may be necessary.

POST-TRAVEL SCREENING AND CARE

The practice of travel medicine goes far beyond pretravel counsel and care. Indeed, practitioners of pediatric travel medicine are often called on to evaluate returned travelers and recently arrived immigrants. While screening tests and medical care should be individualized to each child's particular situation, some general comments can help focus the care of children who have traveled recently across international borders.

Screening of Asymptomatic Individuals

Each returned or immigrating traveler carries a wealth of memories and a growing perspective on life. Sometimes, they also carry health concerns and microbial pathogens. Asymptomatic children returning to their home country following a brief overseas trip rarely need to undergo a medical evaluation or screening procedures. Other travelers coming from a prolonged stay in an area of limited hygiene and nutrition deserve extensive screening.

Medical personnel asked to see a child who has immigrated recently or who has returned from a prolonged stay overseas should help facilitate smooth transitions and adjustments to a new or renewed 'home'. While helping the child sense the importance of past experiences, health care providers can question the child and parent(s) about cultural, linguistic, scholastic, and financial adap-

tation. Further help can be arranged for a child struggling in any of these areas.

Children settling in to a new geographic area should be incorporated into routine health promotion activities with an identified primary care medical home. The family might benefit from education about routine health care and preventive interventions. Vision and hearing screens as well as planned check-ups throughout the school years should be scheduled. Dental problems are common in immigrant children, and dental evaluation is important. Height and weight should be measured, compared to standards for age, and followed over time. Some of these issues are beyond the routine scope of a travel medicine practice, but alert travel medicine practitioners will see that their returned or immigrating travelers are incorporated into these ongoing health maintenance activities.

Immunization schedules vary around the world. A child should generally be updated with immunizations to be current in the site of the new or ongoing residence. If there is any uncertainty about the reliability of the outside immunization records, as there often is for adopted children(Hill, 1998), the 'routine' immunization series should be reinitiated.

Children who have spent more than 3 months in a developing country and children being adopted from situations of uncertain health background can usually benefit from screening procedures. Skin testing for tuberculosis (TB) should be done. Published recommendations help guide the interpretation of results; past receipt of BCG does not exclude the possibility that a positive skin test is due to actual mycobacterial infection (American Academy of Pediatrics, 1997). Children with positive test results (greater than 10 mm of induration following a 5 IU intradermal PPD injection) should have chest radiography. If they are asymptomatic without physical findings of tuberculous infection and with a normal chest X-ray, then preventive therapy would be initiated. If they are coming from an area of low incidence of drug-resistant TB, 9 months of isoniazid ($10 \, mg \, kg^{-1}$ as a daily dose, pyridoxine supplementation if nutritional concerns or other chronic illness) can be given. Children who presumably were exposed to TB in a multidrug-resistant area would use multiple 'preventive' agents. Children with findings of active disease would need further testing and more extensive therapy. A recent case of extensive TB transmission in an immigrant child highlights the need to place and read TB skin tests in immigrants who seem healthy (Curtis *et al.*, 1999).

Laboratory testing might also be helpful for children who have spent more than 3 months overseas. A blood count with a leukocyte differential reading could give a clue of nutritional anemia (low hemoglobin concentration with hypochromic, microcytic red blood cells) or of some parasitic diseases (eosinophilia). Hepatitis B testing could help determine if a vaccine course is actually needed (yes, if negative serology) or if further evaluation is indicated (yes, if positive hepatitis B surface antigen) for chronic active hepatitis or for hepatic tumors. HIV serology would be considered for young children who were born to mothers without known medical history, for children who possibly received nonsterile medical intervention or scarification, and for adolescents with sexual contacts. If recent exposure was possible, a repeat HIV serology might be performed 6 months later so as not to miss a child who was seroconverting at the time the first test was done. Syphilis serology could be done if there is concern about an asymptomatic but untreated congenital infection due to unknown maternal condition.

A urinalysis could give a clue to urinary schistosomiasis (hematuria) in an asymptomatic child returning from a long stay in East Africa or another endemic area. Hepatitis C testing is sometimes recommended for foreign-born adoptees (Miller, 1999). Very young infants and some older children who did not have newborn screening testing might benefit from screening for conditions such as hypothyroidism, galactosemia, phenylketonuria, and hemoglobinopathy.

Stool testing for parasites might uncover silent presymptomatic infection, and it might also help prompt early treatment to stop spread to others. For immigrants from areas where specific pathogens are known to be common, presumptive treatment with an agent such as albendazole is recommended (Muennig *et al.*, 1999) For individual returned travelers who spent months around areas of poor hygiene, microscopic testing of stool is advised. Repeating examinations on three different days increases the yield of positive findings. Young children who have been exposed to nontoilet-trained peers could benefit from specific *Giardia* antigen testing, as these parasites are sometimes missed on stool microscopy. Bacterial stool culture is rarely needed in asymptomatic returned travelers.

Screening tests should be done if they are feasible practically and if a positive finding could result in an intervention that would benefit either the child or the child's contacts. Each returned or immigrating traveler comes with specific risks based on their itinerary, age, medical condition, and exposures. Table 23.4, however, gives some general guidelines that might help a travel medicine practitioner decide on screening tests. Further perspectives are also available in the medical literature (Hayani and Pickering, 1991; American Academy of Pediatrics, 1997; Hill, 1998; Miller, 1999).

Caring for Symptomatic Travelers and Immigrants

Children found to have abnormalities on history, physical examination, or initial screening tests should obviously undergo further evaluation and care. The evaluating health care provider should be cognizant of important 'foreign diseases'. The evaluation and care of ill pediatric travelers has recently been reviewed (Fischer *et al.*, 1998).

Fever is a common symptom in children, but the presence of fever in any child who has been in a malaria-endemic area in recent months should prompt emergent consideration of malaria as a cause of fever. As mentioned, malaria is often a delayed diagnosis in a nonen-

Table 23.4 Screening of asymptomatic returned or immigrating travelers

If brief international trip:
No tests

If more than 3 months in a developing country:
Growth parameters
Developmental screening
Psychosocial, scholastic, and cultural adjustment
TB skin test
Complete blood count
Stool microscopy for parasites (also *Giardia* antigen if young)

If cutaneous exposure to fresh water in an area with schistosomiasis:
Urinalysis (for hematuria)
Stool microscopy
Possibly, schistosomal serology

If risky sexual contact or if received medical care, scarification, body piercings of uncertain sterility:
HIV serology
Hepatitis B serology
Hepatitis C serology

If foreign born, less than 6 months of age, and/or uncertain maternal health history:
'Routine' newborn screening (phenylketonuria, hypothyroidism, galactosemia, hemoglobinopathy, perhaps others)
Syphilis serology

demic region (Emanuel *et al.*, 1993; Viani and Blomberg, 1999). Anemia, thrombocytopenia, and hepatosplenomegaly should prompt ongoing concern for malaria even if the initial malaria smear is negative. Tachypnea is an important finding of severe malaria which can predict a poor outcome; this finding should not be overlooked (Marsh *et al.*, 1995). The laboratory evaluation and medical management of malaria is similar in children as in adults. Doses of antimalarials would be adjusted on the basis of body weight, and tetracyclines are used only if necessary for life-threatening infection in children under 8 years old. Fever could also be due to rickettsial disease of typhoid fever.

Diarrhea persisting for more than 2 weeks should also prompt a search for the etiologic agent. A foul odor with nonbloody but greasy-looking stool and excessive flatulence suggests a diagnosis of giardiasis. Bloody stool in a febrile child suggests a bacterial etiology such as shigellosis. Bloody stool in an afebrile child could represent amebiasis.

ORGANIZING THE CARE OF PEDIATRIC TRAVELERS

Many general physicians are neither comfortable nor competent in caring for international travelers. Some travel medicine specialists are not fully at ease in seeing traveling children. How, then, should pediatric travel medicine services be organized?

One academic center in the United States reported on its experience in caring exclusively for pediatric travelers (Walter and Clements, 1998). Children came after referral from other physicians, but their adult traveling companions were required to obtain pretravel care elsewhere.

Another model is to provide 'full service' pretravel care to travelers of all ages. A recent report describes the combined effort of an academic center and a governmental health department (Christenson et al., 2000). At one setting and at the same time, physicians trained in both pediatrics and travel medicine provided counsel to all members of families and groups traveling with children. Individuals traveling without children were scheduled preferentially to see a different travel medicine specialist who did not have particular pediatric expertise.

Usually, travel medicine specialists provide care for travelers of all ages. They must merely be comfortable with their own limitations and know when to seek outside input on specific patients, be they pediatric, immunocompromised, or otherwise unique.

TRAINING THE NEXT GENERATION

International organizations such as the International Society of Travel Medicine and the American Society of Tropical Medicine and Hygiene have taken a lead in the training and certification of travel medicine specialists. Meanwhile, individual travel medicine practitioners are mentoring the next generation of specialists. International experience by trainees is beneficial in shaping future career interests and styles (Gupta et al., 1999), and guidelines for the implementation of useful overseas rotations for pediatric trainees are available (Torjesen et al., 1999).

CONCLUSION

Karl Neumann, a senior authority in the field of pediatric travel medicine, wrote: 'Children make great travelers. They are inquisitive, fun, and when they choose, inexhaustible. Taking children on trips exposes them to new experiences, sows family togetherness, and builds memories for tomorrow' (Neumann, 1995). This is the truth, yet this is also the goal. Caring for children who travel internationally is a great privilege. As we work to prevent and treat travel-related injury and illness, we can help families maximize the benefits of their international experiences. Together, we can help build favorable memories that will live on through the next generation.

REFERENCES

American Academy of Pediatrics (1996) Practice parameter: the management of acute gastroenteritis in young children. *Pediatrics*, **97**, 424–436.

American Academy of Pediatrics (1997) *1997 Red Book: Report of the Committee on Infectious Diseases*, 24th edn, pp 97, 116–120, 441, 562. Elk Grove Village, Illinois.

Arguin PM, Krebs JW, Mandel E et al. (2000) Survey of rabies preexposure and postexposure prophylaxis among missionary personnel stationed outside the United States. *Journal of Travel Medicine*, **7**, 10–14.

Bowie MD, Hill ID and Mann MD (1995) Loperamide for treatment of acute diarrhoea in infants and young children. A double-blind placebo-controlled trial. *South African Medical Journal*, **85**, 885–887.

Buchanan BJ, Hoagland J and Fischer PR (1999) Pseudoephedrine and air travel-associated ear pain in children. *Archives of Pediatric and Adolescent Medicine*, **153**, 466–468.

Caeiro JP, DuPont HL, Albrecht H et al. (1999) Oral rehydration therapy plus loperamide versus loperamide alone in the treatment of traveler's diarrhea. *Clinical Infectious Diseases*, **28**, 1286–1289.

Campagne G, Garba A, Fabre P et al. (2000) Safety and immunogenicity of three doses of a *Neisseria meningitidis* A + C diphtheria conjugate vaccine in infants from Niger. *Pediatric Infectious Disease Journal*, **19**, 144–150.

CDC (1999a) Press release. October 22, 1999. http://www.cdc.gov/nip/news/rotavirus-pr.htm.

CDC (1999b) *Health Information for International Travel 1999–2000*, p. 212. US Department of Health and Human Services, Atlanta.

Christenson JC, Fischer PR, Hale DC et al. (2000) Pediatric travel consultation in an integrated clinic. *Journal of Travel Medicine*, **8**, 1–5.

Csortan E, Jones J, Haan M et al. (1994) Efficacy of pseudoephedrine for the prevention of barotrauma during air travel. *Annals of Emergency Medicine*, **23**, 1324–1327.

Curtis AB, Ridzon R, Vogel R et al. (1999) Extensive transmission of *Mycobacterium tuberculosis* from a child. *New England Journal of Medicine*, **341**, 1491–1495.

D'Alessandro U, Olaleye BO, McGuire W et al. (1995) Mortality and morbidity from malaria in Gambian children after introduction of an impregnated bednet programme. *Lancet*, **345**, 479–483.

De Meer K, Heymans HS and Zijlstra WG (1995) Physical adaptation of children to life at high altitude. *European Journal of Pediatrics*, **154**, 263–272.

Durmowicz AG, Noordeweir E, Nicholas R et al. (1997) Inflammatory processes may predispose children to high-altitude pulmonary edema. *Journal of Pediatrics*, **130**, 838–840.

Edwards DL and Johnson CE (1987) Insect-repellent-induced toxic encephalopathy in a child. *Clinical Pharmacy*, **6**, 496–498.

Emanuel B, Aronson N and Shulman S (1993) Malaria in children in Chicago. *Pediatrics*, **92**, 83–85.

Fischer PR (1998a) Travel with infants and children. *Infectious Disease Clinics of North America*, **12**, 355–368.

Fischer PR (1998b) Summer, travel, and injuries. *Travel Medicine Advisor Update*, **8**, 25–26.

Fischer PR and Christenson JC (1998) Concentrated DEET safe—and sometimes necessary (letter). *Contemporary Pediatrics*, **15**, 25-28-204.

Fischer PR, Christenson JC and Pavia AT (1998) Pediatric problems during and after international travel. In *Travel Medicine Advisor* (ed. F Bia), TC2.9–2.18. American Health Consultants, Atlanta GA.

Fradin MS (1998) Mosquitoes and mosquito repellents: a clinician's guide. *Annals of Internal Medicine*, **128**, 931–940.

Gattuso JM and Kamm MA (1994) Adverse effects of drugs used in the management of constipation and diarrhea. *Drug Safety*, **10**, 47–65.

Gupta AR, Wells CK, Horwitz RI *et al.* (1999) The international health program: the fifteen-year experience with Yale University's internal medicine residency program. *American Journal of Tropical Medicine and Hygiene*, **61**, 1019–1023.

Habluetzel A, Cuzin N, Diallo DA *et al.* (1999) Insecticide-treated curtains reduce the prevalence and intensity of malaria infection in Burkina Faso. *Tropical Medicine and International Health*, **4**, 557–564.

Hayani KC and Pickering LK (1991) Screening of immigrant children for infectious diseases. *Advances in Pediatric Infection Diseases*, **6**, 91–110.

Heick HMC, Shipman RT, Norman MG *et al.* (1980) Reye-like syndrome associated with use of insect repellent in a presumed heterozygote for ornithine carbamoyl transferase deficiency. *Journal of Pediatrics*, **97**, 471–473.

Hill DR (1998) The health of internationally adopted children. *Travel Medicine Advisor Update*, **8**, 17–20.

Hostetter MK (1999) Epidemiology of travel-related morbidity and mortality in children. *Pediatrics in Review*, **20**, 228–233.

Jick S (1997) Ciprofloxacin safety in a pediatric population. *Pediatric Infectious Disease Journal*, **16**, 130–134.

Khan WA, Seas C, Dhar U *et al.* (1997) Treatment of shigellosis: comparison of azithromycin and ciprofloxacin. *Annals of Internal Medicine*, **126**, 697–703.

Khoury GH and Hawes CR (1963) Primary pulmonary hypertension in children living at high altitude. *Journal of Pediatrics*, **62**, 177–185.

Kim HJ, Ghali FE and Tunnessen WW (1997) Here comes the sun. *Contemporary Pediatrics*, **14**, 41–69.

Knirsch CA (1999) Travel medicine and health issues for families traveling with children. *Advances in Pediatric Infectious Diseases*, **14**, 163–189.

Lange WR and Frame JD (1990) High incidence of viral hepatitis among American missionaries in Africa. *American Journal of Tropical Medicine and Hygiene*, **43**, 527–533.

Lell B, Luckner D, Ndjave M *et al.* (1998) Randomized placebo-controlled study of atovaquone plus proguanil for malaria prophylaxis in children. *Lancet*, **351**, 709–713.

Lipscomb JW, Kramer JE and Leikin JB (1992) Seizure following brief exposure to the insect repellent *N,N*-diethyl-*m*-toluamide. *Annals of Emergency Medicine*, **21**, 315–317.

Marsh K, Forster D, Waruiru C *et al.* (1995) Indicators of life-threatening malaria in African children. *New England Journal of Medicine*, **332**, 1399–1404.

Miller LC (1999) Caring for internationally adopted children. *New England Journal of Medicine*, **341**, 1539–1540.

Muennig P, Pallin D, Sell RL *et al.* (1999) The cost effectiveness of strategies for the treatment of intestinal parasites in immigrants. *New England Journal of Medicine*, **340**, 773–779.

Neumann K (1995) Traveling with infants and young children. *Pediatric Basics*, **73**, 12–20.

Osimitz TG and Murphy JV (1997) Neurological effects associated with use of the insect repellent *N,N*-diethyl-*m*-toluamide (DEET). *Clinical Toxicology*, **35**, 435–441.

Paredes P, Campbell-Forrester S, Mathewson JJ *et al.* (2000) Etiology of travelers' diarrhea on a Caribbean Island. *Journal of Travel Medicine*, **7**, 15–18.

Parkins KJ, Poets CF, O'Brien LM *et al.* (1998) Effect of exposure to 15% oxygen on breathing patterns and oxygen saturation in infants: interventional study. *British Medical Journal*, **316**, 887–894.

Peltola H and Gorbach S (1997) Travelers' diarrhea: epidemiology and clinical aspects. In *Textbook of Travel Medicine and Health* (eds HL DuPont and R Steffen), pp 78–86. Decker, Hamilton, Ontario.

Piazza M, Safary A, Vegnente A *et al.* (1999) Safety and immunogenicity of hepatitis A vaccine in infants: a candidate for inclusion in the childhood vaccination programme. *Vaccine*, **17**, 585–588.

Pitzinger B, Steffen R and Tschopp A (1991) Incidence and clinical features of traveler's diarrhea in infants and children. *Pediatric Infectious Disease Journal*, **10**, 719–723.

Reid D and Keystone JS (1997) Health risks abroad: general considerations. In *Textbook of Travel Medicine and Health* (eds HL DuPont and R Steffen), pp 3–9. Decker, Hamilton, Ontario.

Roland EH, Jan JE and Rigg JM (1985) Toxic encephalopathy in a child after brief exposure to insect repellents. *Canadian Medical Association Journal*, **132**, 155–156.

Sagliocca L, Amoroso P, Stroffolini T *et al.* (1999) Efficacy of hepatitis A vaccine in prevention of secondary hepatitis A infection: a randomised trial. *Lancet*, **353**, 1136–1139.

Schaad UB, Salam MA, Aujard Y *et al.* (1995) Use of fluoroquinolones in pediatrics: consensus report of an International Society of Chemotherapy commission. *Pediatric Infectious Disease Journal*, **14**, 1–9.

Sime F, Banchero N, Penaloza D *et al.* (1963) Pulmonary hypertension in children born and living at high altitudes. *American Journal of Cardiology*, **11**, 143–149.

Steffen R, Collard F, Tornieporth N *et al.* (1999) Epidemiology, etiology, and impact of traveler's diarrhea in Jamaica. *Journal of the American Medical Association*, **281**, 811–817.

Sui GJ, Liu YH, Cheng XS *et al.* (1988) Subacute infantile mountain sickness. *Journal of Pathology*, **155**, 161–170.

Theis MK, Honigman B, Yip R *et al.* (1993) Acute mountain sickness in children at 2835 meters. *American Journal of Diseases of Children*, **147**, 143–145.

Thompson RF, Bass DM and Hoffman SL (1999) Travel vaccines. *Infectious Disease Clinics of North America*, **13**, 149–167.

Torjesen K, Mandalakas A, Kahn R *et al.* (1999) International child health electives for pediatric residents. *Archives of Pediatric Adolescent Medicine*, **153**, 1297–1302.

Trach DD, Clemens JD, Ke NT *et al.* (1997) Field trial of a locally produced, killed, oral cholera vaccine in Vietnam. *Lancet*, **349**, 231–235.

Troisi CL, Hollinger FB, Krause DS *et al.* (1997) Immunization of seronegative infants with hepatitis A vaccine (Havrix; SKB): a comparative study of two dosing schedules. *Vaccine*, **15**, 1613–1617.

Viani RM and Bromberg K (1999) Pediatric imported malaria in New York: delayed diagnosis. *Clinical Pediatrics*, **38**, 333–337.

Walter EB and Clements DA (1998) Travel consultation for children in a university-affiliated primary care setting. *Pediatric Infectious Disease Journal*, **17**, 841–843.

Wiedermann G, Kollaritsch H, Kundi M *et al.* (2000) Double-blind, randomized, placebo controlled pilot study evaluating efficacy and reactogenicity of an oral ETEC B-subunit-inactivated whole cell vaccine against travelers' diarrhea. *Journal of Travel Medicine*, **7**, 27–29.

Yaron M, Waldman N, Niermeyer S *et al.* (1998) The diagnosis of acute mountain sickness in preverbal children. *Archives of Pediatric and Adolescent Medicine*, **152**, 683–687.

Zadikoff CM (1979) Toxic encephalopathy associated with use of insect repellent. *Journal of Pediatrics*, **95**, 140–142.

24

Women's Health and Travel

Susan Anderson

Stanford University, Stanford, California, USA

INTRODUCTION

Travel health issues for women will vary according to the life stage and lifestyle of the women. Considerations will differ, depending on whether, for example, a woman is in her second trimester of pregnancy and about to work in a refugee camp, or is an eighty year old grandmother about to go on her first solo journey around the world. Over the last century women have been striving to prove their equality with men in all arenas: professional, intellectual and physical. During the past few years the field of gender-based research has been developing to address the biological and physiological differences between men and women. These differences could be important for risk assessment with regards to disease susceptibility, response to infection, disease manifestations and treatment recommendations in travel medicine. Examples in the field of travel medicine in which gender issues might be important include the susceptibility of the pregnant women to malaria and the effects of female genital schistosomiasis. Thus to adapt the standard pretravel health recommendations to the needs of a woman traveler one needs to consider potential gender- and age-related questions with regards to susceptibility and long term sequelae of parasitic and other infectious diseases, safety of immunizations and medications during pregnancy and adaptation of the medical kit for health concerns specific to the lifestage of the woman.

Until recently, researchers have paid little attention to either sex or gender issues in the field of tropical medicine. If differences were considered at all, the focus was clearly on the effects of the tropical disease on fertility and pregnancy outcome. There are few data on the effects of tropical disease in the elderly. Gender and lifestage issues are important when considering risks for travel and tropical disease, possible complications, available treatment and response to treatment. They are also important when considering preventative measures, including vaccines and chemoprophylaxis. Biological differences between men and women may affect the course of tropical disease, long-term sequelae or response to treatment.

These issues are important to consider when we counsel our women travelers about risks of disease prior to travel. For example, are the immunizations and medications recommended for a specific itinerary contraindicated in pregnancy? Can women on estrogen (oestrogen) replacement therapy trek safely over a 5500 m pass? Do the antimicrobials prescribed for malaria chemoprophylaxis or for self-treatment of travelers' diarrhea interfere with the efficacy of the oral contraceptive pill? What is a woman's risk of schistosomiasis and future infertility if she is a Peace Corps volunteer working on a water conservation project for 2 years in a schistosomiasis endemic country? The definitive answers to these questions are not known. More research is needed.

Gender-related Issues in Tropical Disease

Although there is a growing amount of research in industrialized countries on the interrelationships between gender and health, few studies in developing countries have focused on the gender differences in the biomedical, social or economic impact of tropical diseases much less their impact at the personal level. For this reason the World Health Organization (WHO) section of the Tropical Disease Research (TDR) programme (TDR) formed the Gender and Tropical Disease Task Force to stimulate evaluation of gender determinants and consequences of tropical disease. These include differences in exposure to disease, intensity of infection and morbidity, length of incapacity, care received or given during an illness, access to and utilization of health services and impact of illness on productive and reproductive capacity, social activities and personal life. The focus of the WHO is on women living in endemic countries. We need to consider the possible gender-related effects of tropical disease on women travelers living in endemic areas for extended periods of time and/or female adventure travelers involved in high-risk activities.

Principles and Practice of Travel Medicine. Edited by Jane N. Zuckerman.

Table 24.1　Pretravel checklist for women travelers

- Pretravel consultation for women travelers should take into account the individual lifestage and the lifestyle of a woman:
    Itinerary
    Age
    Immunization history—need for updates
    Reproductive issues
      Menstruation
      Contraceptive need
        Contraceptive choice
      Emergency contraception
      Pregnancy
        Planned
        Unplanned
      Lactation
      Perimenopausal and menopausal issues
    Sexually transmitted disease risk
      Partners: men, women or both
      Preventative measures/treatment
      HIV past exposure prophylaxis
    Medical issues
      Urinary tract
      Vaginitis
      Other significant past medical history
      Long-term travel—need baseline data
        Pap smear
        Mammogram
        Carry copy of electrocardiogram if over 50
    Psychological issues
      Loneliness
      Depression
      Isolation
- Gender-specific recommendations related to disease exposure according to itinerary
- Gender-specific recommendations related to sports/environment
    Altitude
    Scuba
- Cultural issues
- Personal safety
- Travel medicine kit
- Emergency plans
    Carry copy of medical record
    Emergency resources—medical and evacuation insurance
    Web site
    Mobile phone access

- Carry a menstrual cycle diary for long-term travel.
- Menstrual supplies.
    Consider the advantages and disadvantages of tampons, pads, menstrual cups and alternative products.
    Carry wipes and bags to dispose of sanitary supplies.
- Premenstrual syndrome-cramping, bloating.
    Medication for cramping PMS symptoms.
- Change in menstrual pattern.
    Irregular periods.
    No period (amenorrhea).
- Pregnancy risk/testing.

Between the ages of 10 and 50 +, women menstruate on the average of once a month, with a high degree of variability among women. Women travelers should be prepared to experience changes in their cycle and premenstrual symptoms during travel. The changes in time zones, diet, exercise and sleep patterns that occur during travel can affect the woman's hypothalamic-pituitary axis and cause menses to cease and/or become irregular. It is helpful for women on long-term travel to chart their cycles. Guidelines can be given to a woman to advise her what to do if she becomes amenorrheic or has dysfunctional uterine bleeding while traveling (Nelson, 1998). Women of reproductive age who are sexually active with men should carry pregnancy test kits to diagnose a pregnancy if they miss their menstrual period. Women should be advised to bring adequate supplies of feminine hygiene products as familiar brands of tampons and disposable sanitary napkins might not be available at many travel destinations. The issue of how the products will be disposed of should also be considered and appropriate disposal material included in the medical kit. A number of alternative menstrual products are available. One example is a soft reusable rubber cup that is reported to last 10 years. Women may experience the worst premenstrual symptoms of their lives while traveling, even if they have never experienced symptoms before. Medications for self-treatment of these symptoms should be included in the medical kit (see Table 24.16).

PRETRAVEL ASSESSMENT

Where do we start when addressing women's health needs in a travel context? Table 24.1 outlines a pretravel assessment for women travelers.

MENSTRUATION

Advice to the female traveler, and points she should consider related to her menstruation include:

Controlling the Menstrual Cycle

Some women prefer not to have a menstrual period if they are long-distance trekking, bicycling or undertaking similar activities. These women have can have the option of controlling their menstrual cycle by taking oral contraceptives without a pill-free interval. This option could decrease the need for supplies and reduce premenstrual symptoms. Tricycling involves taking 3–4 cycles continuously without the pill-free days. Women should be warned that a small amount of breakthrough bleeding may occur as the endometrium may not remain stable without the physiologic curettage of the pill-free interval. This option is safe (Guillebaud, 2000; Thomas and Ellertson, 2000).

Self-Diagnostic Pregnancy Tests

For women who are sexually active with men it is important to carry pregnancy tests in the travel medicine kit. The urine pregnancy kits are not always available and the reliability of the kits in some countries is not known so it is important for women to take their own. Pregnancy tests have a limited shelf life: the date must be checked to make sure the test has not expired. Environmental extremes might also affect the accuracy of the test so it is important to keep the test kits in a safe place and to check the manufacturer's recommendations regarding storage. As with most self-diagnostic tests, the procedure should be reviewed with the traveler prior to travel.

Urine pregnancy tests are based on the identification of human chorionic gonadotropin (hCG) metabolites in urine, which consist of the 'beta core', a polypeptide fragment of the beta subunit of hCG. Most urine pregnancy tests today are the ELISA-type kits based on highly specific monoclonal antibodies to the beta subunit of hCG. The sensitivity of most urine tests ranges from 5 to $25\,mIU\,ml^{-1}$ of hCG. Thus urine pregnancy tests can be positive as early as 3–4 days after implantation, and are positive by the expected date of the missed period in almost 100% of normal pregnancies. Use of the first morning urine is recommended for all urine pregnancy tests as it contains the highest concentration of hCG and its metabolites. Urine specimens can be tested at other times of the day but if negative, and the suspicion is still high, the test should be repeated in a day or two with a first morning specimen.

Several factors can affect the performance of the urine pregnancy test. A false negative may result if the date of the last menstrual period was judged to be earlier then it was, so the test was performed too early from the date of conception to be positive. The use of too little or too much urine can lead to false-negative results. Women who are color-blind or visually impaired may have trouble reading the test appropriately. Grossly bloody urine may lead to a false negative (unless it is an ELISA test that can be used with either urine or blood). Most pregnancy tests have to be read within a strict time window so it is helpful to have a timer. Some brands have a built-in timer. Most brands have a negative control (Polaneczky and O'Connor, 1999).

Women travelers should be advised to use the urine pregnancy tests when they are concerned because they have missed their period. The kits might also be helpful in the evaluation of the etiology of abdominal pain to help rule out an ectopic pregnancy.

URINARY TRACT ISSUES

Women are prone to urinary tract infections during travel. Infection can be caused by a number of factors, including dehydration, less frequent urination due to a lack of convenient toilets, fewer available facilities for hygiene, and an increase in sexual activity. Women of all ages should be taught the symptoms of a urinary tract infection and how to treat it with oral antibiotics and a urinary analgesic agent (see Table 24.16).

Measures to prevent urinary tract infections include instructions for female travelers to stay well hydrated and to urinate, whether or not the bladder is full, wherever there is convenient access to a public toilet. Some women find the squatting position, necessary to make use of a pit toilet or the outdoors, to be a difficult maneuver. Women should consider attire that would facilitate this stance and add some privacy, such as a loosely cut skirt. A number of plastic and paper funnels have been designed to assist women to urinate in the standing position. This method requires some practice. The funnels are especially useful in extremes of cold weather and altitude when a woman might not want to wear a skirt or pull down her pants.

To maintain hygiene in unexpected places it is important to carry a supply of paper tissues or toilet paper and some packets of premoistened towelettes.

If an older woman has a problem with stress incontinence or bladder control she should consult with a physician specializing in female urinary tract problems prior to her trip. For minor problems women can be taught to do pelvic floor exercises and advised to take a supply of panty liners. Older women may experience vaginal dryness and urinary frequency or urgency without dysuria. Recent data suggest that estrogen vaginal cream, vaginal rings or even an oral contraceptive pill inserted intravaginally may decrease urogenital dryness and frequency symptoms (Nash et al., 1999; Gass and Rebar, 2000; Rioux et al., 2000).

VAGINAL DISCHARGE/ITCHING

Traveling tends to promote a change in a woman's vaginal ecosystem that may result in increased vaginal discharge and/or itching. One of the most common causes of vaginitis is *Candida albicans*. This organism usually causes a thick cottage cheese discharge with vulvar and vaginal itching. The risk of yeast vaginitis is greater when doxycycline is used for malarial prophylaxis or other antibiotics are used for the treatment of travelers' diarrhea, bronchitis or urinary tract infections. Several intravaginal creams and suppositories are available over the counter (see Table 24.16). Due to the messiness of vaginal creams, some women prefer to use an oral treatment such as fluconazole (Diflucan). Other women prefer the creams, as they help with local itching. Both should be included in the travel medicine kit. A mild hydrocortisone cream may also be included for vaginal itching.

Another common cause of vaginitis is bacterial vaginosis. This is caused by overgrowth of the bacteria in the vagina. The discharge is usually more of a grayish color and has a fishy odor. Bacterial vaginosis is treated with metronidazole or clindamycin vaginal cream or tablets.

Women should be taught self-diagnostic skills and given the appropriate treatment to include in her medical kit. Even if a woman has never had a vaginal infection before she should be prepared for this possibility, especially during extended trips. Women should be advised to seek medical evaluation if the symptoms do not improve with self treatment.

If a woman traveler has a new discharge and pelvic pain following a new sexual encounter she may have a sexually transmitted disease and should be evaluated accordingly.

SEXUALLY TRANSMITTED DISEASES

The importance of safe sex practices and a discussion of the risks associated with the range of sexually transmitted diseases pertinent to the destination should be included as part of the pretravel visit (Hawkes and Hart, 1998). Women should be reminded that they are at a higher risk of acquiring a sexually transmitted disease from an infected partner owing to the fluid dynamics of sex. In general, women suffer disproportionately to men from the long-term complications of sexually transmitted diseases. Complications include pelvic inflammatory disease, chronic pelvic pain and infertility.

To prevent acquisition of sexually transmitted diseases women should avoid casual sex and always practice safe sex by using condoms, no matter what other means of contraception are being used simultaneously. High-quality latex condoms are an essential part of a travelers medical kit, regardless of gender and regardless of whether or not sexual activity is planned. A male or female condom made of polyurethane is an effective alternative for persons allergic to latex.

Women should be advised of a list of screening questions to ask a potential partner prior to sexual exposure. Some couples are being screened for the human immunodeficiency virus (HIV) prior to sex and use a negative result to assume there is no risk. There is a window of somewhere between 3 and 6 months in which a person infected with HIV will not test positive with a screening test. The reliability of these tests in some settings of the world is not known. It is best to for a woman either to insist on the use condoms or to refrain from intercourse.

HIV Prophylaxis

Women should be educated about the availability of postexposure HIV prophylaxis for high-risk sexual exposures or sexual assault. If travel is to a remote area, the initial 2 weeks of treatment should be included in the traveler's medical kit. Travelers should check with the Centers for Communicable Disease or similar source for the latest information on postexposure prophylaxis recommendations. Home testing kits for HIV are available in many countries. The sensitivity and sensitivity of these tests is not known and should be reviewed with a reliable source (Pinkerton et al., 1998; Gerberding and Katz, 1999).

CONTRACEPTION

Contraceptive advice is an important area to address. The number of women travelers who experience an unplanned pregnancy as a result of misuse, failure or lack of contraception remains high. Advice to all women travelers of reproductive age should include recommendations on contraceptive use during travel. Guidelines should be discussed, such as what might be the best contraceptive method depending on the style of travel and itinerary, and what should be done in case of emergencies such as contraceptive failure or loss. Emergency contraception options should be reviewed. Travel medicine providers should have access to reference books and Web-based sites on contraception, as this is a rapidly changing field and options around the world vary (Hatcher et al., 1998; Guillebaud, 1999).

Contraceptive advice should also be included in pretravel counseling for men who might put women at risk for pregnancy. This is particularly important in developing countries where their women partners might not have easy access to contraception.

Options

If a woman is already using a contraceptive method, it should be evaluated for ease of use and reliability, together with any special recommendations concerning its use during travel. If a woman wishes to try a new method, she should begin months prior to travel, especially if she is planning to be overseas on a long-term assignment or in a remote area. Back-up methods should be discussed in case she loses her present method; for example, if she is on an oral contraceptive and loses her packages what can she do? The International Planned Parenthood Federation keeps a worldwide guide to contraceptives and a list of family planning clinics. There are a number of websites that might also be helpful (Table 24.2).

Choosing a Method

The advantages and disadvantages of particular methods are reviewed in Table 24.3. Considerations when choosing a contraceptive method should include length of travel, ease of use considering the itinerary and style of travel (backpacking versus luxury hotels), possible environmental effects on the reliability of the method, such as extreme heat, immersion in water, etc., and accessibility.

A woman traveler should be instructed about the basic types of contraception and how they work (Table 24.3). This information will be helpful if she is trying to choose a new method in another country. For a more indepth review the reader is referred to one of the many excellent texts available (Hatcher et al., 1998; Guillebaud, 1999).

Table 24.2   Resources on reproductive options

Resource	Notes
Center for Reproductive Law and Policy http://www.crlp.org/abortion1__icpd.html	Web site provides a list of countries where abortion is legal (and what restrictions are placed on abortion)
Contraceptive Research and Development (CONRAD) Program http://www.conrad.org/general.html	Primary objective is the development of new or improved contraceptives and methods for prevention of the transmission of sexually transmitted infections that are safe, effective, acceptable, and suitable for use in developed and developing countries Links to sites for general contraceptive information
International Planned Parenthood Federation (IPPF) www.ippf.org	Regent's College Inner Circle Regents Park London W1 4NS, UK Tel + 44 0207 487 7900 Fax + 44 0207 487 7950 E-mail info@ippf.org
Marie Stopes International http://www.mariestopes.org.uk/abortion.html	Web site provides country information on the availability of emergency contraception, contraceptive methods and abortion, with help line numbers for advice and services related to family planning and sexual health
Office of Population Research Emergency Contraception http://ec.princeton.edu/worldwide/default.asp	Web site with information on emergency contraception Click on country of destination to see options that are available in the country Click on 'search EC type' to find out in which countries a particular contraceptive is available
PATH (Program for Appropriate Technology in Health) Consortium for Emergency Contraception http://www.path.org/cec.htm http://path.org/	Health information on emergency contraception for providers and patients. Available in many different languages PATH has been designated the WHO collaborating center on research in human reproduction
WHO Gender and Health Technical Paper http://www.who.int/frh-whd/GandH/GHreport/gendertech.htm	Excellent paper on the importance of gender with regards to all aspects of health including tropical disease

Users of Combined Oral Contraceptives

Women should be advised to take adequate supplies of their oral contraceptives with them, as the same formulation may not be available in the country of destination. An empty package should be retained in case the traveler needs help from a local pharmacist to find an alternative. Many low-income countries have higher dose formulations that are effective in preventing pregnancy but may result in a higher incidence of side-effects.

To maintain effectiveness of the oral contraceptive method, women should be reminded about the factors outlined below.

Changes in Time Zone

Many of the low-dose formulations are time sensitive, so forgetting to take a pill because of time zone changes or a change in schedule could result in ovulation. It is advised that a woman carry a special wristwatch alarm, dedicated to oral contraceptive dosing control for every 24 h. This is important for both the low-dose combined and progestin-only pills.

If Pills are Missed

If a woman misses a pill she should take it as soon as she remembers and then take the next one at it its usual time. If she misses two or more pills and has intercourse she should consider emergency contraception measures and/or using a back-up method for the rest of the month.

Pill Absorption

Another issue is problems with pill absorption due to illness. Nausea, vomiting and/or diarrhea may decrease absorption of the pill. If vomiting occurs within 3 h of taking a pill, another should be taken. If a woman experiences nausea and vomiting or diarrhea and cannot keep a replacement down (equivalent to missing a pill) she should use a back-up method for the rest of the month. Elimination of the pill-free interval and starting the next package right away can also be considered if the missed pill was less than 7 days from the end of the package. For continued nausea and vomiting some clinicians recommend inserting the oral contraceptive pill into the vagina for absorption. New contraceptives in the form of vaginal

Table 24.3a Currently available contraceptive choices for travel

Method	Mechanism	Advantages/disadvantages	Travel issues
Barrier			
Spermicides: creams, jellies, foams, melting suppositories, sponges, foaming tablets, films	Surface-active agents that damage the cell membranes of sperm, bacteria and viruses	Chronic exposure may cause mucosal injury that increases risk of HIV transmission	Easy to carry Readily available Bring own supplies Female controlled
Cap	Mechanical barrier Requires spermacide	Needs fitting by clinician Can use for up to 48 h Needs practice to use	Easy to carry Rubber may deteriorate in heat and humidity
Sponge	Polyurethane sponge containing nonoxynol-9 Protects for 24 h no matter how many times intercourse occurs Leave in place for 6 h after intercourse	One size Over the counter Moisten with water prior to use and insert Loop for removal Do not wear longer than 24–30 h due to risk of toxic shock syndrome	Easy to carry, use Use bottled water for moistening in countries with questionable water supply
Diaphragm	Domed-shaped rubber cup Must use with spermacide Protection for 6 h	Requires fitting by clinician Insert extra spermacide with repeated intercourse After use leave in for 6 h	Carry in climate-resistant case Spermacide may not be available in developing countries
Condom			
Female (Reality)	Polyurethane pouch Spermicide not required One use only	Can be inserted 8 h before intercourse	Female controlled Bring supply from home Does not deteriorate in heat and humidity
Male	Latex	Possible allergy Do not use oil-based lubricants	Male controlled Quality varies country to country
	Polyurethane	Thinner/stronger, more resistant to deterioration Can use oil-based lubricants	Bring supply from home of latex and polyurethane types
	Lambskin/natural	Small pores permit passages of viruses-Hep B, HSV, HIV Use only for contraception Brands and materials differ in quality	May break down in heat and humidity. Carry in special case Use emergency contraception if condom breaks or slips and no back-up method in place (OCP/diaphragm/sponge/etc.) Store in cool, dry place
Hormonal			
Pills			
Progestin only	Inhibition of ovulation (may occasionally ovulate) Thickened and suppressed cervical mucus Suppression of midcycle LH and FSH	Use if can not take oestrogen Take same type of pill every day: no pill-free week Decreased menstrual cramps, less bleeding Can use when breast feeding, older women, smokers	Need to be prepared for irregular bleeding *Must* take pill at same time every day—set alarm watch to help with time zone changes Must use additional method for protection against STDs (condoms, etc.)
Combined pill: oestrogen + progesterone	Inhibition of ovulation Many different types Monophasic (fixed dose of hormones in every pill) Triphasic (dosage of hormones in pills varies week to week)	Increased menstrual cycle regularity Less blood loss Less cramping Fewer ectopic pregnancies Less pelvic inflammatory disease Fewer cysts Fewer fibroids Less endometriosis	Convenient, effective, easy to carry Need to take every 24 h Must use additional method to prevent STDs (condoms, etc.) May use to delay menses by starting next packet of active pills following 3 weeks of previous packet

Table 24.3a (*cont.*)

Method	Mechanism	Advantages/disadvantages	Travel issues
Combined pill: oestrogen + progesterone (*cont.*)		If nausea and vomiting, need to take back-up method or consider placing pill in vagina for absorption May use as emergency contraception; check instructions Contraindications: blood clots	Consider drug interactions Bring supply from home Research availability of OCP and/or other method to use if OCP lost or stolen See IPPF guide to hormonal contraception Check Princeton website for availability http://ec.princeton.edu/world wide/default.asp

Depo-Provera	Intramuscular injection (shot) 150 mg dose administered every 3 months
	Blocks luteinizing hormone surge and prevents ovulation
		Side-effects:
		  Weight gain
		  Menstrual irregularities
		  Acne
		  Mood changes
		  Decreased libido
		  Osteoporosis
		  Good for women who cannot take oestrogen
			Compliance issues
			Good if unable to remember OCP
			Good if travel is for < 3 months
			Need injection every 3 months—may be difficult to get if traveling
			Need to be prepared for irregular bleeding

Norplant 1 and Norplant 2	6 or 2 thin permeable silastic capsules which contain the synthetic progestin levonorgestrel	Menstrual irregularities—varies from unpredictable irregular bleeding to no menstrual period Implants difficult to remove, may be broken No protection against STDs Weight gain, acne, alopecia (hair loss) Contraindications: thrombophlebitis (blood clots in the lower extremities), liver disease, liver tumors, breast cancer, pregnancy	Long-term protection 3–5 years May be difficult to remove when traveling Need to be prepared for irregular bleeding, carry pads/tampons/menstrual cups) Amenorrhea (lack of menses) may be positive side-effect, need fewer menstrual supplies

Intrauterine devices
Only two approved for use in USA
Others worldwide
	Inhibition of sperm migration, fertilization and ovum transport
	Creates environment that is spermicidal by provoking a sterile inflammatory reaction which is toxic to sperm and implantation
		Main risk of IUD-induced infection:
		  at insertion
		  more than one partner increases risk of infection
		Medical risks:
		  hx pelvic inflammatory disease (infection in uterine tubes)
		  STD/HIV risk factors
		  Pregnancy
			Good method for women who have already had children, have one sexual partner
			Good for travel as lasts for 1–10 years depending on type of IUD
			Need to use additional method to prevent STDs (condoms, etc.)
			Need to know how to check for string
			Need to know warning signs and what to do in an emergency

Progesterone T Replace every year	T-shaped IUD composed of ethylene/vinyl copolymer; contains titanium dioxide Vertical stem holds 38 mg of progesterone dispensed in silicone fluid	Abnormal bleeding Impaired immunity History of ectopic pregnancy Impaired coagulation (ITP, warfarin) Anemia < 28% Anatomic difficulty (fibroids, other)	Need to know what to do in case of emergency Back-up method if falls out Need to protect against STDs
Copper T 380A Replace every 10 years	T-shaped polyurethane frame holding 380 mg of exposed surface of copper		Good for 10 years Need fewer supplies, etc.

FSH = follicle-stimulating hormone; Hep B = *Hepatitis B virus*; HIV = *Human immunodeficiency virus*; HSV = *Herpes simplex virus*; ITP = idiopathic thrombocytopenic purpura; LH = luteinizing hormone; OCP = oral contraceptive pill; STD = sexually transmitted disease.

Table 24.3b   Methods of contraception currently in clinical trials and/or available in countries other than the USA

Method	Mechanism and use	Travel issues
Barrier		
Lea's Shield (Available in Canada and Europe)	Silicone rubber cap; one size fits all; oval bowl which looks like a loose fitting cervical cap Recommended for use with spermicidal jelly Does not require fitting by clinician Has a loop for easy removal Should be left in place for at least 8 h after intercourse Can be worn for 48 h Replace once a year	Easy to transport Carry in climate-resistant case Rubber may deteriorate in heat
Fem Cap	Silicone rubber sailor hat-shaped cap; intended for use with or without spermicide Two sizes being tested; fitting by clinician required Can be worn up to 48 h Phase III clinical trials involving 800 women at 10 university health centers 5% failure rate	Easy to carry Use Do not need spermacide
Gyneseal (Made in Australia)	Unique two-part chamber designed in Australia as either a menstrual blood collection device (like a tampon) and/or a contraceptive barrier Inner diaphragm-shaped chamber drains through a one-way valve into an outer collection chamber, which clings by suction to the vaginal vault. The inner part seals to the outer part so that blood or secretions do not stay in contact with the cervix and do not leak into the vaginal vault	Could be used during menstrual periods and for contraception Less to carry!
Oves (Made in France)	Shaped like the Prentiff cervical cap Disposable device made of thinner, softer silicone rubber designed for one-time use with spermicide Dow Chemical recently acquired rights to product May be developed as a vehicle to deliver medicines transvaginally rather then as a contraceptive device Vaginal mucosa provides a good adsorptive surface for administering medicines (used by women taking emergency contraception or chemotherapy who experience so much nausea they cannot take their oral medicines; can place pills high in vagina and achieve good systemic levels)	Disposable Need enough for entire trip May also be used to absorb medicine such as an oral contraceptive pill if have nausea and vomiting. Not FDA approved for this use[a]
Protectaid Sponge (Available in Canada)	Soft polyurethane sponge impregnated with a F-5 gel dispersing agent and 3 spermicides Works as a physical barrier Protecting the cervix Chemical action of spermicides Reservoir of gel (continuous release) Absorption of semen, no leakage Leave in for at least 6 h after intercourse Can be kept in for 12 h May have repeated acts of intercourse during that period	Easy to use Easy to carry in individual packets Available without a prescription
Disposable diaphragms	Two diaphragms which release spermicide are being tested in clinical safety trials They may be used up to 24 h with multiple acts of intercourse	Easy to use No spermacide required
Hormonal		
Transdermal patches	Designed to deliver 1 week's worth of hormone; used 3 weeks on 1 week off	Good alternative method if unable to take pills owing to gastrointestinal illness

Table 24.3b (*cont.*) WOMEN'S HEALTH AND TRAVEL 389

Method	Mechanism and use	Travel issues
Intravaginal rings (Tested in 19 centers worldwide. May be produced by the UK)	Doughnut-shaped rings are composed of soft silastic, slightly smaller than a diaphragm and inserted into the upper vaginal vault Presently being evaluated for use with a number of hormone formulations Release progestin alone Levonorgestrel Desogestrel (Dutch firm Organon) Release a combination of a progestin with an oestrogen for absorption across the vaginal wall	Biggest advantage over the other long-acting sustained release methods is the ease with which woman can insert or remove the ring It can be removed for up to 24 h without losing efficacy, so it can be taken out for intercourse Disadvantage Slightly lower efficacy rate that with injectables, implants or medicated IUDs Increased vaginal discharge, irritation, irregular bleeding with progestin-only rings, expulsion; and partner able to feel it during coitus
IUDs Levonorgestrel IUD—LNg IUS	Available in 14 European and Asian countries Delivers 20 μg of levonorgestrel directly on the inner wall of the uterus for 5 years Dosage is equivalent to taking 2–3 minipills per week Unlike copper IUD, which can increase blood loss by 50%, the LNg IUS reduces blood flow by 90% after one year of use Other health benefits include a reduction in fibroids and menstrual pain Manufactured name 'Levonovas' in Scandinavia and 'Mirena' in Europe and Hong Kong	May be option for traveler if she can find a reliable clinic
Frameless IUD	A frameless IUD would eliminate any pressure against the uterus and thus minimize cramping Polyurethane thread anchors the copper-releasing sleeves in the myometrium at the fundus Another version a biodegradable anchor cone allows insertion immediately postpartum	

*Not tested in women travellers in rapidly changing time zones and with hectic schedules.

Table 24.3c Vaccines/immunocontraceptives*

Immunocontraceptives	Status
For women	Most advanced testing is on human chorionic gonadotropin (hCG)-based approaches either the whole molecue or fragments Both approaches are abortifacients; thus even if efficacy, safety and reproducibility could be demonstrated it is unlikely a company will pursue hCG-based vaccines Other antigens that prevent fertilization may be more promising from a political point of view, and include sperm, ovum, zona pellucida antigens
For men	Luteinizing hormone-releasing hormone (LHRH) or follicle-stimulating hormone (FSH) may be used as potential vaccines for men. A vaccine using LHRH linked to a tetanus toxoid shuts down the testes to eliminate testosterone as well as sperm production. To maintain libido and potency one would have to supplement with testosterone In contrast, FSH vaccines have eliminated sperm while maintaining normal testosterone levels in monkeys. Initial studies are underway in India

*Research in progress. Travel health practitioners may, in the future, be able to give contraceptive vaccines.

Table 24.3d 'Computerized' natural family planning[a]

Product	Description	Availability
Persona	Hand-held monitor. Computer reads, stores and analyzes hormonal cycle data from urine tests to give feedback on safe sex times. Becomes more accurate with time as computer gets to know the women's cycle Uses urine test to monitor hormone level	Available from UK $US185.00
Bioself Fertility Indicator	Electronic fertility indicator Identifies both period of maximum fertility (most favorable days for conceiving a child) and the infertile period during which contraception is not possible	$US100.00
Lady Comp	Microcomputer equipped with a thermic sensor which allows the user to measure the body's basal body temperature in the mouth on rising in the morning A sophisticated program takes charge to determine actual fertility of the day based on the measurement of the last 10 years Provides an indication of current fertility, a prognosis for fertility for the next 6 days, a prognosis for impregnation and prognosis of menstruation	Available for $US700.00 from Germany
Baby Comp	Microcomputer similar to above which can be used for contraceptive purposes by assessing least fertile days or for help in conceiving on most fertile days	$US900.00 from Germany
Clear Plan Fertility Monitor	Identifies a woman's fertile days, about 6 per month Allows women to avoid or maximize chance of pregnancy	$US200.00
PFT 1-2-3-KIT	Combines a powerful compact microscope with multicolored slides to distinguish fertile days from nonfertile days Used to pinpoint ovulation, enabling the woman to avoid or achieve pregnancy	

[a]None of these options have been tested in women travelers in rapidly changing time zones and with hectic schedules.

rings and skin patches are presently being evaluated in research trials. These options may be available in the future for women who cannot absorb their pill from the gastrointestinal tract due to illness. Estrogens are actually absorbed better through the vaginal mucosa than through the gastrointestinal tract (Hatcher *et al.*, 1998; Fraser *et al.*, 2000).

Drug Interactions and Oral Contraceptive Efficacy

A common question is whether antibiotics affect oral contraceptive efficacy. Antibiotics have been shown, in animal studies, to kill intestinal bacteria responsible for the deconjugation of oral contraceptive steroids in the colon. Without such deconjugation and subsequent reabsorption, decreased hormone levels result, leading to a decrease in hormone efficacy. Despite numerous case reports of penicillins, tetracyclines, metronidiazole and nitrofurantoin causing contraceptive failure in humans, no large studies have demonstrated that antibiotics, other than rifampicin, lower steroid blood concentrations (Weaver and Glasier, 1999).

To date there are no known interactions between oral contraceptive pills and malaria chemoprophylaxis.

Emergency Contraception

The potential for becoming a pregnant traveler exists for most women of reproductive age. Contraceptive failures are common. Condoms break, diaphragms slip, contraceptive jelly runs out, oral contraceptive pills may be missed due to changes in time zones, or malabsorption of the pill may occur due to vomiting and diarrhea. Emergency contraceptive options should be taught to every woman traveler of reproductive age.

Emergency contraception is defined as a method of contraception that women can use to prevent pregnancy after unprotected intercourse or contraceptive failure (Table 24.4). Emergency contraception should be used in cases of unprotected intercourse, contraceptive failure or sexual assault. It should be included in every woman's medical kit (Table 24.5). For an excellent review on this topic see the articles by Glasier (Glasier, 1997, 1999) and the emergency contraception web site (see Table 24.2).

The emergency contraception options available in most countries include either two doses of estrogen–progestin combination contraceptive pills or two doses of levonorgestrel pills taken 12 h apart. A variety of pills may be used. Women should be taught the generic names of the formulations so they can obtain more if needed.

Table 24.4 Emergency contraception options

Method	Brand names	Advantage	Disadvantage	Availability
Oestrogen–progestin combination pill	See Table 24.5 Schering PC4 (UK) Tetragynon (Switzerland) Preven (USA)	Established safety and efficacy Can continue as regular contraceptive	Nausea (up to 50%) and vomiting (up to 20%) are common side effects 72 h window	Available worldwide Check web site for availability at destination Availability over the counter in many countries
Progestin only 0.75 mg levonorgestrel given 12 h apart	Postinor: available from pharmacists in eastern Europe, Far East and many developing countries NorLevo (France): available from pharmacists Plan B (USA, Canada)	Well tolerated Fewer side-effects compared with combined pill regimen	72 h window	Worldwide
Oestrogen alone Ethinyl estridiol	Netherlands (called 5 × 5)	Failure rate	Nausea and vomiting	Europe
Antiprogestin Mifepristone	RU-486	Highly efficacious and well tolerated; 100% effective in some studies Can be used up to 5 days after unprotected intercourse Inhibits ovulation and prevents implantation	Menses can be delayed	China France USA
IUD Copper		Can be inserted up to 5 days after uprotected intercourse Can continue as long-term contraception Failure rate less than 1%	IUD limitations[a] Requires office visit Needs strict sterile technique, which may not be available in some countries, and thus not recommended due to risk with insertion	Worldwide

[a]Include the following: should not be used in women with history of a pelvic infection, undiagnosed uterine bleeding, or at risk for sexually transmitted disease.

Mifepristone is an antiprogesterone that is considered to be as effective as the combined pill regimen with fewer side-effects. Recent data demonstrate doses as low as 10 mg to be effective (compared to 600 mg for a medical abortion).

A copper-containing intrauterine device (IUD) is also highly effective. Advantages include its high efficacy, 5 day window for insertion, and ongoing contraceptive benefit if it is kept in place. This method is not recommended for women with more than one partner, at risk for sexually transmitted diseases or who have never been pregnant. Access to a health care facility that can safely insert the IUD is also important.

Options available in other countries and how to access them should also be reviewed. Women can obtain information on what options are available in various countries by checking the emergency contraception web site and typing in her country of destination (see Table 24.2). For information in a variety of languages see the Consortium for Emergency Contraception web site (see Table 24.2).

Unplanned Pregnancy

If a traveler becomes pregnant and wishes to terminate the pregnancy it may be best for her to return home, depending on where she is and where she is going. Over half the countries listed by the International Planned Parenthood Federation prohibit abortion except in extreme cases such as rape and life-threatening illness.

Issues of safety and legality for terminating a pregnancy vary. The Center for Reproductive Law and Policy web site provides a list of countries where abortion is legal (and what restrictions are placed on abortion). Women travelers should be advised to obtain advice regarding the options available. The Marie Stopes International web

Table 24.5   Emergency contraceptive methods for the travel medicine kit

Contraceptive pill	No. of pills per dose	Ethinylestradiol per dose μg	Levonorgestrel per dose μg	Instructions for combined pill regimens
Combined				
Preven Kit	2 light blue	100	0.5	Two doses 12 h apart
Ovral	2 white	100	0.5	Within 72 h of unprotected intercourse
Lo-Ovral	4 white	120	0.6	May need antinausea medication
Nordette	4 orange	120	0.6	
Levelen	4 orange	120	0.6	
Levora	4 white			
TriLevelen	4 yellow	120	0.5	
Triphasil	4 yellow	120	0.5	
Trivora	4 pink			
Alesse	5 pink	100	0.5	
Progestin only[a]				
Plan B	1 pill	0	0.75	Two doses 12 h apart within 72 h
Ovrette	20 pills	0	0.75	Two doses 12 h apart within 72 h
Levonorgestrel (Postinor)	1 pill	0	0.75	Two doses 12 h apart within 72 h
Antiprogestins				
RU-486[b]	1 pill			Within 72 h
IUD	Copper			Insert within 5 days

[a]Much lower incidence of nausea and vomiting compared with pill regimen (*Lancet* 1998, **352**: 428–433).
[b]Available in China, Europe and USA.
Women should know what is available in other countries if your medications are stolen or forgotten. They should consult: Emergency Contraception Web site, http://not-2-late.com; US Emergency Contraception Hotline, 1-888-NOT-2-LATE; IPPF *Directory of Hormonal Contraceptives* 1996.

site gives a list of services available in different countries. This web site provides country-specific information on the availability of emergency contraception, contraceptive methods and abortion, along with helpline numbers for advice and services related to family planning and sexual health (see Table 24.2).

RISK OF VENOUS THROMBOSIS

With Oral Contraceptives

Studies have shown a slight increase in the risk of deep vein thrombosis (DVT) for women on oral contraceptives. The absolute risk of venous thromboembolism is small, ranging from 10 to 30 cases per 100 000 women per year in women using oral contraceptives, versus 4 per 100 000 in nonpregnant women not using oral contraceptives. The risk in pregnancy is much greater, estimated to be 60 per 100 000 pregnant women. Women travelers on oral contraceptives should be advised about this small

risk and taught preventative measures such as exercise and hydration. They can also decrease their risk by avoiding smoking, maintaining a normal blood pressure and normal weight. A woman with a personal history of a venous thrombosis should not take oral contraceptives. A common scenario may involve a woman traveler with a strong family history of venous thrombosis who wants to take oral contraception for an expedition to a remote area with no access to medical care. In this case she might be screened for one of the biochemical or genetic defects associated with an increased risk of venous thrombosis to get a better idea of her actual risk; for example, factor V Leiden mutation or protein C, protein S or antithrombin deficiencies have been associated with venous thrombosis (Vandenbroucke *et al.*, 2001).

Some studies have found no difference in risk for venous thrombosis between the low-dose second- and third-generation oral contraceptive pill formulations containing less than 50 μg ethinylestradiol (Farmer *et al.*, 2000). Newer studies on the effects of the second- and third-generation oral contraceptives show a net prothrombic effect. See the article by Vanderbroucke *et al.* (2001) for an excellent review of the recent data and theories describing possible hemostatic mechanisms relating to the risk of venous thrombosis associated with the use of oral contraceptives. These authors also discuss the pros and cons of screening for genetic defects associated with an increased risk of clotting.

For travel to altitude above 4000 m the risk–benefit ratio should be discussed, as should the possibility of using another method. If a woman insists on continuing her pill and she has no known risk factors she should maintain hydration and takes an aspirin a day. Of the thousands of woman students on oral contraceptives seen over a period of 10 years in one advice center, and trekking to over 4000 m, not one case of DVT was seen. A well-designed study to address this issue needs to be undertaken.

With Emergency Contraception

The risk of venous thrombosis during pregnancy is of the order of 60 per 100 000 per year, which is much higher than the risk for routine oral contraception. The risk of DVT with emergency contraceptive use is thought to be insignificant due to the limited time frame (Glasier, 1997; Vasilakis *et al.*, 1999).

With Pregnancy

Risk of DVT is of the order of 60 per 100 000, as stated above. Risk is increased due to hormonal changes affecting hemostatic coagulability factors and due to the pressure of the uterus on the great vessels, decreasing venous return. Exercise and hydration help to decrease risk.

With Estrogen Replacement Therapy

Current use of estrogen replacement therapy has been associated with a 2–3-fold increase in venous thromboembolism but the absolute risk remains low (Daly *et al.*, 1996; Oger and Scarabin, 1999). For women travelers on estrogen replacement therapy going on long airplane flights, aspirin therapy might help decrease this small risk (Grady *et al.*, 2000).

PREGNANCY

Pretravel Evaluation

See Table 24.6.

Risk Factors Related to Past Medical and Obstetric History

The medical and obstetric history of a pregnant traveler

Table 24.6 Checklist for pregnant travelers

Pretravel risk assessment
Stage of gestation
Obstetric risk factors
Medical risk factors
Destination risk considerations
  Due to infectious disease
    Chloroquine-resistant *Plasmodium falciaprium* malaria
    Outbreak of disease requiring a live virus vaccine
    Outbreak of a disease for which no vaccine is available but has a high risk of maternal and fetal morbidity and mortality
      Due to food water exposure
      Due to insect exposure
  Due to environment
    Sports or exercise risk
    Altitude
    Open water
  Lack of access to care

Travel risk assessment
Mode of travel
Medical services available during transit and at destination
Medical insurance and evacuation coverage
Review emergency signs and symptoms for which care should be sought
  Severe vaginal bleeding, abdominal pain, contractions, proteinuria, severe headache with visual change, severe edema and/or accelerated weight gain
  Rupture of membranes

Recommendations
Immunizations to reflect actual risk of disease and probable benefit
Medications–review safety during pregnancy
Preventative measures to decrease:
  Gestation-related risks
  Typical problems
  Mode of travel risks
  Food-related risk
  Water-related risk
  Insect-related risk
  Environment-related risk
  Sexual-behavior risk
Medical kit adaptations
Postpone travel if risks outweigh benefit

should be reviewed carefully, with particular attention to gestational age and evaluation for high-risk categories, as listed in Table 24.7.

Relative Contraindications for Travel during Pregnancy

Travel should be delayed until after delivery in these categories if possible. If travel is unavoidable, preventative measures should be delineated to decrease risk as much as possible, as outlined below.

Pregnant women should carry a copy of their medical

Table 24.7 Relative contraindications for travel during pregnancy

Medical risk factors
Congenital or acquired heart disease (especially valvular disease or congestive heart failure)
History of thromboembolic disease
Medical disease requiring ongoing assessment and medication
Severe anemia
Chronic lung disease, including asthma

Obstetric risk factors
History of miscarriage
Threatened abortion or vaginal bleeding during present pregnancy
Incompetent cervix
Premature labor, premature rupture of membranes, or placental abruption or seperation with prior pregnancy
History of ectopic pregnancy (should be ruled out prior to travel, using ultrasound)
History of or present placental abnormalities
Multiple gestation in present pregnancy
History of toxemia, hypertension, diabetes with any pregnancy
History of infertility or difficulty becoming pregnant
Primigravida over 35 or under 15 years old

Travel to destination that may be hazardous
High altitude
Scuba diving
Areas endemic for, or where epidemics are occurring of, life-threatening food- or insect-borne infections
Areas where chloroquine-resistant *Plasmodium falciparum* is endemic
Areas where live vaccines are required and recommended

Adapted from the CDC Health Information for International Travel 1999–2000.

record with them in case of an emergency and/or to get general advice in transit or at the destination. This should include a recent evaluation by the women's health clinician. The following should be included: gestational age, presence of an intrauterine pregnancy on ultrasound, fetal growth performance, and appropriate medical and obstetric history. Laboratory data should include blood type and Rh factor. Serology for toxoplasmosis, rubella, measles, chickenpox, cytomegalovirus and hepatitis B should also be considered, if not done previously.

What is the Best Time to Travel?

Women can travel during all stages of their pregnancy, but the safest time is during the second trimester (between 18 and 24 weeks) according to the American College of Obstetricians and Gynecologists. During the first trimester there is a risk of spontaneous miscarriage and the theoretical risk from immunizations, needed medications and/or exposure to infectious disease might have a greater effect on the developing fetus. During the third trimester, preterm labor and/or other complications, such

as hypertension, hyperglycemia or thrombophlebitis, are of greater risk. In fact many obstetricians recommend that pregnant women remain within 500 km of home during their last trimester, especially during the last month of the pregnancy.

Options for Emergency Care?

One of the most important considerations for a pregnant woman planning travel should be the availability of care during transit and at the destination. Although there is no one resource that has all the information, there are a number of Web-based and mobile services that are evolving (Table 24.8).

All pregnant women traveling to a less developed country should purchase a travel health insurance policy that provides a worldwide 24 h medical assistance hotline number. This service would provide telephone contact with medical personnel who can help arrange emergency medical consultation and treatment, monitor care and provide emergency evacuation to a more advanced medical facility if necessary. Each policy must be reviewed carefully to make sure that it covers the expenses associated with a normal pregnancy (such as delivery) together with the possible complications of pregnancy, such as a miscarriage early in pregnancy or pre-eclampsia in the third trimester. The policy should also cover expenses associated with care of the neonate. Worldwide Assistance and AEA/SOS insurance policies cover complications of pregnancy through the third trimester (Table 24.8).

Pregnant women should carry a copy of their medical record and their physician's phone number, fax number and e-mail address. This information may be helpful for routine questions, or if there is an emergency, to help the overseas physicians.

All pregnant women should be taught the warning signs of a potentially serious problem: bleeding, passing tissues or clots, abdominal pain or cramps, rupture of membranes, headache or visual changes.

Transportation Risks/Preventative Measures

Air Travel

For a healthy pregnant women and her fetus, commercial air travel should pose no extra risk. Air cabins of most commercial jetliners are pressurized to 5000–8000 feet (1524–2438 m). The fetal circulation and fetal hemoglobin protect the fetus against desaturation during air flight due to the fetal hemoglobin dissociation curve, which allows a greater extraction of oxygen. The arterial blood Po_2 of a healthy person is estimated to be 55 mmHg at 8000 feet (2438 m). This level of oxygen desaturation can lead to complications during pregnancy if the woman has severe anemia ($< 8.5 \, g \, dl^{-1}$), sickle cell disease or trait, or a history of placental problems. In these instances travel should be deferred or supplemental oxygen should be

Table 24.8 Agencies for Medical Assistance Worldwide

Agency	Address	Comments
SOS/AEA International	4050 Columbia Seafirst 701 5th Ave Seattle, WA 98104-7016, USA Phone: 800 468 5232 206 340 6000 Fax: 206 340 6006 8 Neshaminy Interplex Suite 207 Trevose, PA 19053 6956, USA Phone: 800 523 6586 215 245 4707	Medical evacuation, repatriation, medical referral, 24 h medical services Alarm centers located around the world Subscribers have access to services worldwide Global coverage
Credit card and insurance companies, banks		American Express, Bank America
International Association for Medical Assistance to Travelers (IAMAT)	417 Center Street Lewiston, NY 14092, USA Phone: 716 754 4883 40 Regal Road Guelph, Ontario MGE 1B8, Canada	Directory listing of IAMAT centers throughout the world furnishes the names of physicians
Internet/WWW OBGYN.net	www.obgyn.net/country Europe, South America, USA	Country-specific information on associations, hospitals, research, medical schools, culture and much more Made possible through the efforts of OBGYN.net international representatives
Local US, Canadian or British embassy or consulate	Respective countries	Provide names of physicians in the area
Local medical school or university		For English-speaking physicians
SAFEtrip	PO Box 5375 Timonium, MD 21093, USA Phone: 800 537 2029 410 453 6300 Fax: 410 453 6301 E-mail: medexasst@aol.com	Offered by MEDEX Assistance Corporation Provides emergency assistance, close monitoring of treatment, evacuation, and others
MedicinePlanet	2310 Mason Street 3rd floor San Francisco, CA 94133, USA Phone: 415 362 1444 www.medicineplanet.com	Mobile health resource for travelers, offering valuable information and services before, during and after a trip Developing section focusing on issues pertinent to woman travelers Mobile health offerings, such as the Medicine Translator and regional health news and alerts, provide travelers with access to needed health care tools and services

Adapted from Samuel BU and Barry M (1998) The pregnant traveler. *Infectious Disease Clinics of North America*, **12**, 325–354.

ordered in advance (Bia, 1992).

Pregnancy predisposes pregnant travelers to a risk of superficial and deep vein thrombosis due to alterations in clotting factors and the pressure of the expanding uterus. Preventative measures should include frequent stretching, walking up and down the aisle and isometric leg exercises. An aisle seat would facilitate this activity. Dehydration is a risk for passengers due to the low humidity on pressurized flights (Bia, 1992). Women should be encouraged to drink nonalcoholic beverages to maintain hydration and placental blood flow.

Most airlines have regulations that prevent travel by pregnant women beyond 32–36 weeks of gestation. It is important to check with the airline ahead of time. Pregnant women should always carry a letter from their physician documenting their gestational status and due date.

The radiation exposure associated with a long flight from London to Tokyo has been estimated to be the equivalent of one chest radiograph. For the infrequent flyer this is not of much concern. For pregnant travelers who are aircrew or business frequent flyers this may be a consideration and should be discussed with their physician. Airport security machines are magnetometers and are not harmful to the fetus.

Motor Vehicle Travel

Motor vehicle accidents resulting in blunt trauma are a common cause of maternal and fetal morbidity and mortality in pregnant women. Complications are obviously increased when the women is ejected from the vehicle. Unfortunately, lap belts have been associated with placental and fetal injury. A diagonal shoulder strap with a lap belt provides the best protection, with the straps carefully placed above and below the 'abdominal bulge' to distribute the impact energy over the anterior chest and pelvis. Safety restraints do not exist in most automobiles in many parts of the world. Pregnant women on an extended automobile or bus ride should take frequent exercise breaks and walk for at least 10 min every 2 h to prevent venous stasis and risk of thromoboembolism.

Sea Voyages

The main health risk associated with sea voyages is the exacerbation of the nausea and vomiting associated with pregnancy. Lack of access to medical care in case of an emergency is another issue, especially on sailboats operated by smaller tour companies or in self-designed tours. On the larger cruise carriers pregnant women are allowed to travel until the seventh month. Medical facilities aboard are usually quite well equipped but this should be assessed in advance of travel.

Gestation-related Changes in Immune Status

Data suggest that pregnancy results in a number of changes in the maternal immune system, although research on the immune response during pregnancy is continually evolving. The evidence from a number of studies suggests that there is a reduction in cell-mediated immunity during pregnancy. There is evidence to support this hypothesis. Pregnancy has been found to result in increased susceptibility and/or a predisposition to more severe disease in a number of infections in which the cell-mediated immune response is the most important. Examples of this type include malaria, amebiasis, coccidiomycosis, leishmaniasis, leprosy, listeriosis and tuberculosis (Pedler, 2000). Thus, when the itinerary is being reviewed, risk for these infections should be determined.

By contrast, infections in which the humoral response is the most important show no increase in susceptibility to infection. B-cell numbers and functions do not appear to be reduced during pregnancy.

Immunizations

Ideally all women have had their immunizations updated prior to pregnancy. In fact there has been a recent emphasis on encouraging maternal immunization to protect the newborn against certain childhood diseases (Munoz and Englund, 2000). Advice to pregnant women regarding recommended immunizations should balance the theoretical risk of the immunization against the potential for maternal and fetal illness. The basic questions are:

- What is the real incidence of the vaccine-preventable disease along the pregnant traveler's itinerary?
- What is the real risk to the pregnant traveler or her fetus of acquiring the disease?
- What would be the risk of treatment of the particular disease during pregnancy or fetal development (if there is a treatment)?
- What is the known effectiveness of the vaccine in preventing the disease?
- What is the theoretical risk of the vaccine to the mother or the fetus?

Are Vaccines Safe for the Pregnant Woman and her Fetus?

Vaccines based on inactive viruses, inactivated bacterial toxins (toxoids), inactivated bacteria or bacterial components are thought to be of low risk for the pregnant woman and her fetus (Fischer et al., 1997).

Live attenuated viral vaccines and live bacterial vaccines are not generally recommended to pregnant women due to a theoretical concern secondary to the 'live' components. In general, pregnant women should avoid live vaccines, and women generally should avoid becoming pregnant within 3 months of having received a live vaccine. However, limited data from registries of live vaccines given inadvertently to pregnant women suggest that many of these vaccines may be safe in pregnancy. Until more data are available, live vaccines should be used during pregnancy only if the risk of exposure to a vaccine-preventable disease outweighs a possible theoretical risk of the vaccine (Munoz and Englund, 2000). Ideally it is best to avoid any form of immunization during the first trimester of pregnancy.

Table 24.9 summarizes the latest data. All vaccines are listed as category C under the FDA pregnancy categories (Briggs et al., 1998; Anonymous, 2000a).

FDA has developed a set of guidelines to categorize drugs, vaccines and toxoids with regard to developmental toxicity and adverse fetal outcome. The assessments are based on the degree to which available information has ruled out a risk to the fetus, balanced against the potential benefits to the pregnant women (Table 24.10). Most medications in the US Physicians Desk Reference fall under the FDA category C. Few double-blind studies have been carried out in pregnant women to categorize drugs. Clinicians who want more information can obtain it from teratogen reference systems available around the world (see Additional Resources).

High fevers occurring during the first trimester have been associated with neural tube defects; such fevers may be vaccination-induced. Vaccinations which might cause a febrile response are not recommended during pregnancy.

Live Vaccines or Live Attenuated Vaccines

Measles/Mumps/Rubella (MMR) and Measles

Immunity to measles is essential for all travelers. Many young adults require immunization (or reimmunization) for protection. The specific recommendations for the age groups vary depending on the traveler's country of origin and epidemiology of measles in that country. The measles vaccine as well as the MMR (measles, mumps, rubella combination) are live vaccines and contraindicated in pregnancy. Due to the increased incidence of measles in children in developing countries, its communicability, and its potential for causing serious consequences in pregnancy, some health providers would advise delaying travel of a nonimmune woman until after delivery, when the vaccine can be given. If a documented exposure to measles occurs, immune globulin may be given within a 6 day period to a pregnant woman to prevent disease. It is important to remember that the immune globulin may not be available in many high-risk countries.

Rubella

The Centers for Disease Control and Prevention (CDC) established a registry for women who received the rubella vaccine within 3 months before or after conception. Pregnancy outcomes collected from 1979 to 1998 have not shown any fetal abnormalities or congenital rubella syndrome. Guidelines still state that reasonable precautions should be used to prevent administration during pregnancy. However, inadvertent administration of the rubella vaccine is not considered a reason to terminate the pregnancy because, in cases where rubella vaccine has been accidentally given, no complications have been reported.

Routine prenatal screening for rubella immunity should be emphasized. The vaccine should be administered to susceptible women who are not pregnant.

Varicella

The vaccine manufacturer, in collaboration with the CDC, has established the Varivax Pregnancy Registry to monitor maternal and fetal outcomes of women who are inadvertently immunized with varicella vaccine 3 months or less before pregnancy or anytime during pregnancy (Centers for Disease Control and Prevention, 1996). The registry, which contains data from more than 300 deliveries, indicates no defects compatible with congenital varicella syndrome. However, the small number of pregnancies followed up to date gives low power to detect a rare effect, and the serologic status of the majority of the women was unknown, but the majority were likely to be immune. A 12-month-old infant who developed approximately 30 vesicular lesions after receiving the currently licensed varicella vaccine transmitted vaccine virus to his previously healthy mother, who was 5–6 weeks pregnant. After an elective abortion, polymerase chain reaction testing of fetal tissue did not reveal the virus. Varicella zoster immune globulin should also be given to a nonimmune woman with exposure to varicella within 96 hours of exposure.

Poliomyelitis

It is important for all pregnant women to be protected against polio. Paralytic disease may occur with greater frequency when infection develops during pregnancy. Anoxic fetal damage has been reported, with up to 50% mortality in neonatal infection. If not previously immunized, a pregnant women should have at least two doses of the vaccine prior to travel (day 0 and 1 month). Despite being a live vaccine, the oral polio vaccine is recommended by some experts when immediate protection is needed. The recommendation is for one dose prior to travel, followed by completion postdelivery.

Mass immunization programs, prompted by polio virus epidemics in Finland and Israel, which included thousands of pregnant women failed to show any association between maternal immunization with oral polio vaccine and congenital malformations or adverse perinatal outcomes (Anonymous, 1994). For pregnant women traveling to endemic areas, it is recommended that the inactivated poliovirus (eIPV) be used for routine boosting. If a pregnant woman needs immediate protection for a high-risk area, oral polio vaccine should be used.

Tetanus and Diphtheria

To maintain immunity against diphtheria and tetanus a booster dose of tetanus–diphtheria vaccine (Td for adult use) should be given every 10 years. Women traveling to areas where they may deliver under unhygienic circumstances or surroundings should update their immunity to prevent neonatal tetanus. The WHO, the Advisory Committee on Immunization Practices (ACIP) and the American College of Obstetricians and Gynecologists all endorse tetanus toxoid administration during pregnancy. Immunization of pregnant women with tetanus toxoid at least 6 weeks before delivery effectively provides protection of newborns against neonatal tetanus by stimulating the production of specific IgG antibodies that cross the placenta, while also protecting these women against puerperal tetanus. Maternal immunization with tetanus toxoid is practiced worldwide and has resulted in dramatic decreases in the incidence of neonatal tetanus in many regions, with no evidence of adverse effects to mother or fetus (Munoz and Englund, 2000).

Nonimmunized or incompletely immunized pregnant women should receive one or two properly spaced doses of Td (for adult use) preferably in the last two trimesters. Pregnant women traveling to areas endemic for diphtheria should also be vaccinated. Contraindications to a booster immunization would include a history of a high

Table 24.9   Immunizations during pregnancy

Immunobiologic agent	Type of vaccine	Issues in pregnancy
Measles Mumps Rubella	Live attenuated	Contraindicated Pregnancy should be delayed for 3 months after MMR is given Check titer if immunity unknown May give immune globulin if exposure
Polio	Trivalent live attenuated (OPV)	Avoid in previously nonimmune individuals due to risk of vaccine-associated paralysis ACIP recommends use in outbreak situation
	Killed (eIPV)	Preferred over OPV in pregnancy
Varicella	Live attenuated	Contraindicated in pregnancy Check titer if exposed during pregnancy Give varicella zoster immune globulin if nonimmune If symptoms treat with Aciclovir i.v. or orally
Tetanus–diphtheria	Combined toxoid	Safe in pregnancy Use if lack of primary series or no booster within 10 years
Influenza	Inactivated vaccine	Women in their second or third trimester during influenza season
Pneumococcus	Polysaccharide	Vaccine used only in high-risk pregnancies Postsplenectomy

Meningococcal vaccine
  A,C,Y and W-135
  A, C
B research trials
	Polysaccharide	Administer for high-risk exposure

Haemophilus B conjugate	Polysaccharide	For high-risk persons
Typhoid	Heat/phenol-inactivated, parental	Avoid in pregnancy due to systemic reaction and febrile response
Typhoid (Ty21a)	Live attenuated bacterial, oral	No data in pregnancy Use should reflect acutal risk of disease Avoid in pregnancy on theoretical grounds
Typhoid	V1 capsular polysaccharide, parental	No data in pregnancy Use only if clearly indicated
Hepatitis A	Formalin-inactivated vaccine	Category C drug Use only if clearly indicated Check titer
Hepatitis B	Recombinant, purifed hepatitis B surface antigen	Not contraindicated Pre-exposure and postexposure prophylaxis indicated in pregnant women at risk for infection
Cholera vaccines	Inactivated injectable Oral live Oral killed	Not recommended in pregnancy Practice strict food and water precautions Avoid areas with cholera epidemics Maintain hydation
Yellow fever	Live attenuated	Contraindicated except if exposure unavoidable
Japanese encephalitis (JE)	Killed vaccine	Should reflect actual risk of disease and probable benefit of vaccine JE virus infection acquired during first or second trimester of pregnancy may result in uterine infection and fetal mortality

Table 24.9   *(cont.)*

Immunobiologic agent	Type of vaccine	Issues in pregnancy
Tick-borne encephalitis	Inactivated	Not recommended during pregnancy Practice strict tick-bite precautions
Lyme vaccine	Recombinant outer surface protein A (OspA) vaccine	Not recommended during pregnancy Practice strict avoidance techniques If high-risk exposure treat with antibiotics
Rabies	Killed virus Human dipoid cell rabies vaccine (HDCV) or rabies vaccine adsorbed (RVA)	Pregnancy is not a contraindication for postexposure prophylaxis Pre-exposure prophylaxis only when substanial risk for exposure exists
Immune globulins (IG) Pooled or hyperimmune	Immune globulins or specific antitoxic serum including antivenum for snake bite, spider bite, diphtheria antitoxin, HBIg, rabies Ig, tetanus Ig, RH *(D) Ig, varicella zoster Ig	Give if indicated

Adapted from CDC Information for International Travel 1999–2000 and Samuel BU and Barry M (1998) The pregnant traveller. *Infectious Disease Clinics of North America*, **12**, 325–354.

Table 24.10   FDA use-in-pregnancy categories

FDA Category/Rating	Description
A	Adequate and well-controlled studies in women show no risk to the fetus
B	No evidence of risk in humans. Either studies in animals show risk, but human findings do not, or, in the absence of human studies, animal findings are negative
C	Risk cannot be ruled out. No adequate and well-controlled studies in humans, or animal studies are either positive for fetal risk or lacking as well. Drugs should be given only if the potential benefit justifies the potential risk to the fetus
D	There is positive evidence of human fetal risk. Nevertheless, potential benefits may outweigh the potential risks
X	Contraindicated in pregnancy. Studies in animals or humans or investigational or postmarketing reports have shown fetal risk that far outweighs any potential benefit to the patient

fever (over 39.4 °C) or an Arthrus-type sensitivity reaction, due to concern about the effect of a febrile reaction on the neurological system of a developing fetus.

Influenza

Pregnant women and infants are vulnerable to increased morbidity from influenza virus infection. The risk increases in the third trimester of pregnancy in the presence of other underlying conditions. Inactivated influenza virus vaccine is recommended by the CDC for all pregnant women who will be in the second or third trimester of pregnancy during an influenza season and for those with underlying risk factors, regardless of their stage of pregnancy, such as women with any immunosuppressive disease or pulmonary problems. Maternal immunization with inactivated influenza virus vaccine is considered safe at any stage of pregnancy (Anonymous, 2000c).

Bacterial Polysaccharide Vaccines

In general, polysaccharide vaccines have been given to pregnant women without adverse effects.

Pneumococcal Infection

Vaccine should be given to all pregnant women who would otherwise qualify for special protection against these diseases, such as pregnant women with chronic diseases or pulmonary problems. Another reason to consider is maternal immunization to protect infants under 3 years old who are at risk for severe pnemoncoccal disease.

Meningoccal Meningitis

The bacterial polysaccharide polyvalent meningococcal vaccine may be administered during pregnancy if the woman is entering an area where the disease is epidemic or during an outbreak. The commonly available meningococcal vaccine in the United States is a tetravalent vaccine from groups A, C, Y and W135. In a number of other countries only bivalent vaccine from group A and C is commonly used.

The safety of the vaccine in pregnancy has not been conclusively demonstrated, although a small study published in 1980 showed no birth defects in infants whose mothers were vaccinated during an epidemic in Brazil.

Haemophilus influenzae *Type b*

Haemophilus influenzae type b is an important cause of meningitis and pneumonia in infants in areas of the world where the vaccine is not available. For women traveling to endemic areas to live, the *Haemophilus influenzae* type b (Hib) vaccine could be considered. This vaccine has been a model for the protection of infants from bacterial disease through maternal immunization (Glezen and Alpers, 1999).

In the 1980s Hib capsular polysaccharide vaccines given to women in the third trimester of pregnancy were shown to result in the transmission of vaccine-specific antibodies to the infant serum and maternal breast milk.

Newer conjugate vaccines (Hib-PRP covalently linked to a carrier protein) have been shown to induce the production of IgG_1 antibodies, which are more efficiently transmitted transplacentally than IgG_2 and resulted in a higher level of total protective antibody than the polysaccharide vaccines. Thus maternal immunization with Hib conjugate vaccines should be considered in pregnant women travelers planning to live in endemic areas.

Typhoid

There are three vaccines available for prevention of typhoid; the intramuscularly administered V1 capsular polysaccharide typhoid vaccine (ViCPS, Typhim Vi) is recommended in high-risk exposure. Because it is a polysaccharide vaccine it is less likely to cause a febrile reaction. It is classified as FDA category C and should only be used if clearly indicated. The live oral typhoid vaccine (enteric-coated, lyophilized, Ty21a strain of *Salmonella typhi*) is not recommended during pregnancy as it is a live vaccine. The old subcutaneously administered heat/phenol-activated typhoid vaccine should not be used as it causes a febrile reaction and a sore arm.

Hepatitis A

Pregnant women without immunity to hepatitis A need protection prior to traveling to developing countries. The risk for nonimmune travelers is 3–6/1000 per month. Rates as high as 20/1000 are seen in overland travelers living and eating under poor hygienic conditions. Hepatitis is no more severe during pregnancy then at other times and does not affect the outcome of the pregnancy. There have been reports of acute fulminant disease in pregnant women during the third trimester, when there is also an increased risk of premature labor and fetal death. These events did occur in women from developing countries and may have been related to underlying malnutrition. The hepatitis A virus is rarely transmitted to the fetus but transfer can occur during delivery. Immune globulin is a safe and effective means of preventing hepatitis A but immunization with one of the new hepatitis vaccines gives a more complete and prolonged protection. The effect of the new killed vaccines on fetal development is unknown but the production methods for the vaccines is the same as eIPV, which is considered safe in pregnancy. Thus hepatitis A should be administered to pregnant women when indicated.

Hepatitis B

The hepatitis B vaccine may be administered during pregnancy. Hepatitis B virus infection is a risk for short-term and long-term travelers who may be exposed to blood or body fluids. The risk is increased for travel to Asia, sub-Saharan Africa, the Amazon basin and parts of the Middle East. The main risk factors for a pregnant woman include working in a health care setting, being sexually active with a new partner, planning delivery overseas, or planning extended travel.

Ideally, all pregnant women should be screened for hepatitis B carriage. If a woman is positive for hepatitis B surface antigen (HBsAg) her infant should be given hepatitis immune globulin and hepatitis B vaccine at birth. The hepatitis B vaccine can be administered to pregnant women. It is preferred that it is given after the first trimester (for theoretical reasons) to all women who are at high risk and test negative by serology for past infection.

Immunization for hepatitis B will also prevent hepatitis D infection.

Hepatitis C

Hepatitis C infection is on the rise. Travel-associated risks include exposure to blood that has not been screened, sexual transmission, tattooing and occupational exposures of volunteer health care workers or missionaries to blood products or contaminated needles used for administration of medications or intravenous drug use. There is no evidence that pregnancy alters the natural history of hepatitis C or that it interferes with normal pregnancy, unless the woman already has cirrhosis and its associated complications (Reinus and Leikin, 1999). Vertical transmission is uncommon. Pregnant travelers should be advised of at-risk behaviors to decrease risk of infection. Immune globulin is not thought to be effective postexposure.

Hepatitis E

A new hepatitis E virus (HEV) vaccine is in clinical trials

in Nepal (Shlim and Innis, 2000). HEV is a major cause of hepatitis in Nepal, India, Burma, Pakistan and China, the former Soviet Union and Africa (Ooi, Gawoski et al., 1999). Transmission of the virus occurs through fecal–oral exposure. HEV acquired during pregnancy has a particularly high case fatality rate (15–30%). HEV infection is most common in persons of childbearing age (15–40 years). Clinical illness can range from mild to severe. In the non-pregnant, fulminant disease occurs in less than 1%. In pregnant women the disease may be fulminant in 20–30%. The overall fatality rate for non-pregnant patients is 0.5–4.0%. During pregnancy the fatality rate increases from 1.5% during the first trimester, to 8.5% during the second trimester and 21% during the third trimester (Reinus and Leikin, 1999). The reasons why the infection is more severe in pregnancy are not known. HEV infection acquired during the third trimester is also associated with fetal complications. Fetal mortality is much more common than with the other forms of hepatitis. Most outbreaks occur due to fecal contamination of drinking water.

Prevention of hepatitis E is dependent on strict food and water precautions. Drinking only boiled water and avoidance of local beverages, unpeeled fruit and uncooked vegetables and ice is effective. Administration of HEV-immune serum globulin to persons at risk did not affect disease rates. Pregnant women should not travel to areas where there are known outbreaks of HEV.

Yellow Fever

Yellow fever is increasing worldwide so appropriate immunization is important (Anonymous, 1999). Severe yellow fever has a case fatality rate of between 20 and 50% (Monath, 1999; Tomori, 1999; Anonymous 2000b). Yellow fever vaccine should not be given to a pregnant woman unless travel to an endemic or epidemic area is unavoidable. If travel to a high-risk area cannot be avoided, the benefits of the vaccine far outweigh the small theoretical risk to the fetus (Robert et al., 1999).

The first systemic epidemiological study of yellow fever vaccination in pregnancy found no evidence of congenital infection in 40 exposed infants in Nigeria. The yellow fever vaccine (17d) was given to 101 pregnant women during a yellow fever outbreak in Nigeria. No untoward effects on the mother or infant were noted (Nasidi et al., 1993). Antibody responses of pregnant women and mothers who were vaccinated mainly during the last trimester were much lower than those of yellow fever-vaccinated nonpregnant women in a comparable group. A recent study of women inadvertently immunized during pregnancy found neonates who appeared well but had yellow fever virus-specific IgM antibody, indicating a vaccine-related congenital exposure (Tsai et al., 1993). A small study has found a slight increase in spontaneous abortions during the first trimester but other studies have not (Cobelens, 1998). It is better to give the vaccine during the second or third trimester if possible.

For pregnant women who are traveling or transiting regions within a country where the disease is *not* a current threat but where policy requires a yellow fever certificate, a physician waiver should be carried along with documentation on the immunization record. In general, travel to areas where yellow fever is a risk should be postponed until after delivery, when the vaccine can be administered without concern of fetal toxicity.

A nursing mother traveling to a yellow fever endemic area should also delay travel as a neonate cannot be immunized because of the risk of vaccine-associated encephalitis. Breastfeeding is not a contraindication to the vaccine for the mother.

Japanese Encephalitis

Japanese encephalitis vaccine is an inactivated vaccine but is reactogenic, especially in atopic individuals. To determine whether a pregnant traveler should receive the vaccine, the risk of exposure and infection versus the risk of the vaccine to the fetus or the mother must be weighed carefully. Risk factors for the disease would include the particular location and duration of intended stay, housing conditions, nature of activities, and the possibility of travel to high-risk areas. The safety of this vaccine in pregnancy has not been established and it should only be given after weighing the risks and benefits.

Tick-borne Encephalitis

Tick-borne encephalitis is a virus transmitted by a tick in endemic areas. A number of vaccines are available (Demicheli et al., 2000). Inactivated tick-borne encephalitis vaccine is highly immunogenic and reactive in most studies. There have been no studies in, and it is not recommended for, pregnant women. Strict tick-bite precautions are recommended for women hiking or traveling through an endemic area.

Lyme Disease

Lyme disease is a potentially serious infection that is caused by the spirochete *Borrelia burgdorferi* and transmitted by the bite of infected *Ixodes* ticks. The infection is endemic in certain areas of North America, Europe and Asia. There was a concern about the possiblility of fetal infection and teratogenicity from Lyme disease contracted during pregnancy because of the similarities of disease caused by *B. burgdorferi* to syphilis. Although initial case reports were alarming, more recent prospective data have been reassuring. A study of 2000 pregnant women in Weschester, New York, was carried out to determine if prenatal exposure to Lyme disease was associated with an increased risk of adverse pregnancy outcome. The results demonstrated that Lyme disease was not associated with fetal death, decreased birth weight, or length of gestation at delivery. Tick bites or Lyme disease around the time of conception was not associated with congenital malformations. Maternal exposure to Lyme disease before conception or during pregnancy was not associated with fetal death, prematurity, or congenital malformations. The possibility that exposure to Lyme disease increases the risk of specific malformations or has an effect if a pregnant women's infection is not treated is not known. This study overall supports the benign nature of this infection with respect to the fetus and the pregnant woman (Strobino *et al.*, 1993).

Lyme disease vaccine (LYMErix) is an adjuvanted formulation of the outer surface protein A (OspA) of the causative spirochete. It is effective against the Lyme disease spread by ticks in the USA only. It acts by inducing high titres of anti-OspA antibodies (anti-OspA), which must be present in vaccinated individuals before exposure to *B. burgdorferi* to provide protection against Lyme disease. Efficacy against Lyme disease was 80% for definite and asymptomatic cases and 76% for definite cases at year 2 using the recommended dosage.

This is an example of a vaccine-preventable disease with a vaccine that is only moderately efficacious at 80%. As studies have shown that Lyme disease is not associated with fetal death, prematurity or fetal malformation if treated, the vaccine is not recommended for pregnant women. Preventive measures should be emphasized, such as avoiding heavily wooded areas in endemic areas, wearing protective clothing, and having 'body checks' for ticks to promote early removal and less likelihood of transmission.

Rabies

Pregnancy is not a contraindication for postexposure prophylaxis. Pre-exposure prophylaxis with rabies vaccine should be given if there is substantial risk of exposure.

Use of Medications

All physicians advising pregnant women should have ready access to a reference such as *Drugs in Pregnancy and Lactation* (Briggs *et al.*, 1998), which includes reviews of the reproductive literature relevant to drugs and immunizations. Each medication is categorized by the risk classifications outlined by the FDA. It is difficult to state categorically that any medication used before or during pregnancy is completely safe. As most medications have not been tested in pregnant women, they are classified as category C. For up-to-date information one can consult the teratogen web sites (see Additional Resources).

There are other classification systems (for example in Sweden, Australia, Netherlands, Switzerland and Denmark) that are based on a hierarchy of estimated fetal risk.

General Principles

The following questions should be considered before prescribing a medication to a pregnant woman:

- How does pregnancy affect the pharmacokinetics of the medication?
- Are the side-effects of the medication more severe or more common than in the nonpregnant woman?
- What is the potential risk to the developing fetus?

There are a number of physiological changes during pregnancy that might affect the pharmacokinetics of a particular medication. The volume of distribution of drugs is increased during pregnancy owing to an increase in maternal weight and plasma volume. The result is less drug due to a reduced maternal serum concentration. Drugs that are excreted mainly by the kidney may be influenced by increased renal blood flow and glomerular filtration. The increase in progesterone during pregnancy may lead to an induction of liver metabolism of some medications. A change in gastrointestinal motility may lead to variable and reduced absorption of orally administered agents. Any of these factors could lead to a reduction in the maternal serum level of the drug and failure of the clinical response. The actual clinical significance of these changes is not known.

Most drug transfer across the placenta occurs by simple diffusion. Drugs with low molecular weight, high lipid solubility and low protein binding are most readily transferred. Drug transfer increases with gestation due to reduced thickness of the placenta. To minimize risk to the fetus, doses at the lower end of the therapeutic range should be prescribed.

The typical problems of pregnant travelers are the same as those experienced at home. Appropriate self-management tools should be discussed to address issues such as morning sickness, heartburn, indigestion, constipation, hemorrhoids, frequent urination and leg cramps.

Other medications for treating urinary tract infection, vaginitis, diarrhea and malaria should be reviewed for safety during pregnancy.

Malaria and Pregnancy

Malaria affects between 300 and 500 million people a year, resulting in over 3 million deaths. Morbidity and mortality are the greatest in children and pregnant women and travelers. There is increasing incidence of chloroquine-resistant strains of *Plasmodium faciparum* (CRPF) and *P. vivax* worldwide. A greater effort needs to be made to reach pregnant women who may be returning to a malaria endemic area to see family and friends.

What is the incidence of malaria in pregnant travelers? Preliminary data from the CDC surveillance program during 1997–1999 demonstrates that 3810 cases of malaria were reported to the CDC; of these, 2313 were men, 1279 were women and the sex was not known in 218 people. Sixty-three of the women were reported to be pregnant; 25 of the women were US residents; 36 were foreign residents; others of unknown status (M. Parise, 2000, personal communication).

These data suggest that the highest risk of malaria in pregnant travelers is in those women returning to an endemic area to see their family(18/25 US residents). Travel medicine practitioners should promote chemophylaxis in this high-risk group. Most cases of malaria were acquired in Africa and most cases were falciparum plasmodium. According to the data collected most of the pregnant travelers did not take, or took inappropriate, prophylaxis for the area of destination (20/25 US residents); 47 of the women were hospitalized. Complications during treatment included adult respiratory distress syndrome, renal failure and anemia. None of the cases was fatal.

Malaria acquired during pregnancy has severe consequences. If a woman is pregnant or plans to become pregnant and cannot defer travel to a high-risk area, appropriate chemoprophylaxis is essential. Pregnancy is associated with an increased susceptibility to malaria both during pregnancy and during the postpartum period (Diagne *et al.*, 2000). Pregnancy increases susceptibility and clinical severity of falciparum malaria in women both with and without existing immunity, i.e. women living in and traveling to endemic areas. A pregnant traveler visiting an endemic area is at significant risk for malaria infection and its devastating consequences for her and her fetus.

Most of the studies on malaria occurring during pregnancy have been done on pregnant women living in endemic areas. These studies have demonstrated that women living in such areas have an increased susceptibility to *P. falciparum* infection during pregnancy when compared with local women who are not pregnant. The increase in susceptibility appears to be more during the first pregnancy and to diminish, in some studies, with subsequent pregnancies. For individuals living in endemic areas protective immunity is acquired during childhood. The increased susceptibility to malaria for women during pregnancy has been thought to be due to sequestration of the parasites in the placenta and suppression of selected components of the immune system, associated with the increased production of several hormones and other proteins (Fried and Duffy, 1996; Diagne *et al.*, 1997; Duffy and Fried, 1999; Nahlen, 2000).

Plasmodium vivax *Infection*

Plasmodium vivax is more common than *P. falciparum* as a cause of malaria in many parts of the tropics outside Africa. Most of the studies done on malaria in pregnancy have concentrated on *P. falciparum* infection. The effects of *P. vivax* have not been as well characterized. A study investigated the effects of *P. vivax* infection during pregnancy on women living in camps for displaced people on the western border of Thailand (Nosten *et al.*, 1999a). The women were screened for malaria and anemia each week

of pregnancy until delivery, and pregnancy outcome was recorded. The effect of *P. vivax* infection on anemia and pregnancy outcome were compared with the effect of either *P. falciparum* or the effect of no evidence of malaria infection during the pregnancy. *P. vivax* malaria was not associated with miscarriage, stillbirth or with a shortened duration of pregnancy but it was associated with maternal anemia and low birthweight. The effects of *P. vivax* infection are less striking than those of *P. falciparum* infection but antimalarial prophylaxis against *P. vivax* in pregnancy is still justified (Nathwani *et al.*, 1992; Nosten *et al.*, 1999).

For nonimmune pregnant travelers the risk of contacting any type of malaria during any pregnancy is significant. Maternal malaria is a major cause of pregnancy-related complications, including premature delivery, intrauterine growth retardation and perinatal mortality in the infant and anemia and maternal mortality for the mother. Contraction of malaria by a nonimmune pregnant traveler greatly increases the risk of losing the fetus.

Theories of Pathogenesis of the Malaria Parasite During Pregnancy

Why are women more at risk for malaria during pregnancy? In endemic areas women have, with time, acquired immunity to *P. falciparum* equivalent to their male counterparts. It has been found, however, that pregnant women have a unique susceptibility to malaria, especially with their first pregnancy. This susceptibility to malaria has been found to decrease as the number of pregnancies increases. One theory for an increased risk of malaria during pregnancy has been thought to be due to the immunosuppression of pregnancy necessary to inhibit maternal–fetal placental unit rejection. This is believed to lead to a number of increased infections during pregnancy, including malaria. The fact that this susceptibility is markedly lower in gravid women than it is in primigravid women in endemic countries suggests that immunosuppression cannot entirely explain the phenomenon.

The placenta is a preferential site for sequestration of red blood cells and may have a high density of multiplying parasites, while the peripheral circulation is free of parasites. Thus the peripheral blood smear may be negative, making the diagnosis of malaria difficult. The parasites sequestered in the placenta might be the source of an overwhelming maternal malarial infection if not treated in time. The placental infection leads to fetal growth retardation and may lead to intrauterine fetal death (Matteelli *et al.*, 1997; Steketee *et al.*, 1996).

Guidelines for Prevention

As no antimalarial agent is 100% effective, it is of crucial importance that pregnant women use personal protective measures to avoid and/or minimize mosquito bites when traveling through a malaria endemic area.

A recent study demonstrated that pregnant women might be more attractive to mosquitoes and therefore more at risk for malaria, as well as other mosquito-borne infections such as dengue and yellow fever (Lindsay *et al.*, 2000). The mechanisms underlying an increased attractiveness to mosquitoes during pregnancy are likely to be related to at least two physiological factors. First, women in the advanced stages of pregnancy were found to produce 21% more exhaled breath than their nonpregnant counterparts. There are several hundred different components in human breath, some of which are likely to be used by mosquitoes for detecting a host. At close range, body warmth, moist convection currents, host odors and visual stimuli allow the insect to locate its target. During pregnancy, blood flow to the skin increases, which helps heat dissipation, particularly in the hands and feet. Thus, the second reason for increased attractiveness may be that these hotter pregnant women increase the release of volatile substances from the skin surface and produce a larger host signature that allows mosquitoes to detect them more readily at close range. Not only do pregnant women appear to be physiologically more attractive to mosquitoes, but changes in their behavior can also increase exposure to night-biting mosquitoes. In comparison with the nonpregnant, pregnant women are likely to leave the protection of their bed net at night to urinate twice as frequently. This study demonstrates that pregnant women are at increased risk of malaria, and perhaps other mosquito-borne diseases, and underlines the importance of protecting this vulnerable group against biting by vectors. Pregnant women should be encouraged to use a combination of preventative measures including: permethrin-treated clothing, topical insect repellents and bed nets.

Topical insect repellents—DEET. *N,N*, diethyl-*m*-tolumide (DEET)-containing preparations have been used by millions of people worldwide for 40 years. DEET has a remarkable safety profile. Studies of high doses of DEET administered orally to mice and rats did not reveal any potential in humans for teratogenicity or oncogenicity. Because the reproductive effects of DEET in laboratory animals are conflicting and there are no human data, DEET is currently classified as category B. It has been shown to cross the placental barrier in some studies and not in others; thus pregnant women should avoid the use of highly concentrated DEET-containing repellents. Lower concentrations of DEET, from less than 10% to 35%, may be used sparingly (Fradin, 1998). There is also a new slow-release formula (microcapsule) of DEET that may be safer for use in pregnancy.

Non-DEET topical insect repellents. The safety and efficacy of non-DEET preparations has not been established and cannot be relied upon to prevent malaria in highly endemic areas. For example, one of the brands recommended by the lay press as effective and safe in pregnancy has been shown to be neither safe nor effective; it may be a weak mosquito repellent for 15 min and thus is clearly not indicated for malarial endemic areas.

Chemoprophylaxis

A list of the available antimalarials and their uses and contraindications during pregnancy can be found in Table 24.11. Any medication taken during pregnancy carries some risk. In order to truly evaluate a medication during pregnancy large-scale studies involving hundreds of thousands of pregnant women would have to be undertaken. This has not been done.

Most travel health advisors recommend that pregnant women do not travel to areas where cholorquine-resistant faliciparum malaria occurs because of the potential risk of acquiring the disease and the possible effects from treatment or chemoprophylaxis. This is particularly important in areas of confirmed mefloquine resistance, such as the Thai–Burmese border. However, sometimes a woman *must* travel to an endemic area and it is important for the travel medicine advisor to help a woman appreciate the risk of such a decision and what she can do to decrease that risk if travel is unavoidable. A clinician involved with advising pregnant women will have to consult up-to-date web sites and research centers for the most current data.

Chloroquine-sensitive **P.falciparum** *Malaria*

Although chloroquine crosses the placenta, it has been found to be safe in pregnancy both for chemoprophylaxis and in therapeutic doses for established malaria. Pregnant women have used chloroquine for decades without any documented increase in birth defects. Thus travel by a pregnant woman to an area where chloroquine can be used for prophylaxis can be considered relatively safe. This includes endemic areas in Central America, the Caribbean and the Middle East. In these areas, chloroquine remains the drug of choice. It should be given as the 300 mg base equivalent (equal to 500 mg of chloroquine base salt), starting 1 week prior to travel in an endemic area, continuing weekly while traveling in an endemic area and for 4 weeks after.

P. vivax *and* P. ovale *Malaria*

It is usually recommended that the nonpregnant traveler take a drug called primaquine phosphate for causal prophylaxis to prevent relapse of malaria caused by the liver stage of *P. vivax* or *P. ovale*. However, it is important that primaquine is not given to a pregnant traveler owing to the possibility of a life-threatening hemolytic anemia in the fetus if the fetus is glucose-6-phosphate dehydrogenase (G6PD) deficient. Instead, weekly chloroquine or other appropriate antimalarial agent should be continued until delivery to prevent a febrile episode caused

Table 24.11 Malaria chemoprophylaxis in pregnant travelers

Antimalarials	Dose	Comments
Chloroquine-sensitive areas		
Chloroquine	300 mg base (equal to 500 mg of phosphate salt per week)	Safe Reactions rare
Cholorquine-resistant areas		
Mefloquine	250 mg weekly Start 1 week before travel and continue for 4 weeks after travel to malarious zone	Neuropsychiatric reactions 1 : 15 000–20 000 Safety in first trimester not fully established although CDC approved Possible trend in stillbirths noted in some studies
Atovaquone–proguanil (Malarone)	Atovaquone 500 mg + proguanil 200 mg, or Atovaquone 250 mg + proguanil 100 mg 1 tablet daily for 1–2 days before travel and for 1 week after leaving malarious area	Recommended for individuals who can not take mefloquine Safety of atovaquone in pregnancy *not* established It is not known whether atovaquone is excreted into human milk Proguanil is excreted into human milk in small quantities Based on experience with other antimalarial drugs, the quantity of drug transferred in breast milk is insufficient to provide adequate protection against malaria for the infant Because data are not yet available on safety and efficacy, Malarone should not be given to a woman who breast feeds an infant who weighs less than 11 kg unless the potential benefit to the woman outweighs the potential risk to the child (for example, for a lactating woman who had acquired *P. falciparum* malaria in an area of multidrug resistance who could not tolerate other treatment options)
Proguanil and chloroquine	Proguanil 200 mg per day Chloroquine 300 mg base per week	Anecdotally safe in pregnancy Only 70% effective Folate supplements recommended Limited use due to increasing drug resistence
Pyrimethamine–dapsone (Maloprim)	Pyrimethamine 12.5 mg and dapsone 100 mg, 1 tablet once a week	Pyrimethamine should be avoided in the first trimester Folinic acid supplement needed Side-effects of dapsone include dose-related hemolytic anemia, more severe in G6PD-deficient individuals, methemoglobinemia, agranulocytosis 1 : 20 000 Restricted use only Not FDA approved
Pyrimethamine–sulfadoxine (Fansidar)	Pyrimethamine 25 mg + sulfadoxine 500 mg, 1 tablet once a week	Severe cutaneous reactions 1 : 5000 to 1 : 10 000 Generally *not* recommended
Azithromycin (Zithromax)	250 mg daily	More data needed Effectiveness only 70–80% Not recommended

Adapted from Samuel BU and Barry M (1998) The pregnant traveler. *Infectious Disesase Clinics of North America*, **12**, 325–354.

by symptomatic malaria. After delivery the mother should be tested for G6PD deficiency and given primiquine if she is not G6PD deficient.

Multidrug-resistant Falciparum Malaria

Travel to an area with multidrug-resistant falciparum malaria by pregnant women should be avoided if possible. If travel is unavoidable or if a woman plans to conceive while on an extended stay in a malaria endemic area, the woman should be advised of the risks involved, with emphasis on the importance of preventative measures, and educated about the symptoms of malaria and the need to treat promptly.

The choice of regimen will need to balance the efficacy with the most current knowledge of safety during pregnancy.

Mefloquine. The CDC, WHO and other national expert groups have expanded their indications for mefloquine to include pregnant women in their second and third trimesters (Phillips-Howard *et al.*, 1998; Schlagenhauf, 1999). Mefloquine is not recommended during the first trimester, nor is conception recommended for 2 months after the last dose unless there is high-risk exposure. There have been numerous reported cases of inadvertent use in pregnancy in which there was no increase in congenital malformations. In fact, mefloquine use at any stage of pregnancy is not an indication for an abortion. Large scales studies need to be performed.

Melfloquine use is being monitored by a registry at the CDC. A few studies have suggested a slight increase in the number of stillbirths in the mefloquine group (Nosten *et al.*, 1999b). Another study on the use of mefloquine by the armed forces in Somalia also indicated an increase in spontaneous abortion (Smoak *et al.*, 1997). These studies are small and it is difficult to eliminate other variables, such as nutrition and extreme stress, that may be related to the slight increase in stillbirths. There are also studies demonstrating that pregnant women given mefloquine in their first trimester, followed by weekly prophylaxis, did not experience any significant untoward effects (Na Bangchang *et al.*, 1994; Phillips-Howard *et al.*, 1998).

A more rapid clearance of mefloquine late in pregnancy may necessitate an increase in the dose when the drug is used for prophylaxis. More studies need to be carried out to confirm this effect and to assess whether there would be a toxicity associated with a higher dose.

There are limited data to suggest that late pregnancy is associated with accelerated clearance of mefloquine when the drug is used prophylactically, necessitating an increase in the dose (Nosten *et al.*, 1990) described above. Lactation is not an absolute contraindication to mefloquine use, although low concentrations (3–4%) are excreted in breast milk with a 250 mg dose. Breast milk should not, however, be construed as having enough concentration of mefloquine to protect a newborn.

Other issues with mefloquine relate to its long half-life.

For women of reproductive age it is recommended that they do not become pregnant while taking the drug and for 3 months afterwards.

Alternatives to mefloquine include the following.

Atovaquone with proguanil (Malarone). Malarone has been available in Europe and Canada. It was approved in the USA in 2000. It is listed as FDA pregnancy category C. Data from research trials suggest that atovaquone was not teratogenic and did not cause reproductive toxicity in rats at maternal plasma concentrations up to 5–6.5 times the estimated human exposure during treatment of malaria. The combination of atovaquone and proguanil hydrochloride was not teratogenic in rats at plasma concentrations up to 1.7 times for atovaquone and 0.10 times for proguanil, the estimated human exposure during treatment of malaria. In rabbits, the combination of atovaquone and proguanil hydrochloride was not teratogenic or embryotoxic to rabbit fetuses at plasma concentrations up to 0.34 and 0.82 times, respectively, the estimated human exposure during treatment of malaria.

While there are no adequate and well-controlled studies of atovaquone and/or proguanil hydrochloride in pregnant women, Malarone may be used if the potential benefit justifies the potential risk to the fetus. The proguanil component of malarone acts by inhibiting the parasitic dihydrofolate reductase. To date there are no clinical data indicating that folate supplementation diminishes drug efficacy. Women of childbearing age receiving folate supplements to prevent neural tube birth defects may continue to take these supplements while taking Malarone. In clinical trials, there was only one subject who became pregnant while taking Malarone. She delivered a healthy term infant.

WHO is sponsoring two safety, efficacy and pharmacokinetic studies of Malarone in the treatment of women with symptomatic malaria in the third trimester of pregnancy. One study will be in Thailand, the other in Zambia. These studies will provide important data on which to base further recommendations.

Chloroquine with proguanil. Another option in some areas of the world is a combination of weekly choloquine and the biguanine proguanil daily. Proguanil appears to be safe in pregnancy, however studies are limited. The main concern is that resistance to biguanides and cholorquine is increasing in Southeast Asia, Thailand, Papua New Guinea, parts of Africa, and South America. The other concern is that this combination is less effective than mefloquine: it is estimated to be only 80–85% as effective.

Pyrimethamine with sulfadoxine (Fansidar). Pyrimethamine with sulfadoxine (Fansidar) has been recommended by WHO as a prophylactic and for treatment of malaria at any stage of pregnancy. It is also recommended for stand-by treatment until the traveler can get help. Concerns about this drug in pregnancy were the teratogenic effects of pyrimethamine in rats, preventable by folate supplementation, and hyperbilirubinemia and kericterus in the newborn state due to sulfadoxine near term. Folinic acid should be given and/or continued by the pregnant women to prevent folic acid depletion.

Fansidar is a fixed drug combination consisting of pyrimethamine 25 mg and sulfadoxine 300 mg. In 1984 a series of severe cutaneous reactions were reported to the CDC following the use of Fansidar, thus limiting its use in the USA. *P. falciparum* resistance to Fansidar is developing in areas of South America, Thailand, Myanmar, Cambodia and parts of sub-Saharan Africa, limiting its use. It is not recommended as a first-line agent for chemoprophylaxis or treatment.

Pyrithamine and dapsone (Maloprim).

Another combination drug consists of pyrimethamine in a fixed dose combination with dapsone and is marketed as Maloprim. Pyrimethamine should be avoided in the first trimester owing to concerns about teratogenicity. Dapsone has been established as safe during pregnancy in leprosy patients. The FDA has not approved this drug but it may be considered for use as a back-up method for travelers to high-risk areas.

Amodiaquine.

Amodiaquine (related to chloroquine) is considered safe for chemoprophylaxis in pregnant women; however, concerns about agranulocytosis and increasing drug resistance preclude its use for chemosuppression.

Quinine and Quinidine.

The cinchona alkaloids quinine and quinidine can be used as a life-saving measure in pregnant women severely infected with malaria. These drugs belong to the FDA category X. Stillbirths, congenital malformations, including auditory nerve hypoplasia and limb abnormalities, have been described. Neonatal thrombocytpenia and hemolytic anemia in G6PD-deficient newborns have been described with quinine. These quinine derivatives should be used for life-threatening illness in a pregnant women but they are not recommended for prophylaxis.

Areas of confirmed mefloquine resistance such as Thai–Burma and Thai–Cambodia borders.

Doxycycline is the drug of choice, but is contraindicated in pregnancy. Travel to the Thai–Burma or Thai–Cambodia areas with multidrug resistant strains of *P. falciparum* should be strongly discouraged for the pregnant woman as she will have no good option for chemoprophylaxis. If travel is unavoidable, the combination of sulfisoxasole and proguanil can be considered for prophylaxis in the second and third trimesters; however, the effectiveness of this drug combination is much less than that of doxycycline.

Artemisinin (qinghaosu) and its derivatives (artmether, arteether, artesunate) belong to the first generation endoperoxide class of antimalarials with a novel mode of action. They are potent blood schizotocides that rapidly reduce the parasitemia and the clinical symptoms. These drugs are not good for prophylaxis due to their short half-life. They have been used in the second and third trimester of pregnancy for treatment of severe malaria.

The new combination chemoprophylaxis option of proguanil and atovaquone (Malarone) seems to be as effective as mefloquine and may be of potential use in pregnant travelers. Atovaquone is categorized as a category C drug. Its safety and efficacy in pregnant women has not been established.

Treatment

Any pregnant traveler with a fever who has traveled from an endemic area should be treated as an emergency. No chemotherapeutic agent is 100% effective: pregnant travelers must be advised about the symptoms of malaria so that immediate presumptive treatment can be given, even on return. Pregnant travelers should also be given stand-by treatment to use if they become ill while they are in transit or away from health care resources. As the field of malaria treatment is rapidly changing, the travel health advisor and the pregnant women should contact one of the malaria centers to check for up-to-date recommendations for treatment of malaria acquired at a particular destination (CDC, WHO, London School of Tropical Medicine, etc.).

Fever is a prominent feature of malaria in a nonimmune pregnant traveler. Any fever, especially within the first 3 months after return from a malarious area, should prompt quick evaluation of a blood smear.

Travel to a chloroquine-sensitive area.

Treatment for travel to a choloquine-sensitive area is chloroquine. For severely ill pregnant travelers with life-threatening infections, intravenous quinine or quinidine gluconate is the drug of choice. Hypoglycemia must watched for and prevented. In areas of pyrimethamine/sulfadoxine-sensitive malaria this combination is an option for pregnant women if they are not allergic to either component. Although not first line, mefloquine may be given in doses of 750–1250 mg as single dose for treatment. Malarone may also be used for treatment.

Patients who develop malaria while on mefloquine.

Treatment must be individualized according to the travel itinerary, the drug sensitivity pattern of the malarial parasite in the areas visited by the patient and the balance of the adverse effects of several combination antimalarial drugs.

The combination of atovaquone (1000 mg) and proguanil (400 mg) once a day for 3–7 days achieves consistently high cure rates in adult patients with *P. falciparum* infection. Although there are no adequate controlled studies to date using atovaqone in pregnant women, this combination is an option for multidrug resistant *P. falciparum* infection.

Stand-by treatment is the use of antimalarials for self-administration when fever or 'flu-like symptoms occur and prompt medical attention is not available. It has been considered for pregnant travelers but is generally not recommended because inappropriate use can expose the mother and child to significant drug toxicity. Factors determining the choice of a suitable stand-by treatment include the level of malaria transmission, the degree and nature of drug resistance, the efficacy and toxicity profile of agents used and the ease of administration.

The appropriate use of stand-by treatment for malaria by travelers depends on their knowledge of malaria, attitudes and awareness. This is an ideal area for the development of better educational tools, guidelines and self-diagnostic kits. As the self-diagnostic tests become more reliable they will aid in this process.

Summary

Malaria during pregnancy can lead to serious morbidity and mortality for the infant and the mother. The decision to travel to a malaria endemic area while pregnant should be weighed carefully by each woman and her clinician. If she must travel to a high-risk area, the pregnant traveler should be prepared with adequate preventative measures, chemoprophylaxis, stand-by treatments and an emergency plan for evacuation or treatment at a local hospital. Each pregnant woman should weigh carefully how she might feel if she acquired a severe case of malaria which resulted in a poor fetal outcome that could have been prevented.

Travel-related Diarrheal Illness

The main concern with travelers' diarrhea during pregnancy is the prevention of dehydration, which can lead to decreased placental blood flow, premature labor and shock. Pregnant women may be at greater risk of contracting diarrhea owing to decreased gastric acidity and increased transit time of food through the intestine. Treatment for fluid loss should be started promptly. For travel to rural areas, pregnant travelers should carry oral rehydration packets.

Chemoprophylaxis for mild travelers' diarrhea is not recommended for pregnant travelers. To control frequency of bowel movements, loperamide or diphenoxylate are two antimotility drugs (category B) that may be used with severe diarrhea. Antibiotics commonly used to treat diarrhea, such as ciprofloxacin and tetracycline, are contraindicated in pregnancy; however, for severe diarrhea a few days of a quinolone antibiotic should be considered. Quniolones are category C drugs: adverse effects have been seen in animals but not in humans. A limited dose would be unlikely to affect the fetus. Although many enteric pathogens are resistant to ampicillin/amoxicillin, they may be tried in pregnant woman who are not allergic to penicillin. Erythromycin and azithromycin are safe to take during pregnancy and are especially effective in treating *Campylobacter*-induced

travelers' diarrhea. Second- or third-generation cephalosporins have also been suggested as alternatives.

Several medications commonly used to treat travelers' diarrhea have limitations to use during pregnancy. Ciprofloxacin, trimethoprim-sulfamethoxazole (except during the second trimester), doxycycline and tetracycline are contraindicated, although the short courses (1–3 days) recommended for treatment of travelers' diarrhea are not likely to cause problems. Actually, there are no known problems with ciprofloxacin, but there are inadequate data to evaluate the risk. Ampicillin can be used for travelers' diarrhea, although resistance is becoming widespread. Erythromycin is safe but does not have the best spectrum of action for enteric pathogens. Loperamide is safe. Metronidazole may be taken if there is a strong indication. Paromomycin can be used for amebiasis. If possible, treat giardiasis after delivery; if necessary, treat with paromomycin or furazolidone. Pregnant travelers with persistant diarrhea post-travel may need an extensive evaluation to determine the etiologic agent before therapy is instituted.

The best recommendation for a pregnant traveler is to maintain strict food and water precautions and adequate hydration to maintain placental blood flow. If the diarrhea is severe and incapacitating, alternative measures could include an antiperistaltic agent plus one of the antibiotics suggested for use during pregnancy. Iodine for water disinfection is safe for short-term use up to a few weeks, but prolonged use (months) could contribute to neonatal goiter. Better options are chlorination or filters containing three elements: microfiltration, iodine resin and activated charcoal.

GENDER-RELATED ISSUES IN TROPICAL DISEASE

Gender-related issues in tropical medicine have not been addressed on a large scale until recently. WHO has formed the Gender Task Force of the WHO Tropical Disease Research Programme (TDR), which is evaluating the gender-related biological, behavioral and cultural factors that might affect the epidemiology, diagnosis, treatment and/or outcome of a particular tropical disease (Vlassoff, 1997).

Parasitic Infection

Parasitic infections are common throughout the world but until recently differences between effects on women and men have not been studied. Due to the increase in international travel and the immigration of people from tropical areas to more developed countries, physicians are likely to see an increase in tropical disease with both common and uncommon presentations.

Pretravel advice for women should include a risk assessment as to potential exposure to parasitic disease. Knowledge about how a particular disease might affect

Table 24.12 Potential effects of parasitic infection on reproduction

Parasites	Impaired fertility	Failure to carry to term	Fetal infection
Protozoans			
Entamoeba histolytica	×	×	
Giardia lamblia	x	×	
Leishmania spp	×	×	×
Plasmodium spp	×	×	×
Trypanosoma spp	×	×	×
Toxoplasma gondii		×	×
Pneumocystis carinii		×	×
Intestinal nematodes			
Ascaris lumbricoides	×	×	×
Enterobius vermicularis (pinworm)	×		
Trichuris trichiura (whipworm) Hookworm	×	×	×
Extraintestinal nematodes			
Strongyloides stercoralis	×	×	
Trichinella spiralis	×	×	×
Filaria spp	×	×	×
Trematodes			
Schistosoma spp	×	×	
Clonhorchis sinensis	×	×	
Paragonimus westermani		×	
Cestodes			
Echinococcus spp	×	×	
Taenia spp	×	×	

Adapted from Lee RV (1988) *Medical Complications During Pregnancy* (eds GN Burrow and TF Ferris). WB Saunders, Philadelphia; and Manuel, Elaine C. Jong and Mcmullen Russel (eds) (1995) *Travel and Tropical Medicine*, p. 156. WB Saunders, Philadelphia.

her long-term fertility or pregnancy outcome might make a difference to a traveler's compliance with preventative measures or bring about a change in itinerary so as to avoid the risk of exposure (Table 24.12).

After travel, women should be asked about travel history if they have recurrent gynecological symptoms or are in the process of an infertility workup or breast-mass evaluation. Parasitic worms such as *Ascaris* spp. and *Enterobius vermicularis* have been found on Pap smear results. Amebiasis can result in ulcerating lesions and unusual vaginal disharge in some cases (Hammill, 1989). Breast masses are not always malignant: they can be parasitic in a woman with the appropriate travel history (Sloan *et al.*, 1996; Perez *et al.*, 1997).

Parasitic infection as the only or concomitant cause of infertility in Caucasian women is rare to date; however, with the burgeoning increase in travel for work and play, parasitic causes of infertility will increase. Parasitic infections may be found in unusual places if there is an index of suspicion. An interesting case of microfilariae in follicular fluid was recently described in a case report (Goverde *et al.*, 1996). The case involved an infertile woman undergoing *in vitro* fertilization. Her infertiliy was presumed to be due to *Chlamydia trachomatis* but moving microfilariae of *Mansonella perstans* were found in the aspirated follicular fluid during the *in vitro* fertilization procedure. The woman was also found to have schistosomal infection. Although the authors do not believe a case similar to this has been reported, it is probably because microfilariae and other parasites have not been looked for routinely in the female genital tract.

Thus, physicians evaluating women immigrants or world travelers for infertility and other gynecologic problems should consider parasitic infections in the differential diagnosis (Balasch *et al.*, 1995). Clinicians evaluating pregnant women should also review past travel history during their prenatal visit owing to the risk of an accelerated course of some tropical diseases during pregnancy and/or congenital transmission.

Parasitic diseases in women may have effects on fertility, during pregnancy and throughout the life stages as a result of a variety of mechanisms (Stray-Pedersen, 2000).

The infecting parasite may cause anatomic or functional changes in the genital tract so that conception or implantation does not occur, owing to scarring and inflammation of the fallopian tubes or infiltration of the uterine lining. The parasitic infection may be severe enough to affect maternal health adversely during pregnancy, to the point that pregnancy termination is required. The parasites may infect and cross the placenta

Table 24.13 Tropical parasitic infections: issues specific to women

Parasite/Infection	Issues specific to women	Prevention	Treatment
Intestinal nematodes			
Ascariasis	Adult worms can invade the female genital tract and cause tubo-ovarian abscess, pelvic pain and infertility	Food and water precautions	Pyrantel pamoate Treat in pregnancy only if severe infection Mebendazole Albendazole
Enterobiasis (pinworm)	Pinworms can migrate and ascend the genital tract causing vaginitis and pelvic inflammatory disease Pregnancy can exacerbate the symptoms of vaginitis and pruritus vulva	Good personal hygiene	Mebendazole Albendazole Pyrantel pamote Treat only if severe infection
Hookworm *Ancylostoma duodenalis* Necator	Can cause severe anemia, causing intrauterine growth retardation during pregnancy	Do not walk barefoot	Mild cases treat with iron, vitamins, protein Severe cases pyrantel pamoate $11\,mg^{-1}\,kg^{-1}$ daily for 3 days
Strongylodiasis	Hyperinfection can occur during pregnancy due to immunosuppression Lactation is contraindicated until after treatment as larvae may be passed in milk to infant	Do not walk barefoot	Postpone treatment in asymptomatic women until after delivery Severe infection thiabendazole, ivermectin
Tissue nematodes			
Wucheria bancrofti	Adult worms inhabit lymphatics and regional lymph nodes. Acute and chronic inflammation can lead to obstruction of the lymphatics and edema of the breast, vulva and pelvic organs	Avoid mosquito bites	Treatment should be avoided until after delivery; diethylcarbamazine
Brugia malayi	Adverse effect on fertility and lactation Elephantitis of vulva may obstruct labor and necessitate C-section Pregnancy may exacerbate edema and chyluria May be associated with hydramnios Microfilaria can invade placenta and fetus	Avoid mosquito bites	Treatment should be avoiled until after delivery; diethylcarbamazine
Trichinella spiralis	May disrupt menstrual cycle May cause abortion, premature labor, stillbirth ? Intrauterine infection	Avoid eating pork, boar or bear	Pyrantel pamoate active against ingested larve Once tissue invasion need thiabendazole
Trematodes			
Schistosomiasis (Female genital schistosomiasis, FGS)	The female genital may be infected with eggs of *S. mansoni* and *S. haematobium* Acute and chronic inflammation of the fallopian tubes and ovaries can lead to salpingitis, infertility, ectopic pregnancies Lesions of the cervix, vagina, vulva may ulcerate and be painful with intercourse May facilitate transmission of HIV from infected men to uninfected women May need surgery prior to vaginal delivery Schistosomiasis may affect the placenta and the fetus; however, there is no evidence of growth retardation or preterm delivery to date No evidence that pregnancy accelerates the development or increases the severity in the mother	Avoid water, infested areas	Praziquantel May treat if necessary during pregnancy

Table 24.14 Indications for treatment of intestinal nematodes during pregnancy

Parasite	Infective state	Mode of transmission	Adult habitat	Indications for prescription in pregnancy
Enterobius vermicularis (pinworm)	Egg	Ingestion	Cecum	None
Trichuris	Egg	Ingestion	Colon	Rectal prolapse, blood loss
Ascaris	Mature egg	Ingestion	Small intestines	Worm obstruction
Strongyloides stercoralis	Larvae	Skin or colon mucosa penetration	Small intestine	Presence of infection
Hookworm (*Necator Americanus*, *Ancylostoma duodenale*)	Larvae	Skin penetration	Small intestine	Heavy worm load, anemia

Adapted from Lee RV (1988) *Medical Complications During Pregnancy* (eds GN Burrow and TF Ferris). WB Saunders, Philadelphia.

and cause intrauterine growth restriction, miscarriage, stillbirth and fetal and congenital infection. The infection may cause problems during the perimenopause and menopausal era that have not been studied.

If infection occurs during pregnancy or immediately prior to pregnancy, the effect on maternal health and the developing fetus depends on the type of parasitic infection, the natural immunity to the infection and the parasitic load. Diagnosis is often based on a high index of suspicion due to the patient having traveled to or from an endemic area or to the presence of certain diseases in the local community.

All travel health clinicians should develop an understanding of the most common parasitic diseases, their mode of transmission, clinical manifestations, diagnosis and how the infection might affect a pregnancy or lead to changes in the female genital tract. This information will be helpful for both pretravel and post-travel assessments (Tables 24.12 and 24.13). Most of the work on the effects of tropical disease in women has been done on women that live in developing countries. There may be a range of effects, from asymptomatic to more devastating, due to differences in immunity between women living in endemic countries and women traveling to or working in them. Hopefully, by developing a better understanding of the range of effects, all women can be helped.

When to Treat a Parasitic Disease in Pregnancy

The decision of when to treat a parasitic infection during a pregnancy is difficult but should be based on knowledge of the maternal and fetal effects of the disease balanced with the toxic effects of the antiparasitic drug on the developing fetus. Table 24.14 summarizes the use of antiparasitic agents in pregnancy.

Therapeutic Recommendations for Individual Conditions

Virtually all the important helminth infections in humans can be treated with one of five anthelmintics currently in use: albendazole, mebendazole, diethylcarbamazine, ivermectin and praziquantel (de Silva *et al.*, 1997). These drugs are vital not only for the treatment of individual infections but are also useful in controlling transmission of the more common infections. This article reviews briefly the pharmacology of these five drugs, and then discusses current issues in the use of anthelmintics in the treatment and/or control of soil-transmitted nematode infections, filariasis, onchocerciasis, schistosomiasis (and other trematode infections), neurocysticercosis and hydatidosis.

Mebendazole and albendazole are most effective against intestinal nematodes, but are contraindicated during the first trimester of pregnancy. The efficacy of prolonged therapy with these two drugs for treatment of larval cestode infections has not yet been established. Diethylcarbamazine is widely used to treat and control lymphatic filariasis, but adverse effects related to death of microfilariae or damage to adult worms may be marked. While ivermectin has been used in the treatment of patients with onchocerciasis, it is also undergoing investigation for use against lymphatic filariae. Praziquantel, used to treat schistosome infections, is also effective in other trematode infections and adult cestode infections (de Silva *et al.*, 1997).

Ivermectin is the drug of choice for onchocerciasis. A small study demonstrated no increased incidence of birth defects when it was given inadvertently to pregnant women (Pacque *et al.*, 1990).

Intestinal protozoan disease diagnosed in pregnant women is mostly controlled by symptomatic treatment. Specific therapy can be delayed until after delivery. Only severe cases, i.e. continued diarrhea leading to malnutrition of either mother or fetus, require an immediate specific drug therapy, which might be harmful to the fetus due to toxic and teratogenic potentials. Vertical transmission of intestinal protozoa has not been described. Invasive protozoan infections can be lethal to the mother, making immediate drug therapy mandatory, even if the potentials of fetotoxicity or teratogenicity are known. Vertical transmission occurs independent of maternal symptoms, causing clinical disease in the child either directly after birth or during the first months of life. Knowledge of endemic regions and of the maternal travel history is essential for early diagnosis and treatment of protozoan disease in pregnancy and of congenital protozoan infections (Bialek and Knobloch, 1999).

Prevention is the key concept, owing to the potential adverse effects resulting from the parasite or its treatment. it requires a basic knowledge of the life cycle of the parasite.

Parasitic infection during pregnancy is common. With most parasites, primary prevention is very effective in avoiding infestation. With the exceptions of malaria, toxoplasmosis and African trypanosomiasis, when infection does occur treatment decisions should be based on the impact of the infection on the patient and her fetus on an individual basis. When treatment is indicated, selection of medications with the least potential to harm the mother, and more particularly the developing fetus, is essential (Tietze and Jones, 1991).

Female Genital Schistosomiasis

The recent explosion in the number of women exposed to schistosomiasis, either through adventure travel and/or from working for a relief organization in endemic areas, may increase the numbers of infections (Centron et al., 1996). Thus it is important to review some of the recent studies describing the long-term effects on a women's reproductive tract. This information can be used to educate women before travel about the risks of exposure.

Female genital schistosomiasis (FGS) is characterized by the presence of schistosome eggs or worms in the upper or lower genital tract (Poggensee et al., 2000). The original description dates back to Egypt in 1899, when a tumorous growth was observed in the vagina of a young woman and was found to consist of numerous egg granulomas. Since then schistosoma ova and adult worms have been detected throughout the female genital tract, from the vulva to the ovaries, in many of the countries where urinary schistosomiasis is endemic (Feldmeier et al., 1995). Clinically apparent vulvar, vaginal and cervical schistosomiasis has been reported from both endemic and nonendemic areas due to the increase in travel and migration. This has lead the Gender Task Force of the WHO-TDR to include FGS in a list of scientific areas that deserve a high research priority (Poggensee et al., 1999).

Pathophysiological Basis

Copulating adult worms have been found in histological sections of the vulva, cervix, uterus and fallopian tubes. The specific vasculature of the small pelvis allows the adult worms to migrate and can cause schistosomal eggs to be transferred to the genital organs. Anastomoses between the different venous plexes of the small pelvis, the veins, which are almost without valves and allow blood to flow in either direction, as well as portosystemic anastomoses present a network of routes for the migration of worms and/or the embolization of eggs. Adaptive vascular changes at puberty and changes in the venous blood flow during pregnancy can increase the risk of ectopic vascularization.

Prevalence

Until recently the occurrence of FGS was estimated from postmortem studies in endemic areas. Frequencies of anywhere from 7 to 100% for lesions in the lower reproductive tract, and 2 to 83% for lesions in the upper reproductive tract, were observed (Feldmeier et al., 1995). More research needs to be done on the effects of and immune reponse to schistosome infection in both women and men.

Natural History

The natural history of egg-induced lesions remains unclear. There are two distinct tissue patterns: a strong inflammatory reaction around viable eggs, and fibrous tissue reaction around nonviable eggs or fragments.

FGS symptoms and signs are nonspecfic and may be confounded by those of other pelvic disease: irregular menstruation, pelvic pain, vaginal discharge. Lesions can grow for months and years. If in the vagina or vulva they may lead to hypertrophy and obstruction. They can be painful or painless.

Public Health

FGS may be an important factor in the spread of sexually transmitted diseases, especially AIDS.
Because lesions tend to bleed easily, HIV in semen would have access to the blood circulation via ulcerative lesions, and thence to regional lymph nodes.

Infertility and Pregnancy-related Disorders

Functional and anatomic disorders caused by ovarian, tubal and uterine schistosomiasis include fibrosis of the ovaries and tubal occlusion, which can lead to ectopic pregnancies and infertility. Infection of the placenta may cause stillbirths.

Table 24.15 Consequences of female genital schistosomiasis

Organ affected	Possible consequences
Vulva/vagina	Destruction of clitoris/hymen
Cervix	Anemia due to chronic blood loss
	Carcinoma, may be cofactor with
	human papillomavirus
	May increase risk for STD
Uterus	Anemia due to blood loss
	Metaplasia
	Miscarriage
	Preterm delivery
Tubes	Ectopic/tubal pregnancy
	Secondary infertility
Ovaries	Hypogonadism
	Infertility primary or secondary

Diagnosis

The gold standard is biopsy of the lower genital tract but diagnostic means suitable for fieldwork are still lacking. The aim is the development of assays for detection of indirect disease markers or schistosome antigen from swab eluates that women can do themselves. Until recently, diagnosis of upper tract FGS was incidental.

This is an example of how a tropical disease such as schistosomiasis can have severe consequences in women (Table 24.15). Much more research is needed. There may be difference in immune status between women who live in endemic countries and women who travel to them. It is not known what to do if there is positive serology in an asymptomatic person. Treatment is recommended. If the woman is treated, how will we measure the endpoint? New preventative measures and methods for early diagnosis and treatment need to be developed.

Amebiasis

It has been estimated that 500 million people are infected with either *Entamoeba histolytica* or *E. dispar*, with *E. dispar* infection probably 10-fold more common than *E. histolytica* infection. Among individuals infected with *E. histolytica*, 40 million people develop disabling colitis or extraintestinal abscesses, resulting in 40 000 deaths annually. Among parasitic diseases, only malaria and schistosomiasis result in more deaths than amebiasis. Although amebiasis is found worldwide, the highest prevalence rates are in developing countries. High rates of amebic infection (both *E. histolytica* and *E. dispar*) have been reported from the Indian subcontinent and Indonesia, the sub-Saharan and tropical regions of Africa, and areas of Central and South America.

The prevalence of colonic disease is equal in men and women, but amebic liver abscesses and other extraintestinal disease is 3–10 times more common in men. Children, especially neonates, pregnant women and women in the postpartum period have an increased risk

for severe disease and death (Li and Stanley, 1996). Pregnancy may predispose to the development of fulminant colitis in patients with amebic dysentery. One study reported that two-thirds of the fatal cases of amebiasis occured in pregnant women (Abioye, 1973). Increased circulating cholesterol during pregnancy may be a growth substrate for the amebae and is thought to be one explanation for the fulminant course. The frequency of liver abscesses is thought to be a consequence of a protective effect of estrogen (Ravdin, 1995). Other risk factors for severe disease include treatment with corticosteroids, malignancy and malnutrition. There is no evidence that *E. histolytica* is associated with an intrauterine infection; however, infection during delivery or during the neonatal period, from mother to infant, does occur.

Treatment during pregnancy depends on the symptoms. There is currently no drug that is active against amebic cysts. Antimicrobial therapy is directed against the trophozoite stage. For asymptomatic cases the intraluminal stage can be treated with paromomycin, an oral aminoglycoside. Paromomycin is poorly absorbed from the gastrointestinal tract and is thus considered safe in pregnancy. Metronidazole has broad activity against amebiasis. It is also effective against giardiasis and trichomoniasis. It passes freely through the placental barrier and animal studies to date indicate that it is nonteratogenic. The drug, classified as FDA pregnancy category B, is regarded as safe in pregnant women as no teratogenic effect in humans has been documented (Burtin, 1995). For amebic abscess the treatment of choice is metronidazole followed by paromoycin.

Giardiasis

Although maternal giardiasis does not affect the fetus directly, it may cause growth retardation and impair fertility as a result of malabsorption and nutritional deprivation. Pregnant women should only be treated if they are symptomatic. The treatment of choice is metroniadazole 400 mg t.i.d. for 7 days. Do not use a 2 g dose during pregnancy. Paromomycin, a poorly absorbed aminoglycoside, could be used at a dose of 10 mg kg^{-1} three times a day for 5–10 days.

Trypanosomiasis

Chagas disease is a tropical disease now making its appearance in the USA as immigration from Latin America increases. Pregnant women with chronic *Trypanosoma cruzi* infection may present with cardiac or gastrointestinal symptoms and transmit the infection to their fetuses (Gilson *et al.*, 1995).

African trypanosomiasis is a rare but well-documented cause of fever in US travelers returning from areas where it is endemic. Recently, two cases were diagnosed in tourists who went on safari in Tanzania (Sinha *et al.*, 1999). A comrehensive review of the cases occurring in the USA suggests that disease in returning American travelers is nearly always of the East African form, a fulminant illness for which prompt diagnosis is necessary. Timely and appropriate therapy for this disease in the USA has resulted in favorable outcomes for most patients. Chemoprophylaxis for East African trypanosomiasis is not recommended, but travelers visiting areas of endemicity should undertake appropriate measures to prevent tsetse fly bites.

Toxoplasmosis

Toxoplasma gondii is an intracellular coccidian parasite found throughout the world. Infection is spread through the ingestion of oocysts in undercooked meat, by exposure through handling cat litter, or by consumption of foodstuffs contaminated with oocysts. The most important factor is eating raw or undercooked meat. Cats excrete up to 10 million oocysts a day for up to 2 weeks postinfection. Oocysts become infective 1–5 days after excretion, are spread by surface water and can survive for more than 1 year. Thus contact with soil and water and eating undercooked meat are greater risk factors than exposure to cats.

Fetal infection occurs as a result of *primary* maternal infection. Infection acquired prior to conception is not considered a risk. The risk during pregnancy is that the infection will cross the placenta and cause spontaneous abortion, stillbirth, hydrops fetalis or congenital infection. Risk of fetal infection increases with length of gestation but severity of infection is decreased.

Preventative measures are important: avoid contact with cat feces, wear gloves when gardening, employ high standards of hygiene when preparing food, avoid eating raw or undercooked meat, wash vegetables and salads thoroughly.

Helminth Infections

Disease and morbidity are a function of the number of worms in the body. In the pregnant woman, low worm loads can wait until after delivery for treatment.

Ascariasis

Ascaris lumbricoides is the most common helminth infection of humans, with an estimated 1 billion cases worldwide. Transmission usually occurs from hand to mouth. Ova are ingested from a contaminated environment; larva are released into stomach, penetrate the gut wall and enter the circulation, on reaching the lung, larva cross the alveoli and are transported to the trachea by coughing and muciliary function. They are swallowed and reach the small bowel, where they stay, developing into sexually active forms. Adult worms have an average lifespan of 1–2 years, grow up to 35 cm long and lay 200 000 eggs a year.

Complications of ascariasis include bowel obstruction, appendicitis, peritonitis and pancreatitis. There are rare reports of congenital infection, ascribed to placental transmission. Maternal ascariasis leads to a risk of intrauterine growth retardation. Mebendazole, pyrantel and levamisole are all effective but are not recommended during pregnancy. Piperazine may be given to gravidas after the first trimester.

Enterobiasis

Infection with pinworm is common in temperate climates. There is frequently perianal and perineal itching. The worms may migrate into the genital area, producing chronic vaginitis and on occasion pelvic inflammatory disease.

Leishmaniasis

Each year 500 000 new infections with visceral leishmaniasis occur. According to WHO, the ratio of subclinical to clinical infections is 5:1.14. A study from Kenya suggested that asymptomatic persons can be a reservoir of leishmaniasis for extended periods. People can develop the disease even decades after traveling to endemic areas.

Women become immunosupressed during pregnancy, with a shift from cell-mediated to humoral immunity, which has been described in mice as well as humans. Therefore, women may also have a higher susceptibility to leishmanisis during pregnancy, as has been shown in mice. Pregnancy may trigger the (re)activation of disease. A recent report describes a leishmaniasis infection of an infant determined to have been infected by his mother, who had must have had a subclinical infection that was reactivated by pregnancy (Meinecke *et al.*, 1999). The mother had traveled to the Mediterranean areas of Portugal, Malta and Corsica years previously. Thus leishmaniasis can be transmitted congenitally from asymptomatic mother to child. Women who have lived in endemic areas for extended periods of time should be evaluated for asymptomatic disease. Asymptomatic leishmanaisis should be considered in the prenatal evaluation of women who have lived in endemic countries and may not be symptomatic.

Visceral leishmaniasis is endemic to several tropical and subtropical countries, but also to the Mediterranean region. It is transmitted by the sand fly (*Phlebotomus* and *Lutzomyia* spp). Occasional nonvector transmissions have also been reported, through blood transfusions, sexual intercourse, organ transplants and dog excrements, and sporadically outside endemic areas.

GENDER-RELATED ISSUES IN SPORTS AND ADVENTURE ACTIVITIES

Exercise during Pregnancy and Travel

Exercise during pregnancy has become the norm for most women. Pregnant women may plan to trek at altitude, ski or go on extended bicycle trips. The potential benefits and possible risks of particular exercises have been reviewed in the literature (Clapp, 1994; Artal, 1996). There are both benefits and risks that must be weighed and discussed. Pregnant women who take holidays and vacations expect to take part in all the sports and activities that elective travel allows them. Women without any medical problems can indulge in numerous recreational activities throughout their pregnancy. The usual cautions about exercise in pregnancy hold true

The physician and the pregnant woman should discuss her history, overall fitness, previous level of activity and signs that portend discontinuation of the activity. They should develop a program that is acceptable and enjoyable but not hazardous to the fetus or the mother.

Exercise and Activity Guidelines

For a woman with a normal pregnancy there are no known contraindications to exercise during the pregnancy. Recent reviews have documented the benefits of exercise during pregnancy (Agnostini, 1994; Artal, 1996; Clapp, 2000). The incidence of infertility, spontaneous abortion, congenital malformation and placental abnormalities is not increased in women who continue a strenuous weight-bearing type of exercise (running, aerobics, crosscountry skiing, stair stepping, and so forth) throughout early pregnancy. The concern that continuing a strenuous exercise program or beginning to exercise in mid to late pregnancy might lead to preterm labor or premature rupture of the membranes is not supported by current data. Previous concern about exercise during pregnancy has been related to the hypothetical risks of strenuous maternal exercise, including resulting in fetal stress, competing for blood flow and depriving the fetus of oxygen, fetal hypoxia and thermal stress resulting in neural tube abnormalities (Backer, 1997). Thus pregnant women should be warned to avoid hypoglycemia, hyperthermia and dehydration while exercising.

Studies to date have confirmed the benefits of aerobic exercise. The effects of anaerobic training is not known. Thus the data available indicate that healthy fit women with normal pregnancies can begin or continue a regular program of exercise during pregnancy. In fact, improved outcomes for mother and fetus are associated with regular weight-bearing exercise. Regular exercise appears to enhance placental growth.

The ACOG Guidelines (ACOG, 1994) may be too restrictive for some women who exercise on a regular basis. Most researchers support a more flexible approach to exercise, for both the regular and the elite athlete, during a normal pregnancy.

Temperature control in important. A pregnant woman should avoid extreme exercise in a hot and humid climate because of the possible effect of raising the maternal and fetal temperature. The concern is of an increase in neural tube defects. Hot tubs and saunas should be avoided for the same reason.

A woman's previous level of exercise and endurance should be considered when planning an adventure. Common sense should be used. For example, a pregnant traveler who wants to go on a ski vacation should consider the fact that changes in her body's center of gravity and increased joint laxity may put her at risk of an accident due to a change in balance. Even an expert skier could fall under these circumstances, resulting in trauma to the fetus and the mother. It is probably best not to ski or trek at high altitudes due to the lack of access to care if an emergency should occur.

Limitations and/or contraindications to an exercise program during pregnancy would include any of the following problems: a history of spontaneous abortion or miscarriage, premature labor, multiple gestation, incompetent cervix, unusual bleeding, placenta previa or severe cardiac or pulmonary disease.

Altitude

Advice to pregnant women wishing to exercise at altitude is based on isolated observations and a handful of systematic studies. Few studies have explored the limits of combined exercise and altitude exposure in human pregnancy (i.e. at maximal exercise and maximal altitude). Guidelines must therefore be based on a variety of sources, including the physiology of permanent residence at high altitude, in particular the degree of (and hence requirement for) adaptations specific to pregnancy over and above simple altitude acclimatization, and data from the few systematic studies in human pregnancy under conditions of short-term altitude exposure with or without exercise.

Because the effects of altitude and exercise may be synergistic rather than additive, and because individual altitude tolerance and exercise capacity cannot be reliably determined at sea level, advice should err on the side of caution.

An altitude of 2500 m should not be exceeded in the first 4–5 days of short-term exposure. If exercise is performed directly after exposure, this should take place at correspondingly lower altitude, especially in the first few days. Compounding risks, for example, maternal smoking, anemia or fetal growth retardation, must be carefully excluded (Huch, 1996).

Two studies, at 1800 and 2225 m above sea level, in healthy but sedentary women in late pregnancy, who resided at sea level, indicate that short bouts of moderate-to high-intensity cycle ergotomy are well tolerated by the mother and fetus (Baumann et al., 1985; Artal et al., 1995). Normal adults can easily maintain their Po_2 levels to 3000 m, thus delivery of oxygen to the placenta should be

Table 24.16   Medical kit for women

Categories	Options
Menstrual supplies	
Calender to keep track of menses	
Supplies/devices: pads, tampons, menstrual cups, Keeper towelettes/plastic disposal bags	
PMS medication	
NSAIDS	Ibuprofen, other
Dysfunctional uterine bleeding medication	
Guidelines	Premarin 2.5 mg tablets,
	Premarin 1.25, estradiol 2 mg
	Oral contraceptive pills
	NSAIDS—iboprofen, other
Urinary tract infections	
Antibiotic	Ciprofloxacin 250 mg b.i.d. × 3
Urinary analgesic	Pyridium 200 mg t.i.d. for dysuria
Optional screening	Urinary dipstick to check for leukocytes and nitrites
test	
Pyelonephritis—if fever, nausea and flank pain suspect upper tract disease	
Antibiotic	Ciprofloxacin 250 mg b.i.d. × 14 days
Urinary voiding supplies	
Toilet tissue, towelettes	
Funnels—paper or plastic	
Vaginitis—candidasis	
Self-diagnosis tool pH paper: pH < 4.5 acidophilic	
Vaginal creams—*Candida*	Monistat vaginal cream
Vaginal suppositories	Nystatin
Oral medication	Fluconazole 150 mg × 1
Mild soaps	
Pruritus	Hydrocortisone cream for pruritus
Loosey airy clothes	
Bacterial vaginosis	
Self-diagnosis tool	pH paper: Ph > 4.7
Vaginal creams	Metrogel, clindamycin
Oral antibiotics	Metronidazole, clindamycin
Trichomoniasis	
Metroniadazole	
Contraception	
Chart—to keep track of pills if using them, menstrual periods	
Timer—special wrist watch 'alarm' to use for oral contraceptive pill dosing when changing time zones, traveling	
Male/female condoms	
Diaphragm/cap/sponge	
Spermicides—contraceptive creams, jellies, films	
Review options in country of destination	
Emergency contraception	
Combined pill regimen or levonorgestrel regimen	
Antinausea pills—phenergan 25 mg per rectum	
New method of contraception to be used	
Misopristone (RU-486) China, some European countries, USA (just approved)	
Emergency postexposure HIV prophylaxis for high-risk unprotected sexual encounter	
Check latest	Zidovudine 200 mg t.i.d. for 4 weeks
recommendations	Lamivudine 150 mg b.i.d. for 4 weeks
	Add indinavir 800 mg t.i.d./nefinavir for high-risk exposure or if zidovudine-resistant HIV strains present or suspected

Table 24.16 *(cont.)*

Categories	Options
Try to begin regimen within 2 h of exposure	
Pregnancy tests	
Carry extras, depending on length of trip	
Sexually transmitted infections	
Preventative barrier measures—condoms, dental dams, saran wrap, gloves, barrier methods	
Magnifying glass	
Chart—for identifying basics—recommendations for treatment	
Medicine for treatment—Zithromax, cipro/orofloxin, aciclovir/famciclovir	
Perimenopausal/menopausal issues	
Vaginal dryness	Oestrogen creams, rings, patches
Menstrual cycle	Consider low dose oral contraceptive pill
Irregularity	
Stress incontinence	Vaginal moisturizers and lubricants, Kegal exercises
Hot flushes and	0.3 mg conjugated oestrogens
night sweats	0.5 mg estradiol
	0.025 mg transdermal 17β-estradiol
	As levels decrease, will need to increase oestrogen and add progesterone
	Layered clothing
	Vitamin E
	Clonidine patch or pill
Insomnia	Avoid stimulus (caffeine, other), exercise, eat food with tryptophan
Irritability/moodiness	Exercise, oestrogen replacement therapy, antidepressants
Osteoporosis	Weight-bearing exercise, calcium, vitamin D
Alternative products	Unclear benefit, studies underway (quai, ginseng, black cohash, vitex/chasteberry, melatonin, St John's wort, wild yams (contain diosgenin, the starting point for the synthesis for progestins; human body does not have enzyme to convert progesterone from yams)
Pregnancy supplies	
Blood pressure cuff	
Urine protein/glucose strips	
Leukocyte esterase strips	
Antinausea medications	
Supplies for lactation	
Breast pump	
Nipple cream	
Antibiotics to treat mastitis	
Personal safety	
(Lessons in self-defense prior to trip)	
Alarms	
New hand-held personal alarms	
Pepper spray	

unchanged. Changes in fetal hemoglobin shift the oxygen dissociation curve to the left, which improves cord blood oxygen saturation and reduces the risk to the fetus. Thus risk to the fetus should be insignificant during the short term and at moderate altitudes (Barry and Bia, 1989).

It is reassuring that there have been no reports of injury or pregnancy complications or losses associated with exercise at altitude (skiing, running, mountain bicycling, trekking, etc.). The studies to date have been conducted at moderate altitudes for short periods and low intensities; we need data on pregnant women who perform various recreational activities at altitudes over 2400 m. Fetal bradycardia has been seen with exposure to extreme altitudes. Thus, until more data are available, it is recommended that pregnant women avoid the hypoxic stress of extreme altitude, but moderate altitude is not a significant risk if there is access to care.

Studies on pregnant women at altitude show that the human fetus develops normally under low-oxygen conditions. Exposure of a pregnant woman to the hypoxia of high altitude results in acclimatization responses, which act to preserve the fetal oxygen supply. The fetus also utilizes several compensatory mechanisms to survive brief periods of hypoxia. While fetal heart rate monitoring during air travel suggests no compromise of fetal oxygenation, exercise at high altitude may place further stress on oxygen delivery to the fetus. Thus a pregnant woman who goes to altitude must take time to acclimatize. Low oxygen tension and pressure changes result in intrauterine growth retardation and an increased risk of premature labor in women who spend most of their pregnancy above 2400 m (Ali *et al.*, 1996).

The limited data on maternal exercise at high altitude suggest good tolerance in most pregnancies; however, short-term abnormalities in fetal heart rate and subsequent pregnancy complications have been observed. A survey of Colorado obstetric care providers yielded the consensus that preterm labor and bleeding complications of pregnancy are the most commonly encountered pregnancy complications among high-altitude pregnant visitors (Clapp, 2000). The fact that pregnancy complications are much higher and birth weights lower at altitudes above 3000 m suggests that exposure to the additional physiological stress produced by exercising at high altitudes may not be wise.

Dehydration, engaging in strenuous exercise before acclimatization, and participation in activities with high risk of trauma are behaviors that may increase the risk of pregnancy complications. Medical and obstetric conditions that impair oxygen transfer between the environment and fetal tissue at any point may compromise fetal oxygenation. Knowledge of the medical, obstetric and behavioral risk factors during pregnancy at high altitude can help the pregnant visitor to high altitude to avoid such complications. Short-term travel to a favorite mountain escape with adequate resources may be safe for a pregnant adventurer. More research is needed to evaluate the risks of intense exercise at altitude during pregnancy (Artal *et al.*, 1995).

Water Sports during Pregnancy

Swimming and snorkeling are safe during pregnancy, as long as marine envenemation is avoided. Water skiing, jet skiing and other water sports that might force water up into the vagina and through the cervix, causing a risk of miscarriage or peritonitis, are not recommended during pregnancy (MacLeod, 1992).

Scuba Diving during Pregnancy

More women of reproductive age are scuba diving. Diving vacations to exotic locales are becoming popular. This raises the question of the safety of diving for women who are pregnant or who are planning to become pregnant. Most international federations and the Undersea and Hyperbaric Medical Society advise against scuba diving for pregnant women or those planning a pregnancy, but no randomized trials provide a solid scientific basis. The fetal circulation is characterized by the exclusion of the pulmonary circulation by two right-to-left shunts. As the lung appears to act as a filter against the progression of microbubbles to the main circulation, the fetus may be particularly exposed to gas emboli (Morales *et al.*, 1999). The effects of scuba diving on pregnancy have been reviewed in detail (Camporesi, 1996). The review summarizes physiological changes induced by immersion diving and decompression effects on male and female divers. The study concluded that there is no contraindication to diving for the nonpregnant woman; however, pregnant women should refrain from diving, owing to a risk of fetal malformation and gas embolism following possible decompression disease. The advice for a woman who finds she was pregnant during the time she was diving is not to terminate the pregnancy. There are case reports of normal pregnancies in spite of continued diving.

A few researchers have suggested that shallow diving, not requiring decompression (less than 10 m, where risk of venous air embolism is low), is not associated with abnormal outcome unless frequent and occupationally related. In women who dive regularly there is evidence of a 3–6-fold increase in incidence of spontaneous abortion and congenital malformation. Some recommend that pregnant women limit their dives to 10 m and, if they go deeper, extend their decompression times by a minimum of 50%. However, no safe depth/time profiles have been established.

Until more data are available, scuba diving should not be recommended during pregnancy.

CULTURAL AND SAFETY ISSUES

The issue of global violence is not routinely addressed in the travel medicine literature. Statistics are alarming. WHO estimates that between 20–50% of women in the world have been physically or sexually assaulted by a man at some point in their lives. What does this mean for the woman traveler? Be prepared! Women travelers should research as much as they can about the countries and the cultures along their itinerary.

It is particularly important to find out as much as possible about the roles of both women and men in the places they plan to visit. Harassment exists everywhere. Women should be prepared for the potential of sexual harassment and intimidation. Women travelers should avoid wearing provocative, form-fitting clothing as a general rule. They should always travel with minimal luggage and have an arm free. In some male-dominated cultures, it is considered incorrect for a woman to travel alone. In some areas of the world, if a woman goes out at night on her own it means that she is 'available'. There is an excellent review of these issues in *Her Own Way—Advice for the Woman Traveler* (see Additional Resources).

All women should learn basic self-defense techniques. Travel medicine advisers should stay abreast of new developments in the area of personal alarm and personal security systems that could promote safety for women.

MEDICAL KIT

See Table 24.16.

CONCLUSION

Travel medicine advisors should be able to address the key travel health issues for women across the life span during the pretravel assessment. Pretravel advice should include information on contraception, emergency contraception and prevention of sexually transmitted disease, if appropriate. The woman traveler's itinerary should be carefully evaluated for exposure to any travel or tropical disease that might have long-term consequences. There is a need for appreciation of gender-related issues in travel and tropical medicine and a need for further research.

REFERENCES

Abioye AA (1973) Fatal amoebic colitis in pregnancy and the puerperium: a new clinico-pathological entity. *Journal of Tropical Medicine and Hygiene*, **76**, 97–100.

ACOG (1994) Exercise during pregnancy and the postpartum period. *American College of Obstetricians and Gynecologists* technical bulletin no. 189.

Agnostini R (1994) *Medical and Orthopedic Issues of Active and Athletic Women*. Hanley and Belfus, Philadelphia.

Ali KZ, Ali ME *et al.* (1996) High altitude and spontaneous preterm birth. *International Journal of Gynaecology and Obstetrics*, **54**, 11–15.

Anonymous (1994) From the Centers for Disease Control: progress toward global eradication of poliomyelitis. *Journal of the American Medical Association*, **272**, 345.

Anonymous (1999) Need for vaccination against yellow fever. *Communicable Disease Report Weekly*, **9**(33), 289, 292.

Anonymous (2000a) *Drug Facts and Comparisons*. Wolters Kluwer, St Louis.

Anonymous (2000b) Fatal yellow fever in a traveler returning from Venezuela, 1999. *MMWR Morbidity and Mortality Weekly Report*, **49**, 303–305.

Anonymous (2000c) Statement on influenza vaccination for the 2000–2001 season. An Advisory Committee Statement (ASC). National Advisory Committee on Immunization (NACI). *Canadian Communicable Disease Report*, **26**, 1–16.

Artal R (1996) Exercise in pregnancy. *Seminars in Perinatology*, **20**, 211.

Artal R, Fortunato V *et al.* (1995) A comparison of cardiopulmonary adaptations to exercise in pregnancy at sea level and altitude (see comments). *American Journal of Obstetrics and Gynecology*, **172**, 1170–1178; discussion 1178–1180.

Backer H (1997) Travel related emergencies. *Emergency Medicine Clinics of North America*, **15**(1).

Balasch J, Martinez-Roman S *et al.* (1995). Schistosomiasis: an unusual cause of tubal infertility. *Human Reproduction*, **10**, 1725–1227.

Barry M and Bia F (1989) Pregnancy and travel. *Journal of the American Medical Association*, **261**, 728–731.

Baumann H, Bung p *et al.* (1985) Reaction of mother and fetus to physical activity at altitude. *Geburtshilfe und Frauenheilkunde*, **45**, 869.

Bia FJ (1992) Medical considerations for the pregnant traveler. *Infectious Disease Clinics of North America*, **6**, 371–388.

Bialek R and Knobloch J (1999) Parasitic infections in pregnancy and congenital protozoan infections. Part I: Protozoan infections. *Zeitschrift für Geburtshilfe und Neonatologie*, **203**(2), 55–62.

Briggs GG, Freeman RK *et al.* (1998) *Drugs in Pregnancy and Lactation*. Williams and Wilkins, Baltimore.

Burtin PTA, Ariburnu O *et al.* (1995) Safety of metroniadazole in pregnancy. A meta-analysis. *American Journal of Obstetrics and Gynecology*, **172**, 525.

Camporesi EM (1996) Diving and pregnancy. *Seminars in Perinatology*, **20**, 292–302.

Centers for Disease Control and Prevention (1996). Establishment of VARAVAX pregnancy registry. *Journal of the American Medical Association*, **275**, 173.

Cetron MS, Chitsulo L *et al.* (1996) Schistosomiasis in Lake Malawi. *Lancet*, 348, 1274–1278.

Clapp JF 3rd (1994) A clinical approach to exercise during pregnancy. *Clinics in Sports Medicine*, **13**, 443–458.

Clapp JF 3rd (2000) Exercise during pregnancy. A clinical update. *Clinics in Sports Medicine*, **19**, 273–286.

Cobelens FG (1998) Yellow fever vaccination and risk of spontaneous abortion (letter; comment). *Tropical Medicine and International Health*, **3**, 687.

Daly E, Vessey MP *et al.* (1996) Risk of venous thromboembolism in users of hormone replacement therapy (see comments). *Lancet*, **348**, 977–980.

Demicheli V, Graves P *et al.* (2000) Vaccines for preventing tick-borne encephalitis. *Cochrane Database System Review*, **2**, CD000977.

de Silva N, Guyatt H *et al.* (1997). Anthelmintics: a comparative review of their clinical pharmacology. *Drugs*, **53**, 769–788.

Diagne N, Rogier C *et al.* (1997) Incidence of clinical malaria in pregnant women exposed to intense perennial transmission (see comments). *Transactions of the Royal Society of Tropical Medicine and Hygiene*, **91**, 166–170.

Diagne N, Rogier C *et al.* (2000). Increased susceptibility to malaria during the early postpartum period (see comments). *New England Journal of Medicine*, **343**, 598–603.

Duffy PE and Fried M (1999) Malaria during pregnancy: parasites, antibodies and chondroitin sulphate A. *Biochemical Society Transactions*, **27**, 478–482.

Farmer RD, Lawrenson RA *et al.* (2000) A comparison of the risks of venous thromboembolic disease in association with different combined oral contraceptives. *British Journal of Clinical Pharmacology*, **49**, 580–590.

Feldmeier H, Poggensee G *et al.* (1995) Female genital schistosomiasis: new challenges from a gender perspective. *Tropical and Geographical Medicine*, **47**(Suppl. 2), S2–15.

Fischer GW, Ottolini MG and Mond JJ (1997) Prospects for

vaccines during pregnancy and the perinatal period. *Clinical Perinatology*, **24**, 231–249.

Fradin M (1998) Mosquitoes and mosquito repellants: a clinicians guide. *Annals Internal Medicine*, **128**, 931–940.

Fraser IS, Lacarra M et al. (2000) Vaginal epithelial surface appearances in women using vaginal rings for contraception. *Contraception*, **61**, 131–138.

Fried M and Duffy PE (1996) Adherence of *Plasmodium falciparum* to chondroitin sulfate A in the human placenta (see comments). *Science*, **272**, 1502–1504.

Gass M and Rebar R (2000) Hormone replacement for the new millennium. *Obstetric and Gynecology Clinics of North America*, **27**, 611–623.

Gerberding JL and Katz MH (1999) Post-exposure prophylaxis for HIV. *Advances in Experimental Medicine and Biology*, **458**, 213–222.

Gilson GJ, Harner KA et al. (1995) Chagas disease in pregnancy. *Obstetrics and Gynecology*, **86**, 646–647.

Glasier A (1997) Emergency postcoital contraception (see comments). *New England Journal of Medicine*, **337**, 1058–1064.

Glasier A (1999) Emergency contraception in a travel context (editorial; comment). *Journal of Travel Medicine*, **6**, 1–2.

Glezen WP and Alpers M (1999) Maternal immunization. *Clinical Infectious Diseases*, **28**, 219–224.

Goverde AJ, Schats R et al. (1996) An unexpected guest in follicular fluid. *Human Reproduction*, **11**, 531–532.

Grady D, Wenger NK et al. (2000) Postmenopausal hormone therapy increases risk for venous thromboembolic disease. The Heart and Estrogen/progestin Replacement Study. *Annals of Internal Medicine*, **132**(9), 689–696.

Guillebaud J (1999) *Contraception: Your Questions Answered.* Churchill-Livinstone, Edinburgh.

Guillebaud J (2000) Reducing withdrawal bleeds (letter). *Lancet*, **355**, 2168–2169.

Hammill HA (1989) Unusual causes of vaginitis (excluding trichomonas, bacterial vaginosis, and *Candida albicans*). *Obstetrics and Gynecology Clinics of North America*, **16**, 337–345.

Hatcher R, Trussell J et al. (1998). *Contraceptive Technology.* Ardent Media, New York.

Hawkes S and Hart G (1998) The sexual health of travelers. *Infectious Disease Clinics of North America*, **12**, 413–430.

Huch R (1996) Physical activity at altitude in pregnancy. *Seminars in Perinatology*, **20**, 303–314.

Li E and Stanley SL Jr (1996) Protozoa. Amebiasis (Review; 154 references). *Gastroenterology Clinics of North America*, **25**, 471–492.

Lindsay S, Ansell J et al. (2000) Effect of pregnancy on exposure to malaria mosquitoes (letter). *Lancet*, **355**, 1972.

MacLeod CL (1992) The pregnant traveler.' *Medical Clinics of North America*, **76**, 1313–1326.

Matteeli A, Caligaris S et al. (1997) The placenta and malaria. *Annals of Tropical Medicine and Parasitology*, **91**(7), 803–810.

Meinecke CK, Schottelius J et al. (1999) Congenital transmission of visceral leishmaniasis (kala azar) from an asymptomatic mother to her child. *Pediatrics*, **104**, e65.

Monath TP (1999) Facing up to re-emergence of urban yellow fever (comment). *Lancet*, **353**, 1541.

Morales M, Dumps P et al. (1999) Pregnancy and scuba diving: what precautions? *Journal of Gynecology, Obstetrics and Biological Reproduction (Paris)*, **28**, 118–123.

Munoz FM and Englund JA (2000) A step ahead: infant protection through maternal immunization. *Pediatric Clinics of North America*, **47**, 449–463.

Na Bangchang K, Davis TM et al. (1994) Mefloquine pharmacokinetics in pregnant women with acute falciparum malaria. *Transactions of the Royal Society of Tropical Medicine and Hygiene*, **88**, 321–323.

Nahlen BL (2000) Rolling back malaria in pregnancy (comment) (editorial). *New England Journal of Medicine*, **343**, 651–652.

Nash HA, Alvarez-Sanchez F et al. (1999) Estradiol-delivering vaginal rings for hormone replacement therapy. *American Journal of Obstetrics and Gynecology*, **181**, 1400–1406.

Nasidi A, Monath TP et al. (1993) Yellow fever vaccination and pregnancy: a four-year prospective study. *Transactions of the Royal Society of Tropical Medicine and Hygiene*, **87**, 337–339.

Nathwani D, Currie PF et al. (1992) *Plasmodium falciparum* malaria in pregnancy: a review. *British Journal of Obstetrics and Gynaecology*, **99**, 118–121.

Nelson AL (1998) Menstrual problems and common gynecological concerns. In *Contraceptive Technology* (eds RA Hatcher, J Trussell and F Stewart), pp 95–140. Ardent Media, New York.

Nosten F et al. (1990) Mefloguine antimalarial prophylaxis in pregnancy. Dose finding and pharmacokinetics study. *British Journal of Clinical Pharmacology*, **30**, 79.

Nosten F, McGready R et al. (1999a) Effects of *Plasmodium vivax* malaria in pregnancy. *Lancet*, **354**, 546–549.

Nosten F, Vincenti M et al. (1999) The effects of mefloquine treatment in pregnancy. *Clinical Infectious Diseases*, **28**, 808–815.

Oger E and Scarabin PY (1999) Assessment of the risk for venous thromboembolism among users of hormone replacement therapy. *Drugs and Aging*, **14**, 55–61.

Ooi WW, Gawoski JM et al. (1999) Hepatitis E seroconversion in United States travelers abroad. *American Journal of Tropical Medicine and Hygiene*, **61**, 822–824.

Pacque M, Munoz B et al. (1990) Pregnancy outcome after inadvertent ivermectin treatment during community-based distribution. *Lancet*, **336**, 1486–1489.

Pedler SJ (2000) Bacterial, fungal and parasitic infections. In *Medical Disorders During Pregnancy* (ed. LM Barron), pp 411–465. Mosby, St Louis.

Perez JA, Castillo P et al. (1997) Breast hydatid cyst. A case report. *Revista Medica de Chile*, **125**, 66–70.

Phillips-Howard PA, Steffen R et al. (1998) Safety of mefloquine and other antimalarial agents in the first trimester of pregnancy. *Journal of Travel Medicine*, **5**, 121–126.

Pinkerton SD, Holtgrave DR et al. (1998) Cost-effectiveness of post-exposure prophylaxis following sexual exposure to HIV. *AIDS*, **12**, 1067–1078.

Poggensee G, Feldmeier H et al. (1999) Schistosomiasis of the female genital tract: public health aspects. *Parasitology Today*, **15**, 378–381.

Poggensee G, Krantz G et al. (2000) Screening of Tanzanian women of childbearing age for urinary schistosomiasis: validity of urine reagent strip readings and self-reported symptoms. *Bulletin of the World Health Organization*, **78**, 542–548.

Polaneczky M and O'Connor K (1999) Pregnancy in the adolescent patient:screening diagnosis, and Initial management. *Pediatric Clinics of North America*, **46**, 649–670.

Ravdin J (1995) Amebiasis. *Clinical Infectious Diseases*, **20**, 1453–1466.

Reinus J and Leikin E (1999) Pregnancy and liver disease: viral hepatitis in pregnancy. *Clinics in Liver Disease*, **3**, 116–130.

Rioux JE, Devlin C et al. (2000) 17beta-estradiol vaginal tablet versus conjugated equine estrogen vaginal cream to relieve menopausal atrophic vaginitis (see comments). *Menopause*, **7**, 156–161.

Robert E, Vial T et al. (1999) Exposure to yellow fever vaccine in early pregnancy. *Vaccine*, **17**, 283–285.

Schlagenhauf P (1999) Mefloquine for malaria chemoprophylaxis 1992–1998: a review. *Journal of Travel Medicine*, **6**, 122–133.

Shlim DR and Innis BL (2000) Hepatitis E vaccine for travelers? *Journal of Travel Medicine*, **7**, 167–169.

Sinha A, Grace C *et al.* (1999) African trypanosomiasis in two travelers from the United States. *Clinical Infectious Diseases*, **29**, 840–844.

Sloan BS, Rickman LS *et al.* (1996) Schistosomiasis masquerading as carcinoma of the breast. *Southern Medical Journal*, **89**, 345–347.

Smoak BL, Writer JV *et al.* (1997) The effects of inadvertent exposure of mefloquine chemoprophylaxis on pregnancy outcomes and infants of US Army servicewomen. *Journal of Infectious Diseases*, **176**, 831–833.

Steketee RW, Wirima JJ *et al.* (1996) The problem of malaria and malaria control in pregnancy in sub-Saharan Africa. *American Journal of Tropical Medicine and Hygiene*, **55**(suppl. 1), 2–7.

Stray-Pedersen B (2000) Parasitic infections. In *Cherry and Merkatz's Complications of Pregnancy* (eds R Wayne, MD Cohen, H Sheldon *et al.*), pp 693–833. Lippincott Williams and Wilkins, Philadelphia.

Strobino BA, Williams CL *et al.* (1993) Lyme disease and pregnancy outcome: a prospective study of two thousand prenatal patients. *American Journal of Obstetrics and Gynecology*, **169**, 367–374.

Thomas SL and Ellertson C (2000) Nuisance or natural and healthy: should monthly menstruation be optional for women? *Lancet*, **355**, 922–924.

Tietze PE and Jones JE (1991) Parasites during pregnancy. *Primary Care: Clinics in Office Practice*, **18**, 75–99.

Tomori O (1999) Impact of yellow fever on the developing world. *Advances in Virus Research*, **53**, 5–34.

Tsai TF, Paul R *et al.* (1993) Congenital yellow fever virus infection after immunization in pregnancy (see comments). *Journal of Infectious Diseases*, **168**, 1520–1523.

Vandenbroucke JP *et al.* (2001) Medical progress: oral contraceptives and risk of venous thrombosis. *New England Journal of Medicine*, **334**(20), 1527–1535.

Vasilakis C, Jick SS *et al.* (1999) The risk of venous thromboembolism in users of postcoital contraceptive pills. *Contraception*, **59**, 79–83.

Vlassoff C (1997) Gender and Tropical Disease Task Force of TDR: achievements and challenges. *Acta Tropica*, **67**(3): 173–180.

Weaver K and Glasier A (1999) Interaction between broad-spectrum antibiotics and the combined oral contraceptive pill: a literature review. *Contraception*, **59**, 71–78.

ADDITIONAL RESOURCES

Consortium for Emergency Contraception
(http://www.path.org/cec.htm)

List of Countries for which Emergency Contraception has been Registered as a Dedicated Product

Argentina	Immediate Yuzpe regimen
Brazil	Postinor 2 approved 1999
Bulgaria	Postinor 4 and Postinor 10 levonorgestrel regimens
Czech Republic	Postinor 4 and Postinor 10 levonorgestrel regimens
Denmark	Tetragynon Yuzpe regimen
Finland	NeoPrimovlar Yuzpe regimen
France	Tetragynon Yuzpe regimen approved 1998 Levonorgestrel regimen approved 1998
Germany	Tetragynon Yuzpe regimen approved 1998
Hong Kong	Postinor 4 and Postinor 10 levonorgestrel regimens
Hungary	Postinor 4, Postinor 10 and Postinor 2 levonorgestrel regimens
Jamaica	Postinor 4 and Postinor 10 levonorgestrel regimens
Kenya	Postinor 4 and Postinor 10 levonorgestrel regimens
Malaysia	Postinor 4 and Postinor 10 levonorgestrel regimens
Netherland	Lynohigh-dose oestrogen regimens
New Zealand	PC-4 Yupze regimen marketed but then withdrawn due to legislative need for a physician prescription
Nigeria	Postinor 4 and Postinor 10 levonorgestrel regimens
Norway	Tetragynon Yuzpe regimen
Pakistan	Postinor 4 and Postinor 10 levonorgestrel regimens
Poland	Postinor 4 and Postinor 10 levonorgestrel regimens
Singapore	Postinor 4 and Postinor 10 levonorgestrel regimens
Slovakia	Postinor 4 and Postinor 10 levonorgestrel regimens
South Africa	E-Gen-C Yuzpe regimen launched August 1997, Levonorgestrel regimen expected early 1999
Soviet Union (former)	Postinor 4 and Postinor 10 levonorgestrel regimens
Sei Lanka	Postinor 2 levonorgestrel regimen launched 1998
Sweden	Tetragynon Yuzpe regimen
Thailand	Tetragynon Yuzpe regimen
United Kingdom	PC-4 Yuzpe regimen launched 1985
Uruguay	Postinor 4 and Postinor 10 levonorgestrel regimens
USA	Preven Yuzpe regimen launched Sept 1998 Plan B (levonorgestrel)
Vietnam	Postinor 4 and Postinor 10 levonorgestrel regimen

Note

- Countries that support an emergency contraception program in official guidelines include Brazil, Educator, Ethiopia, Honduras, India, Indonesia, Kenya, USA.
- WHO includes Yuzpe regimen for emergency contraception as essential drug list (will consider adding levonorgestrel-only regimen at next meeting).
- Consortium for Emergency Contraception is introducing a specially packaged levonorgestrel roduct, Postinor 2, manufactured by Gedeon Richter in Hungary. Product will be marketed in Indonesia, Mexico, Kenya, Sri Lanka. Lessons learned from introductory experiences will be written up.
- Population Services International is conducting projects in Nigeria, Pakistan, Uganda, Venezuela.
- Population Council and WHO have been introducing an emergency contraception program in Zambia: 'Emergency Contraception in Zambia: setting a new agenda for research and action'.
- In countries where no dedicated product is available (and even in countries where a product is marketed), many service providers use regular combined oral contraceptives. The obvious drawback tot this approach is that there is room for error in the selection of pills (placebo versus hormone, selecting the correct pills from multiphasic packs, and dosage. In addition combination oral contraceptives do not come with special instructions. Despite this availability, emergency contraception is largely unknown to women in developing countries and many women in developed countries.

Teratogen Reference Resources

Books

Briggs GG, Freeman RK *et al.* (1998) *Drugs in Pregnancy and Lactation: A Reference Guide to Fetal and Neonatal Risk.* Williams and Wilkins, Baltimore

Information Centers

Organization of Teratology Information Services (OTIS) Information Pregnancy Riskline, Box 1444270, Salt Lake City 84111-4270, USA
Tel: 801 328 BABY
Fax: 801 538 6510
http://orpheus.ucsd.edu/ctis/index.html

Electronic

National Library of Medicine, MEDLARS Service Desk (Grateful med TOXLINE, TOXNET, DART and Medline—sources for bibliographic search) Bethesda, MD 800-638-8480, USA
http://www.nlm.nih.gov/pubs/factsheets/toxlinfs.html
http://www.nlm.nih,gov/pubs/factsheets/darfs.html
http://www.nlm.gov/pubs/factsheets/toxnetfs.html

Teratogen Information System (TERIS and Shepard Catalogue of teratogenic agents) University of Washington, Seattle, WA 206-543-2465, USA
http://weber.u.washington.edu/~terisweb/teris/index.html
http://weber.u.washington.edu/~terisweb/computer_info.html
Micromedix, Inc (Reprorisk-CD-ROM system including the following teratogenic catalogs: Reprotext, Reprotox, Shepard catalogue of Teratogenic Agents and TERIS) Englewood, CO 800-293-5137, USA

Her Own Way—Advice for the Woman Traveler

To obtain addtional free copies of this booklet, write to:
Enquiries Service
Department of Foreign Affairs and International Trade
125 Sussex Drive
Ottawa, ON K1A 0G2, Canada
or call 1-800-267-8376 (in Canada) or (613) 944-4000
The Department is on the Internet at:
http://www.dfait-maeci.gc.ca/

This publication in alternative formats upon request.
© Department of Foreign Affairs and International Trade
November 1999
Cat. No.: E2-172/1999E-1
ISBN 0-662-28092-X

25

The Immunocompromised Traveller

Robert J. Ligthelm

Havenziekenhuis and Institute for Tropical Diseases, Rotterdam, The Netherlands

Pieter-Paul A.M. van Thiel

Academic Medical Center, University of Amsterdam, The Netherlands

INTRODUCTION

Several potential problems need to be considered in travellers who are immunocompromised, depending on the type of disorder in their defence system. Apart from the fact that these travellers are at a greater risk of certain infections in a tropical environment during travel, pre-travel advice needs to be tailored specifically. In general, immunocompromised travellers can have a decreased immunological reaction to vaccines compared with the immunologically healthy traveller. Furthermore, depending on the type of immunodeficiency, they may react differently to the administration of vaccines, especially live attenuated vaccines. In certain types of immunocompromised travellers, additional vaccinations need to be considered and a stricter malaria protection might be necessary. During travel, antibiotic prophylaxis against certain tropical infections might be indicated. In this chapter the additional measures to be taken in the immunocompromised traveller will be discussed. The usual pretravel advice given to any traveller will not be considered. It is advisable for any traveller with a specific medical problem to carry a medical alert card or disc summarising the medical history, condition and current treatment. In the case of any complex medical problem the traveller will benefit from carrying a copy of the last full medical report. Entry to a foreign country while carrying drugs for a specific medical condition during travel warrants a 'To whom it may concern' note from the attending physician. In most western countries, lists of recognised clinics are available to hand out to the traveller so that he or she may seek advice at the most appropriate institution in case of emergencies. Lists are, for instance, available of diabetic and dialysis clinics. The International Society of Travel Medicine also provides lists with the addresses of clinics run by their members. Travellers should be made aware of the fact that this information is available to them before travel.

The following categories of immunocompromised travellers may be recognised:

- Non-HIV-related immune deficiencies
- HIV-related immune deficiency
- The pregnant traveller (see also Chapter 24).

NON-HIV-RELATED IMMUNE DEFICIENCIES

This group of travellers can be subdivided for practical purposes into three categories:

- The traveller with chronic disease (Table 25.1)
- The traveller with a congenital immune deficiency due to a cellular immune deficiency or a humoral immune deficiency (Table 25.2)
- The traveller with an acquired immune deficiency due to splenectomy, malignancy, an autoimmune disease or immunosuppressive medication (Table 25.3).

Chronic Disease

In general, the patient with chronic disease will be, both at home and abroad, at a greater risk of acquiring upper respiratory infections, especially pneumococcal infections and influenza. This applies especially to those patients with diabetes mellitus, chronic pulmonary disease and cardiovascular disease. Vaccination against pneumococcal disease is still under discussion in the western world, but has no direct relation to travel. The efficacy of pneumococcal vaccines is still under consideration for this category of patients. In patients not vaccinated against

Principles and Practice of Travel Medicine. Edited by Jane N. Zuckerman.
© 2001 John Wiley & Sons Ltd.

Table 25.1 The traveller with chronic disease

Chronic coronary disease
Chronic congestive cardiac failure
Chronic obstructive lung disease
Chronic renal insufficiency
Nephrotic syndrome
Liver cirrhosis
Alcoholism or alcoholic liver disease
Diabetes mellitus

Table 25.2 The traveller with a congenital immune deficiency

T-cell deficiency: severe combined immune deficiency (SCID)
B-cell deficiency: common variable immunodeficiency (CVI),
IgA deficiency, X-linked agammaglobulinaemia, X-linked
immune deficiency with hyper IgM
Phagocytes deficiency: chronic granulomatous disease (CGD),
cyclic neutropenia
Complement deficiencies
Congenital asplenia

Table 25.3 The traveller with an acquired immune deficiency

Malignancy: leukaemias, lymphomas, metastatic solid tumour
disease
Splenectomy or functional hyposplenia
Drug-induced immune suppression
Autoimmune diseases

Case History
A 64-year-old women with a 30 year history of insulin-dependent diabetes mellitus is seen pre-travel. She is planning to visit her son and daughter-in-law who are in Harare, Zimbabwe. She will be travelling during June and July. They are planning to take her on a 2 week trip through Southern Africa. She will finally return via Cape Town, where she plans to have a short stay with friends. A mild nephropathy and retinopathy are complicating factors of her diabetes mellitus. The last three winters she has suffered from upper respiratory tract infections. She has never been vaccinated before. Apart from the usual vaccinations (diphtheria-tetanus, polio, typhoid fever and hepatitis A), she was advised to have influenza vaccine. Three weeks after arrival during a camping trip she developed a rigor and fever about 12 h after a barbecue. This was followed by watery diarrhoea. None of the accompanying persons were affected, although all took the same food. She started the standby-prescribed ciprofloxacin immediately. Further, as advised, she used oral rehydration salts. Nonetheless, 12 h later, still running a fever and with frequent watery stools, she becomes somnolent and is found to be hyperglycaemic. On admission to a local hospital the blood glucose level was 26 mmol l^{-1} and a blood culture indicated *Shigella sonnei*, sensitive to ciprofloxacin. On questioning she was found to have missed two of her short-acting insulin dosages because of no food intake. She recovered within a few days with appropriate treatment.

influenza travelling in summer to the other hemisphere, vaccination should be considered. However, availability of the vaccine could be a practical problem, and it might not be the most efficacious protection for the country of destination.

Prescribing antibiotics for these patients during travel is advisable. These are to be taken in the event of a respiratory tract infection or diarrhoea presenting with fever. Co-amoxiclav (or a cephalosporin in case of penicillin allergy) and ciprofloxacin, respectively, are the preferred choice under these circumstances.

Apart from the increased incidence of diarrhoea in these patients owing to their immunological problem, several of these conditions will lead to more severe illness in diarrhoea due to nonimmunological causes. Water-salt balance, in chronic congestive heart failure for instance, can be severely disturbed because of diarrhoea. Dehydration due to this cause in diabetics can lead to severe glucose metabolism disturbance. These considerations are important reasons to provide additional pre-travel advice for these travellers.

Congenital Immune Deficiency Due to a Cellular or Humoral Immune Deficiency

Although this is a group of rare disorders, from time to time patients with one of these conditions, needing special consideration before travelling, will be encountered. Table 25.2 lists the conditions seen most frequently. A few will be discussed here.

Severe combined immune deficiency (SCID) is a rare T-cell disorder, which usually presents within the first months of life. In addition, B-cell function is mostly compromised, leading to both cell-mediated and humoral deficiencies. Life expectancy will generally be short; however, if these patients reach travelling age, travel should be discouraged because of disseminated or persistent infection after live attenuated vaccines. This has been described after BCG and oral polio vaccination, but the same can be expected after oral typhoid vaccine and yellow fever vaccine.

In the group of B-cell and humoral immune deficiencies, the age of onset is early, usually before the age of

2, for the rarely seen X-linked agammaglobulinaemia. Other types do not usually become clinically relevant until the third decade. The presenting infections are predominantly with encapsulated bacteria such as pneumococci, meningococci and *Haemophilus influenzae*. Common variable immunodeficiency (CVI) and, to a lesser extent, IgA deficiency are a heterogeneous group of diseases that share the features of hypogammaglobulinaemia and an increased susceptibility to chronic enteric infections with *Giardia lamblia*, *Campylobacter* spp and disseminated echoviral infections, in addition to sinopulmonary bacterial infections. IgA also plays a role as an antiadhesive agent for *H. influenzae B* and meningococci. A person with one of these conditions travelling to less hygienic destinations need specifically to be protected by vaccination against pneumococci, common meningococci and *H. influenzae*. Response to vaccination will usually be diminished and ideally seroconversion should be checked. Special attention needs to be given to infections such as typhoid fever (vaccination) but also the standby treatment for infections with *Shigella*, *Salmonella* and *Campylobacter* spp (all can be treated with ciprofloxacin) and *G. lamblia* (tinidazole).

Immune deficiency disorder due to insufficient phagocytosis is a rare life-threatening condition and will not be discussed here.

A problem in the complement-mediated immunity is that the clinical presentation (with certain bacterial systemic infections) can be as late as young adulthood. This might not even be known to the traveller. The clinical picture depends on the deficient complement. For instance, late complement defects (C5–C9) are associated with recurrent *Neisseria* spp. (bacteraemia and meningitis); early complement pathway defects are associated with bacterial pneumonia. As soon as the complement defect has become obvious, these patients should be vaccinated against *Neisseria* spp or pneumococci. It is essential that these vaccinations be checked before travel. In addition, antibiotics need to be prescribed for standby treatment in case of respiratory tract infection with fever (co-amoxiclav).

Congenital asplenia and its consequences for travel will be discussed in the next section.

Case History

A 24-year-old man came for advice before trekking through India and Nepal. He had an IgA deficiency, and had been treated on and off until the age of 18 by a paediatrician with several experimental treatments. He had to be treated regularly for respiratory tract infections and had been plagued by chronic nasal congestion. As a child he had received the usual vaccinations without problems. He received diphtheria-tetanus and polio boosters, typhoid fever vaccine, hepatitis A vaccine, meningococcal A/C vaccine and *Haemophilus influenzae* vaccine. Instructions were given on the use of standby treatment consisting of co-amoxiclav,

---

ciprofloxacin and tinidazole. Of course malaria prophylaxis was included.

After 4 weeks in India he entered Nepal, where he developed watery diarrhoea, bloating of the abdomen and nausea. He suspected according to his instructions, *Giardia lamblia* infection and took tinidazole 4 tablets of 500 mg once. He recovered over the succeeding days, but gradually developed intermittent diarrhoea with nausea and weight loss of 6 kg over 6 weeks. On return home he was diagnosed again with *G. lamblia* in his stool, but also *Plesiomonas shigelloides*, a bacterium more often found in immunocompromised patients. After adequate treatment he recovered fully.

Acquired Immune Deficiency

In haematological malignancies it is obvious that immune deficiency can occur because of either T- and/or B-cell impairment. Depending upon the clinical situation, travel should be discouraged or appropriate measures should be in place, as mentioned above. Metastatic solid tumour disease will lead to immune suppression, depending on the type and measure of progressive disease. Advice on travel should be in relation to the patient's condition (Karnofski scale). The level of immune deficiency in these patients is often difficult to establish. When travel is considered in such patients, common sense should prevail.

The spleen provides a multitude of important host defence functions. Surgical removal of the spleen, or splenic dysfunction because of disease, results in a heightened predisposition to sepsis caused by *pneumococci* and other *streptococci*, *H. influenzae*, *meningococci* and a variety of other encapsulated bacteria, such as *Capnocytophaga canimorsus*. Splenic hypo- or nonfunction also predisposes to severe infection with intraerythrocytic parasites such as *Plasmodium falciparum*, and *Babesia microti* (after dog bites).

The risk of acquiring these infections in these patients is determined largely by the age at which the splenectomy was performed and the reason for it. If splenectomy is carried out above the age of 5, acquired immunity leads to reduced risk of infectious problems. It is suggested that in post-traumatic splenectomy, splenic cells adhere to the peritoneum and might partially take over splenic function. There is no evidence for this hypothesis. However, the risk of postsplenectomy sepsis after splenectomy for splenic trauma appears to be lower than that found in patients who were splenectomised for other reasons, such as a haematological disorders (malignancy, idiopathic thrombocytopenia, hereditary spherocytosis, etc.). In general, after any splenectomy the risk of developing fulminant sepsis decreases after 2–3 years, but a lifelong increased risk of a serious course of certain infections will exist.

The same problem can be seen in the hypofunctional

spleen, as occurs in sickle cell disease, thalassaemia, certain lymphoid malignancies and irradiated spleens. Before travel, patients without a functioning spleen, or who have undergone splenectomy, need to be protected sufficiently against encapsulated bacteria and malaria. Ideally, before splenectomy, patients should have received pneumococcal vaccination, as the response to pneumococcal vaccine is reduced thereafter. Whether this also applies to other vaccinations is unknown. In pretravel advice these patients should be given adequate vaccination coverage against pneumococci, meningococci A/C, *H. influenzae B*.

Malaria prophylaxis needs to be optimal, and standby treatment should be available in case of an unexpected breakthrough. Travel to multiresistant malaria falciparum areas without adequate medical facilities should be discouraged. Antimosquito measures are self-evident. In case of fever with or without signs of respiratory tract infection, penicillin treatment (or a macrolide in the case of penicillin allergy) should be started promptly. A thick blood film to exclude malaria should be done without delay at the same time. After bites by dogs or cats immediate prophylactic antibiotic treatment must be initiated, with co-amoxiclav (7 days) or, in case of penicillin allergy, clindamycin (300 mg thrice daily for 7 days).

Case History

A 24-year-old nurse was engaged at short notice to start work for a nongovernmental organisation (NGO) in a malarial area of Ethiopia. Her parents' general practitioner, who was not aware of her personal medical history, gave pretravel advice. She was given adequate malaria prophylaxis, consisting of mefloquine and the usual vaccines for a healthy traveller. Two weeks after arrival at the site she experienced the first of several prolonged periods of febrile illness. *Plasmodium falciparum* was diagnosed once and treated, and a second time treated as such without laboratory investigation. Recovery every time, however, was of limited duration. After a short recovery she was treated for pneumonia, which was diagnosed on physical examination. After a stay of 4 months she still experienced physical unfitness and was unable to work. At this time she was fully examined by the visiting doctor of her NGO. He noted a large abdominal scar. On questioning she mentioned a laparotomy because of intra-abdominal bleeding after a motorcycle accident at the age of 11. The physician decided to repatriate her. On admission to a hospital of tropical diseases in her native country she was found to have no spleen. Pneumococcal pneumonia was diagnosed. She also had serological evidence of a recent Epstein–Barr viral infection. On the planned day of hospital discharge, 3 weeks after arriving from the endemic malaria area in Ethiopia, she developed rigor and high fever. Her blood film showed *P. falciparum* trophozoites.

After treatment she had an uneventful recovery. Because she was eager to continue work in developing countries, all necessary vaccinations and precautions indicated for the splenectomised patient were given. In the following years she was seen twice for a check-up. She had worked in refugee camps in the Middle East and in a public health project in Cameroon, so far without any further problems.

Drug-induced Immune Suppression

The drugs responsible most frequently for serious immune suppression are listed in Table 25.4. The exact amount of systemic glucocorticosteroids and the duration of administration needed to suppress immunity are not known. Controlled randomised studies indicated that the rate of infectious complications in patients given a daily dose of less than 10 mg prednisone or a cumulative dose of less than 700 mg prednisone was not increased compared with that of controls.

As a general rule, it is accepted that immune suppression caused by drugs continues for 3 months after the drugs are stopped. It should not be forgotten that these drugs are often prescribed in diseases with an inherent immune deficiency. In general, all of them have the potential to cause serious immune suppression. With patients using them for a short period, postponement of travel should therefore be discussed. Live attenuated vaccines cannot be administered to patients using drugs that cause serious immune suppression. These vaccines may induce disseminated infection. Therefore generally BCG, MMR, yellow fever, oral typhoid fever and oral polio vaccines are contraindicated. Not all drugs of this type cause immune suppression to the same extent, and much depends on the dose and the duration of treatment. The literature does not provide good data. The use of live vaccines should therefore be applied with common sense.

The second problem in administering these vaccines is the diminished immune response. In serious immune suppression, serological tests should be carried out before and after vaccination in the case of hepatitis A, hepatitis B, rabies and tick-borne encephalitis. In all these diseases, if seroconversion has not been achieved by vaccination,

Table 25.4 Immunosuppressive and cytotoxic drugs

Alkylating agents: chlorambucil, cyclophosphamide, estramustine, bisulfan, treosulfan, mustine and procarbazine
Antimetabolites: methotrexate, mercaptopurine and tioguanine
Glucocorticosteroids: > 10 mg prednisone daily, for more than 2 weeks; or < 10 mg prednisone daily but > 700 mg totally in continuous use
Others: hydroxycarbamide; azathioprine and mycophenolate mofetil; ciclosporin and tacrolimus

---

protection with specific immune globulins is possible in case of the risk of infection. Patients receiving these drugs do not run a higher risk of contracting malaria.

Case History

A 57-year-old man is planning to make a trip through Southeast Asia. At the age of 50 he developed a nephropathy with proteinuria due to Henoch–Schönlein disease. He gradually developed end-stage renal insufficiency for which, after 2 years of dialysis, he received a kidney transplant. Since the transplant 1 year ago, he has been treated with mycophenolate mofetil (500 mg t.d.s.) and prednisolone (10 mg o.d.). He is in good general condition with only an unchanging mild renal insufficiency. He is advised to have malaria prophylaxis with mefloquine, in adjusted dosage according to the level of renal insufficiency. Mefloquine does not interact with mycophenolate mofetil or prednisolone. He had a diphtheria-tetanus and polio booster 8 years ago just before the onset of the kidney problem. He is advised to have vaccination against typhoid fever, and antibodies against hepatitis A are also measured. In the case of a negative serology result, immunoglobulin will be administered just before departure, as this will avoid the problem of insufficient antibody response after hepatitis A vaccine. He receives instructions about the use of antibiotics in the case of invasive diarrhoeal disease. Japanese encephalitis could be a risk because of his itinerary. As there are no data on the safety of the live attenuated Japanese encephalitis vaccine, he is instructed to take antimosquito measures.

HIV-RELATED IMMUNE DEFICIENCY

Infection with the human immunodeficiency virus (HIV) causes a gradual decrease of CD4+ T lymphocytes. Because of the main role in the human defence system of these cells, not only the cellular but also the humoral defence system is diminished, leading to increased vulnerability to opportunistic infections. A less effective immune response to immunisation and an increased risk of complications after administration of live attenuated vaccines are then seen. In daily practice, the number of CD4+ cells in the peripheral blood is a measure of the level of immune suppression by HIV.

CD4+ counts above 500 mm^{-3} correspond with a normal immune state. Counts between 200 and 499 mm^{-3} indicate a moderate immune suppression, while a CD4+ level below 200 mm^{-3} indicates a severe suppression of the immune system. The lower the CD4+ count the greater the risk of opportunistic infections. This correlates reciprocally with the amount of viral load in these patients. When highly active antiretroviral therapy

(HAART) is taken, usually a combination of HIV reverse transcriptase and protease inhibitors, viral replication is inhibited and the CD4+ level increases. However, it is not known whether this also indicates a recovery of T and B cell function. The lowest CD4+ count before HAART therapy is the point of reference for establishing the immune status of the patient.

In advising HIV-infected travellers several issues are important for consideration: the increased vulnerability to infection; the decreased efficacy of or contraindications for vaccines; interaction of anti-HIV drugs with, most importantly, the antimalarial prophylactic drugs; and, lastly, practical problems encountered at the borders of many countries. The availability of treatment in many parts of the world and corresponding insurance difficulties should also be considered carefully.

Table 25.5 summarises the risk of infection, the use and side-effects of vaccines and other advice necessary in HIV-infected patients.

In HIV infection an increased risk of a fulminant course of malaria has never been established. All malaria prophylactic drugs can be used in HIV-infected patients, but interaction with drugs used in HAART should be considered and be monitored before travel. Interaction between mefloquine and chloroquine and HIV protease inhibitors is known to exist. Depending on the type of enzymatic change induced in the liver, the doses of mefloquine and chloroquine can either be raised or lowered. On theoretical grounds interaction with proguanil and quinine is also possible but insufficient data are available to determine whether this constitutes a problem. New anti-HIV drugs become available rapidly and therefore a full discussion of the specific interactions of these drugs and antimalarial prophylactic drugs is indicated. In patients using several anti-HIV drugs, thorough advice from the hospital pharmacist should be sought. If anti-HIV drugs interfere with appropriate antimalarial prophylaxis, adjustment of the travel itinerary to nonmalarious areas should be considered. Mefloquine and chloroquine should be used with reservation in HIV patients who have been treated for cerebral space-occupying lesions such as non-Hodgkin lymphoma and toxoplasmosis. In these cases the drugs have the potential to induce seizures.

Ciprofloxacin and doxycycline, used respectively for travellers' diarrhoea and antimalarial prophylaxis, also interfere with reverse transcriptase inhibitors (e.g. didanosine) and need to be given 2 h before or 6 h after these drugs.

In every pretravel consultation with an HIV-infected traveller the following items should be considered in order to ensure tailor-made advice:

• What is the travellers degree of immune suppression?
• What are the risks of (tropical) infection during this particular journey?
• Which advice on hygiene is indicated?
• Which contraindications for live attenuated vaccines are present?

Table 25.5 Considerations in pre- and post-travel advice to HIV-infected travellers

Degree of immune suppression	CD4 count mm^{-3}	Infection risk	Vaccinations + decreased efficacy	Contraindication to vaccinations	Extra vaccinations	Extra advice
Mild	> 500	None	None	BCG	Pneumococci Influenza MMR[b]	Diarrhoea: none Tuberculosis[a]
Moderate	200–499	Pneumococci *Haemophilus influenzae* *Campylobacter jejuni* *Shigella* spp *Salmonella* (nontyphi) *Mycobacterium tuberculosis* Visceral leishmaniasis Measles	All vaccines Consider serotitre control after hepatitis A/B, CETE and rabies vaccination	Oral typhoid fever Oral polio BCG Yellow fever MMR	As above	Diarrhoea > 2 days blood or fever: antibiotics Tuberculosis[a]
Severe	< 200	The above plus *Cryptosporidium* spp. *Isospora belli* *Giardia lamblia* *Histoplasma capsulatum* *Coccidioides immitis* *Penicillium marneffi* *Strongyloides* spp.	As above	As above	As above	Every diarrhoea: antibiotics (consider prophylaxis) Tuberculosis[a]

CETE = Central European tick-borne encephalitis; MMR = measles, mumps, rubella.
[a]Tuberculosis post-travel check-up for travellers who are abroad for more than 6 weeks, and/or have close contact with local populations.

- Which other vaccines should be advised?
- Is there a need for antibody tests after vaccination?
- Is there a need for standby medication in case of diarrhoea, malaria or other conditions?
- Is instruction needed for the time of administration of HAART when passing to other time zones?
- Is it necessary to consider interaction between HAART and prophylactic medication (and standby treatment)?
- Is there any need for medical check-up during travel?

Case History
A 60-year-old HIV-positive patient planned to travel to Tanzania for a visit to relatives. Before starting HAART his lowest CD4+ count was 10 mm^{-3}, and has now risen to 280 mm^{-3}, with a viral load between 500 and 1000 copies mm^{-3}. The course of his HIV infection was complicated 3–4 years ago by *Pneumocystis carinii* pneumonia. Co-trimoxazole was discontinued recently when his CD4+ count rose above 200 mm^{-3}. His medication consists of abacavir, stavudine, lamivudine and evavirenz, of which two are newly introduced

protease inhibitors. He was started on mefloquine treatment 6 weeks before travel, and weekly mefloquine blood levels were measured and were found to be within the normal range. He was given diphtheria-tetanus and inactivated polio booster plus immunoglobulin before departure. Since there was a high risk for yellow fever, he was immunised because the CD4+ count was expected to be sufficient to counteract a complicating viraemia and also sufficient to lead to adequate immune response. His yellow fever IgG titre 4 weeks after vaccination, compared with the prevaccination titre, was found to be protective. The vaccine caused no side-effects.

THE PREGNANT TRAVELLER

Very often it is forgotten that the pregnant woman is immune compromised to some degree. In pregnancy the risk of complications with certain infections is increased. The risk is not only confined to the pregnant woman but

Table 25.6 Antimalarial drugs during pregnancy

Antimalarial drugs	First trimester	2nd/3rd trimester	Breast feeding
Quinolone derivates			
Quinine	+	+	+
Chloroquine	+	+	+
Mefloquine	?	+	+
Primaquine	−	−	−
Folic acid antagonists			
Proguanil	+	+	+
Pyrimethamine	+	+	?
Sulphonamides			
Sulfa drugs	−	+	?
Dapsone	+	+	−
Antibiotics			
Tetracycline	−	−	−
Doxycycline	−	−	−
Clindamycin	−	−	?
Other drugs			
Atoquavone + proguanil	?	?	?
Artemisinin	?	?	?

+ = Safe; − = harmful; ? = no data available.

also threatens the fetus. Infections increase further the risk of premature delivery. It is therefore important to weigh the risks of travel to the tropics for the pregnant woman.

The pregnant woman is immunocompromised because of physiological changes in cortisol levels and a decreased cellular immunity. In the specific case of malaria in pregnancy, the maternal anaemia contributes to a more serious course. Infection with malaria of the placenta causes obstetric problems and the nonimmune pregnant woman also seems to be more susceptible to a serious course of malarial infection. Every pregnancy runs some risk of early activity of the uterus in case of fever, whatever the course. In nonimmune women, 10% who contract falciparum malaria during pregnancy die. The course and treatment of falciparum malaria in pregnant women is complicated by acute oedema of the lungs, secondary bacterial infections and hypoglycaemia. In 50% of patients, labour starts during the malarial infection, leading to stillbirth, premature birth and low birthweight.

Prevention and treatment of malaria in pregnancy is complicated by the fact that several medications generally used are either contraindicated in pregnancy or have not been tested (Table 25.6).

Another problem in pregnant women is the theoretical contraindication against giving live attenuated vaccinations. In the case of yellow fever and oral polio vaccines, there is evidence from case reports that harm to the fetus is extremely unlikely. If the risk of acquiring yellow fever is nonexistent, a letter of contraindication should be given for immigration purposes. There are few case reports concerning oral typhoid vaccine and this is better avoided therefore in pregnancy. With modern vaccines such as hepatitis A and hepatitis B there have been no formal studies into any effect on the fetus, but these are killed vaccines. Nevertheless, if indicated, inactivated vaccines such as hepatitis B, influenza, diphtheria and tetanus can be administered to the pregnant woman under the same circumstances as those in which they would be given to nonpregnant travellers. Japanese encephalitis vaccine has never been studied in pregnant women; however, data from case reports and accidental vaccinations show it to be safe. There are few data for hepatitis A vaccine. In general, vaccinations in pregnant women should be avoided and the traveller and her physician should weigh the pros and cons in every case.

Concerning the risk of life attenuated vaccines to the children of breast-feeding women, even less data are available. The mother herself is considered to have regained her normal immune status soon after giving birth. Both in the pregnant and the breast-feeding female traveller, administration of immunoglobulin, toxoid vaccines and killed or inactivated vaccines are certainly not contraindicated.

Altogether, advice against travel should be considered regularly in pregnant women especially, when travelling to West Africa for leisure. The obligatory yellow fever vaccination, the high risk of acquiring falciparum malaria and other febrile illnesses are sufficient reasons to consider postponing this kind of travel.

FURTHER READING

Driessen SO, Cobelens FGJ and Ligthelm RJ (1999) Travel-related morbidity in travelers with insulin-dependent diabetes mellitus. *Journal of Travel Medicine*, **6**, 12–15.

Janeway C (1996) *Immunobiology: The Immune System in Health and Disease*. Current Biology, London.

Kroon FP (1999) Humoral immune response to vaccinations in HIV-infected individuals. Thesis, University of Leiden, The Netherlands.

Mandell GL, Bennett JE and Dolin R (1995) *Principles and Practice of Infectious Diseases*. Churchill Livingstone, New York.

Nossal GJV (1997) Host immunobiology and vaccine development. *Lancet*, **350**, 1316–1319.

Phillips-Howard PA, Steffen R, Kerr L *et al.* (1998) Safety of mefloquine and other antimalarial agents in the first trimester of pregnancy. *Journal of Travel Medicine*, **5**, 121–126.

Pirofski LA and Casadevall A (1998) Use of licensed vaccines for active immunisation of the immunocompromised host. *Clinical Microbiology Reviews*, **11**, 954–963.

Plotkin SA and Orenstein WA (1999) *Vaccines*. WB Saunders, Philadelphia.

Samuel BU and Barry M (1998) The pregnant traveller. *Infectious Disease Clinics of North America*, **12**(2), 325–354.

Silver HM (1997) Malarial infection during pregnancy. *Infectious Disease Clinics of North America*, **11**(1)1, 99–107.

Sneller MC, Strober E, Eisenstein E *et al.* (1993) The new insights into common variable immunodeficiency. *Annals of International Medicine*, **118**, 720–730.

Stuck AE, Minder CE and Frey FJ (1989) Risk of infectious complications in patients taking glucocorticosteroids. *Review of Infectious Diseases*, **11**, 954–963.

26

Special High-risk Travel Groups: Immunocompromised, Older, Disabled and Chronically Ill Travelers

Maria D. Mileno

Miriam Hospital, Brown University School of Medicine, Providence, Rhode Island, USA

Kathryn N. Suh

Queen's University, Kingston, Canada

Jay S. Keystone

University of Toronto, Toronto, Canada

Frank J. Bia

Yale University School of Medicine, New Haven, Connecticut, USA

INTRODUCTION

More than ever before the benefits of travel are readily accessible to persons with physical limitations of all varieties. Individuals with compromised immune systems due to HIV disease, asplenia, cancer chemotherapy, or other conditions often present challenging questions to primary care physicians and travel medicine experts regarding their potential travel risks. The elderly and chronically ill account for an increasing number of the approximately 500 million travelers who cross international boundaries each year.

The consequences of any illness acquired during travel can be more severe in the elderly, who may have underlying medical conditions. Furthermore, morbidity and mortality from noninfectious health problems are increased in these travelers, even in those with no identifiable health problems. Issues surrounding travel risks for these special travelers, and focused advice for each group, will be addressed in this chapter.

GENERAL ADVICE

A general medical check-up should be performed to de-termine any individual's fitness for travel, and to identify those unsuspected health problems that may prevent travel. There are few, albeit absolute, medical contraindications to travel, which are listed in Table 26.1. There is evidence that some pre-existing illnesses may actually abate or improve with travel (Dessery *et al.*, 1997). Many relative contraindications are remediable with appropriate medical therapy. Some specific considerations for travelers with underlying medical conditions include precautions every travel medicine expert should know, such as the contraindication to mefloquine use for persons with neuropsychiatric disorders, including seizures, and general avoidance of live vaccines in persons who are immunocompromised. There is an absolute contraindication to hyoscine (scopolamine) use in persons with visual disorders such as glaucoma and retinal disease. Less well-known precautions include hyoscine use in persons with hypertrophy of the prostate gland, who may develop acute urinary retention. Thus a fairly complete medical history must be reviewed prior to making recommendations, even for those conditions which may seem benign to comment upon and prescribe for, such as motion sickness.

If a significant increase in physical activity is expected during travel, a conditioning program, started 1 or 2

Principles and Practice of Travel Medicine. Edited by Jane N. Zuckerman.
© 2001 John Wiley & Sons Ltd.

Table 26.1 Medical contraindications to air travel

Absolute contraindications
Pneumothorax or pneumomediastinum
Thoracic, cardiac, abdominal, middle-ear surgery within previous 3 weeks
Acute myocardial infarction, uncontrolled angina, congestive heart failure, or dysrhythmia within 4 weeks
Cerebrovascular infarction within 2 weeks

Relative contraindications[a]
Respiratory tract infection, including sinusitis, otitis, pnuemonia
Cyanosis or dyspnea at rest or with exercise
Active uncontrolled bronchospasm
Inadequate pulmonary function as indicated by one or more of the following:
    Vital capacity, diffusing capacity, or maximum voluntary ventilation < 50% of predicted
    Hypercapnia ($P_{CO_2} > 50$ mmHg)
    Hypoxemia ($P_{O_2} < 55$ mmHg on room air)
    Hemoglobin < 7.5 g dl^{-1} (75 g l^{-1}) or sickle cell anemia

Adapted from Gong (1991) and Jong and Benson (1997). [a]Relative contra-indications can usually be improved or corrected prior to travel.

months before travel, can increase cardiovascular fitness and muscular strength, and identify potential limitations or problems. Exercise stress testing for asymptomatic individuals may be considered in men over 40 years of age and women over 50 who are beginning vigorous exercise, and for older travelers planning remote or lengthy treks, particularly those with a prior history of cardiac disease (Hultgren, 1990; Backer, 1997).

Certain needs, such as special meals and inflight oxygen, should be arranged with the carrier at least 48 h prior to departure. Aisle or bulkhead seats allow greater leg room and comfort, and can be requested at the time of booking. Intestinal gas expands with altitude; avoidance of food or beverages that cause bloating is advisable. Alcohol and excessive caffeine may lead to dehydration and worsen fatigue or jet lag.

Trip Cancellations and Medical Insurance

Travelers should verify the extent of medical coverage that their health insurance provider offers for travel outside their home country and ensure that any supplemental medical insurance, if required, is purchased prior to departure. Insurance should be sufficient to cover the costs of emergency medical care, as well as evacuation and repatriation costs. There may be restrictions as to what conditions will be covered by supplemental insurance, and this should be clarified with the insurance carrier. For many out-of-country medical services the traveler will be required to pay at the time the service is provided, with subsequent reimbursement from the insurance company.

Medications and Medical Supplies

An adequate supply of all medications, enough for the entire trip plus several extra days' worth, plus other essential medical supplies (e.g. alcohol pads, syringes, needles) should be carried with the traveler or in hand luggage—not in checked baggage—so as to prevent theft or loss. Duplications of some medications may be critical. Commonly used nonprescription medications such as analgesics, antiemetics, antacids, laxatives, and hydrocortisone cream may also be useful. Certain medications such as insulin may ultimately require long-term refrigeration; the availability of suitable storage facilities at the destination should be confirmed. Medications such as sublingual nitroglycerine, which may be ineffective when expired, should be refilled prior to travel. Because the composition and potency of some medications may vary according to manufacturer, and not all medications are available in every country, loss of such medications can pose significant problems.

Written prescriptions for all medications (generic names) and special supplies, with indications for them, should be carried with the traveler. Prescriptions that can be presented to customs and law enforcement officials provide legitimate documentation of needs for specific medications (e.g. narcotics, needles, and syringes) which might otherwise hinder travel across international borders. Furthermore, they can be filled abroad when needed. A letter from the traveler's physician outlining these needs may be of additional benefit. Some prescription medications may be prohibited in certain countries (e.g. amphetamines cannot be brought into Singapore). Administration times of medications should be altered gradually, over several days, when multiple time zones are crossed. Modification of insulin dosing is outlined in the section on diabetes.

Approach to Travelers' Diarrhea

Perhaps the most common problem about which a traveler should be well versed is an approach to travelers' diarrhea. The older traveler is somewhat more predisposed to developing travelers' diarrhea, but complications such as dehydration and electrolyte imbalances are more poorly tolerated and may result in serious morbidity, especially in those with underlying cardiac, renal, gastrointestinal, or immune disorders.

Preventive measures and supportive therapy should be reviewed, as well as the indications for empiric antimicrobial therapy. Antimotility agents such as loperamide and diphenoxylate can improve diarrhea, but should not be used if dysentery or fever is present. Anticholinergic effects may lead paradoxically to abdominal distension, constipation, or paralytic ileus. The older traveler may be wise to begin antimicrobial therapy early in an illness in order to minimize the risk of complications. A fluoroquinolone is the treatment of choice; the dose must be reduced if renal failure is present, and caution is advised with coadministration of theophylline preparations because the quinolones increase serum theophylline levels.

Prophylactic antimicrobial agents for travelers' diarrhea are generally not recommended for the healthy traveler; exceptions include those who cannot afford to be ill during travel and those with a bad 'track record' for travelers' diarrhea. Many travelers, often older persons, are at increased risk of acquiring travelers' diarrhea due to reduced gastric acidity from achlorhydria, gastrectomy, or H_2 blockers. Others are at increased risk of developing disseminated infection from travelers' diarrhea, such as individuals with congenital and acquired immunodeficiency states. Both of these groups should be advised to take a daily dose of a fluoroquinolone. In addition, this approach should be considered for persons who have underlying illnesses that may flare or lead to severe consequences in the face of dehydration, such as inflammatory bowel disease, chronic renal failure, known cardiac ischemia or failure, and poorly controlled diabetes. Chemoprophylaxis should begin 1 day before departure and continue until 2 days after the last exposure, for a maximum of 3 weeks (Tellier and Keystone, 1992).

Medical Records

A summary of any significant past medical problems, including known allergies, should be carried by the traveler. A recent electrocardiogram for those with cardiac disease is advisable, especially recordings with and without pacing for travelers who have pacemakers. The make, model, and lot number of implanted devices (e.g. pacemakers, defibrillators, and prosthetic cardiac valves or joints) and date of insertion should be recorded. Copies of other significant and relevant laboratory results should also be carried. For serious medical conditions, especially those that may result in an altered level of consciousness, a medical bracelet can allow rapid identification of these problems and could be life saving.

Medical Services Abroad

Travelers should carry the name and telephone number of their physician(s), as well as those of a family member or friend to contact in the event of an emergency. They must be advised to seek medical attention urgently if a febrile illness develops or persists after they have returned home. Selected resources for travelers, including those with special needs, as discussed below, are listed at the end of the chapter

When ongoing medical care such as hemodialysis is required during travel, arrangements should be made in advance by having the traveler's physician contact an appropriate specialist at the destination. A list of English-speaking physicians throughout the world is available from the International Association for Medical Assistance to Travelers (IAMAT). Personal Physicians World-

wide will locate an appropriate English-speaking physician abroad and arrange medical appointments for the traveler. Subscribers to Shoreland's EnCompass service, a web-based travel medicine resource, have access to information concerning health care facilities in a number of developing countries.

Last but not least of these general considerations: all travelers should confirm their travel schedules prior to departure, and allow adequate time for travel to the terminal and for check-in. Arrangements for extra assistance or wheelchairs should be made in advance if possible, but help is often readily available within the terminal. Wheeled luggage requires less effort to transport and may be preferable for some travelers.

IMMUNOCOMPROMISED TRAVELERS

An important part of advising any immunocompromised traveler is providing detailed education about the risks of their particular journey. They should know how some risks could be avoided, such as receiving advice about drinking water, and they should be instructed about when and how to seek medical help. There are few absolute contraindications to their travel plans, however each person should be counseled on an individual basis. Attention to PPD skin testing upon return of all travelers who spend time in endemic regions for tuberculosis is of paramount importance. Other chapters in this book are dedicated to an approach to other important immunocompromised groups, such as pregnant travelers, and HIV-infected travelers (Mileno and Bia, 1998). Here we address an approach to persons with immunologic compromise from asplenia, transplantation, cancer chemotherapy, high-dose corticosteroid use, diabetes mellitus, and chronic renal or liver failure.

Asplenic Travelers

Once considered a nonessential organ, it is now known that the spleen plays a central immunologic role. It actively facilitates phagocytosis, removing blood-borne bacteria, intraerythrocytic parasites, and immune complexes. It also serves as a site for the genesis of both humoral and cellular immunity. Defensive host factors such as cytokine synthesis, natural killer cell function, and complement activation may be diminished after splenectomy.

Splenectomy has been estimated to carry a lifetime risk for overwhelming sepsis of up to 5%, with the highest risk within the first 2 years after splenectomy (O'Neal et al., 1981). The risk for children reaches 8.1% and is higher than for adults (1.9%), which may be related to adults having prior exposure to encapsulated organisms. Death rates from overwhelming postsplenectomy infections (OPSI) are thought to be up to 600 times greater than in the general population (Lynch and Kapila, 1996). Most of the risk relates to an increased susceptibility to pneumococcal infection, although other encapsulated bacteria such as *Haemophilus influenzae* and *Neisseria meningitides* are also risks.

Whether functionally or anatomically impaired, splenic dysfunction is a risk for travelers. Functional asplenia occurs in association with a number of conditions including sickle cell anemia, hemoglobin sickle cell disease, splenic atrophy or congenital asplenia, and even in such varied diseases as systemic amyloidosis, lupus erythematosus or rheumatoid arthritis. Common indications for splenectomy in children relate to malignancies such as Hodgkin's lymphoma and other hematological disorders, while adults more often require splenectomy because of trauma or hypersplenism. The reasons for splenectomy may affect the subsequent risk of sepsis in a given individual. Patients who undergo splenectomy for hematological disease may be at greater risk of infection than those who have splenectomy following trauma. There is no evidence that splenic tissue left in the peritoneal cavity following trauma surgery provides any useful splenic function. However, patients undergoing splenectomy for hematological and reticuloendothelial diseases or for portal hypertension have been shown to have a higher incidence of subsequent sepsis than those undergoing splenectomy for trauma (Lynch and Kapila, 1996). Moreover, increased mortality occurs in those with underlying reticuloendothelial disease and in patients treated with chemotherapy or radiation. Lifetime sepsis incidence rates of up to 25% reported after childhood splenectomy for hematological disorders warrant vigilance in the education and evaluation of such persons who anticipate travel, not only in the first 2 years after splenectomy but for a lifetime.

There is no evidence that live vaccines pose any increased risk to asplenic individuals (Conlon, 2000). Although such individuals generally respond poorly to polysaccharide vaccines, with resulting low antibody titers that wane unpredictably, a serious attempt should be made to immunize asplenic travelers. Ideally, such travelers were previously immunized with the pneumococcal vaccine 2 weeks prior to splenectomy. We recommend a pneumococcal booster dose after 5 years, and would suggest meningococcal immunization along with other routine travel immunizations.

Recently, seven-valent pneumococcal conjugate vaccines have been produced by linking polysaccharide to protein carrier molecules, thus stimulating T and B cells in a concerted fashion. Conjugation results in increased immunogenicity and the ability to prime for a booster response. This vaccine is currently indicated for infants at birth and for children up to 59 months of age. It has been shown to be immunogenic in very young infants, and may have a preventive role in the asplenic individual (Kobel *et al.*, 2000). Given the worldwide emergence of drug-resistant *Streptococcus pneumoniae* and the continued observation of severe invasive pneumococcal infections (Kobel *et al.*, 2000), we also offer a course of amoxicillin to take if such travelers become ill when abroad. They are advised to seek medical help using the suggested resources at the end of this chapter.

There are no data to confirm any increased risk of severe malaria in asplenic individuals, although it is theoretically possible. Fatal malaria has been reported in some asplenic patients (Styrt, 1996). There is known susceptibility of asplenic individuals to overwhelming infection caused by *Babesia* species, the erythrocyte parasitic infection that occurs along the eastern seaboard of the United States and in some parts Europe. There are no case-controlled studies comparing normal hosts and asplenics with regard to parasite clearance times or incidence of clinical reactivation. Malaria prevention advice should be no different than for other travelers to malarious regions, and must include a rigorous discussion of personal protection measures in addition to chemoprophylaxis. The importance of urgent evaluation for fever cannot be overemphasized, along with a thoughtful discussion about potentially avoiding travel to areas where transmission rates of malaria are high.

Transplant Recipients

Immunosuppressive agents, particularly cyclosporine and tacrolimus used to prevent graft rejection in transplant recipients, have profound effects on T cells. Azathioprine and corticosteroids may also be part of an immunosuppressive regimen and further impair neutrophil function. Intracellular pathogens pose the greatest risk to these individuals. Persons who have undergone allogeneic bone marrow transplantation (e.g. for leukemia) have more severe immunosuppression than solid organ recipients, and are functionally asplenic. Live virus vaccines should be avoided because there is a risk that disease with a vaccine strain of yellow fever or poliomyelitis might emerge. Overall, transplant recipients have weaker and less durable antibody responses than normal individuals. Fortunately, there is no evidence to suggest that immunizations lead to a greater risk of graft rejection. Recent evidence shows that the hepatitis A vaccine is both safe and immunogenic in liver and renal transplant recipients (Stark *et al.*, 1999). Inactivated polio vaccine can be used when necessary, but travelers to countries requiring yellow fever vaccination should be provided with a waiver letter addressed to the embassy of the country to be visited.

Increased risk of bacteremia during episodes of gastroenteritis caused by *Salmonella* or *Campylobacter* spp warrants empiric treatment for all transplant recipients with a quinolone antibiotic. Malaria advice should not be different from usual, although the effects of antimalarials such as chloroquine or mefloquine upon levels of immunosuppressive medications are not fully known. We suggest that documenting such levels during antimalarial prophylaxis would be prudent prior to travel. Transplant recipients have an increased risk of skin cancers, and this risk may be increased by exposure to sunlight. Specific advice concerning hats and sunblocking agents with UVA and UVB protection is warranted.

Cancer Chemotherapy

While hematological malignancies lead to immunosuppression beyond that caused by the chemotherapeutic regimen used to treat them, solid organ tumors may lead to more subtle immune defects. These patients respond less well than do normal hosts to immunizations after cancer chemotherapy, with the poorest responses occurring in those with primary hematological malignancies. Live virus vaccines should be avoided until at least 3 months following completion of chemotherapy. It is likely that responses to other travel immunizations will also be poor. Persons with chronic lymphocytic leukemia or myeloma are functionally antibody-deficient and will not produce useful responses to immunizations. It is better to provide these patients with empiric antibiotics for use if they become febrile while abroad. In addition, standard malaria advice is indicated.

Corticosteroid Usage

Increasing numbers of travelers are using high-dose steroids or other agents such as methotrexate and cyclophosphamide for connective tissue diseases and other immune-mediated disorders. The defects in cell-mediated immunity result in weakened responses to immunizations (McDonald et al., 1984). As with recipients of solid organ transplants, live vaccines should be avoided and a standby course of antibiotics should be given should they develop fever.

Hepatic Cirrhosis

Mefloquine is metabolized in the liver and should be avoided in persons with significant liver impairment. Travelers' diarrhea may lead to serious dehydration and loss of intravascular volume and empiric antibiotics are warranted. In addition, travelers with cirrhosis are at increased risk of acquiring severe gastrointestinal or cutaneous *Vibrio vulnificus* infections from seafood or saltwater exposure, particularly along the Atlantic and Gulf coasts in the United States.

Renal Disease

Travelers with chronic renal disorders should also be offered empiric antimicrobial chemoprophylaxis against travelers' diarrhea, with appropriate dose adjustments. Dehydration may worsen chronic renal failure and precipitate nephrolithiasis; adequate hydration in warm climates is advised.

Proguanil is an older antimalarial that is being used more often for prophylaxis; it undergoes renal excretion. Renal impairment may lead to its accumulation, which in turn may lead to folate deficiency. Patients with creatinine clearances below 50 ml min^{-1} should take half the normal proguanil dose after the first 4 weeks of prophy-laxis, and all patients with renal impairment should take folic acid supplements when using proguanil (Conlon, 2000).

Dialysis should not preclude travel, but advanced planning is essential. Peritoneal dialysis can be managed with relative ease during travel, provided the necessary equipment and dialysis solutions can be transported and/or delivered reliably. Hemodialysis is available worldwide, but several months' notice may be required for scheduling. Some units will require hepatitis B, hepatitis C, and HIV testing to be performed, and may refuse to dialyze hepatitis B surface antigen carriers.

Careful scrutiny of which dialysis center to choose is important, as blood-borne pathogens may be easily transmissible in a dialysis unit if there is a break in technique or repeat exposure to blood products. Epidemic transmission of HIV in renal dialysis centers in Egypt was reported 7 years after the documented event (El Sayed et al., 2000). Hepatitis B vaccination using a high-dose vaccine should be ensured in nonimmune hemodialysis patients prior to travel. The traveler's dialysis unit and local branches of the Kidney Foundation should be able to provide information and help arrangements. A list of dialysis centers throughout the world can be obtained from Creative Age Publications in the United States, or the International Dialysis Organization in Europe. Some travel and cruise companies also offer trips specifically tailored for dialysis patients.

THE DIABETIC TRAVELER

The problems encountered by patients traveling with diabetes have not been given the attention they warrant, and much of what influences their lives is not yet appearing in the travel medicine literature (Dewey and Riley, 1999). One group from The Netherlands (Driessen et al., 1999) studied traveling diabetics in a small exploratory, retrospective cohort study, using telephone interviews of all patients with insulin-dependent diabetes mellitus (IDDM) advised in their travel clinic over a 12 month period. Unfortunately, respondents did not increase their frequency of blood glucose monitoring during travel. Several reported febrile illnesses with adverse consequences for control of glycemia, while others experienced difficulty with insulin dosage adjustments in the tropics. More than 50% of respondents reported more glycemic dysregulation than in the preceding time period at home. Travel through several time zones was associated with dysregulation in two patients, and one even experienced difficulty at customs when carrying injection materials. Clearly there are problems (Mileno and Bia, 1998).

Preparations for Travel

Safe drinking water and prevention of enteric infections are particularly important for younger patients with

IDDM traveling in developing countries. Chronic *Helicobacter pylori* infection, in particular, has been associated with increased insulin requirements and poor diabetes control in children with IDDM. Safe drinking water should decrease *H. pylori* seroconversion rates as well as other acute enteric infections.

If either the traveler or health provider has not yet joined their national diabetes association, trip preparation would be an excellent time to join, taking advantage of their resources for the traveling diabetic. The American Diabetes Association (ADA) publishes at least three patient monographs, useful for travel. They include *A Guide to Eating Out*, *All About Insulin*, and *On the Go?* The ADA also publishes a 'Buyer's Guide to Diabetes Supplies', which includes manufactured insulin in the United States and abroad, insulin delivery systems, injections aids for visually impaired patients, syringe magnifiers, needle guides, vial stabilizers, glucose meters, data management systems, ADA publications, products for treating reactions, medical identification products, carrying cases and suppliers.

The ADA suggests each physician provide two documents for traveling diabetics. One is a letter listing supplies, medications, and any drug allergies. The second is a prescription for emergency use in case medications are lost. The traveler and health provider should write for a list of International Diabetes Federation groups at the IDF, 40 Washington St, B-1050, Brussels, Belgium. An identity bracelet is important for identifying the traveler as diabetic in an emergency, and the ADA affiliates have Diabetes Identity Cards available in several languages.

Insulin Products for Travel

There are over 30 types of insulin manufactured in the United States alone, which are potential sources of confusion and error while abroad. Insulin preparations in the United States are now all U-100 strength, but they can still be sold as U-40 or -80 abroad. Use of a U-100 syringe with these preparations would result in underdosing insulin.

Insulin's onset of action may vary with the site injected, in addition to the type of insulin preparation. The abdomen injection site produces the fastest insulin response, then upper arms, followed by nonexercised thighs and buttocks. Insulin is absorbed more quickly from all injection sites in hotter climates.

Patient and physician should discuss the objectives of insulin therapy during long, complicated flights and foreign travel. Should they aim for very tight glycemic control (*intensive insulin therapy*) during the trip, with the potential for hypoglycemia? Or should they settle for *conventional therapy* with programmed dosing throughout the day, based upon the length of day and other factors related to travel?

Lifestyles vary. Not all traveling diabetic patients are the same, nor do they travel for the same reasons. The spectrum of travelers who are diabetic also includes some populations that have a relatively high prevalence of this disease. One in five Indo-Asians over the age of 65 is diabetic (Roshan *et al.*, 1996), with a high prevalence of obesity, insulin resistance and complications, including diabetic nephropathy and myocardial infarction. During travel they may also be fasting for religious reasons.

During their fasting Muslims, some Sikhs and some Hindus abstain from food between sunrise and sunset, which can be as long as 18 h. Abstention includes injections and medicines, and only one large meal taken at sunset with a smaller one at sunrise. Patients with IDDM cannot fast in this manner, and patients with noninsulin-dependent diabetes mellitus (NIDDM) may require a short-acting insulin or sulfonylurea to cover the meal at sunset, which breaks the daily fast.

New Insulin Delivery Systems for Travelers

Some diabetic patients use insulin pumps but most do not. Insulin delivery systems in the form of convenient, easy-to-carry, profiled pens may offer diabetics tremendous advantages during travel. The manufacturers of insulin in the United States produce regular insulin and mixtures of 70/30 (NPH/regular) insulin among others, which are available in cartridge pen systems. Either the entire pen can be disposed of when the insulin has been used, or a new cartridge can be inserted in a nondisposable unit. The insulin is stable, even if not refrigerated for 1 week (70/30 mixtures), or up to a month (regular insulin). With a traveler able to carry these devices as simply as a pen, compliance increases.

Control of glycemia, whether individuals are traveling or not, also relates to the often mistimed usage of regular insulin before meals. This is a difficult area for compliance because regular insulin must be given 30–45 min before a meal. Usually it is not. Compliance has been made much easier with the availability of rapidly acting insulin lispro.

There are several advantages for travelers who gain familiarity with this rapidly acting insulin (Noble *et al.*, 1998). Because there is a strong tendency for travelers with diabetes to take their insulin *immediately* before a meal, rather than the 30–45 min before a meal required for regular insulin to become absorbed, the inconvenience of timed administration leads to poor control of glycemia. There is a mismatch between postprandial carbohydrate absorption and the 2–4 h postinjection peaking of regular insulin. In addition, there will still be circulating insulin present as the peripheral blood glucose is falling. This predisposes such patients, particularly those who exercise, to late postprandial hypoglycemia.

Regular human insulin is absorbed slowly because it consists of hexamers of insulin that are crystallized around zinc molecules. To be absorbed from its subcutaneous injection site, it must first dissociate into monomers and dimers. Insulin lispro derives its name from the switching of two amino acids, proline and lysine, within the β chain of insulin. After subcutaneous injection, this insulin dissociates more rapidly into dimers and monomers. The peak serum concentrations of insulin lispro occur within 30–90 min following administration, regardless of the site of administration. There is a better match between carbohydrate absorption and insulin availability with less chance for late-peaking regular insulin to cause postprandial hypoglycemia.

Holleman and Hoekstra (1997) have summarized the potential advantages of insulin lispro. They include a reduction of postprandial increases in blood glucose concentrations, a reduced frequency of hypoglycemia prior to the next meal in patients with IDDM, and greater convenience for patients who wish to administer insulin immediately before a meal. Active traveling patients would benefit from both the convenience and the short action profile of insulin lispro (Medical Letter, 1996).

Travel Across Time Zones

With the general availability of small, portable glucometers for monitoring blood glucose, convenient insulin delivery devices, and rapidly acting insulin lispro, older guidelines for management of insulin administration could be altered to include more frequent monitoring and less rigid formulae for insulin administration.

Suggested regimens had become excessively complicated in well-meaning attempts to achieve nearly perfect glycemic control during travel. We prefer the method outlined by Sane et al. (1990). It calls for a 2–4% adjustment in insulin dosing for each time zone crossed. For instance, a traveler going west over 10 time zones would have his or her day lengthened and require about a 30% increase in long-acting insulin dose. Adjustments to that regimen can be more finely tuned using insulin lispro as needed, based upon more frequent blood glucose monitoring. Individualization of advice by expert nursing personnel, informing airlines about diabetes and the potential for hypoglycemia, carrying carbohydrates during flights, avoiding airlines' largely nonstandardized diabetic meals, frequent monitoring of blood glucose, and detailed tips for planning insulin regimens are all useful. Unexpected delays during trips should be anticipated, such that extra food and insulin doses are carried.

New Technological Advances

Personal laser lancing devices for obtaining capillary blood samples became available in 1999. Since a beam of light, rather than a lancet, penetrates the skin, sharps disposal is eliminated and pain is reduced. Skin patch systems for glucose monitoring on the forearm are also under development. Monitors that read the patch test results and can store months' worth of data, by time and date, will be paired with such patch monitoring systems. A new formulation of glucagon, based upon recombinant DNA technology, eliminates dependency on animal pancreas glands for manufacture. Generalized allergic reactions and nausea/vomiting, which occurred using previous animal glucagon formulations, may still occur with the new product formulation but at a reduced rate.

All glucose pumps for subcutaneous infusion of insulin were not created equal. On at least three occasions one system had delivered 150–200 IU of extra insulin during long airline flights, causing nearly catastrophic hypoglycemia (Midthjell et al., 1994). Low atmospheric pressure on an airtight pump system had produced suction of the piston within insulin cartridges. Whatever pump system is used, carrying emergency intravenous glucose administration equipment, while informing fellow travelers and airline personnel may be prudent, even if the infusion system has clearly been tested and guaranteed for equilibration of pressures at higher altitudes.

Diabetes, Ocular Disease and Travel

Some forms of diabetic retinal disease and surgery could be relative contraindications to prolonged flights requiring pressurized cabins. Daniele and Daniele (1995) reported a 62-year-old woman who had bilateral panretinal laser treatment (argon photocoagulation) for diabetic retinopathy and cystoid macular degeneration. Prolonged flights, totaling 42 h, may have severely exacerbated retinal hypoxia and cystoid macular degeneration. The authors postulated an inability of the diabetic retina to respond to hypoxia nearly 1 year after laser treatments. These authors also warn that recent operations on cornea, retina or cataracts must be closely monitored. Cases of central retinal vein occlusion and other forms of chorioretinopathy have been linked to air travel.

High Altitude: An Issue for the Traveling Diabetic?

If oxygen delivery to the retina is compromised both by high altitude and diabetes, what are the implications for pre-existing retinopathy? There is a known high incidence of retinal hemorrhages in climbers, observed at about 18 000 feet (5500 m), suggesting the combination of diabetic retinopathy and high altitude could have serious implications for a diabetic climber. Interactions, if any, are unclear, but any diabetic traveler must not ignore visual symptoms at high altitude that suggest hemorrhage.

Giordano et al. (1989) tested the performance of seven commercial blood glucose testing systems at high elevations (6800 feet (2100 m) and higher). Both relative humidity and partial pressure of oxygen (altitude) seriously altered their performance. Six of seven tested systems underestimated true blood glucose enough to prompt a patient response. Patients monitoring blood glucose must correct for such errors by testing their glucose standards and correcting measured blood values during flights and while on high-altitude treks.

Common Infections in the Traveling Diabetic

Diabetic travelers are at risk for other serious infections while traveling abroad on the basis of their predilection for cutaneous Gram-positive infections, neuropathies, vascular compromise, and abnormal phagocytic cell function. Unnoticed foot trauma from new footwear or hiking shoes may lead to diabetic foot ulcers and osteomyelitis. Careful instructions regarding local care of early ulcers, changes of socks to avoid persistent pressure points, and careful wound dressings at night to supplement the use of antibiotics are necessary to prevent cellulitis and lymphangitis. Both staphylococci and Group B streptococci are important pathogens under these circumstances.

Pyomyositis. The diabetic who engages in strenuous sports or long arduous treks adds additional risk factors for the development of serious skeletal muscle infection with *Staphylococcus aureus*. Strenuous muscle activity, local abrasions, cutaneous infections during travel, infected insect bites, and muscle trauma in particular (Belsky *et al.*, 1994), can predispose to muscle infection in diabetic patients. The same is true for the HIV-infected patient. Pathogens are predominately *S. aureus* but also include other species such as groups B, C and G streptococci, and occasionally facultative Gram-negative organisms or anaerobes.

Urinary tract infections are more common in women with diabetes, particularly if fluid intake has been decreased. Risk during travel may be associated with increased sexual activity on vacation: Gram-negative enteric flora or enterococci are the major offenders, unless there has been prior use of antibiotics or vaginal candidasis is present. Upper tract disease (renal carbuncle, perinephric abscess or renal papillary necrosis) occurs more commonly in diabetic patients. It should be anticipated by utilization of a 2 week antibiotic regimen for such infections, rather than short-course therapy.

Community-acquired pneumonia may be more severe in diabetic patients and it may require both hospitalization and broader antibiotic coverage for other organisms which are less common in nondiabetics, such as *S. aureus*, Gram-negative organisms, or even *Mycobacterium tuberculosis*. Oral antibiotics may not always prove to be adequate for all infections in diabetics. Nephrotoxic agents must be avoided, particularly when renal insufficiency is already present, as should the additional burden of ototoxic drugs in patients who already have the potential for impaired vision from diabetes.

Immunizations should include annual influenza vaccine and pneumococcal vaccine, in addition to purified protein derivative (PPD) skin testing *before and after* any travel that includes added tuberculosis risk, such as medical work in endemic regions. The risk of tuberculosis for diabetics is also several-fold higher than that of the general population.

Candidasis. Diabetics readily colonize and develop clinical infections with *Candida* spp. Patients receiving oral doxycycline for malaria prophylaxis would be at particu-larly increased risk, and should be prepared to treat the first appearances of candidal infections.

Melioidosis, insulin and the diabetes connection. The medical literature originating from geographic areas where melioidosis is an endemic disease, such as Southeast Asia and northern Australia, makes frequent reference to its clinical associations with diabetes mellitus. The causative organism, *Burkholderia pseudomallei*, has a unique ability to bind human insulin, and this bacterial property may underlie a remarkable biological and clinical relationship, with important implications for diabetics traveling to endemic areas (Woods *et al.*, 1993). The geographic distribution of this disease is wider than we had appreciated in the past.

The causative organism gained notoriety during both the French and American involvement in Indo-China, such that by 1973 over 340 cases had been described among American soldiers fighting in Vietnam, with helicopter pilots at greater risk of infection from soil blown around by rotor blades. The geographic extent of disease distribution was later found to reach the northern rice-growing regions of Thailand, Australia and even the Caribbean basin. It continues to expand (Dance, 1999).

B. (formerly *Pseudomonas*) *pseudomallei* can be isolated from both soil and water, and it is particularly prevalent in rice paddies during the rainy season. Infections seem to be acquired by several routes, including inoculation and inhalation. Melioidosis is a seasonal disease, with a majority of cases occurring during the rainy seasons among those who are regularly in contact with soil and water. Males predominate and the peak age incidence ranges from ages 40 to 60.

In endemic regions, melioidosis accounts for an unusually high proportion of community-acquired sepsis, being the most common source of fatal community-acquired sepsis in the northern territories of Australia. Most patients have an underlying metabolic or disease process such as alcohol abuse, an immunosuppressive disorder, diabetes mellitus, renal disease, liver disease or pregnancy, although melioidosis does not appear to be an AIDS-associated opportunistic infection. Melioidosis may be localized or disseminated and might only present clinically after many years of bacterial latency.

Travel medicine consultants should be aware that all diabetics (both type I and type II) with the appropriate exposure to infected soil and water are clearly predisposed to severe melioidosis when physiologic insulin levels are not maintained. Although type I diabetes and insulin deficiency do not fully explain the predisposition of all diabetics for melioidosis, human insulin levels do appear to play a unique role in modulating the pathogenesis of infection and septicemia associated with melioidosis. Review such emerging epidemiological data and advise travelers, particularly diabetic patients, of the risks of acquiring melioidosis during their travel to endemic regions as this information is further refined.

SPECIAL CONSIDERATIONS FOR OLDER TRAVELERS

Although pretravel counseling usually emphasizes the prevention of infectious and tropical diseases—and certainly these should be addressed in the elderly—it is important to realize that travelers rarely die from these illnesses (Guptill *et al.*, 1991; Hargarten *et al.*, 1991). Almost 75% of deaths in travelers result from cardiovascular disease and injury (Hargarten *et al.*, 1991). Pretravel advice for elderly travelers, even those in excellent health, and those with chronic medical conditions must therefore include risk reduction strategies for noninfectious health problems, as well as education regarding the management of the potential medical complications of travel.

Health care standards during travel may differ from those of industrialized nations. Illness or hospitalization in foreign countries, where communication can be difficult, may be particularly stressful for the elderly, and stress can often be prevented with appropriate advice (Patterson, 1992). Some simple but easily overlooked preparations prior to travel will eliminate unnecessary delays and contribute to a healthy, enjoyable travel experience.

Motion Sickness

Nonpharmacological methods to reduce motion sickness include closing the eyes, focusing on the horizon, and limiting head and neck movements. Medications such as dimenhydrinate, diphenhydramine, and hyoscine can provide symptomatic relief but cause anticholinergic and other side-effects, such as drowsiness and confusion, with increased frequency in elderly travelers. Hyoscine inhibits sweating and can contribute to heatstroke, particularly in warm climates; it is contraindicated in individuals with glaucoma and prostatic hypertrophy.

Jet Lag

The elderly may be more susceptible to jet lag. A well-rested state and adaptation of normal routines to the current time of day upon arrival at the destination can aid in reducing jet lag. Benzodiazepines, while providing some relief from sleep disturbances, may cause drowsiness, impaired memory, and fatigue with increased frequency in the older traveler unaccustomed to taking these medications. Melatonin is of unclear benefit for the treatment of jet lag (Spitzer *et al.*, 1999).

Heatstroke and Hypothermia

The elderly are also more susceptible to the effects of extreme temperatures. Adapting to a different climate may take several days, during which limitation of outdoor activity is advisable. Gradual acclimatization before travel, if possible, facilitates this adjustment. Adequate hydration and appropriate clothing are essential in both hot and cold climates. In hot climates, anticholinergic agents as well as beta blockers, calcium antagonists, diuretics, antihistamines, and tricyclic antidepressants may impair thermoregulation, worsen dehydration, or precipitate heatstroke.

Thromboembolic Disease

Individuals with known venous disorders (venous stasis, prior episodes of venous thrombosis) and cardiac disease may have an increased risk of venous thrombosis, with or without pulmonary embolism, during travel. Dehydration and prolonged immobilization alone may be sufficient stimuli for these to occur in some travelers (Cruickshank *et al.*, 1988; Bia and Barry, 1992). Symptoms may develop during flight, or not until several days later.

Contracting leg muscles frequently while seated, frequent short walks, when safe to do so, and adequate hydration with nonalcoholic beverages may help reduce the risk of thromboembolic disease. Compression stockings and pharmacological prophylaxis (aspirin or subcutaneous heparin) may be indicated for high-risk patients, but are not recommended for most travelers.

Injuries and Accidents

Injury is the second most common cause of death overall in Americans traveling outside the United States; only cardiovascular deaths occur more frequently (Hargarten *et al.*, 1991; Paixao *et al.*, 1991; Sniezek and Smith, 1991; Prociv, 1995). At some travel destinations, however, Americans die primarily as a result of injury, and usually without ever reaching a hospital (Guptill *et al.*, 1991). Even if transport to a hospital occurs, many will not have adequate trauma facilities and evacuation may be required. Leading causes of deaths due to injury include car accidents, drowning, and homicides (Hargarten *et al.*, 1991). Elderly travelers may be at higher risk for car accidents and other injuries due to slower reaction times, visual and/or auditory impairments, and adverse effects of medications.

Malaria

The incidence of severe illness and death due to malaria increases with age (Dessery *et al.*, 1997). Personal protective measures apply to the elderly as they would to younger travelers. Potential neurotoxicity from DEET (*N,N*-diethyl-3-methylbenzamide) is not of concern for the elderly (Veltri, 1994; Fradin, 1998). Chemoprophylactic agents can be safely administered in the healthy older traveler and may in fact be better tolerated than in younger travelers (Dessery *et al.*, 1997).

Mefloquine should be used with caution in the presence of cardiac conduction defects (such as bifascicular block), and is contraindicated in those with seizure disorders and psychiatric disturbances. Mefloquine is no longer contraindicated in those taking beta blockers and/or calcium antagonists. No dose adjustment is required for travelers with renal failure.

Chloroquine has been reported to cause irreversible retinal damage when used in the presence of known retinal disorders. Severe, irreversible hearing loss has also occurred with brief exposure in individuals with pre-existing auditory disturbances. Alternatives should be considered.

Vaccine-Preventable Illnesses

Routine immunizations (measles/mumps/rubella, polio, tetanus toxoid, varicella, if appropriate) should be updated prior to travel. One dose of 23-valent pneumococcal vaccine and annual influenza immunization are recommended for healthy adults 65 years and older, and for high-risk individuals below age 65.

Age alone is not a contraindication to any vaccine, although seroconversion rates may decrease with age. For the healthy older traveler, general recommendations for both routine and travel vaccines apply. Hepatitis A seropositivity rates are higher in older travelers who have lived in or traveled extensively to endemic areas, or have a prior history of jaundice; serologic hepatitis A antibody screening prior to immunization in these individuals may be cost-effective (Castelli *et al.*, 1996; Schwartz and Raveh, 1998).

Live vaccines (oral typhoid, oral polio, varicella, yellow fever) should not be given routinely to immunocompromised travelers. Elderly travelers are at higher risk of adverse events related to yellow fever vaccine (Martin *et al.*, 1999). Immunologically impaired individuals, including those on hemodialysis, require a higher vaccine dose for hepatitis B (usually double, but consult the manufacturer's recommendations).

ADVICE FOR THE DISABLED TRAVELER

The Visually Impaired Traveler

Travelers needing eyeglasses should take an extra pair during travel, as well as a copy of their current prescription. Tools for emergency eyeglass repairs, sold in pharmacies or at opticians' offices, may come in handy.

Contact lens wearers should take all required equipment and solutions with them, as well as an extra pair of glasses. Iodine-purified water should *not* be used for lens care as it will permanently stain lenses. Daily disposable contact lenses are an attractive, relatively inexpensive, maintenance-free alternative to conventional contact lenses.

Blind travelers may prefer to travel with a companion, who may be eligible for discounted fares. If this is not possible, special arrangements can be made ahead of time to facilitate check-in, transfers, etc. Inquiries should be made at the time of booking. International travel with guide dogs can be a problem; certain countries will impose quarantine for imported animals. Travelers should contact the embassy or consulate of their destination(s) if considering travel with a guide dog, and should remember to inquire at home about restrictions for re-entry after travel.

The Hearing-Impaired Traveler

Travelers who rely on hearing aids should carry extra batteries for their units. Hearing impaired and deaf travelers may also benefit from traveling with a companion and discount airfares may apply. They should inform transportation carriers of their hearing impairment if overhead announcements are likely to go unheard, and can request that information be delivered to them individually.

The Physically Disabled Traveler

The physically disabled traveler should discuss his or her specific needs with the travel agent. Facilities and assistance that can be provided during travel and at the destination(s) should be confirmed prior to booking. Help with boarding and disembarking may be requested and/or required. Disabled travelers should not expect flight attendants to help them with eating, administering medications, or providing assistance in washrooms. If the degree of assistance required during travel is beyond that which can be provided by flight attendants, the carrier may not allow travel unless the individual is accompanied by a companion. Discount fares for travel companions are often available. A recent ruling states that cruise ships, whether registered in the United States or abroad, must accommodate disabled travelers under the Americans with Disabilities Act.

Personal mobility devices, including wheelchairs, canes, crutches, and folding walkers, can usually be stored in the aircraft cabin. Transfer to smaller wheelchairs, which should be provided by the airline, may be required to board certain aircraft. Wheelchairs cannot yet be accommodated in most aircraft washrooms; the carrier can provide details regarding washroom space, if requested.

Wheelchair batteries may be damaged in baggage compartments. It is the airline's responsibility to transport mobility devices intact. If any device is damaged in transit, the carrier is obliged to pay for repairs or replace it with a similar model, and to provide a temporary replacement if needed. To avoid these problems, lightweight or smaller sized, nonmotorized wheelchairs may be preferable for travel. Tools for emergency repairs may be invaluable.

CONSIDERATIONS FOR TRAVELERS WITH OTHER CHRONIC MEDICAL CONDITIONS

Cardiovascular Disease

Cardiovascular diseases, including myocardial infarction and cerebrovascular events, are the leading causes of death, accounting for 49% of all deaths in American travelers outside the United States; most occur in those 55 years of age and older (Hargarten *et al.*, 1991; Paixao *et al.*, 1991; Sneizek and Smith, 1991; Prociv, 1995). Cardiac events accounted for 11% of medical emergencies in travelers at the Seattle-Tacoma International Airport over a 1 year period, occurring both within the airport, where they accounted for 7% of all airport emergencies, and in the air, where they accounted for 20% of all inflight emergencies (Cummins and Schubach, 1989).

Cummins *et al.* (1988) reviewed 577 deaths which occurred during flight between the years 1977 and 1984, of which 56% were attributed to cardiac events. Most (66%) occurred in men, with a mean age of about 54 years. Strikingly, cardiac deaths in apparently healthy travelers were common, accounting for 63% of all deaths in this group and 78% of all sudden cardiac deaths. Sudden cardiac events during flight frequently necessitate unscheduled landings, which can be especially problematic during overseas flights.

For individuals with cardiovascular disease, contraindications to air travel include myocardial infarction, uncontrolled angina, congestive heart failure, and/or significant dysrhythmias within the previous month, or cerebrovascular infarction within the past 2 weeks (Table 26.1). Implanted cardiac devices are not contraindications to flying. Proper functioning of such devices should be ensured prior to travel, and batteries replaced if needed. Electronic pacemaker checks by phone cannot yet be relayed by satellite from overseas destinations, but relay will soon be available aboard aircraft (Micromedical Biolog monitors). It may be prudent to determine the facility closest to the travel destination that is best equipped to service travelers with such devices in the event of an emergency. It is important to note that portable security magnets may interfere with the functioning of an implantable defibrillator; a physician's letter may be useful for such travelers. Supplemental oxygen may be required for some travelers with cardiovascular disease. Guidelines for assessing oxygen requirements are discussed in the following section.

Pulmonary Disease

Most commercial aircraft cruise at altitudes between 22 000 and 44 000 feet (6706 to 13 411 m) above sea level. Cabin pressure equivalent to sea-level pressure can be maintained up to an altitude of roughly 22 500 feet (6858 m). Above this altitude, the partial pressure of oxygen begins to fall and active cabin pressurization is required, resulting in an atmosphere equivalent to that found between 5000 and 8000 feet (1529 and 2438 m) above sea level.

Active cabin pressurization can adversely affect sinusitis and otitis. Air travel is contraindicated in those with pneumothorax or pneumomediastinum, and should be delayed for several weeks following middle-ear or thoracic surgery (Gong, 1991). The reduction in atmospheric oxygen during flight, while well tolerated by healthy travelers, can lead to marked hypoxemia in travelers with cardiopulmonary compromise, although the clinical significance of this is not completely clear (Gong, 1992). Dillard *et al.* (1991) found that pulmonary symptoms, including dyspnea, edema, wheezing, chest pain, and cyanosis, worsened during flight in 8 of 44 travelers (18.2%) with chronic obstructive lung disease. Assessment of the need for supplemental oxygen is therefore recommended in travelers with underlying cardiopulmonary disease.

The minimum desired PaO_2 during flight is 50 mmHg, and supplemental oxygen should be used if the predicted PaO_2 will be below this level. Using a hypoxia–altitude simulation test (HAST), Gong *et al.* (1984) determined that the arterial oxygen tension (PaO_2) measured at sea level in normocapnic individuals with chronic airway obstruction is the best predictor of the resting PaO_2 at a given altitude. They developed a nomogram that can be used to predict the estimated PaO_2 during flight (Figure 26.1). Using the HAST, a sea level PaO_2 of 72 mmHg correlates to a PaO_2 of at least 50 mmHg in a cabin altitude of 8000 feet (2438 m) in most normocapnic individuals.

The inspired oxygen concentration (FiO_2) required during flight can be estimated using several methods. For travelers who do not require supplemental oxygen on land, an FiO_2 of 30% (2 l min^{-1}) should be adequate. The HAST nomogram can be used, with baseline PaO_2 measured using supplemental oxygen. Alternatively, Dillard *et al.* (1989) devised a formula which also incorporates the measured forced expiratory volume in the first second (FEV_1):

$$PaO_2 \text{ (at 8000 feet)} = [0.519(PaO_2 \text{ at sea level})] + [11.855(FEV_1 \text{ in litres})] - 1.760$$

Regardless of the method used, the PaO_2 (and FEV_1, if used) should be measured within 2 weeks of scheduled travel (Gong, 1989).

Pulmonary function should be optimized prior to and during flight by using bronchodilators and/or corticosteroids, if indicated. If oxygen is required, provide the airline with at least 48 h notice prior to scheduled departure. A prescription for oxygen (indicating the flow rate or FiO_2, and specifying continuous versus intermittent oxygen) is required, as is a physician's letter outlining the individual's fitness to travel. Inflight oxygen and equipment will be supplied by the carrier, at a cost to the traveler, usually based on flight segments and/or the number of oxygen canisters required. Check with the air carrier for charges, and be aware that delivery systems

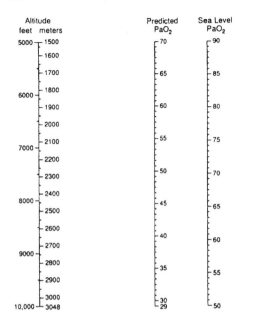

Figure 26.1 Nomogram for predicting altitude Pao_2 (mmHg) between 5000 and 10 000 feet (1524 and 3048 m) in normocapnic patients with chronic airway obstruction at sea level. A straight line connecting sea-level Pao_2 and the anticipated altitude will intersect the altitude Pao_2 at the appropriate value. Reproduced with permission from Gong H *et al.* (1984) Hypoxia-altitude simulation test. Evaluation of patients with chronic airway obstruction. *American Review of Respiratory Diseases*, **130**, 980–986. Official Journal of the American Thoracic Society. © American Lung Association

may vary. Airline attendants can provide basic assistance such as changing canisters, but should not be expected to assist if mechanical problems arise. If oxygen is required during layovers or at the final destination(s), delivery should be arranged well in advance. The traveler's regular oxygen vendor should be able to assist with these arrangements. Payment may be required when services are delivered, and may or may not be reimbursed by insurance plans.

On any flight where smoking is still permitted, seating away from the smoking section should be requested. Adequate hydration will facilitate the clearance of pulmonary secretions in bronchitic travelers. Tracheostomies should not be expected to pose significant problems during travel; the traveler should bring any equipment required for care.

Gastrointestinal Disorders

Travelers with reduced gastric acidity or inflammatory bowel disease may benefit from travelers' diarrhea prophylaxis. Because intestinal gas expands with altitude, air travel following abdominal surgery should be delayed for

several weeks if possible. Travelers with colostomies should use a larger bag and have an extra bag on hand for the same reason.

Anemia

Hypoxemia with altitude may adversely affect travelers with severe anemia (hemoglobin less that $7.5\,g\,dL^{-1}$ or $75\,g\,L^{-1}$) and sickle cell disease. If anemia is not correctable with red blood cell transfusion, supplemental oxygen should be used during flight.

Orthopedic Conditions

Travelers with lower extremity fractures should keep the leg elevated as much as possible, to reduce swelling and circulatory impairment. A bivalved cast that can accommodate some limb expansion may also be helpful. Some orthopedic fixation devices can trigger security alarms at airports. A physician's letter outlining the presence of the device can be useful if this occurs.

Neuropsychiatric Disorders

Air travel is not contraindicated in individuals with seizure disorders, but seizures should be well controlled. Modification of therapy prior to travel is probably unnecessary, contrary to many airlines' recommendations (Nassar *et al.*, 1998). Epileptic travelers should inform flight attendants of their disorder, and emergency medications with instructions for their use should be carried with the traveler. Mefloquine is contraindicated in those with known seizure and psychiatric disorders.

Individuals with increased intracranial pressure should be advised against air travel. Rarely, undiagnosed cerebral mass lesions have presented during flight (Shlim and Meijer, 1991).

In summary, organized, tailored advice may enable persons with complicated medical issues to embark safely upon their ever-increasing opportunities to travel to potentially risky parts of the world.

REFERENCES

Backer H (1997) Medical limitations to wilderness travel. *Emergency Medicine Clinics of North America*, **15**, 17–41.

Belsky DS, Teates CD and Hartman ML (1994) Case report: diabetes mellitus as a predisposing factor in the development of pyomyositis. *American Journal of Medical Sciences*, **308**, 251–254.

Bia FJ and Barry M (1992) Special health considerations for travelers. *Medical Clinics of North America*, **76**, 1295–1312.

Castelli F, Carosi G, Tebaldi A *et al.* (1996) Age-specific anti-hepatitis A virus seroepidemiology in Italian travelers: indications for anti-hepatitis A vaccination. *Journal of Travel Medicine*, **3**, 214–218.

Conlon CP (2000) Travel and the immunocompromised host. *Hospital Medicine*, **61**, 167–170.

Cruickshank JM, Gorlin R and Jennett B (1988) Air travel and thrombotic episodes: the economy class syndrome. *Lancet*, **ii**, 497–498.

Cummins RO and Schubach JA (1989) Frequency and types of medical emergencies among commercial air travelers. *Journal of the American Medical Association*, **261**, 1295–1299.

Cummins RO, Chapman PJC, Chamberlain DA et al. (1988) In-flight deaths during commercial air travel. How big is the problem? *Journal of the American Medical Association*, **259**, 1983–1988.

Dance DAB (1999) Melioidosis. In *Tropical Infectious Diseases. Principles, Pathogens and Practice* (eds RL Guerrant, DH Walker and PF Weller), pp 430–437. Churchill Livingstone, Philadelphia.

Daniele S and Daniele C (1995) Aggravation of laser-treated diabetic cystoid macular edema after prolonged flight: a case report. *Aviation, Space and Environmental Medicine*, **66**, 440–442.

Dessery BL, Robin MR and Pasini W (1997) In *Textbook of Travel Medicine and Health* (eds HL DuPont and R Steffen), pp 320–328. Decker, Hamilton, Ontario.

Dewey CM and Riley WJ (1999) Have diabetes, will travel. *Postgraduate Medicine*, **105**, 111–126.

Dillard TA, Berg BW, Rajagopal KR et al. (1989) Hypoxemia during air travel in patients with chronic obstructive pulmonary disease. *Annals of Internal Medicine*, **111**, 362–367.

Dillard TA, Beninati WA and Berg BW (1991) Air travel in patients with chronic obstructive pulmonary disease. *Archives of Internal Medicine*, **151**, 1793–1795.

Driessen SL, Cobelens FGJ and Litghelm RJ (1999) Travel-related morbidity in travelers with insulin-dependent diabetes mellitus. *Journal of Travel Medicine*, **6**, 12–15.

El Sayed NM, Gomatos, PJ, Beck-Sagué CM et al. (2000) Epidemic transmission of human immunodeficiency virus in renal dialysis centers in Egypt. *Journal of Infectious Diseases*, **181**, 91–97.

Fradin MS (1998) Mosquitoes and mosquito repellents: a clinician's guide. *Annals of Internal Medicine*, **128**, 931–940.

Giordano BP, Thrash W, Hollenbaugh L et al. (1989) Performance of seven blood glucose testing systems at high altitude. *Diabetes Educator*, **15**, 444–448.

Gong H (1989) Advising patients with pulmonary diseases on air travel. *Annals of Internal Medicine*, **111**, 349–351.

Gong H (1991) Air travel and patients with pulmonary and allergic conditions. *Journal of Allergy and Clinical Immunology*, **87**, 879–885.

Gong H (1992) Air travel and oxygen therapy in cardiopulmonary patients. *Chest*, **101**, 1104–1113.

Gong H, Tashkin DP, Lee EY et al. (1984) Hypoxia-altitude simulation test. Evaluation of patients with chronic airway obstruction. *American Review of Respiratory Diseases*, **130**, 980–986.

Guptill KS, Hargarten SW and Baker TD (1991) American travel deaths in Mexico. Causes and prevention strategies. *Western Journal of Medicine*, **154**, 169–171.

Hargarten SW, Baker TD and Guptill K (1991) Overseas fatalities of United States citizen travelers: an analysis of deaths related to international travel. *Annals of Emergency Medicine*, **20**, 622–626.

Holleman F and Hoekstra JBL (1997) Insulin lispro. *New England Journal of Medicine*, **337**, 176–183.

Hultgren NH (1990) Coronary heart disease and trekking. *Journal of Wilderness Medicine*, **1**, 154–161.

Jong EC and Benson EA (1997) Travel with chronic medical conditions. In *The Travel and Tropical Medicine Manual* (eds EC Jong and R McMullen), 2nd edn, pp 142–150. WB Saunders Company, Philadelphia.

Kobel D-E, Friedel A, Cerny T et al. (2000) Pneumococcal vaccine in patients with absent or dysfunctional spleen. *Mayo Clinic Proceedings*, **75**, 749–753.

Lynch AM and Kapila R (1996) Overwhelming postsplenectomy infection. *Infectious Disease Clinics of North America*, **10**, 693–707.

McDonald E, Jarrell MP, Schiffman G et al. (1984) Persistence of pneumococcal antibodies after immunization in patients with systemic lupus erythematosus. *Journal of Rheumatology*, **11**, 306–308.

Martin M, Letteau L, Steele S et al. (1999) Advanced age as a risk factor for serious adverse events due to yellow fever vaccine. *Program of the 6th Conference of the International Society of Travel Medicine*, Montreal, Quebec, p. 74 (abstract A-12).

Medical Letter (1996) Lispro, a rapid-onset insulin. *Medical Letter*, **38**, 97–98.

Midthjell K, Kapelrud H, Bjørnerud A et al. (1994) Severe or life-threatening hypoglycemia in insulin pump treatment. *Diabetes Care*, **17**, 1235–1236 and letter (comment) **18**, 1201.

Mileno MD and Bia FJ (1998) The compromised traveler. *Infectious Disease Clinics of North America*, **12**, 369–412.

Nassar NN, Keiser P and Gregg CR (1998) Keeping travelers healthy. *American Journal of the Medical Sciences*, **315**, 327–336.

Noble SL, Johnston E and Walton B (1998) Insulin lispro: a fast-acting insulin analog. *American Family Physician*, **57**, 279–286.

O'Neal BJ and McDonald JC (1981) The risk of sepsis in the asplenic adult. *Annals of Surgery*, **194**, 775–778.

Paixao MLT, Dewar RD, Cossar JH et al. (1991) What do Scots die of when abroad? *Scottish Medical Journal*, **36**, 114–116.

Patterson JE (1992) The pre-travel medical evaluation: the traveler with chronic illness and the geriatric traveler. *Yale Journal of Biology and Medicine*, **65**, 317–327.

Prociv P (1995) Deaths of Australian travellers overseas. *Medical Journal of Australia*, **163**, 27–30.

Roshan M, Burden R and Murden M (1996) Indo-Asians with diabetes: a special case. *Practitioner*, **240**, 120–124.

Sane T, Kovisto VA, Nikkanen P et al. (1990) Adjustment of insulin doses of diabetic patients during long distance flights. *BMJ*, **301**, 421–422.

Schwartz E and Raveh D (1998) The prevalence of hepatitis A antibodies among Israeli travellers and the economic feasibility of screening before vaccination. *International Journal of Epidemiology*, **27**, 118–120.

Shlim DR and Meijer HJ (1991) Suddenly symptomatic brain tumors at altitude. *Annals of Emergency Medicine*, **20**, 315–316.

Sniezek JE and Smith SM (1991) Injury mortality among non-US residents in the United States, 1977–1984. *International Journal of Epidemiology*, **19**, 225–229.

Spitzer RL, Terman M, Williams JB et al. (1999) Jet lag: clinical features, validation of a new syndrome-specific scale, and lack of response to melatonin in a randomized, double-blind trial. *American Journal of Psychiatry*, **156**, 1392–1396.

Stark K, Gunther M, Neuhaus R et al. (1999) Immunogenicity and safety of hepatitis A vaccine in liver and renal transplant recipients. *Journal of Infectious Diseases*, **180**, 2014–2017.

Styrt BA (1996) Risks of infection and protective strategies for the asplenic patient. *Infectious Diseases in Clinical Practice*, **5**, 94–100.

Tellier R and Keystone JS (1992) Prevention of traveler's diarrhea. *Infectious Disease Clinics of North America*, **6**, 333–354.

Veltri JC, Osimitz TG, Bradford DC *et al.* (1994) Retrospective analysis of calls to poison control centers resulting from exposure to the insect repellent *N,N*-diethyl-*m*-toluamide (DEET) from 1985–1989. *Journal of Toxicology and Clinical Toxicology*, **32**, 1–16.

Woods DE, Jones AL and Hill PJ (1993) Interaction of insulin with *Pseudomonas pseudomallei*. *Infection and Immunity*, **61**, 4045–4050.

ADDITIONAL RESOURCES

General Travel Information

Rose SR (1998) *International Travel Health Guide, 10th* edn. Available in bookstores, or from Travel Medicine, Inc.
Tel: (800) 872 8633 or (413) 584 0381
Web site: www.travmed.com
e-mail: travmed@travmed.com

Centers for Disease Control and Prevention International Travelers' Hotline
Tel: (404) 639 8105
Web site: www.cdc.gov

World Health Organization Headquarters
Avenue Appia 20
1211 Geneva 27, Switzerland
Tel: + 41 22 791 2111
Web site: www.who.int
e-mail: info@who.ch

Medical Services

Medic Alert Foundation
2323 Colorado Avenue
Turlock, CA 95382-2018, USA
Tel: (800) 432 5378
Web site: www.medicalert.org
e-mail: customer__service@medicalert.org

250 Ferrand Drive, Suite 301
Toronto, ON M3C 3G8, Canada
Tel: (800) 668 1507

International Association for Medical Assistance to Travelers (IAMAT)
417 Center Street
Lewiston, NY 14092, USA
Tel: (716) 754 4883
Web site: www.sentex.net/~iamat
e-mail: iamat@sentex.net

40 Regal Road
Guelph, ON N1K 1B5, Canada
Tel: (519) 836 0102

Personal Physicians Worldwide
815 Connecticut Avenue NW
Washington, DC 20006, USA
Tel: (888) 657 8114 (from the USA) or (301) 657 8114
Web site: www.executivephysicians.com
e-mail: doctors@executivephysicians.com

Shoreland's EnCompass
Web site: www.shoreland.com

Medical Travel Insurance

International SOS
PO Box 11568
Philadelphia, PA 31685, USA
Tel: (800) 523 8930
Web site: www.internationalsos.com

Worldwide Assistance Services
1133 15th Street NW, Suite 400
Washington, DC 20005, USA
Tel: (800) 821 2828 or (202) 331 1609

TravMed
Box 10623
Baltimore, MD 21285-0623, USA
Tel: (800) 732 5309 or (410) 296 5225

HealthCare Abroad
243 Church Street NW, Suite 100-D
Vienna, VA 22180, USA
Tel: (800) 237 6615 or (703) 281 9500

Major Credit Card Companies (e.g. American Express, Visa)

Visually Impaired Travelers

American Council of the Blind
1155 15th Street NW, Suite 1004
Washington, DC 20005, USA
Tel: (800) 424 8666 or (202) 467 5081
Web site: www.acb.org
e-mail: info@acb.org

Canadian National Institute for the Blind (Head Office)
1929 Bayview Avenue
Toronto, ON M4G 3E8, Canada
Tel: (416) 480 7580
Web site: www.cnib.ca

Hearing-Impaired Travelers

Alexander Graham Bell Association for the Deaf
3417 Volta Place NW
Washington, DC 20007-2778, USA
Tel: (202) 337 5220
TTY: (202) 337 5221
Web site: www.agbell.org

National Association for the Deaf
814 Thayer Avenue
Silver Spring, MD 20910, USA
Tel: (301) 587 1788
TTY: (301) 587 1789

Web site: www.nad.org
e-mail: NADinfo@nad.org

Travelers on Hemodialysis

Creative Age Publications (publishes list of dialysis centers worldwide for $US10)
7628 Densmore Avenue
Van Nuys, CA 91406, USA
Tel: (800) 442 5667 (from the USA) or (818) 782 7328

International Dialysis Organization
153 rue du Port
69390 Fernaison, France
Tel: + 33 72301230

Dialysis Traveler/Dialysis at Sea Cruises
801 West Bay Drive
Largo, FL 33770, USA
Tel: (800) 544 7604 or (727) 518 7311
Web site: www.dialysis-at-sea.com
e-mail: dasc@dialysis-at-sea.com

Dialysis Travel and Vacations
7969 Engineer Road, Suite 105
San Diego, CA 92111, USA
Tel: (800) 771 4878
Web site: www.dtv.tierranet.com

Physically Disabled Travelers

Society for Advancement of Travel for the Handicapped
347 Fifth Avenue, Suite 610
New York, NY 10016, USA
Tel: (212) 447 0027
Web site: www.trav.org/sath

Canadian Transportation Agency
Tel: (800) 883 1813 or (819) 997 6828
TTY: (800) 669 5575 or (819) 953 9705
Web site: www.cta-otc.gc.ca

Mobility International
25 rue de Manchester
B-1070 Brussels, Belgium

27

Aid Workers, Expatriates and Travel

Kenneth L. Gamble

Missionary Health Institute, Toronto, Canada

Debbie Lovell

University of Oxford, Oxford, UK

Ted Lankester

InterHealth, London, UK

Jay S. Keystone

University of Toronto, Toronto, Canada

INTRODUCTION

Expatriates, defined as individuals who go overseas to accomplish a job-related goal, make up a heterogeneous and poorly defined subset of international travelers; however, other definitions could expand the scope of membership into this community and thus there is no published census that has delineated its size. The United States alone has more than 3500 multinational companies, 25 000 companies with overseas branches and more than 40 000 companies doing business abroad on a sporadic basis. In North America it is estimated that more than 150 000 missionary personnel from various faith backgrounds work in international settings. In the UK two major multinational companies contribute more than 200 000 employees to the pool of 'not home country employees' and in 1996 a survey of 116 aid agencies found that between them they received over 3000 enquiries per week about work opportunities abroad. To this, one would add a variety of other disciplines such as explorers, geologists, miners, ambassadors, military and embassy personnel.

As diverse as the background are the risk factors that impact health. Assignments range from less than 3 months, to permanent contracts. While some enjoy ready access to sophisticated and well-funded medical care, others will live in primitive settings with a minimum of support. Some expatriates, although isolated from amenities found in industrialized countries, live in a relatively simple, predictable and controlled environment. Others

live and work in affluent environments with modern amenities, yet embark on risk-taking diversions throughout their sojourn.

As early as the 1890s mission societies were utilizing medical screening to determine who was 'fit' for international assignments, while instructing those who were hired to pack their belongings in a coffin, so common was the risk of death from infectious diseases, which, with malaria alone, claimed the lives of 60% of missionaries in West Africa during the nineteenth century (Greenwood, 1991).

Added to this were losses from premature attrition related to psychosocial stress. In 1913, Price wrote a paper entitled 'Discussion on the Causes of Invaliding from the Tropics', documenting attrition rates of 40%, the majority (20.6%) 'invalid' because of nervous conditions of a neurasthenia type. Attempting to reduce the rate of premature attrition, many agencies established a health appraisal process that was intended to screen out candidates who might be ill suited for the challenge. In 1920, Culpin introduced psychological screening for employees of the Anglo-Persian oil company and reduced repatriation from 20 to 4% over 5 years. Later, others concluded that the efforts were often in vain (Gordon, 1967).

Risk of illness among expatriates is influenced by a variety of factors that can be extrapolated from those identified among other travelers, including age, sex, behaviour, climate, environment, accidental injury and infectious diseases. However, the complexity of crosscul-

Principles and Practice of Travel Medicine. Edited by Jane N. Zuckerman.

tural assignments and the varied physical and emotional responses to those challenges appears to predispose expatriates to ailments that are not shared by the short-term traveler (Lange et al., 1994a). In 1678, Yohannis Hofer following a study of veterans of the Thirty Years' War, described a series of psychiatric presentations cured by returning home. In 1963, Useem coined the term 'Binational Third Culture' to depict the culture that bridges the Western culture to the host culture in the physical setting of a non-Western society. The children became known as 'Third Culture Kids' or TCKs in recognition of the transcendent culture that they shared with other children who spend or have spent a portion of their developmental years in a culture that was not their own.

Despite a longstanding acceptance of medical and psychological testing, there are relatively little modern published data to improve our understanding of the health risks of expatriates, especially data that would distinguish the physical health risks of this community from risks identified in the short-term traveler. However, there are ample data to demonstrate the impact of crosscultural stress that adds to the diversity and complexity of international assignments. It has been estimated that 60% of all referrals for medical treatment in the Foreign Service has a stress-related basis; therefore it is prudent for health care providers to recognize the factors that could influence both the medical and psychological health status of expatriate personnel (Karson and O'Dell, 1987). In fact the burden of suffering related to the psychosocial burden is more significant than that related to infectious diseases. Frequently, the medical and psychological dimensions are intertwined, making it mandatory to consider a multi-disciplinary approach if care to enhance effectiveness is one of the goals of the health care professional. To that end, both disciplines will be addressed in concert throughout this chapter as the data on morbidity, screening, preparation, care during the international assignment and re-entry are examined.

MORBIDITY, ATTRITION AND MORTALITY AMONG EXPATRIATES

Morbidity

Expatriates are often at increased risk of illness and injury because of conditions and inadequate medical facilities in the areas in which they work, although studies documenting morbidity and mortality among expatriates are too limited to differentiate all of the risks experienced by different subsets. The Peace Corps is the only international agency that published data from a formal epidemiologic surveillance system, which was developed in 1985 to monitor health trends in over 5500 volunteers. The most commonly reported health problems were diarrhea (48 cases per 100 per year), injuries (20 cases per 100 per year) and skin conditions (19 cases per 100 per year). The surveillance data in Peace Corps volunteers 25 years earlier was comparable, although in that series respir-

atory illnesses were also significant (27 cases per 100 per year) (Bernard et al., 1989).

Lange et al. (1994b) looked at morbidity of refugee relief workers in Somalia, Ethiopia and Malaysia. Thirty-eight staff serving the equivalent of 46 person-years reported a total of 49 health problems that resulted in time lost from service. Infectious diseases accounted for the majority of reported illnesses; 57% were related to food-borne agents. The infectious disease experience mirrored that of Peace Corps volunteers.

There is insufficient data to determine the impact of age, sex and geographic location on the burden of illness, although there is a trend toward a greater burden of illness in West Africa. There have been little published data on the rate of repatriation for medical reasons, although it appears to vary widely from one region to another and ranges between 1 and 5% (Peppiatt and Byass, 1991). Psychiatric illness appears to be among the more common causes. The quality of local facilities is likely to account for some of the geographic variance, although that is not well documented.

Prevalence of Psychological Problems among Expatriates

Many describe their time overseas as enjoyable and fulfilling. Making new friends and job satisfaction are usually reported as the best part of the experience (Lovell, 1997). Nevertheless, expatriates as a group encounter a variety of potentially stressful experiences. Difficulties commonly reported include crosscultural adjustment, loneliness, communication problems, unpredictable circumstances, role ambiguity, long working hours, little opportunity to relax or socialize, overwhelming responsibility, ethical dilemmas, and powerlessness. In some countries there are extreme temperatures to contend with, and the living and working conditions may be uncomfortable or dangerous. Some expatriates encounter widescale poverty, injustice, suffering, despair and death. Many do not have any access to any form of psychological support.

In guidelines produced by the International Committee of the Red Cross (ICRC), it is stated that 'Cumulative stress ... affects health personnel and humanitarian workers in particular, as they always have to perform in overwhelming situations, where the demands are such that they can never be met' (ICRC, 1994, p.10).

Expatriates tend to have high ideals and expectations, which may put them at particular risk of experiencing emotional exhaustion or 'burnout' (Chester, 1983; Richardson, 1992). They tend to work very long hours, perhaps because they feel guilty about taking time off when the needs are great, or because they feel that there is little to do in their new environment apart from work. In one study of 200 aid workers, 50% claimed they regularly worked more than 60 h a week. One respondent said that, in retrospect, 'more breaks and less work would have been more efficient, as we were all burnt out' (Macnair, 1995, p. 23).

Given the magnitude of stressors that expatriates may experience, and the lack of help received in coping with these, one might expect to find psychological difficulties among this group. Clinical observation and surveys have supported this hypothesis (Dye, 1974; Austin and Beyer, 1984; Foyle, 1987). In a survey of 390 missionaries, Parshall (1988) found that 97% reported experiencing tension, 88% found anger to be a frequent or occasional problem, and 20% had taken tranquilizers since becoming missionaries. Donovan (1992) stated that 25% of missionaries return home prematurely and 50% were likely to work with reduced efficiency because of stress.

Depression is probably the most common form of psychopathology found among expatriates (Richardson, 1992; Lovell, 1997). Clinicians have suggested that other common reactions include anxiety disorders (including post-traumatic stress disorder, PTSD), drug/alcohol abuse, loss of self-esteem, anger problems, chronic fatigue syndrome and psychosomatic problems (Foyle, 1987; Donovan, 1992; Richardson, 1992; Carr, 1994; Lovell, 1999a).

A few empirical studies have been conducted on the psychological adjustment of expatriates. In a longitudinal study, Paton and Purvis (1995) administered the General Health Questionnaire (GHQ-30) (Goldberg et al., 1976) to a group of 18 nurses before they went to work in Romanian orphanages for 3 months, and again on their return. The nurses were also administered the Impact of Event Scale (IES), Horowitz et al., 1979) on their return. GHQ-30 scores increased significantly during the time in Romania, indicating an increase in health-related problems. On the IES, the nurses reported symptoms of intrusive thoughts and avoidance that resembled those of clinical trauma patients. These symptoms were maintained at 1 month follow-up. In addition, 56% of the nurses reported that they had experienced depression (although this probably indicated low mood rather than clinical depression), and 22% reported sleeping difficulties.

Paton (1992) also found high levels of symptomatology among relief workers in El Salvador, Armenia, Iran and the Philippines. Among those who had worked in Armenia, 75% reported depression.

In another study (Lovell, 1997), aid workers representing 62 different organizations completed questionnaires after returning to their home country. Participants were recruited randomly, and the response rate was remarkably high (82%), with 145 individuals completing the questionnaires. The mean time spent as expatriates was 51 months, although there was a wide range. Forty-six percent of these respondents reported that they had experienced a psychological illness of clinical severity, either while they were away or on their return home. In 87% of cases the primary diagnosis was depression, with another 7% having been clinically diagnosed as having chronic fatigue syndrome, 4% PTSD, and 2% other diagnoses. These figures were based on self-report of clinical diagnoses, but as the responses were anonymous and the sample appeared to be reasonably representative; there is no particular reason to doubt these figures.

In Lovell's (1997) study, expatriates who reported psychological problems were found to have spent significantly longer overseas than those who did not report such problems. This suggests that it might be worth considering shorter contracts (e.g. for 3 years) for expatriates, so that there would be less time for stress to accumulate, and readjustment on return might be easier. Contracts could be renewed after psychological reassessment for those who wished to continue the work.

Another issue raised by Lovell (1997) was that sending agencies were only aware of about one in six of the cases of psychological difficulties among their workers. Many workers chose not to disclose their difficulties to their organization, as they feared that this would interfere with their chances of going overseas again, or of getting promotion or a good reference for another job.

Premature Attrition

Premature attrition was addressed as early as the 1920s and continues to be a major concern. The published data from a global survey conducted among missionary personnel indicate an attrition rate of 3–8% per year in larger organizations, and up to 60% of agencies that have fewer than 10 employees (Brierley, 1997). Health reasons are cited as the most common of the personal reasons for attrition, although the stated reason may not always correspond to the real reason (Gardner, 1984). Not all expatriates are aid workers. Although there has been little research on the mental health of other groups of expatriates, Deshpande and Viswesvaran (1992) stated that an average of 20–40% of all expatriate managers returned home early due to poor performance or an inability to adjust to the new culture. Moreover, nearly half of those who did not return early were reported to function below their normal level of productivity.

Harzing (1995) questioned the high expatriate failure rates that had been reported, stating that there had been few reliable large-scale studies. Perhaps the figures have been exaggerated, but it certainly seems clear that the vast majority of American multinational companies see more than 10% of their expatriates return home prematurely (Tung, 1988). The rate may be much higher among expatriates sent to the countries that are culturally the most different from the USA.

Mortality Data

Studies have found the mortality rate to be doubled among aid and development workers compared with colleagues remaining at home, despite medical selection of healthy applicants for aid work (Schouten and Borgdorff, 1995). In contrast, the adjusted rate among missionary personnel was 40% lower than would be expected in a comparable US population, although mortality risks from homicides and complications of pregnancy were greater (Frame et al., 1992). Suicide emerged as significant in Peace Corps personnel, accounting for 13% of reported deaths compared with < 1% among missionary personnel. Both North American missionaries and Peace Corps personnel were at greatest risk from motor vehicle accidents, with motorcycles accounting for a disproportionate number of deaths (Hargarten and Baker, 1985; Frame *et al.*, 1992). From 1970 to 1985, the rate of death from infectious diseases approximated that reported in the USA; this may change now that HIV exposure has been found to be an occupational risk for aid workers in some parts of the world (Schouten and Borgdorff, 1995).

PREDEPARTURE ASSESSMENT

Purpose of Predeparture Screening

It is estimated that premature attrition could cost the sending agency up to $500 000 per family, more if the assigned task is very specialized. Thus, at a very basic level, predeparture screening could be viewed as a way of protecting that investment, hoping to avert unnecessary premature attrition. However, like alchemists of old, the quest for a universal screening tool that would predict for success has ended in frustration. Legal constraints in many countries prevent employment discrimination based on physical impairment, whereas the laws of host cultures often impose medical restrictions for employment visas. Environmental, climactic and political upheaval could pose other threats that would eliminate some applicants.

Ultimately, from an ethical perspective, one could propose that a thorough health assessment provides baseline data upon which care and health management strategies are founded. The 'Code of Best Practice' established by aid agencies in the UK asserts that the aid worker is the agency's most valuable resource and thus those who ascribe to this code affirm their commitment to maintain and enhance the well-being of their international employees (Davidson, 1997).

Medical Assessment

Medical screening that is limited to a 'complete medical' with a 'pass/fail' outcome has been abandoned in favor of a more selective approach to the prevention and detection of health problems (American College of Physicians, 1981). Protocols based on practice guidelines for preventive care ensure that appropriate general and selective interventions are part of the evaluation while excluding routine testing that has no proven merit (Hayward *et al*, 1991). Many will present for a preassignment medical assessment without a travel history that would prompt screening for geographic specific risk factors: therefore it is sufficient to follow national guidelines that set forth the appropriate general and selective interventions.

General Interventions

General interventions have been defined as services offered to persons who have neither symptoms of, nor risk factors for, a target condition (Hayward *et al.*, 1991). From a cost: benefit perspective, a comprehensive history is the most essential component. From a qualitative perspective, a structured questionnaire will serve to reduce inconsistencies based on external constraints and should:

1. Delineate current health issues that require attention prior to deployment.
2. Identify long-term problems where management issues are significant and could jeopardize the well-being of the individual or compromise the assignment.
3. Determine the risk factors that could predispose one to develop certain conditions during the tenure of service.

There are very few conditions that absolutely contraindicate a crosscultural assignment, particularly if a person is stable medically. The majority of persons will recognize health conditions that are obviously a contraindication and will not embark on such an adventure. However, there are many pre-existing health conditions that could be exacerbated by environmental conditions or other geographic specific risks, and thereby place the individual at greater risk for some illnesses such as cardiac or infectious diseases. After being appraised of the risks the management team and the applicant may re-evaluate their options. For example, an aid worker with reactive airway disease might be assigned to a remote region where access to pharmaceuticals is limited and houses are heated with a low-grade coal. The history reveals that chemical irritants trigger his reactive airway disease. Understanding those risks, the employee might reconsider his placement, or the management team could develop contingency plans in the event that his condition deteriorates.

The physical assessment and laboratory testing should focus on age- and gender-specific risk factors. The outcome of these evaluations could prompt a need for more selective interventions.

Selective Interventions

Selective interventions are services offered to asymptomatic persons with one or more risk factors for a target condition, if there is a significant burden of suffering and if treatment at a preclinical stage offers a better outcome than waiting until after the disease manifests itself. Pulmonary function tests would clearly be justified for the individual noted above because the findings will further clarify the risk, which in turn could impact decisions made by the client and management team.

Appropriate selective interventions for other target conditions, such as diabetes mellitus, coronary artery disease, some types of cancer, osteoporosis and sexually transmitted diseases, should be recommended in accordance to the standard of care in the applicant's country of

Table 27.1 Routine and selective laboratory investigations

Routine tests	Complete blood count
	Urine chemistry test: glucose, blood, protein
Selective screening based on symptoms or identified risk factors	Chest X-ray
	ECG/stress testing
	Glucose
	Hepatitis serology
	Liver function tests
	Sexually transmitted disease screen/HIV
	Thyroid-stimulating hormone
Selective screening based on age- and sex-specific risk factors	Bone density studies
	Cholesterol, triglycerides
	Colon cancer screen
	Mammogram
	Papanicolaou test
	Prostrate-specific antigen
Selective screening based on identified risk factors for parasitic and tropical diseases	Schistosomiasis serology
	Stool for ova and parasites (one)
	Strongyloides serology
	Filaria serology

origin. Understandably, these guidelines vary. Recommendations for colorectal cancer surveillance range from a colonoscopy for all persons over the age of 40 to national guidelines that limit colonoscopy to persons with additional risk factors (Hayward et al., 1991) (Table 27.1).

It is folly to assume that all primary care physicians have already uniformly applied these standards for all of their patients. T.L. Dwelle (personal communication, 1996) evaluated the files of 204 missionaries who were assigned to an international setting and determined that 88% of the records did not have evidence to confirm that the applicant had been appropriately screened for cancer in accordance to the USA guidelines. Furthermore, one could overlook the significance of an equivocal finding in a client who will be living in a remote setting where follow-up testing is both costly and disruptive. Thus, the consultation serves the applicant by apprising him or her of the health risks and serves the agency by delineating the responsibilities that they should assume in the context of placement, services and support.

Psychological Assessment

What sort of person would apply for a job far from family and friends, leaving the comfort of home, their belongings and all that is familiar, to work in a place where he or she would have to learn new skills, customs and maybe even a language, perhaps in an extreme climate? Are some people drawn to expatriate work because of pre-existing problems or a desire to escape? Engel (1980, p. 304) wrote, 'there is a tendency for individuals with personality problems to volunteer for the tropics'. Smith et al. (1996,

p. 398) reported: 'relief workers themselves have used phrases such as *martyr*, *misfit*, *masochist*, or *running away from bad relationships* to categorize the motivations of others around them, perhaps not their own, for entering relief work' (italics in original).

Paluszny and Zrull (1971) studied 50 applicants for missionary service. They found that, although the majority appeared to be well adjusted, seven (14%) had significant psychological difficulties. One anonymous aid organization admitted in a survey that: 'Some situations require people who can destroy themselves and thrive on chaos . . . at times we have employed workaholics and alcoholics' (McCall and Salama, 1999, p. 114).

A small proportion of the people who apply to go overseas as aid workers or expatriates do so because of emotional difficulties, perhaps being motivated by guilt or a desire to escape from their current situation. The vast majority, on the other hand, are psychologically healthy (Lovell, 1997). Among those with no current difficulties, some are more vulnerable than others to experiencing difficulty in adjusting to the demands of the new culture. Those who cannot work effectively in the new culture may suffer from a loss of self-esteem and from stress-related problems. They may have to return home early, which can cause family problems and career difficulties. Their colleagues may also be adversely affected. Recruiting people for positions overseas, training them, and transporting them abroad is a costly business. Difficulties carry a financial cost, as well as an emotional one. Moreover, if an organization is perceived as having inadequate selection or support procedures, they may in future be refused entry visas or funding (Fawcett, 1999).

In an attempt to reduce such problems, many organizations now include psychological screening in the selection process. Researchers have generated long lists of qualities that are desirable among expatriates, which have been summarized as follows:

he should have the stamina of an Olympic runner, the mental agility of an Einstein, the conversational skill of a professor of languages, the detachment of a judge, the tact of a diplomat, and the perseverance of an Egyptian pyramid builder . . . he should also have a feeling for culture; his moral judgment should not be too rigid; he should be able to merge with the local environment with a chameleon-like ease; and he should show no signs of prejudice (Oates, 1970, p. 24).

Given that no one could possibly meet these criteria, what type of psychological screening will provide the most useful predictive information about how the individual will adjust, cope and perform overseas?

Psychometric Tests

It is rare for an expatriate assignment to 'fail' due to lack of skill or ability: 80% of 'failed' assignments are due to adjustment difficulties (Holmes and Piker, 1980). Therefore, the focus here will be on tests that help to assess the presence and severity of psychological difficulties, and measures which give an indication of personality characteristics, as these may help to predict adjustment.

There are three main advantages of psychometric testing. First, the candidate's score can be compared with standardized scores; therefore, a test score may be perceived as more objective than a judgment based on 'intuition' during an interview. Second, test results may pick up indications of, for example, a personality disorder that might not have been apparent during an interview. The third advantage is that some psychometric tests are cost-effective, especially if they can be sent to the candidate for completion and scored relatively quickly. A major disadvantage is that tests can provide a false sense of security. Many factors interact to influence how an expatriate will adjust and perform overseas, and no single test measures all of these factors.

Little research has been conducted on the effectiveness of psychometric tests for predicting expatriate adjustment. The limited research, which has been published, has mainly concerned the use of the Minnesota Multiphasic Personality Inventory (MMPI, and the revised version MMPI-2) (Hathaway and McKinley, 1989). The MMPI is the most widely used personality test. It was originally developed to diagnose psychological disorders, but has been revised and standardized on normal populations, and has been used effectively in some areas of personnel selection (Westefeld and Maples, 1998). The MMPI has been described as 'the "gold standard" for detection of personality disorders' (Schubert, 1992, p.85). It also provides a broad range of information about other psychological disorders, and normal personality traits. Norms exist for people of different backgrounds and cultures (Butcher, 1996). Although computer programs are available to assist in the rapid scoring of responses, someone who has appropriate training and expertise should interpret the results.

Research suggests that the MMPI has some use in the prediction of expatriate adjustment (Guthrie and Zektick, 1967; Dicken, 1969; Dillon, 1983; Schnurr et al., 1993). Schubert and Ganter (1996) conducted a double-blind study of 129 missionary candidates (or couples). They concluded that the MMPI was inadequate as a sole instrument in evaluating candidates, but had a high potential for use in combination with an in-depth psychological interview. Schubert (1999, p. 88) stated: 'The MMPI allows insight into unconscious issues . . . and vulnerable underlying personality traits not apparent in clinical interviews alone. . . . [Certain subscales] appear to tap some unconscious aspects of personality which are helpful in cross-cultural predictions'. Schubert's research was based on the original MMPI, and not the MMPI-2. There are advantages and disadvantages to using each of these measures (Hargrave et al., 1994; Westefeld and Maples, 1998; Schubert, 1999).

Despite the attention paid to the MMPI, it is not necessarily the most appropriate measure. It is important to choose a test that is not only reliable, valid and standardized, but will also answer the questions of interest. A test that is useful for one type of post may be of little value for another position (Doll et al., 1969). Some people want a test that can help screen out applicants with psychological disorders, while others are interested in one that could help to identify strengths and weaknesses, or interests and values. The latter can assist in deciding where an individual will best be placed, in terms of both location and role.

Ones and Viswesvaran (1997) reviewed the literature on personality-related predictors of expatriate 'success', and recommended that the 'big five' dimensions of personality should be considered (emotional stability, extraversion, openness to experience, agreeableness, and conscientiousness). A number of questionnaires consider such dimensions. Discussion with a psychologist can assist in ascertaining which test is most appropriate for a particular organization.

It is not difficult for intelligent candidates to modify their responses to hide symptoms of depression or other difficulties, and even the validity scales of the MMPI-2, which are sensitive to global deception or defensiveness, can miss subtle 'toning down' of responses. Therefore, it is important that psychological tests, if used, are taken in combination with a clinical interview. The interview may uncover difficulties that were not apparent from questionnaire scores. In cases where the questionnaire results appear abnormal, the interview provides an opportunity to assess why. It is possible that an unusual profile is a sign of creativity or cultural difference, rather than psychopathology. Psychometric tests are of greatest use if they are appropriate for the applicant's culture, selected carefully to answer specific questions, interpreted skilfully, and used in combination with a psychological interview.

Psychological Assessment Interview

It is recommended that every applicant for an expatriate post receive an in-depth psychological assessment interview. Ideally, a psychiatrist or clinical psychologist, who is able to assess the candidate's mental state, should conduct this interview. A skilled interviewer should be able to put the candidate at ease and elicit honest responses, or at least detect when a candidate is being defensive or dishonest. The manner in which people speak about their experiences, and what they choose not to say, can be just as important as what they say.

The interview should include a life history covering the candidate's childhood and adolescence, and education and employment up to the present. The interviewer should attempt to build up a picture of the candidate's strengths and weaknesses. It is important to consider what causes candidates stress and how they handle it; how they deal with anger and frustration; how resilient, resourceful and flexible they are, and where they get their support from. Their motivation for applying for a post overseas should be explored, and interviewers should assess how realistic their expectations are, and discuss any previous experience of working overseas. As interpersonal problems are a major cause of stress and possibly of premature return home (Lovell, 1997; Carter, 1999), it is also important to assess how they relate to other people.

The interviewer should also take a detailed history of any experience of traumatic incidents (including abuse), and any personal or family history of psychological problems. Where there is a vulnerability to psychological disorders, this should be carefully assessed. Foyle *et al.* (1998) found that affective disorders among expatriates were associated with a past personal history of depressed mood, and a family psychiatric history. They concluded (p. 282):

Those with heavily loaded family and personal psychiatric histories should not be accepted for overseas service unless there is clear evidence that they have remained well for several years, have a good work record in their home country, and have shown a capacity for coping in general, and for maintaining good interpersonal relationships. There must also be good personal and medical support in the locations to which they will go (italics in original).

A psychological assessment can be used not only to say 'yes' or 'no' but to provide recommendations that will help to maximize the probability that the candidate will adjust well. Knowledge of vulnerabilities can highlight any special support that might be beneficial. In some cases it is wise to advise delaying overseas work until there has been time to engage in personal or marital therapy. It may also be advisable to recommend a delay if the candidate has suffered from a recent bereavement or relationship breakdown.

If a couple will be moving overseas together, both partners should be interviewed separately, even if only one of them will be working. One of the predictors of an expatriate's adjustment is the spouse's adjustment (Stroh *et al.*, 1994), and there is a strong relationship between marital satisfaction and depression among expatriate couples (Sweatman, 1999). If the couple have children, it is useful to assess the whole family. Concern about children is a common cause of early return, and potential problems might be identified during the assessment, avoiding much distress later (Foyle, 1994).

The effectiveness of a psychological interview depends to a large extent on the skill and experience of the interviewer. Fisher *et al.* (1967) found that assessment ratings made by more experienced psychiatrists correlated significantly and positively with the later performance of Peace Corps volunteers, while the ratings of less experienced interviewers did not. Likewise, Gunderson and Kapfer (1966) found that the psychological interview had a weak predictive validity when the interviewer was poorly informed about the placement environment, but better predictions were made when interviewers were provided with more information.

Even if the applicant has worked overseas previously, there should be a brief reassessment before every new assignment. It is not rare for applicants with psychiatric disorders to be accepted for reassignments without further psychological screening, to the detriment of themselves and those who have to support them in their post (Lovell, 1997).

Other Forms of Psychological Assessment

Some agencies use simulation activities as part of their assessment (Fawcett, 1999). Some organizations inform candidates that their entire period of training is a prolonged assessment period. Additional assessment such as this may have value, but as yet research on such activities is lacking, and so they should only be used in addition to a psychological interview, and not in place of one.

Conclusions Concerning Psychological Assessment

It is recommended that a psychological assessment interview should be part of the selection procedure for every assignment and reassignment. The interviewer should have some knowledge of expatriate life and the relevant environment. A major purpose of the interview is to check whether the candidate is currently suffering from any psychological disorder, and to assess areas of vulnerability. If more detailed information is desired, a carefully selected psychometric test might provide this.

PREDEPARTURE: PREPARATION

Many of the guidelines for predeparture preparation will also apply to the short-term traveller and thus will be dealt with in more detail in other chapters. Suffice it to say that one cannot assume that the organization's guidelines will be in accordance with current standards of care, nor can one assume that the person has been adequately prepared if he or she has seen the local health practitioner (Beallor *et al.*, 1997; Dwelle, 1995; Lange *et al.*, 1987).

Immunizations

Immunization advice is thoroughly addressed elsewhere; however, there are some risk factors that are particularly significant for the expatriate community and will be briefly addressed.

Hepatitis B

Hepatitis B is an established risk for expatriates, in part related to unprotected intercourse in nonmonogamous relationships and in part related to inadvertent exposure in communities where the prevalence of hepatitis B is high. Given the potential for adverse outcomes, the efficacy of the vaccine and the relatively low cost, universal immunization for the expatriate task force can readily be justified (Lange and Frame, 1990; Smalligan *et al.*, 1995).

Japanese Encephalitis B

Japanese encephalitis B vaccine is one of few vaccines

where there is potential for harm to the recipient. However, clinical disease is associated with a mortality rate ranging from 10 to 25%, with up to 50% of survivors demonstrating permanent psychoneurological sequelae (Vaughn and Hoke, 1992). Although persons in urban settings are usually exempt, one should determine if the cumulative risk could exceed 4 weeks during the proposed assignment (CDC, 1993).

Rabies

It is difficult to assess the risk of exposure to rabies but the rate of postexposure treatment closely approximates 1 per 1000 volunteers per month among expatriates living in rabies enzootic regions (Arguin et al., 2000; Bernard and Fishbein, 1991; Bjorvatn and Gundersen, 1980; Hatz et al., 1994; LeGuerrier et al., 1996). The risk of children being bitten is conservatively estimated to be four times greater than that of adults (LeGuerrier et al., 1996). Furthermore, bites in children are usually higher on the trunk or face and are more severe or, conversely, minimized and neglected.

Dogs are usually the source of risk. Often pets are involved but it is disturbing to note that many expatriates keep pets that are not appropriately vaccinated against rabies. Postexposure treatments are often delayed, biologics may not be available in less affluent countries and frequently management is not in accordance to World Health Organization (WHO) guidelines (Arguin et al., 2000).

There are two options for the prevention of rabies: pre-exposure rabies immunization with three doses of a tissue culture rabies vaccine; or relying exclusively on postexposure immunization. Pre-exposure immunization does not eliminate the need for careful wound management and immunization with two doses of a potent tissue culture; it obviates the need for rabies immune globulin (RIG).

Expatriates residing in rabies enzootic countries with limited access to rabies biologics, particularly RIG, are at greater than average risk for contracting rabies should they be exposed. For postexposure vaccination to work and be cost-effective, it is essential that medical expertise be available on an urgent basis and that there be access to tissue culture vaccines plus RIG or purified equine RIG.

Given that rabies prevention for persons previously immunized with a cell culture vaccine relies on the anamnestic response to the two postexposure doses of the vaccine, routine booster doses are not required for expatriates unless there is judged to be a significant risk for inadvertent exposure, or there is a likelihood that access to care will be limited so as to prevent timely administration of the postexposure doses. Persons at risk for inadvertent exposure must follow the usual guidelines for serological testing and booster doses (ACIP, 1999).

Cholera

Routine immunization against cholera is not recommended; however, the oral cholera vaccine effectively reduces the volume of fluid loss and therefore is recommended for persons residing in endemic areas where access to rehydration therapy may be limited (Advisory Committee Statement, 1998).

Tick-borne Encephalitis

In terms of aid workers and the military, tick-borne encephalitis vaccine is an important issue, given the need for ongoing aid and peacekeeping in the Balkans, and for long-term health and development programs in eastern Europe and in the endemic band, which runs across the former Soviet Union.

On balance, aid workers, expatriates, longer term travelers and environmentalists should consider having this vaccine if spending significant time in rural settings, especially in forested areas in late spring and summer in pockets where the disease is known to exist (Department of Health, 1996).

Malaria

Risk Factors

Malaria was the leading cause of death among expatriates who died from infectious diseases (Frame et al., 1992) and continues to pose a threat in sub-Saharan Africa, where the rate of malaria is at least 10-fold greater than in other malarious countries (Adera et al., 1995), with the exception of Papua New Guinea and Irian Jaya (Ohrt et al., 1997). The true incidence of malaria in expatriates is difficult to determine but rough estimates range from 31 per 1000 per year in Asia to 209 per 1000 per year in West Africa (Schneider, 1998; Peppiatt and Byass, 1990; Phillips-Howard et al., 1990). The majority make the diagnosis based on the presence of fever or are diagnosed by laboratories where the false-positive rate could be as high as 75% (Lobel et al., 1998).

The risk of malaria appears to increase over time, particularly evident in persons who resided in malaria-endemic regions for 2–3 years or longer (Adera et al., 1995; Schneider, 1998). In sub-Saharan Africa, children, persons who do not take antimalarial prophylaxis and persons living and working in rural areas are at greater risk for contracting malaria. Environmental factors that have been found to be protective are altitudes above 2000 m and arid climates (World Health Organization, 1997).

Chemoprophylaxis

Guidelines on the prevention of malaria in expatriates

should not deviate significantly from standard guidelines (Chapter 8). The lack of international consensus on chemoprophylaxis is problematic for the expatriate community. From the descriptive data available, it becomes evident that the practice guidelines may bear little influence on the behavior and practice of the expatriate and underscores the importance of meticulous advice when preparing expatriates who anticipate living in malaria-endemic regions.

Most would concede that mefloquine is the preferred antimalarial for chloroquine-resistant areas when convenience, cost and efficacy are the primary considerations. Failure of mefloquine prophylaxis is due primarily to noncompliance (Lobel *et al*, 1998). Studies on Peace Corps volunteers have demonstrated that mefloquine is safe and well tolerated by most individuals who have continued to use it over extended periods of time (Lobel *et al.*, 1991, 1993; Schlagenhauf *et al.*, 1996). However, in a study that involved 1200 persons from a broader sector of the expatriate community working in sub-Saharan Africa, only 3% continued to use mefloquine, primarily because of concerns regarding neuropsychiatric side-effects. Of those who were initially prescribed mefloquine, 28% noted that colleagues or health workers influenced them to change; 20% changed to another prophylaxis regimen because of side-effects, although only half of those were classified as neuropsychiatric in nature (Schneider, 1998).

Chloroquine and proguanil resistance is known to be widespread throughout sub-Saharan Africa, yet it was found to be the favored antimalarial regimen for 55% of the persons included in this large cross-section of expatriate workers. Chloroquine alone or proguanil alone was utilized by about 20% (Schneider, 1998).

Maloprim, a combination of dapsone and pyrimethamine, or pyrimethamine alone was the choice for another 20%. A Canadian missionary in Malawi, using dapsone and pyrimethamine for malaria prophylaxis, died in 1999 from complications related to malaria, underscoring concerns regarding resistance (Kain *et al.*, 2000). Agranulocytosis developed in 1:2000 when the dose of dapsone and pyrimethamine was increased to improve efficacy (Friman *et al.*, 1983). Doxycycline has been recommended as an alternative to mefloquine, yet it is not widely utilized by members of this community, in part because of concerns regarding safety and tolerance. However, tetracycline derivatives have been utilized from long-term treatment of other disorders such as acne.

Compliance

Compliance is generally poor. As noted above, the choice of antimalarial medication does not necessarily conform to the standard guidelines. Furthermore, half of the study participants adjusted their regimen, independent of medical counsel, after their arrival. In sub-Saharan Africa only 75% of expatriates use regular chemoprophylaxis, in Asia about 28% and in the Pacific about 35%. Although personal protection measures have proven to be effective,

only 38% of expatriates screened doors and windows, 53% used mosquito netting and only one in five participants treated their nets with insecticides (Schneider, 1998).

Self-Diagnosis and Self-Treatment

Self-diagnostic kits are now available and have proven to be very accurate and reliable in the hands of laboratory workers (Banchongaksorn *et al.*, 1996; Pieroni *et al.*, 1998; Mills *et al.*, 1999) but they do not appear to be very accurate in the hands of travelers (Funk *et al.*, 1999; Trachsler *et el.*, 1999). Without training, there is no reason to believe that the efficacy will be any better in the expatriate community, although to date there are no published studies. However, given that expatriates represent a reasonably finite group, training may prove to be efficient and effective. Self-diagnostic kits that require refrigeration will limit access to this technology in some regions.

Of the drugs available for self-treatment, the combination of atovaquone and proguanil appears to be the most promising: it is easy to administer, it is relatively well tolerated, it has no known severe adverse reactions and it has an efficacy rate close to 100% (Kremsner *et al.*, 1999). Pyrimethamine with sulfadoxine (Fansidar) is no longer an effective antimalarial agent in many parts of Southeast Asia, Africa and the Amazon region of South America. Halofantrine is still available in many international settings, although it is no longer recommended because of the potential for cardiac complications. The artemether derivatives are now widely available and are used by expatriates for self-treatment; however, the dose is often suboptimal and they are frequently utilized as a single agent, thereby increasing the potential for treatment failures.

Malaria and Pregnancy

Women have to understand that there is an increased risk of severe malaria during pregnancy, which may result in maternal and neonatal death, miscarriage and stillbirth. Special care should be taken to avoid mosquito bites, and chemoprophylaxis should be used.

The use of doxycycline and primaquine are contraindicated in pregnancy. Chloroquine and proguanil are considered to be safe in pregnancy, although they are not as efficacious as mefloquine in preventing drug-resistant *Plasmodium falciparum* infection. Based on current data, mefloquine is also believed safe and should be considered the drug of first choice in regions where the attack rate and chloroquine resistance is high (Kain and Keystone, 1998).

Malaria Prevention in Children

With the exception of doxycycline, antimalarials, including primaquine, are safe for children when administered at the prescribed dose. Children and adolescents are at special risk of malaria, perhaps because of poor compliance or inaccurate calculation of the dose (Adera *et al.*, 1995), and they may rapidly become seriously ill. Babies, including breast-fed infants, and children should be well protected against mosquito bites and receive malaria chemoprophylaxis. Children are at greater risk than adults for *N,N*-diethyl-*m*-toluamide (DEET) toxicity, which includes seizures among other central nervous system abnormalities.

Tuberculosis

Tuberculosis is not only spreading, but the proportion of multidrug-resistant cases is rising, in some areas explosively. It is estimated that between the years 2000 and 2020 nearly 1 billion people will be newly infected and 70 million will die if control is not strengthened (World Health Organization, WHO, 1998).

Many expatriates, particularly aid workers and missionaries, have a significant risk of being exposed to tuberculosis. This includes those working in refugee camps, in long-term health and development, in urban health programs, amongst communities that also have a high level of HIV disease.

Opinions differ as to the value of routine BCG immunization for those who are tuberculin negative (Chapter 11). Current advice in the UK would be to offer BCG to those without contraindications or a previous exposure or immunization, going to a developing country or high-risk location or occupation for more than 1 month (Department of Health, 1996). In North America, BCG is not usually recommended for adults; however, many advocate the immunization of children under 5, primarily to prevent disseminated disease. Recent studies suggest that current strains of BCG have been overattenuated and thus may be less effective than they were during earlier trials (Behr and Small, 1997).

Diarrheal Diseases

Diarrheal diseases related to bacterial infections account for the majority of illnesses among expatriates (Bernard *et al.*, 1989). There is both a seasonal variation and a significant variation from one region to another. Foods cooked earlier in the day, such as lasagna and quiche, as well as blended fruit and yogurt drinks have recently been identified as risk factors. Other dominant risk factors include: younger age, shorter duration of stay and eating in restaurants. Although the severity of diarrhea in expatriates may be somewhat less than that found among short-term travelers, the morbidity is still significant and remains so for up to 2 years (Hoge *et al.*, 1996; Shlim *et al.*, 1999).

Handwashing for household food handlers and employees should be emphasized in addition to standard advice regarding water purification and food precautions.

The expatriate families should be instructed in self-treatment protocols. In contrast to the short-term traveler, they should be familiar with the varied presentations and seasonality to ensure that the most appropriate regimen is applied to their situation.

Risk Behavior

Excessive alcohol consumption and a high rate of extramarital sexual activity are common among certain groups of expatriates (Lange and McCune, 1989; Macnair, 1995; De Graaf *et al.*, 1998a). In some cases these behaviors are related to peer pressure and expectations, while in other instances they are a consequence of stress, or an attempt to avoid unpleasant thoughts and feelings, or a result of loneliness and separation from the social support network (perhaps including the spouse). Boredom and a lack of opportunity for recreational activities may also be a factor. In many cases expatriates do not use condoms during sexual activity (Moore *et al.*, 1995), increasing the risk of HIV infection and other sexually transmitted diseases.

Sexually Transmitted Diseases

Sexually transmitted diseases have been associated with travelers since they were first described and are a well-documented risk in the expatriate community (Bonneux *et al.*, 1988; Rowbottom, 1993; Mabey, 1995; De Graaf *et al.*, 1998b). A study of approximately 900 Dutch expatriates living in four different geographic regions showed that 41% of males and 31% of females reported having sex with casual or steady local partners, and 11% of males and 24% of females acknowledged that they had casual or steady expatriate partners during an average stay of 26 months. Consistent condom use with steady local or expatriate partners was noted by 69% in these study participants, compared with 21% reported in an earlier study (De Graaf *et al.*, 1997).

HIV

There is little doubt that human immunodeficiency virus (HIV) transmission is primarily related to sexual activity and occupational hazards. Of the 2000 Dutch expatriates working in sub-Saharan Africa, 0.4% of men and 0.1% of women contracted HIV. One case related to occupational exposure (Houweling and Coutinho, 1991).

There is less known about the incidence of HIV amongst aid and relief workers (Lange *et al.*, 1989; Lange and Frame, 1991). Although extremely rare in some groups, Schouten and Bordoff (1995) confirm that cases are occurring and Dutch medics in HIV/AIDS endemic areas were found to have a mean occupational risk of HIV of 0.11% per person per year. Elsewhere, 1.1% of Belgian advisers working in Africa and 0.9% of European expatriates living in Africa were found to be HIV-positive in a voluntary screening program (Bonneux et al., 1988). We can expect the number of reported cases to increase, given the explosive increase in HIV infection in many parts of the world where aid workers are posted and expatriates live (World Health Organization, 1999).

Aid workers and expatriates may need predeparture testing for the following reasons: visa applications; eligibility to join a Trusted Donor Blood Group (Walking Blood Bank); to assess employer liability if personnel return HIV-positive after their assignment; to provide health counsel for management of unique health risks, especially as it pertains to opportunistic infections and live vaccines; and to offer treatment to persons found to be HIV-positive.

There remains the vexed issue of postexposure prophylaxis following an occupational health exposure (or sexual assault). Kits are increasingly available—made up in 7 or 28 day packs and comprising two or three antiretroviral drugs, commonly comprising zidovudine, lamivudine and sometimes a protease inhibitor such as indinavir. These kits are largely designed for aid workers perceived to have a high occupational risk of HIV exposure, including doctors, nurses and medical students. An increasing number of agencies are now providing these kits. Detailed guidelines and instructions about the best ways of using these are currently being hammered out in the hopes that a degree of consensus will emerge. The area is fraught with medical, financial, logistical and moral issues. Some agencies including Médicins sans Frontières are following clearly defined and managed protocols (Médecins sans Frontières, 1997; and revised draft 2000).

Psychological Training and Preparation

Many people who show no particular signs of vulnerability at assessment go on to develop difficulties while overseas, or return home early because of stress (Christy and Rasmussen, 1963; Dally, 1985). Can adequate training and preparation make a difference?

Tung (1988) investigated why the rate of premature repatriation was more than twice as high among expatriates from the USA compared with those from Europe or Japan. Tung found that American companies were much less likely than European or Japanese companies to provide formal training for crosscultural posts.

Not all groups of American expatriates have a high attrition rate, and so the difference cannot be explained in terms cultural differences in expectations or attitudes. Henry (1965, p. 18) observed that only 3–4% of American Peace Corps volunteers were sent home early as 'out-and-out selection errors', compared with 30% of expatriates sent abroad by American companies. One of the major differences between the groups was the 3 month training course received by the Peace Corps volunteers.

Deshpande and Viswesvaran (1992), in a meta-analysis of 21 studies, concluded that crosscultural training had a strong and positive effect on crosscultural adjustment,

job performance, and crosscultural skills development. Holmes and Piker (1980) estimated that expatriate attrition averaged around 40% among companies who neither screened candidates for cultural adaptability nor provided cultural orientation, compared with 25% among those with orientation programs only, and 5–10% among those using both screening and orientation programs.

An important part of the preparation package should be to explain what to expect in terms of culture shock, and the longer-term adjustment process. It is not unusual for expatriates to have stress-related symptoms at some point. Those who have been informed that this often happens tend to be able to normalize their symptoms. Those who have not been informed about normal symptoms of stress may worry that they are 'over-reacting'. This is likely to add to their distress and to maintain and intensify the symptoms (Lovell, 1997).

Aid workers have a greater tendency to deny stress-related symptoms than other people in helping professions (Chester, 1983). Some believe that they have been 'trained to be tough and not to let certain feelings affect them' (Grant, 1995, p. 75). Teaching them the benefits of gaining relief through sharing concerns may help them to cope better in the long run.

Perhaps a parallel can be drawn with marriage preparation. If a couple have been helped to prepare, they are more likely to perceive difficulties as a normal part of married life, and to cope with them and remain together. Likewise, expatriates are likely to face difficulties at times. If they have received adequate preparation, they are more likely to be able to cope with the problems and resolve them. A lack of preparation may result in them giving up, or else developing stress-related symptoms.

As part of stress management training, expatriates should be given information about the importance of taking sufficient time to rest and relax. Excessive working hours contribute to the difficulties that can cause premature return (Lovell, 1999a). Couples and families benefit from scheduling sufficient quality time together. Discussing how to create and maintain a strong social support network can also take place at the preparation stage.

Some organizations have found it beneficial to provide training in 'team building', and to teach expatriates about personality differences, in order to help team members to understand each other better. Acquiring an understanding of differences can be extended to understanding crosscultural differences. The preparation package should include ample opportunity to learn about the relevant culture, so that unrealistic expectations can be exchanged for realistic ones. Unmet expectations are a common cause of frustration, and modifying them in advance can reduce difficulties later on.

It is important that training does not focus on crises to the exclusion of other potential stressors. Many expatriates cope well with political instability and war situations because the conflict is external and not aimed at them personally. Personal criticism and relationship conflict can be more detrimental (Lovell, 1997). Ongoing frustrations may be more harmful psychologically than short-lived traumatic events, as they can be a cause of chronic stress. Training in problem-solving skills, negotiation techniques and conflict resolution can help to reduce stress.

Many expatriates report feeling underprepared for their assignment (Dunbar and Ehrlich, 1993), which adds to their levels of stress and uncertainty. A comprehensive preparation program, including the components described above, could help to reduce both emotional problems and attrition among expatriates.

Safety While Abroad

Training in crisis management may also be appropriate (Goode, 1995). Many expatriates are at increased risk of experiencing traumatic incidents, perhaps related to terrorist bombing, war situations, evacuations, hostage taking, rape, robbery, riots, traffic accidents, land mines, natural disasters, or illness epidemics. A crisis management package should include a security briefing covering measures to prevent crises wherever possible, by being alert to potential danger and taking precautions to enhance safety. The package should also provide information about established policies. Training can also be given in the importance of not abandoning hope during a crisis, but rather trying to engage in active problem solving, as this is associated with a reduction in negative psychological after-effects (Ehlers et al., 1998).

In some areas, expatriates are targeted for hostage taking or assassination (Slim, 1995; Rogers, 1998). Expatriates who are involved with humanitarian work in conflict zones may face particularly severe difficulties. Helping people on one side can be perceived as being an enemy of the other side. People suspected of war crimes may attempt to kill expatriates, fearing that they might speak out at criminal tribunals. Although the survival rates among expatriates taken hostage mirrors that of the general population, fatalities are not rare. It is reported that at least 160 United Nations civilian personnel were killed in the 7 years leading up to 1999 (Editorial, 1999), and the UN is only one of many organizations working in such areas.

Kidnapping often follows cycles of terrorism, at times involving multiple victims. Unlike random crimes, kidnapping usually involves preselected targets. Crisis management and contingency preparation seminars are now available and it is prudent for those orientating and caring for expatriates to become familiar with risk management principles.

CARING FOR EXPATRIATES IN INTERNATIONAL SETTINGS

Sieveking et al. (1981, pp 101–102) remind us that, 'Regardless of how valid our selection is, and how thorough our orientation, most any employee will encounter difficulties . . . we can never leave even the best employee alone'.

As part of the preparation package, expatriates should receive information about where they can go for help should they have health problems or other difficulties overseas. Sending agencies should have a policy on this issue. For mild difficulties, information may be sufficient. In more severe cases, consultation with a health professional should be arranged. Ideally, organizations should obtain information about health services in the area, and how they can be accessed, before the expatriate arrives.

Ongoing contact from the sending agency can reduce the sense of isolation and anxiety, including anxiety about what will happen when they return home. Aycan (1997, p. 33) reported that, 'expatriates who feel confident about company support are likely to adjust better than those who experience uncertainty and stress about their future'. It can be useful to check that they are not working excessively long hours, and that they are taking days off regularly. They should be informed about how they can provide feedback, make requests or ask for help (practical or emotional) at any time should they require it. Adequate supervision should be provided. Inviting their suggestions for changes and improvements can foster job satisfaction. Chronic stress problems are less likely to materialize in an environment where people feel free to acknowledge difficulties and request help at an early stage.

Very little has been written about models of care that can be provided in international settings and there are no data in the literature that would distinguish one model of care as being more effective than another. The possibilities include: (1) self-reliant staff who develop their own network and health care providers; (2) national staff who have received international training who are familiar with the culture of the home country; (3) international clinics staffed by persons who are also members of that expatriate community; (4) clinics staffed by members of the same organization; and (5) reliance on networks that have been established by the embassy for their personnel.

Although 'self-care' is necessary, it appears that most do seek help from health care professionals for more complex medical problems. Professional help should also be sought in cases of psychosis, severe depression, suicidal ideation, anorexia nervosa, PTSD, serious difficulties with a child (including the possibility of abuse), or any mental health problem that appears to be getting worse. Organizations could increase the potential for more effective care by fostering a culture that promotes help-seeking behaviour (MMWR, 1999).

Future Trends

Expatriates can feel isolated and undervalued if they are not asked periodically how their workload is, and how they are coping personally. Even without sophisticated technology, satellite telephones and e-mail links will often provide timely counsel for persons in remote regions.

Self-care is often strengthened by access to reputable web sites, many of which have been developed for travelers who do not have formal medical training. Patients now have the potential to access their medical records via the Internet. Although care through electronic mediums is often limited to general advice rather than formulation of a specific diagnosis and management plan, one can often provide guidance that will help expatriates to determine an appropriate course of action. Results of laboratory testing can be faxed, and good quality films from a variety of diagnostic imaging services can be couriered to a tertiary care center for a fraction of the cost of repatriation.

Soon that will seem archaic. With technology that is currently available, telemedicine is experiencing a resurgence of interest. Several models of medical care have been developed that can serve as practical examples, such as the Yale Telemedicine Center which has created links with physicians in Saudi Arabia. It is probable that the military will establish a number of precedents, given their established communication links. When utilizing telemedicine it is difficult to know the limits of medical licensure and difficult to determine medical–legal boundaries. Many are critical of endorsement without careful attention being given to the standards of care and the appraisal process.

What To Do if Difficulties Develop while Overseas

If appropriate treatment is not available locally, or the expatriate is unwilling to accept it, there may be a need for repatriation. A local medical professional may be able to liaise with the organization in such cases. The expatriate should be helped to accept that repatriation is not a sign of failure. Comprehensive travel insurance includes cover for emergency repatriation (Medivac). By accessing the company's helpline (given on the insurance documents), travel arrangements will be made by the assistance company.

A common situation is evacuation due to deterioration in the security situation. It is very helpful if organizations have clear evacuation policies, which expatriates are asked to adhere to as a condition of their contract. It is not uncommon for expatriates to refuse to follow an evacuation policy, perhaps because they do not believe that there is any danger, or because in the heat of a crisis they develop a 'martyr instinct' and insist that they will not abandon their local friends. Expatriates who have consented to a policy before going overseas, having been informed of the reasons for it, are more likely to adhere to it later. Organizations should also have policies on such issues as abuse and hostage situations.

If an expatriate does experience evacuation or any other traumatic incident, it may be appropriate to offer critical incident stress debriefing (CISD) (Mitchell, 1983). If there are several expatriates working in close proximity, it may be beneficial to ensure that at least one of them is trained in such debriefing. CISD was proposed originally as an intervention where groups of people who had experienced a traumatic incident would meet together 24–72 h after the incident, and describe in a structured way the facts about what had happened, and then their thoughts, followed by their feelings. Participants would then be helped to normalize their reactions, and then to move towards future planning.

There is currently considerable debate about the effectiveness of CISD. No randomized controlled trials have been conducted for CISD in groups, and there have only been six such trials using CISD with individuals (Rose and Bisson, 1998). These six trials had mixed results, possibly due to methodological shortcomings. It appears from the literature that most people who receive CISD report finding it helpful, although it is not clear whether it actually leads to a reduction in post-traumatic symptoms. Further research will hopefully add further insight to this debate.

After any traumatic incident, it is wise to ensure that there is adequate time to rest. Accidents are more common following a stressful experience, and so the individual should be encouraged to take particular care, especially when driving. PTSD can develop months or even years after a traumatic event, perhaps being triggered by a subsequent event, and so follow-up support should be offered should the expatriate wish to receive it at any point.

HEALTH SCREENING AND CARE ON RETURN

The Context

Expatriates will generally be exposed to similar pathogens as other travelers. Of course they may be exposed to more of them and they may be exposed over a longer period of time.

Longer-term expatriates will have often developed different ways of perceiving themselves, their lives and the world. They may have collected a medical worry list because of local health care they perceive to be inadequate. They may be suffering from acute, or more probably a degree of, cumulative stress. These factors can cause or confound their medical symptoms. As a result, some will be introspectively concerned about what is going on in their bodies (and their minds), and may have consulted a range of friends.

The different mindset of longer-term expatriates means that a purely mechanistic, evidence-based approach to screening is, on its own, woefully inadequate. Many expatriates will need to unravel concerns and bid into an action plan of which they feel ownership. We must be prepared to think in either postmodern or modern paradigms with this subgroup of travelers, without losing our evidence-based, cost-effective approach as the foundation of what we advise and recommend.

Purpose of Postreturn Screening and Care

What we mean by screening in this section is the following: to diagnose, treat and manage any real or perceived problem in the returning traveler that has a significant physical or mental health component. Most readers will recognize this as being radically different from the technical definition used by epidemiologists: 'The systematic application of a test or enquiry, to identify individuals at sufficient risk of a specific disorder to warrant further investigations or direct preventive action, amongst persons who have not sought medical attention on account of symptoms of that disorder' (Department of Health, 1997).

In practice, the 'tropical check-up' is a hybrid, a combination of screening and case finding in such a way that the needs of both practitioner and patient are met, within the limits of an affordable system. Churchill et al. (1993) begin pointing us to a model beyond that of classical, mechanistic screening. Patients' perceptions and wishes should be guiding factors which lead us to define two particular subgroups: returnees concerned that they may have latent infections that could cause problems later, and those wishing to have retrospective diagnoses of illness suffered abroad.

Evidence for the Validity of Screening

This continues to generate a great deal of debate (Conlon, 1993; Genton and Gehri, 1999; Okereke and Gelletie, 1999). A major problem is the definition of validity, which will be defined differently by the practitioner, epidemiologist, health economist and client.

A few papers have been written on the value of screening longer-term travelers, or indeed of the major health problems they suffer while abroad. One reason is the difficulty of monitoring or remembering episodes of illness or threats to health that may have occurred many months ago. The only way to investigate such health problems reliably is to provide regular and systematic monitoring of expatriates' health while they are overseas. Without the bedrock knowledge of what illnesses have occurred abroad, health screening on return gives only a patchy idea of the expatriates' overall state of health during their overseas assignment.

The screening of the returned traveler is covered in Chapter 12. In this section we will refer only to more recent papers concerned with aid workers and expatriates.

Carroll et al. (1993) looked at a mixed group of travelers including diplomats, long-term volunteers and trekkers. The authors concluded that screening was useful but could be largely conducted through structured history taking and relevant laboratory tests: specialist examination added little. One in four of those screened had an abnormal result. In addition, nontropical abnormalities where found in a significant number, reflecting the value to the individual of opportunistic screening for problems unrelated to travel. Eosinophilia was found in 67 out of 852 samples, positive schistosomal antibodies in 10.7%; 18.7% had abnormalities on stool tests. Although eosinophilia is often an important marker of helminth infection, its significance should be interpreted in the context of other risk factors and the absence of eosinophilia does not rule out helminth infection (Libman et al., 1993; MacLean and Libman, 1998; Moore and Nutman, 1998).

Peppiatt and Byass (1991) looked at the health of 212 returning missionaries serving in 27 countries for 488 person-years: 6.5% of adults had a raised eosinophil count, but only 13 out of 157 had cysts of pathogenic organisms on stool test, lower than in many reported studies. Self-reporting from overseas showed malaria, diarrhea and giardia infection to be the most common perceived illnesses, but psychiatric illness accounted for nearly 110 episodes per 1000 person years, underlining the need for careful assessment and stress management seminars before leaving, and appropriate debriefing and counseling on return.

The screening of children returning from the tropics has been studied by Brouwer el al. (1999). They looked at 282 check-ups of children, aged from 3 months to 16 years, with stays ranging from 3 months to 13 years. Of these, 62% were on children who had lived in sub-Saharan Africa; 156 diagnoses of travel-related infectious and parasitic illnesses were found. Quoting from figures in this paper from asymptomatic cases: 23% of check-ups showed asymptomatic giardiasis, 10% eosinophilia and 8% schistosomiasis. The jury is still out on the value and cost-effectiveness of screening asymptomatic children. However, a holistic paradigm, which takes into account the broader picture of parental concern and perceived public health risks in the schools they join, probably tilts the balance in favor of screening.

Who Needs a Medical Check-up?

In a postmodern culture, practitioners are expected to be facilitators, placing evidence and benefits before their patients and their sending agencies, so both can make informed choices; however, some will wish to consult in a more classical paradigm. Equally there will be some employers, including the military, certain companies and many relief agencies, that will have strict pre-employment protocols that must be adhered to.

The following outline underscores the variety of reasons for medical consultations on return from overseas:

- Significant symptoms or concerns
- Significant exposure to serious diseases
- Being fit on return but subsequently developing symptoms
- Somatization, with the client blaming parasites for worsening or recurrent symptoms
- Establishing a diagnosis for illness experienced abroad
- Medical assessment and/or psychological debriefing

following high-risk assignments
• Screening asymptomatic personnel returning from long-term assignment (> 6 months).

Almost any problem, worry or symptom can be presented, often representing a life crisis or chronic personal dilemma. There may be unresolved problems from overseas or from before the assignment, including a myriad of nontropical ailments such as failed birth control, an alcoholic spouse, unexplained exhaustion, worries about debt, loss of role, temporary unemployment, a failing marriage, undisclosed rape or tormented dreams.

Health care practitioners may well be the only person travelers have the courage to speak to about such issues. For some, quick, firm reassurance may be all that is needed; but, for others, referrals or a broader, multidisciplinary team, including ministers of religion, counsellors or group therapy with other individuals experiencing similar situations may be required.

What Should Screening Consist Of?

History

To consult effectively we will need to have a wide understanding of both world geography and world news so that we can make 'informed leaps of faith' into our client's situation.

Medical history taken for expatriates needs some exploration of specific components. These include any unusual health and safety risks, psychosocial factors, failed expectations, causes of sleep disturbance, signs of abnormal stress, sexual health risks, alcohol consumption, risks specific to hostile or dangerous environments and occupational health risks from HIV, hepatitis B or hepatitis C. Structured questionnaires or protocols can provide the majority of the information and make the consultation more effective.

Carrying Out the Examination

The clinical examination seeks to substantiate the findings discovered in the history and identify signs that were not revealed by the history and investigations: this is especially important with the skin, lymph nodes, liver and spleen.

Laboratory Investigations

There are two mistakes to avoid: doing too few tests, and doing too many. The minimalists risk leaving their patients dissatisfied and missing important pathology. The maximalists may do unnecessary tests out of clinical insecurity, for research interests or for medicolegal reasons. In overtesting, they risk making the tropical check-up so expensive that companies and voluntary agencies will vote with their feet and stop referring their employees (Libman *et al.*, 1993).

In practice we should do the minimum tests necessary consistent with evidence-based medicine, our professional judgment and the concerns of the traveler. Selective interventions are based on risk factors identified during the general assessment phase of the evaluation (Table 27.1). There is a growing body of literature that will help the pratitioner to distinguish the appropriate tests (MacLean and Libman, 1998; MacPherson, 1999).

Postassignment HIV Screening

Questions surrounding HIV testing on return are somewhat different. Aid workers may qualify for screening because of occupational and sometimes lifestyle risk. Many returning aid workers and expatriates are worried about risks, even if they are negligible. Sensitive pretest counseling is a prerequisite to testing, and a strategy for follow-up counseling for persons found to be seropositive is essential.

Tuberculosis Surveillance

An equally important issue is to monitor travelers exposed to tuberculosis, to detect whether they have been infected before any signs of active infection develop. Standard screening involves tuberculin tests with purified protein derivative (PPD) before and after possible exposure to tuberculosis. In the UK, PPD is often administered as a Heaf test. In North America, the Mantoux skin test with 5 tuberculin units of PPD administered intradermally is the standard protocol.

Tuberculin skin testing has many practical drawbacks. Many aid workers are on short-term contracts, and return to their home countries every 3, 6 or 12 months. Many are poorly compliant with preventative health measures, and some are on relief registers and have to respond rapidly when called. Arranging routine pre- and postassignment tuberculin skin testing is difficult and is likely to have low compliance. For those on longer assignments and with more time to prepare, tuberculin skin testing remains a workable option.

Recently a blood test has become available which detects IgC antibodies to *Mycobacterium tuberculosis* and is claimed to detect active infection (Desem and Jones, 1998; Streeton *et al.*, 1998). Further validation is required but initial research is promising.

Concluding the Consultation

At the end of the consultation, we need to make sure that the patient does not leave in a confused muddle, especially as many issues may have been touched on and plans suggested. Furthermore, the mobile nature of this community can make follow-up communication a logistical nightmare.

Patients will need to be clear about the following:

- How and when results will be relayed to them
- How to determine the results of confidential testing, such as for HIV
- Whether any counseling or debriefing is agreed to
- Action to be taken if symptoms suggestive of malaria arise over the coming weeks.

Reporting

A report summarizing health problems noted in the history and examination, copies of all investigations, and details regarding action plans may be necessary for many expatriates, especially those returning to an international assignment. If a report is to be sent to the agency, one should determine the reason for the report, the detail required and who will be the recipient of the confidential information. Larger organizations may have a medical director and thus more explicit detail may be expected. Other organizations may have limited medical expertise and thus only need to be apprised of the detail that could impact management decisions. In both cases permission for release of information is mandatory.

Re-entry Issues

For some expatriates, the most disturbing part of their experience comes when they return to their home country. Some expatriates suppress their emotions while they are overseas, in order to cope, and on return home experience extreme emotional reactions, as they begin to confront their feelings (Smith *et al.*, 1996).

Macnair (1995) found that 75% of 200 returned aid workers reported difficulty readjusting on their return. The main difficulties reported were feelings of disorientation (33%), problems getting a job (24%), lack of understanding from family and friends (17%) and financial difficulties (15%). McConnan (1992) found that 73% of aid workers felt inadequately debriefed and supported on their return to the sending country. Many were not informed about sources of help available or encouraged to make use of these.

In another study (Lovell, 1997), 60% of returned aid workers reported feeling predominantly negative emotions on their return home. The most common experiences were feeling disorientated and confused, and feeling devastated and bereaved, having left friends overseas. Some described their experience vividly, for example:

The feeling of hollowness and absolutely 'gutted-loss' when returning to the UK just doesn't bear thinking about. Quite literally the worst experiences of my life were leaving India.

For some of us this is not a homecoming but the beginning of exile. We become displaced persons (p. 25).

Expatriates and their families should be helped to pre-

pare for their return home, several months before they actually return. Preparation should include information about 'reverse culture shock'. A book such as *Re-entry* (Jordan, 1992) may be helpful. Assistance with practical and employment concerns is also greatly appreciated.

Debriefing: A Reflective Pause

It is good practice routinely to offer personal debriefing to all expatriates when they return to their home country, preferably between 1 and 3 weeks after their return. Offering debriefing routinely rather than on request is preferable, as many people do not feel that they will benefit from it until after they have received it. Moreover, some people are concerned that requesting debriefing might be taken as a sign of weakness and affect future employment prospects.

While operational debriefing focuses on tasks, personal debriefing is concerned with how expatriates have been affected personally. A structured approach can be used, along the lines of the CISD model, modified for use with an individual after multiple stressors (Armstrong *et al.*, 1995, 1998). Debriefing should not be rushed. The expatriate should be invited to reflect on the whole experience, paying particular attention to any traumatic incidents or longer-term stressors. Each incident or stressor can be explored using the CISD model. The expatriate should be asked about the worst part of the experience, but they do not need to describe this in graphic detail. He or she should also be asked what the best parts of the experience were, and what has been learned, to help integrate the experience as a whole and find meaning in it. There should be an opportunity to discuss how the expatriate feel about being back 'home', and for the debriefer to provide information about the readjustment process.

Personal debriefing should help the expatriate to normalize any symptoms of stress, and move on towards thinking about the future. Information should be given about sources of further help should he or she wish to take this up, and a follow-up appointment should be arranged if this is desired. Debriefing along these lines can also be offered to groups (Fawcett, 1999). The process can be used with families, and it is certainly important to include older teenagers.

Approximately 25% of returned aid workers report clinically significant symptoms of avoidance and intrusive thoughts months after returning from a post overseas (Lovell, 1997). Although they do not necessarily meet the diagnostic criteria for PTSD, such symptoms are distressing and can interfere with normal functioning. One study indicated that after a single session of personal debriefing, lasting on average about 2 h, only 7% of aid workers reported clinically significant levels of avoidance or intrusion (Lovell, 1999b). This suggests that personal debriefing may play an important role in preventing the development of PTSD-related symptoms.

Debriefing may also help to prevent depression.

Approximately 36% of aid workers report developing depression shortly after their return home (Lovell, 1997). In many cases this is related to difficulty readjusting to life at home, or to a sense of meaninglessness. A skilled debriefer can guide the expatriate towards identifying a sense of meaning in the overseas experience, and help to normalize the adjustment process. People who have received debriefing may also be more likely to accept further help, such as counselling, if this is required.

Expatriates generally feel very tired when they return home, and benefit from ample time to rest before resuming work. For longer-term expatriates, it might take months to fully adjust (Lovell, 1997). Care should be taken to support them through this transition period, and not put pressure on them to prepare quickly for another overseas assignment.

CONCLUSIONS

The vast majority of expatriates enjoy their time overseas, despite the inevitable difficulties that they meet along the way. In order to help maximize both their productivity and their satisfaction, it is useful to follow certain guidelines. First, selection methods should be chosen carefully, and should include a medical review and a psychological assessment interview. Such assessments can help in placing expatriates appropriately and can serve to enhance care by ensuring that the agency assumes appropriate responsibility for the needs of their personnel.

Second, training should prepare personnel to recognize common medical problems, apprise them of the appropriate preventive strategies and equip them to recognize signs of illness and how to deal with emergencies. There should also be teaching that covers techniques of stress management, problem solving, safety, crisis management and coping strategies aimed at helping expatriates acknowledge, normalize and request help for any stress-related problems that may develop.

While overseas, the expatriate should continue to receive support, and procedures should be in place for ensuring that help is available should problems develop. The expatriate should be offered help in preparing for the return home. Personal debriefing after return should be routine and an opportunity should be provided for an independent medical assessment, with further support as necessary. Sufficient time should be provided for rest and readjustment. If a partner or family are involved, support should also be available for them.

Finally, there is a need for further research in this area, appraising critically the value of screening, the impact of prevention strategies, the effects of training, the efficacy and extent to which one can become meaningfully involved with telecommunication, the role and value of health assessments upon return and an evaluation of the effects of debriefing among different types of expatriate groups. This will help to ensure that we focus on the appropriate issues in a cost-sensitive manner and that we

do all that we can to help take care of expatriates' psychological and physical health in every stage of their journey.

REFERENCES

ACIP (1999) Human rabies pevention—United States. Recommendations of the Advisory Committee on Immunization Practices. *Morbidity and Mortality Weekly Report*, **48**, (no. RR-1).

Adera T, Wolfe MS, McGuire-Rugh K *et al.* (1995) Risk factors for malaria among expatriates living in Kampala, Uganda: the need for adherence to chemoprophylactic regimens. *American Journal of Tropical Medicine*, **52**, 207–212.

Advisory Committee Statement (1998) Statement on oral cholera vaccination. *Canada Communicable Disease Report*, **24** (ACS-5), 1–4.

American College of Physicians (1981) Periodic health examination: a guide for designing individualized preventive health care in the asymptomatic patient. Medical Practice Committee, ACP. *Annals of Internal Medicine*, **95**, 729–732.

Arguin PM, Krebs JW, Mandel E *et al.* (2000) Survey of rabies preexposure and postexposure prophylaxis among missionary personnel stationed outside the United States. *Journal of Travel Medicine*, **7**, 10–14.

Armstrong KR, Lund PE, Townsend McWright L *et al.* (1995) Multiple stressor debriefing and the American Red Cross: the East Bay Hills fire experience. *Social Work*, **40**, 83–90.

Armstrong KR, Zatzick D, Metzler T *et al.* (1998) Debriefing of American Red Cross personnel: pilot study on participants' evaluations and case examples from the 1994 Los Angeles earthquake relief operation. *Social Work in Health Care*, **27**, 33–50.

Austin CN and Beyer J (1984) Missionary repatriation: an introduction to the literature. *International Bulletin of Missionary Research*, **4**, 68–70.

Aycan Z (1997) Acculturation of expatriate managers: a process model of adjustment and performance. In *New Approaches to Employee Management*, vol. 4, *Expatriate Management: Theory and Research* (ed. Z. Aycan), pp 1–40. Jai Press, Greenwich CT.

Banchongaksorn T, Yomokgul P, Panyim S *et al.* (1996) A field trial of the *Para*Sight—F test for the diagnosis of *Plasmodium falciparum* infection. *Transactions of the Royal Society of Tropical Medicine and Hygiene*, **90**, 244–245.

Deallor C, Gamble K and Keystone J (1997) Travel health recommendations provided by family physicians—are they adequate? *Fifth International Conference on Travel Medicine*, Geneva.

Behr MA and Small PM (1997) Has BCG attenuated to impotence? *Nature*, **389**, 133–134.

Bernard KW and Fishbein DB (1991) Pre-exposure rabies prophylaxis for travellers: are the benefits worth the cost? *Vaccine*, **9**, 833–836.

Bernard KW, Graitcer PL, van der Vlugt T *et al.* (1989) Epidemiological surveillance in Peace Corps volunteers: a model for monitoring health in temporary residents of developing countries. *International Journal of Epidemiology*, **18**, 220–226.

Bjorvatn B and Gundersen SG (1980) Rabies exposure among Norwegian missionaries working abroad. *Scandinavian Journal of Infectious Diseases*, **12**, 257–264.

Bonneux L, Van der Stuyft P, Taelman H *et al.* (988) Risk factors for infection with human immunodeficiency virus among European expatriates in Africa. *British Medical Journal*, **297**, 581–584.

Brierley PW (1997) Missionary attrition: The ReMAP Research Report *Too Valuable to Lose* (ed. WD Taylor), pp 85–102. William Carey Library, Pasadena CA.

Brouwer ML, Tolboom JM and Hardeman JH (1999) Routine screening of children returning home from the tropics: retrospective study. *British Medical Journal*, **318**, 568–569.

Butcher JN (1996) *International Adaptations of the MMPI-2.* University of Minnesota Press, Minneapolis.

Carr K (1994) Trauma and post-traumatic stress disorder among missionaries. *Evangelical Missions Quarterly*, **30**, 246–253.

Carroll B, Dow C, Snashall D *et al.* (1993) Post-tropical screening: how useful is it? *British Medical Journal*, **307**, 541.

Carter J (1999) Missionary stressors and implications for care. *Journal of Psychology and Theology*, **27**, 171–180.

CDC (1993) Inactivated Japanese encephalitis virus vaccine. recommendations of the Advisory Committee on Immunization Practices (ACIP). *Morbidity and Mortality Weekly Report*, **42** (RR-1), 1–15.

Chester RM (1983) Stress on missionary families living in 'other culture' situations. *Journal of Psychology and Christianity*, **2**, 30–37.

Christy RL and Rasmussen JE (1963) Human reliability implications of the US Navy's experience in screening and selection procedures. *American Journal of Psychiatry*, **120**, 540–547.

Churchill DR, Chiodini PL and McAdam K P (1993) Screening the returned traveller. *British Medical Bulletin*, **49**, 465–474.

Conlon CP (1993) Post-tropical screening. Is of little value . . . *British Medical Journal*, **307**, 1008.

Dally P (1985) Psychiatric illness in expatriates. *Journal of the Royal College of Physicians of London*, **19**, 103–104.

Davidson S (1997) People-in-aid code of best practice in the management and support of aid personnel. Overseas Development Institute, London. Available from aidpeople@aol.com.

De Graaf R, van Zessen G, Houweling H *et al.* (1997) Sexual risk of HIV infection among expatriates posted in AIDS endemic areas. *AIDS*, **11**, 1173–1181.

De Graff R, van Zessen G and Houweling H (1998a) Underlying reasons for sexual conduct and condom use among expatriates posted in AIDS endemic areas. *AIDS Care*, **10**, 651–665.

De Graaf R, Houweling H and van Zessen G (1998b) Occupational risk of HIV infection among western health care professionals posted in AIDS endemic areas. *AIDS Care*, **4**, 441–452.

Department of Health (1996) *Immunization against Infectious Disease.* Stationery Office, London.

Department of Health (1997) *Annual Report of the National Screening Committee.* DOH, London.

Desem N and Jones SL (1998) Development of a human gamma interferon enzyme immunoassay and comparison with tuberculin skin testing for detection of *Mycobacterium tuberculosis* infection. *Clinical and Diagnostic Laboratory Immunology*, **5**, 531–536.

Deshpande SP and Viswesvaran C (1992) Is cross-cultural training of expatriate managers effective: a meta analysis. *International Journal of Intercultural Relations*, **16**, 295–310.

Dicken C (1969) Predicting the success of peace corps community development workers. *Journal of Consulting and Clinical Psychology*, **33**, 597–606.

Dillon DE (1983) Personality characteristics of evangelical missionaries as measured by the MMPI. *Journal of Psychology and Theology*, **11**, 213–217.

Doll RE, Gunderson EKE and Ryman DH (1969) Relative predictability of occupational groups and performance criteria in an extreme environment. *Journal of Clinical Psychology*, **25**, 399–402.

Donovan K (1992) *The Pastoral Care of Missionaries*, Commo-

dore Press, Lilydale.

Dunbar E and Ehrlich MH (1993) Preparation of the international employee: career and consultation needs. *Consulting Psychology Journal*, **45**, 18–24.

Dwelle TL (1995) Inadequate basic preventive health measures: survey of missionary children in sub-Saharan Africa. *Pediatrics*, **95**, 733–737.

Dye SF (1974) Decreasing fatigue and illness in field-work. *Missiology*, **2**, 79–109.

Editorial (1999) Targeting the helpers. *Refugees*, **114**.

Ehlers A, Clark DM, Dunmore E *et al.* (1998) Predicting response to exposure treatment in PTSD: the role of mental defeat and alienation. *Journal of Traumatic Stress*, **11**, 457–471.

Engel HO (1980) Fitness for work abroad. *Journal of the Royal Society of Medicine*, **73**, 303–304.

Fawcett G (1999) *Ad-Mission: The Briefing and Debriefing of Teams of Missionaries and Aid Workers.* Self-published: Harpenden, England.

Fisher J, Epstein LJ and Harris MR (1967) Validity of the psychiatric interview. Predicting the effectiveness of the first Peace Corps volunteers in Ghana. *Archives of General Psychiatry*, **17**, 744–750.

Foyle MF (1987) *Honourably Wounded.* MARC Europe, Bromley, Kent.

Foyle MF (1994) Expatriate children: selection, preparation, and typical needs. *Travel Medicine International*, **12**, 93–97.

Foyle MF, Beer MD and Watson JP (1998) Expatriate mental health. *Acta Psychiatrica Scandinavica*, **97**, 278–283.

Frame JD, Lange WR and Frankenfield DL (1992) Mortality trends of American missionaries in Africa, 1945–1985. *American Society of Tropical Medicine and Hygiene*, **46**, 686–690.

Friman G, Nystrom-Rosander C, Jonsell G *et al.* (1983) Agranulocytosis associated with malaria prophylaxis with Maloprim. *British Medical Journal*, **286**, 1244–1245.

Funk M, Schlagenhauf P, Tschopp A *et al.* (1999) MalaQuick versus ParaSight F as a diagnostic aid in travellers' malaria. *Transactions of the Royal Society of Tropical Medicine and Hygiene*, **93**, 268–272.

Gardner LM (1984) A study of missionary terminations to determine predictability and preventability factors. DMin thesis, Conservative Baptist Seminary, Denver, Colorado.

Genton B and Gehri M (1999) Routine screening of children returning home from the tropics. Authors' definition of asymptomatic children is not the one usually accepted. *British Medical Journal*, **319**, 121–122.

Goldberg DP, Rickels K, Downing R *et al.* (1976) A comparison of two psychiatric screening tests. *British Journal of Psychiatry*, **129**, 61–67.

Goode GS (1995) Guidelines for crisis and contingency management. *International Journal of Frontier Missions*, **12**, 211–216.

Gordon LV (1967) Clinical, psychometric, and work-sample approaches in the prediction of success in Peace Corps training. *Journal of Applied Psychology*, **51**, 111–119.

Grant R (1995) Trauma in missionary life. *Missiology*, **23**, 71–83.

Greenwood BM (1991) Malaria chemoprophylaxis in endemic regions. In Malaria: Waiting for the Vaccine. *London School of Hygiene and Tropical Medicine, First Annual Public Health Forum* (ed. GA Targett. Wiley, Chichester.

Gunderson EK and Kapfer EL (1966) The predictive validity of clinical ratings for an extreme environment. *British Journal of Psychiatry*, **112**, 405–412.

Guthrie GM and Zektick IN (1967) Predicting performance in the Peace Corps. *Journal of Social Psychology*, **71**, 11–21.

Hargarten SW and Baker SP (1985) Fatalities in the Peace

Corps. A retrospective study: 1962 through 1983. *Journal of the American Medical Association*, **254**, 1326–1329.

Hargrave GE, Hiatt D, Ogard EM *et al.* (1994) Comparison of the MMPI and the MMPI-2 for a sample of peace offers. *Psychological Assessment*, **6**, 27–32.

Harzing AK (1995) The persistent myth of high expatriate failure rates. *International Journal of Human Resource Management*, **6**, 457–473.

Hathaway SR and McKinley JC (1989) *Minnesota Multiphasic Personality Inventory-2*, University of Minnesota Press, Minneapolis.

Hatz CF, Bidaux JM, Eichenberger K *et al.* (1994) Circumstances and management of 72 animal bites among long-term residents in the tropics. *Vaccine*, **13**, 811–815.

Hayward SA, Steinberg EP, Ford DE *et al.* (1991) Preventive care guidelines: 1991. *Annals of Internal Medicine*, **114**, 758–783.

Henry ER (1965) What business can learn from Peace Corps selection and training. *Personnel*, **42**, 17–25.

Hoge CW, Shlim DR, Echeverria P *et al.* (1996) Epidemiology of diarrhea among expatriate residents living in a highly endemic environment. *Journal of the American Medical Association*, **275**, 533–538.

Holmes WF and Piker FK (1980) Expatriate failure—prevention rather than cure. *Personnel Management*, **12**, 30–32.

Horowitz MJ, Wilner N and Alvarez W (1979) Impact of event scales: a measure of subjective distress. *Psychosomatic Medicine*, **41**, 209–218.

Houweling H and Coutinho RA (1991) Risk of HIV infection among Dutch expatriates in sub-Saharan Africa. *International Journal of STD and AIDS*, **4**, 252–257.

ICRC (1994) *Humanitarian Action in Conflict Zones: Coping with Stress*, ICRC Guidelines. Comrex, Geneva.

Jordan P (1992) *Re-entry*. YWAM Publishing, Seattle.

Kain KC and Keystone JS (1998) Malaria in travelers. Epidemiology, disease, and prevention. *Infectious Disease Clinics of North America*, **12**, 267–284.

Kain KC, MacPherson D, Kelton T *et al.* (2001) Malaria deaths in visitors to Canada and in Canadian travellers: a case series. *CMAJ*, **164**, 654–659.

Karson S and O'Dell JW (1987) Personality profiles in the US Foreign Service. In *Advances in Personality Assessment* eds JN Butcher and CD Spielberger, pp 1–12. Laurence Earlbaum, Hillsdale NJ.

Kremsner PG, Lovareesuwan S and Chulay J (1999) Atovaquone and proguanil hydrochloride for treatment of malaria. *Journal of Travel Medicine*, **6** (Suppl. 1), S18–S20.

Lange WR and Frame JD (1990) High incidence of viral hepatitis among American missionaries in Africa. *American Journal of Tropical Medicine and Hygiene*, **43**, 527–533.

Lange WR and Frame JD (1991) Assessment of risk for HIV-1 infection for missionaries in sub-Saharan Africa. *Southern Medical Journal*, **84**, 193–197.

Lange WR and McCune BA (1989) Substance abuse and international travel. *Advances in Alcohol and Substance Abuse*, **8**, 37–51.

Lange WR, Kreider SD, Kaczaniuk MA *et al.* (1987) Missionary health: the great omission. *American Journal of Preventive Medicine*, **6**, 332–338.

Lange WR, Dax EM, Kovacs R *et al.* (1989) Are missionaries at risk for AIDS? Evaluation for HIV antibodies in 3207 protestant missionaries. *Southern Medical Journal*, **82**, 1075–1078.

Lange WR, Frankenfield D and Contoreggi CS (1994a) Psychological concerns of overseas employees and families. *Travel Medicine International*, **12**, 176–181.

Lange WR, Frankenfield DL and Frame JD (1994b) Morbidity among refugee relief workers. *Journal of Travel Medicine*, **1**, 111–112.

LeGuerrier P, Pilon P and Deshaies D (1996) Pre-exposure rabies prophylaxis for the international traveller: a decision analysis. *Vaccine*, **14**, 167–176.

Libman MD, MacLean JD and Gyorkos TW (1993) Screening for schistosomiasis, filariasis, and strongyloidiasis among expatriates returning from the tropics. *Clinical Infectious Diseases*, **17**, 353–359.

Lobel HO, Bernard KW, Williams SL *et al.* (1991) Effectiveness and tolerance of long-term malaria prophylaxis with mefloquine. Need for a better dosing regimen. *Journal of the American Medical Association*, **265**, 361–364.

Lobel HO, Miani M, Eng T *et al.* (1993) Long-term malaria prophylaxis with weekly mefloquine. *Lancet*, **341**, 848–851.

Lobel HO, Varma JK, Miani M *et al.* (1998) Monitoring for mefloquine-resistant *Plasmodium falciparum* in Africa: implications for travellers' health. *American Journal of Tropical Medicine and Hygiene*, **59**, 129–132.

Lovell DM (1997) *Psychological adjustment among returned overseas aid workers*. DClinPsy Thesis, University of Wales, Bangor.

Lovell DM (1999a) Chronic fatigue syndrome among overseas development workers: a qualitative study. *Journal of Travel Medicine*, **6**, 16–23.

Lovell DM (1999b) *Evaluation of Tearfund's critical incident debriefing process*. Tearfund, Teddington.

Mabey D (1995) Sex and travel. *British Journal of Hospital Medicine*, **54**, 264–266, 275.

McCall M and Salama P (1999) Selection, training and support of relief workers: An occupational health issue. *British Medical Journal*, **318**, 113–116.

McConnan I (1992) *Recruiting Health Workers for Emergencies and Disaster Relief in Developing Countries*. International Health Exchange, London.

MacLean JD and Libman M (1998) Screening returning travelers. *Infectious Disease Clinics of North America*, **12**, 431–443.

Macnair R (1995) *Room for Improvement: The Management and Support of Relief and Development Workers*. Overseas Development Institute, London.

MacPherson DW (1999) Intestinal parasites in returned travelers. *Medical Clinics of North America*, **83**, 1053–1075.

Médicins Sans Frontières (1997) Procedures to be followed after an accidental exposure to blood *MSF Holland*. These guidelines are subject to regular review and update.

Mills CD, Burgess DCH, Taylor HJ *et al.* (1999) Evaluation of a rapid and inexpensive dipstick assay for the diagnosis of *Plasmodium falciparum* malaria. *Bulletin of the World Health Organization*, **77**, 553–559.

Mitchell JT (1983) When disaster strikes. *Journal of Emergency Medical Services*, **8**, 36–39.

MMWR (1999) Suicide prevention among active duty air force personnel: United States, 1990–1999. *Morbidity and Mortality Weekly Report*, **48** (no. 46).

Moore J, Beeker C, Harrison J *et al.* (1995) HIV risk behavior among Peace Corps Volunteers. *AIDS*, **9**, 795–799.

Moore TA and Nutman TB (1998) Eosinophilia in the returning traveler. *Infectious Disease Clinics of North America*, **12**, 503–521.

Oates D (1970) What it takes to work abroad. *International Management*, **10**, 24–27.

Ohrt C, Richie Tl, Widjaja H *et al.* (1997) Mefloquine compared with doxycycline for the prophylaxis of malaria in Indonesian soldiers. *Annals of Internal Medicine*, **126**, 963–672.

Okereke E and Gelletie R (1999) Letter. *British Medical Journal*, **319**, 121–122.

Ones DZ and Viswesvaran C (1997) Personality determinants in the prediction of aspects of expatriate job success. In *New Approaches to Employment Management*, vol. 4, *Expatriate Management: Theory and Research* (ed. Z Aycan, pp 63–92. Jai Press, Greenwich CT.

Paluszny M and Zrull JP (1971) The new missionary: a review of 50 candidates. *Archives of General Psychiatry*, **24**, 363–366.

Parshall P (1988) How spiritual are missionaries? In *Helping Missionaries Grow: Readings in Mental Health and Missions*, (eds KS O'Donnell and ML O'Donnell, pp 75–82. William Carey Library, Pasadena CA.

Paton D (1992) International disasters: issues in the management and preparation of relief workers. *Disaster Management*, **4**, 183–190.

Paton D and Purvis C (1995) Nursing in the aftermath of disaster: orphanage relief work in Romania. *Disaster Prevention and Management*, **4**, 45–54.

Peppiatt R and Byass P (1990) Risk factors for malaria among British missionaries living in tropical countries. *Journal of Tropical Medicine and Hygiene*, **93**, 397–402.

Peppiatt R and Byass P (1991) A survey of the health of British missionaries. *British Journal of General Practice*, **41**, 159–162.

Phillips-Howard P, Radalowicz F, Mitchell J *et al.* (1990) Risk of malaria in British residents returning from malarious areas. *British Medical Journal*, **300**, 499–503.

Pieroni P, Mills CD, Ohrt C *et al.* (1998) Comparison of the *Para*Sight-F test and the ICT Malaria Pf test with the polymerase chain reaction for the diagnosis of *Plasmodium falciparum* malaria in travellers. *Transactions of the Royal Society of Tropical Medicine and Hygiene*, **92**, 166–169.

Richardson J (1992) Psychopathology in missionary personnel. In *Missionary Care* (eds K O'Donnell and ML O'Donnell, pp 89–109. William Carey Library, Pasadena CA.

Rogers C (1998) The changing shape of security for NGO field workers. *Together*, 9–11.

Rose S and Bisson J (1998) Brief early interventions following trauma: a systematic review of the literature. *Journal of Traumatic Stress*, **11**, 697–710.

Rowbottom J (1993) STDs and the overseas traveller. *Australian Family Physician*, **22**, 125–131.

Schlagenhauf P, Steffen R, Lobel H *et al.* (1996) Mefloquine tolerability during chemoprophylaxis: focus on adverse event assessments, stereochemistry and compliance. *Tropical Medicine and International Health*, **4**, 485–494.

Schneider G (1998) Malaria prevention for long-term workers overseas. Choice or necessary evil? MSc thesis, University of London.

Schnurr PP, Friedman MD and Rosenberg SD (1993) Premilitary MMPI scores as predictors of combat-related PTSD symptoms. *American Journal of Psychiatry*, **150**, 479–483.

Schouten EJ and Borgdorff MW (1995) Increased mortality among Dutch development workers. *British Medical Journal*, **311**, 1343–1344.

Schubert E (1992) Current issues in screening and selection. In *Missionary Care* (eds K O'Donnell and ML O'Donnell), pp 74–88. William Carey Library, Pasadena, CA.

Schubert E (1999) A suggested prefield process for missionary candidates. *Journal of Psychology and Theology*, **27**, 87–97.

Schubert E and Ganter K (1996) The MMPI as a predictive tool for missionary candidates. *Journal of Psychology and Theology*, **24**, 124–132.

Shlim DR, Hoge CW, Rajah R *et al.* (1999) Persistent high risk of diarrhea among foreigners in Nepal during the first 2 years of residence. *Clinical Infectious Diseases*, **29**, 613–616.

Sieveking N, Anchor K and Marston RC (1981) Selecting and preparing expatriate employees. *Personnel Journal*, **60**, 197–202.

Slim H (1995) The continuing metamorphosis of the humanitarian practitioner: some new colours for an endangered chameleon. *Disasters*, **19**, 110–126.

Smalligan RD, Lange WR, Frame JD *et al.* (1995) The risk of viral hepatitis A, B, C, and E among North American missionaries. *American Journal of Tropical Medicine and Hygiene*, **3**, 233–236.

Smith B, Agger I, Danieli Y *et al.* (1996) Health activities across traumatized populations: emotional responses of international humanitarian aid workers. In *International Responses to Traumatic Stress: Humanitarian, Human Rights, Justice, Peace and Development Contributions, Collaborative Actions and Future Initiatives* (eds Y Danieli, NS Rodley and L Weisaeth), pp 397–422. Baywood, New York.

Streeton JA, Desem N and Jones SL (1998) Sensitivity and specificity of a gamma interferon blood test for tuberculosis infection. *International Journal Tuberculosis and Lung Disease*, **2**, 443–450.

Stroh LK, Dennis LE and Cramer TC (1994) Predictors of expatriate adjustment. *International Journal of Organizational Analysis*, **2**, 176–192.

Sweatman SM (1999) Marital satisfaction, cross-cultural adjustment stress, and the psychological sequelae. *Journal of Psychology and Theology*, **27**, 154–162.

Trachsler M, Schlagenhauf P and Steffen R (1999) Feasibility of a rapid dipstick antigen-capture assay for self-testing of travellers' malaria. *Tropical Medicine and International Health*, **4**, 442–447.

Tung RL (1988) *The New Expatriates: Managing Human Resources Abroad*. Ballinger, Cambridge MA.

Vaughn D and Hoke C (1992) The epidemiology of Japanese encephalitis: prospects for prevention. *Epidemiologic Reviews*, **14**, 197–221.

Westefeld JS and Maples M (1998) The MMPI-2 and vocational assessment: a brief report. *Journal of Career Assessment*, **6**, 107–113.

World Health Organization (1997) World Malaria Situation in 1994. *Weekly Epidemiological Report*, **36**, 269–273.

World Health Organization (1998) Tuberculosis. Fact sheet no. 104. WHO, Geneva.

World Health Organization (1999) AIDS not losing momentum. WHO Press Release, **66**, Geneva.

28

The Health of Migrants and Refugees

Louis Loutan

University Hospital of Geneva, Geneva, Switzerland

INTRODUCTION

Traditionally, individuals or populations on the move are referred to as either travellers or migrants. International *travellers* number nearly 1 billion persons per year. Their journey involves the crossing of international borders on a two-way ticket and their travel is often between rich countries, or from rich to poor countries. The duration of these journeys is often limited. Their contact with foreign populations is frequently sporadic, and may occur in comfortable hotels, although there is an increase in 'exotic' or wilderness travel. These travellers may be exposed to poor hygiene and foreign pathogens and have some risk of bringing the consequences of that exposure home with them. However, as a whole, the experience is often considered recreational, and consequently even illness acquired in this manner may not be perceived as a significant hardship (Loutan and Gushulak, 1999).

Migrants number approximately 2–4 million persons per year. They travel primarily on a one way ticket, usually from poor to richer countries, carrying with them the specific burdens of their country of origin. Their conditions of travel often include journeys of much longer duration than those of tourists. Migrants tend to have prolonged contact with new populations, experience new cultural practices and suffer some restriction in access to traditional health care at their new destination. There are several 'sub-categories' of migrants and travellers, including tourists, business travellers, humanitarian workers, students, military personnel, immigrants, refugees, asylum seekers, illegal migrants and others. Each category can be defined according to some specific characteristics but they all share common factors related to travel and the risk of some health consequences resulting from that movement process.

WORLD MIGRATION: NUMBERS AND TRENDS

In today's globalised world, a growing number of people seek to migrate, searching for a better life or escaping war, human rights violations, poverty or environmental disasters. International migration is a worldwide phenomenon, not one that is restricted to industrialised nations. According to the United Nations Population Division there were 120 million international migrants in the world in 1990, rising from 75 million in 1965, with an annual growth rate of 1.9% (WHO, 1998). In 1990, international migrants accounted for 2.3% of the world population. They made up 18% of the total population in Australia and New Zealand; nearly 11% in western Asia; less than 9% in North America; over 6% in western Europe; and less than 2.5% in Asia, Africa and Latin America. Net international migration contributed to 45% of the population growth in the developed world in 1990–1995. In Europe, it contributed to almost 88% of the population growth during this period. The number of refugees has increased markedly, reaching a maximum in 1993 at 18.2 million. Since then, the number of refugees has been decreasing, to 13.2 million in 1996, a decline due to major repatriations [United Nations High Commissioner for Refugees (UNHCR) 1997]. By January 2000, the total number of persons (including internally displaced persons) of concern to the UNHCR (2000) was 22.3 million. The number of persons seeking asylum also increased drastically until 1992, then stabilised due to more restrictive policies of the receiving countries. Between 1985 and 1995, over 5 million asylum applications were registered in the industrialised states. In 1998 and 1999, due to the increasing instability and then war in Kosovo, the number of refugees fleeing the Balkans and seeking asylum rose drastically in Europe, with 473 000 new applications in 1999, a 19.1% increase over 1998 (UNHCR, 2000). As asylum is granted only to a minority of candidates, between 10 and 15%, the majority live in very precarious conditions, some being deported back to their country of origin, others becoming illegal residents or seeking asylum in other European countries.

As the tide of refugees and migrants increases, with a growing influx seeking refuge or better life opportunities in industrialised countries, strengthened border controls

Principles and Practice of Travel Medicine. Edited by Jane N. Zuckerman.

Table 28.1 Persons of concern to UNHCR (at 1 January 2000, by category and region)

Region	Refugees	Asylum seekers	returned refugees	IDPs and others of concern	Total
Africa	3 523 250	61 110	933 890	1 732 290	6 250 540
Asia	4 781 750	24 750	617 620	1 884 740	7 308 860
Europe	2 608 380	473 060	952 060	3 252 300	7 285 800
Latin America and Caribbean	61 200	1 510	6 260	21 200	90 170
North America	636 300	605 630	—	—	1 241 930
Oceania	64 500	15 540	—	—	80 040
Total	11 675 380	1 181 600	2 509 830	6 890 530	22 257 340

IDPs = internally displaced persons.
Adapted from United Nations High Commissioner for Refugees (2000).

and more stringent administrative barriers are being implemented to contain this influx of newcomers. This has resulted in a significant increase of irregular migration and human trafficking of migrants. The United Nations estimates that 4 million persons are victims of international trafficking each year (Gushulak and MacPherson, 2000a). Of these, 700 000 are women or children, of whom 175 000 are estimated to come from the former Soviet bloc; approximately 45 000–50 000 arrive in the United States. There are an estimated 5 million irregular migrants in the USA and 3 million in western Europe (Ghosh, 1998). Trafficking in migrants has become a very lucrative illegal market, with worldwide ramifications. Having no legal status and living with the constant fear of being deported, illegal migrants represent a very vulnerable population with very little access to health care. Table 28.1 gives statistics on persons of concern to the UNHCR for 1999.

As economic inequalities between the developing world and industrialised countries, between the East and the West, are not levelling rapidly, migration pressure will not diminish in the near future. Simultaneously, the ageing of the population of the western world coupled to low fertility rates will lead to negative demographic trends. Policies encouraging selective and controlled migration into Europe can be anticipated in order to counterbalance these demographic trends, leading to new influxes of migrants.

THE MIGRATION PROCESS AND HEALTH

Migrant populations are very heterogeneous in origin, in experienced exposure to risk factors, conditions of living in the host country and access to health care services. No doubt these many factors will influence their health status. One way of looking at the health of migrants is to consider it in relation with the very process of migration.

Taking into account the successive stages of the migratory steps allows for a more systematic analysis of the factors influencing the present health condition of an individual or a community. The successive and interconnected steps are the predeparture phase, the journey phase of migration, the arrival and settling phase and for some migrants the returning phase. At each of these steps of the migratory process, several specific factors may have consequences and influence the final outcome.

The predeparture phase. This is characterised by the influences on health of the environment in which one individual or a group of migrants has lived. This refers to a broad spectrum of factors. One thinks immediately of exposure to endemic diseases such as malaria, tuberculosis, intestinal parasites or hepatitis. Nutritional factors such as sufficient intake of micronutrients, vitamins and proteins will shape the nutritional status and normal growth of children. Social and economic factors such as poverty, illiteracy, unemployment, occupational hazards, poor housing and unhygienic living conditions are among key factors shaping the future health status of migrants, as will exposure to insecurity, war, violence, torture and other human rights violations. Religion and cultural background are of course of key importance in influencing health belief and behaviours. Finally, experiences encountered in contact with the medical services in the country of origin and with other traditional and lay medical providers will also influence expectations of and rapport with medical services in the country of settlement.

The journey phase of migration. This may be very short and uneventful in the case of a regular flight to the new destination. For many refugees and migrants the journey may be a long process, characterised by uncertainty, deprivation, insecurity, abuse, trauma and sometimes life-threatening events. This may be particularly the case for illegal migrants smuggled into a new country. Several tragedies have been reported: for instance, drowning of migrants crossing the Gibraltar straits or off the coast of Florida; the recent discovery of 50 Chinese migrants found dead from suffocation in a trailer in Dover; and those frozen after a intercontinental flight hidden in the wheel compartment of an aeroplane. Women being sexually abused, repeated threats of being denounced to the local police, and the very process of being trafficked without proper documents, completely dependent on Mafia networks, place illegal migrants under great physical and psychological strain.

The postmigration environment. This may differ greatly according to the legal status of a particular person or community. The level of education, professional skills, language and communication skills will influence the capacity of migrants to adjust to the new cultural, professional and social environment and progressively interact with and integrate into the new society. Previous exposure to violence and trauma may pose a serious barrier to adaptation, as persons suffering from post-traumatic stress disorder (PTSD) may avoid contacts or over-react to new unexpected constraints or situations. Living conditions, such as overcrowding or isolation, may accelerate the transmission of diseases such as tuberculosis and varicella, or may have an important psychological impact. Restrictive policies aimed at discouraging newcomers from seeking asylum may have also a deleterious effect on the mental health of asylum seekers or migrants (Silove *et al.*, 2000). Access to health services may be restricted. Arriving in the receiving country may also be a relief and gives the opportunity to start a new life, with access to services and better living conditions influencing positively the health of newcomers.

The return back home. This is being experienced by a growing number of migrants. Recently, a large proportion of refugees having fled the war in Kosovo have been given incentives to return home. Those who were not willing have been put under strong pressure to comply with this policy, some being deported against their will. The return to a country under reconstruction, where insecurity still prevails, with the possibility of retaliation towards those who have fled abroad, may pose specific risks to these persons.

In taking into account the successive steps of the migratory process, it is possible to build a clearer view of potential exposures and risk factors that may influence the present health condition of specific persons or a community. This can help primary care providers to identify the present complaint or illness with the previous events related to the person's migration process.

Thus, the health of migrants is largely influenced by specific living conditions, previous exposure to communicable diseases, deprivation or violence, professional risks, the degree of integration in the new society, the access to health care, the capability to communicate and the presence or absence of a community or family safety net. At present, most of the data on migration and health come from surveys on specific groups of migrants or services, or through medical screening programmes at the time of entry into the host country. Routinely gathered data on the health of ethnic minorities or of foreign-born residents are often lacking in this area. Thus caution should be exercised in extrapolating the conclusions of specific studies to all migrants and, in so doing, contributing to the negative perception of migrants and to some indirect form of discrimination.

A recent review of health issues and problems of migrants in the European Union found that, compared with the host population, migrants have less access to health services and often have a higher rate of certain conditions such as tuberculosis, HIV, hepatitis B, accidental injuries, psychosomatic problems and depression (Carballo *et al.*, 1998). Does migration in itself constitute an unhealthy process and put people on the move at higher risk of disease? Do we have a biased view on the health of migrants from studies uncontrolled for socioeconomic disadvantages or unequal access to health services? (Junghaus, 1998). Migration is a very selective process and those arriving in industrialised nations as immigrants, refugees or asylum seekers may not be representative of the population from which they come. They are probably the stronger, mentally and physically.

FIRST ENCOUNTER WITH HEALTH SERVICES

The introduction of communicable diseases by foreigners and travellers has always been of concern to health authorities. International regulations, quarantine procedures and medical screening have been designed to control the spread of diseases. At a time of worldwide mobility of millions of travellers, medical screening is still implemented for immigrants and refugees before or at the time of entry in the receiving country. It is most frequently mandatory and in some instances it determines acceptance for entering the country. No doubt migrants may be afraid that such a medical examination that may hinder them from reaching their destination. Medical screening is aimed mainly at identifying communicable diseases such as tuberculosis, hepatitis B, syphilis, HIV or other health conditions that may cause a financial burden on the receiving country. Preventive measures such as vaccinations are often implemented at that time. Much of the data available on the health of migrants are drawn from medical screening at time of entry.

Obviously, mandatory medical screening is the result of public health concern both for protecting the host population and identifying sick individuals in order to provide them with care. This is not patient-centred medicine. Immigrants and refugees have health needs that often are not met by medical screening and many health professionals question its medical soundness, moving towards a normal medical interview and examination, promoting access to local medical facilities and responding to specific health needs individual migrants have.

Furthermore, the diminishing impact of classical infectious diseases in a globally mobile world forces us to explore new approaches and responses. Until recently, most of the emphasis has been put on the diseases responsible for epidemics (yellow fever, cholera, smallpox). Access to clean water, immunisation and use of antibiotics have reduced drastically their prevalence and population health impact, thus reducing the effectiveness and need for mass medical screening (Gushulak and MacPherson, 2000b). With mobile populations becoming a larger component of societies, diseases with long latency periods or subclinical or chronic stable infectious periods pose problems not solved by screening at the time of entry. Chronic infectious diseases, such as tuberculosis, hepatitis B or C, schistosomiasis or diseases with a long latency such as malaria vivax, will often be recognised after many months in the host country. Even in the case of tuberculosis, 47% of cases recorded in foreign-born people in the USA are detected more than 5 years after their arrival (Binkin *et al.*, 1996). This shift towards chronic diseases creates a situation where the first interaction with the health care system is likely to be at community level with primary care providers. This has direct implications on how and where to reinforce surveillance systems and provide the family doctors with adequate knowledge and training in recognising and managing diseases they are not familiar with.

CARE OF MIGRANTS AT THE PRACTITIONER'S OFFICE

Primary care providers and travel medicine professionals may frequently see foreign-born patients of diverse origins, both for treatment and for preventive measures such as immunisation. They need to be able to recognise diseases that are more 'exotic' than those prevalent in the local native population. They should also be aware of long-term effects of exposure to violence, as many refugees and immigrants come from war-torn regions of the world. They also need to develop cultural competence to communicate with patients and identify clearly their concerns, their health beliefs and how to address their needs in a culturally sensitive manner.

Infectious Diseases

Coming from regions where many cosmopolitan or tropical communicable diseases are more prevalent, a significant proportion of migrants may have been in contact with, may be infected with or may be a carrier of some specific disease. This is particularly the case with tuberculosis.

Tuberculosis

Tuberculosis is a disease that is increasing worldwide as a result of population growth, as a coinfection with HIV and with insufficient access to adequate treatment leading to the spread of resistant strains. Although in North America and Europe there has been a steady decrease in cases of tuberculosis, there is an increase in the proportion of cases diagnosed in the foreign born (Rieder *et al.*, 1994; Zuber *et al.*, 1997). In Denmark, the proportion of foreign-born cases has risen from 18% in 1986 to 60% in 1996 (Carballo *et al.*, 1998). The incidence in foreign-born children was very high, probably due to intrafamilial transmission (Mortensen *et al.*, 1989). In Switzerland the incidence of tuberculosis in native Swiss is 7.8 per 100 000; it is 24.7 per 100 000 in foreign-born residents of European origin; and 147 per 100 000 for asylum seekers (Zellweger, 1996). In England, travellers visiting friends and relatives in Asia accounted for 20% of all notifications, with 80% reported within 3 years of return to the UK, suggesting a significant risk of transmission, in particular for children returning to their country of origin (McCarthy, 1984). Pulmonary symptoms lasting more than 2 weeks, fatigue and weight loss should always raise the possibility of an underlying tuberculosis. In patients coming from countries of endemicity, a significant proportion of cases of tuberculosis are extrapulmonary and this should be looked for. In a recent survey of cases of tuberculosis in illegal migrants in Geneva, 36% had an isolated extrapulmonary lesion (Aebischer Perone *et al.*, 1999). Resistant strains of tuberculosis are emerging all over the world, including in industrialised countries. In areas where access to treatment is inadequate, there has been a marked increase in the appearance of drug resistance. Of particular concern are some east European countries.

Hepatitis

Hepatitis A is highly prevalent in the developing world. In general, by the age of 10, the vast majority of children have been exposed and have lifelong protective antibodies. Sometimes, child refugees, some incubating the disease, have caused limited outbreaks in persons having close contacts with them (Castelli *et al.*, 1999). In Asia and Africa, the endemicity of hepatitis B is high, with over 5% carriers of hepatitis B surface antigen. Table 28.2 shows the seroprevalence of hepatitis B in asylum seekers screened in Switzerland at the time of arrival, according to their origin (Raeber *et al.*, 1990). This illustrates its variability as the result of the level of endemicity in their country of origin; it is also related to some selection inherent in the migratory process. Counselling and providing medical care to those who are chronically infected, and immunising relatives to prevent intrafamilial infection, should be carried out by medical providers. Hepatitis C is also of concern, with high prevalence rates (> 10%) in the developing world.

Table 28.2 Results of hepatitis B screening in asylum seekers

Country	HBsAg			Anti-HBs			HBeAg	
	n	Pos	%	n	Pos	%	n	Pos
Turkey	5091	573	11.3	4304	2205	51.2	497	71
Sri Lanka	2643	11	0.4	2355	201	8.5	20	1
Iran	1324	14	1.1	633	121	19.1	3	1
Pakistan	676	29	4.3	563	210	37.3	32	3
Zaire	538	27	5.0	525	265	50.6	44	4
Chile	443	0	0	361	32	8.9	2	0
India	393	10	2.5	284	58	20.4	9	0
Ethiopia	343	14	4.1	312	113	36.2	14	1
Angola	323	24	7.4	316	147	46.5	21	1
Ghana	240	23	9.6	211	120	56.9	26	10
Lebanon	216	5	2.3	46	12	26.1	1	0
Other countries	1443	97	6.7	1228	439	37.7	86	23
Total	13673	827	6.0	11137	3923	35.2	755	115

Pos = positive.
HBeAg tested only in a limited sample of HBsAg-positive persons (756/827).
Adapted from Raeber *et al.* (1990).

Malaria

Plasmodium falciparum malaria does not have a long incubation period. In the vast majority of cases, the disease become clinically apparent less than 1 month after an infective mosquito bite. For other types of malaria, such as *P. vivax*, *P. ovale* and *P. malariae*, the latent phase can last for several months, even years, after contamination. Thus, fever in a patient who originated from a tropical country should always trigger the possibility of malaria. In many European countries, an increased proportion of cases of malaria is seen in patients of foreign origin. In northen Italy, the proportion rose from 34.4% in 1991 to 59.9% in 1995 (Matteelli *et al.*, 1999). In England, between 1987 and 1992, 49% of 8355 cases of malaria occurred in ethnic minority travellers visiting friends and relatives. Visitors and immigrants constituted 19% and 11%, respectively (Behrens, 1995). In comparing ethnic minority travellers with UK tourists with imported malaria, 51% versus 20%, respectively, were not taking any prophylaxis. It is possible that risk perception in these two groups may be very different. The former may believe they have retained some immunity, having lived at their destination, and are thus not seeking pretravel health advice and not taking prophylaxis. The attack rate of those visiting West Africa was three time higher compared with business travellers or tourists. This may be related to a higher rate of transmission in the places visited, rural versus urban, unprotected houses versus air-conditioned hotels, with less protection.

HIV/AIDS and Sexually Transmitted Diseases

Migrants coming from regions where the epidemic is common may have been infected, although asymptomatic at time of arrival. In Switzerland, the incidence rate of newly diagnosed cases is much higher in residents from sub-Saharan Africa (> 500 versus 12 per 100000 per year) (Swiss Office for Public Health, 2000). Voluntary screening, counselling, information on the disease and prevention should be encouraged in potentially at-risk groups. Access to therapy may be problematic, particularly for illegal migrants with no insurance cover. Nevertheless, many migrants come from areas of the world where the HIV/AIDS infection is much less prevalent than in the industrialised western countries and thus become at higher risk of contamination in the new host country. Targeted prevention programmes should be implemented at the time of arrival. Mandatory screening for HIV has often been considered unethical and discriminatory.

Sexually transmitted disease is on the increase in certain countries, such as Russia, in the context of serious social and economic disruptions. Testing for syphilis is still mandatory for entry to some countries as a refugee or an immigrant. In testing for VDRL/TPHA in more than 13000 asylum seekers arriving in Switzerland, only 0.6% were positive (Raeber *et al.*, 1990). Many of these may have been infected with some endemic treponematosis prevalent in many parts of the world, and not the sexually transmitted syphilis.

Parasitic Infections

Intestinal infection due to protozoans and worms is very common in arriving migrants. The proportion of persons infected varies greatly according to origin (10–40%) (Raeber *et al.*, 1990). Most of the time they are asymptomatic and some programmes have proposed systematic anthelmintic treatment with mebendazole or albendazole. Helminth infection can last for years. It may cause growth retardation and anaemia in children and should be sought for.

Clinical presentation is often aspecific, but eosinophilia should prompt a search for looking for helmintic parasites. *Strongyloides stercoralis* can remain for decades, causing marked eosinophilia, cutaneous larva currens and pulmonary symptoms in relation to periodic autoreinfection. Schistosomiasis can also persist for more than 20 years, causing potentially local complications such as uretheral stricture, bladder fibrosis and possibly cancer. In patients coming from areas of hyperendemicity, haematuria may be considered as normal: being experienced by every child, it may not be reported. There are many other systemic parasitic diseases that physicians should be aware of, understanding their specific geographical distribution and its relationship to the patient's origin and journey; for example, neurocysticercosis, echinococcosis, filariasis, onchocerciasis and paragonimiasis. Strongyloidiasis, leishmaniasis and American trypanosomiasis should be remembered as they can resurface in immunocompromised patients.

Other Infectious Diseases

The recent outbreak of menigococcal meningitis W135 that took place in Mecca in the Spring of 2000, with imported cases and transmission to relatives in several European countries, reminds us that mobile populations can be at risk and emphasises the importance of effective surveillance mechanisms. Migrants are not always the introducers disease. They may arrive unprotected against common diseases in European and North American countries. This is the case with varicella, a disease much less prevalent in certain tropical regions. Epidemics have been recorded in European countries (Kjersem and Jepsen, 1990), and immunisation should be considered, as varicella can be a very serious disease in unprotected adults.

Noninfectious Diseases

There is often a tendency to look at migrant health only from an infectious diseases perspective. Noninfectious diseases should not be forgotten, as the world is changing rapidly. Cardiovascular diseases, diabetes, asthma, respiratory diseases linked with smoking, cancers, occupational diseases and injuries, exposure to environmental hazards, mental disorders are on the increase in the developing world, as a result of rapid urbanisation, socioeconomic and behavioural changes (WHO, 1998). The recent Kosovo crisis revealed the burden of chronic diseases in the refugee population. Surveys have shown that, as a result of lifestyle changes, the incidence of cardiovascular diseases in immigrants to Canada or USA tend to

adjust with time to those observed in the local population (Kliever, 1992). Thus, epidemiological data on migrants should be integrated in a dynamic way, as their migratory journey evolves. Doctors should also look at the short- and long-term effects of protein or vitamin deficiencies leading to osteomalacia and bone deformation, iron deficiency and anaemia. Anaemia can result also from genetic traits, such as glucose-6-phosphate dehydrogenase deficiency or thalassaemia. Both are quite common in ethnic minorities in England: 3–10% in Indians, 10–14% in Afro-Caribbeans, 20–25% in West Africans (Modell and Modell, 1990). Oral health is often a forgotten problem of particular concern in children, who may show a high proportion of dental carries, with long-term consequences.

Caring for migrants is not only a matter of looking for infectious diseases. Chronic noninfectious diseases are of growing importance, posing difficult challenges to health care providers in promoting changes in behaviour and adequate compliance to treatment in patients of different cultural origin.

Mental Health and Violence

Recently, the mental health of refugees and other migrants affected by conflicts has attracted more attention and become a priority for WHO (Brundtland, 2000). Studies conducted in the field have shown a high prevalence of traumatic events with high levels of mental morbidity (50%) and PTSD symptoms (De Jong et al., 2000; Lopes Cardozo et al., 2000). In refugees and asylum seekers arriving in European countries, similar rates have been observed. Over 60% of asylum seekers arriving in Geneva, Switzerland reported having been exposed to trauma, 18% to torture and 37% reported at least one severe symptom during the previous week, most often of a psychological nature, such as sadness most of the time, insomnia, nightmares and anxiety (Loutan et al., 1999). Exposure to war-related trauma or torture may jeopardise seriously their capability to adjust to a new environment and a new society. Adaptation difficulties can be numerous and the administrative status may or may not facilitate this process. Concern has been expressed about the impact on mental health of restrictive policies: not allowing asylum seekers to work; and maintaining them in a high level of uncertainty about their future, with pending demands for asylum lasting for years (Silove et al., 2000). At present there is much debate on the validity of western classification of mental and psychiatric symptomatology across the cultural diversity of societies from various origins. This has led to much confusion for both researchers and primary care providers on how to identify and characterise mental health problems in different communities and persons, and how to address these problems and provide support to those suffering in an adequate manner. Some authors are looking at the various adaptive systems in response to exposure to human rights violations and trauma to propose new frameworks for adequate care (Silove, 1999).

Primary care physicians should be aware of possible previous exposure to war, torture or other trauma and its impact on health. Recognising physical and psychological symptoms related to rape or to various forms of physical abuse, symptoms of PTSD or depression, and how there are being expressed in a specific society or ethnic group, is of prime importance. Very often, victims of organised violence will not present to doctors as such, but will come with common unspecific symptoms, such as headache, fatigue and general pain. It is only when trust, confidence and empathy are established, when the patient feels that the physician or the nurse is open to listening, that he or she will talk about traumatic experiences and then allow the therapeutic process to start.

ACQUIRING CULTURAL COMPETENCE

As medical providers and travel medicine physicians provide care for patients of diverse sociocultural backgrounds, it is essential to acquire cultural competence. Patient satisfaction and compliance with medical recommendations and treatment are closely related to the effectiveness of communication and the quality of the patient–doctor relationship. Physicians need to understand how each patient's sociocultural background affects his or her health beliefs and behaviour. Much work has already been done in proposing ways for doctors to recognize cultural differences and to understand better how patients perceive and experience their health condition or illness.

Eliciting the patient's (explanatory) model gives the physician knowledge of the beliefs the patient holds about his illness, the personal and social meaning attached to his disorder, his expectations about what will happen to him and what the doctor will do, and his own therapeutic goals. Comparing the patient model with the doctor's model enables the clinician to identify major discrepancies that may cause problems for clinical management (Kleinman et al., 1978).

Acknowledgement and discussion of differences and similarities between the two models leads to a negotiation process to reach a satisfactory solution. A set of questions to help the clinician to elicit the patient model is given in Table 28.3. Language barriers may be such that working with interpreters and bilingual cultural mediators is a necessity. They can play a central role in helping medical providers to understand the cultural differences to be taken into account for adequate management of patients (Loutan, 1999).

To develop cultural competence, medical providers need to integrate health-related beliefs and cultural values, disease incidence and prevalence, and treatment efficacy (Lavizzo-Mourey and MacKenzie, 1996). To understand the patient model and expectations, an epidemiological perspective, as illustrated above for refugees and migrants of different origin, should be included. In the case of travel medicine, much emphasis has been put

Table 28.3 A few questions to elicit the patient's explanatory model

1. What do you think has caused your problem?
2. Why do you think it started when it did?
3. What do you think your sickness does to you? How does it work?
4. How severe is your sickness? Will it have a short or long course?
5. What kind of treatment do you think you should receive?
6. What are the most important results you hope to receive from this treatment?
7. What are the chief problems your sickness has caused for you?
8. What do you fear most about your sickness?

Adapted from Kleinman et al. (1978).

on quantifying risks of acquiring diseases according to destination, for proposing both preventive and therapeutic measures. How travellers and other mobile populations perceive risk, comply with prophylactic procedures, and how much health beliefs influence their behaviour, is still largely unknown.

Efficacy of treatment and population-specific pharmacological variations have been recognised. Response to angiotensin-converting enzyme inhibitors, diuretics and beta blockers differs according to race. Reduced metabolism of diazepam derivatives is more frequent in certain populations in Asia. Caring for migrants implies the ability to develop these skills to provide effective services to migrants (Carillo et al., 1999).

TOWARDS A CONCEPT OF GLOBAL MOBILITY

As the world continues to experience the effects of globalisation, distinctions between traditional travellers and migrants are becoming less clear, as the groups share more and more in common. Thus, in an attempt to understand better the implications of mobility, it will be necessary to examine both the differences and the common characteristics, risk factors and consequences of international movement for both traditional travellers and migrants.

One of the basic health concepts of international mobility is traversing geobiological boundaries during the journey. This can be explained as a process of leaving one specific biological environment (with its own climate, temperature, pathogens and vectors), for which a certain degree of adaptation exists, and moving to other locations where the traveller is exposed to different biological characteristics. In today's world this process is resulting in an increasing number of persons being exposed to new environmental stresses that have potential health consequences. Crossing these epidemiological boundaries is also associated with an increased circulation of pathogens and vectors worldwide, resulting in the increased exposure of both the newcomers and the receiving populations to new disease challenges (Loutan and Gushulak, 1999).

The movements of individuals and populations also imply crossing sociocultural boundaries. Leaving family and community to move to another sociocultural environment has extensive implications, both for the person moving and for the receiving population. Knowledge, beliefs and attitudes towards disease and health, the expectations of and perceived needs for medical services and access to health services or information may be very different between the traveller's origin and destination. These differences can affect importantly the process of adaptation to a new environment for the newcomer and can influence the effectiveness of health care providers who serve migrants and travellers.

The health aspects of the movements of persons are often perceived in terms limited to the risks of importing or exposure to communicable diseases. However, moving also implies changes in lifestyle, food habits, exercise; it imposes psychological stress and a certain degree of isolation. Each of these factors can affect the health and well-being of the migrant traveller and can have potential consequences on physical and mental health. These various factors have a definite impact on the use of medical services, with direct consequences on the cost of the services provided and their adequacy. Medical providers and travel medicine physicians need to acquire the appropriate skills to respond to this new demand. They face today the challenge of caring for patients from many cultures who have different languages and socioeconomic status and unique ways of understanding illness and health care. Primary care providers need to know more about exotic diseases that they are not familiar with, and travel medicine physicians need to acquire more cultural competence to be applied to the provision of adequate prevention measures and care when the traveller returns. Close collaboration between the different types of medical professional will raise the quality of care provided to these global travellers.

REFERENCES

Aebischer Perone S, Loutan L, Bovier P *et al.* (1999) Tuberculosis in illegal residents of Geneva (1994–1998). In *Proceedings of the Annual Congress of Swiss Society of Tropical Medicine and Parasitology*, 4–5 November 1999, Solothurn, Switzerland (abstract 21).

Behrens RH (1995) Travel morbidity in ethnic minority travellers. In *Travel-associated Disease* (ed. GC Cook), pp 93–100. Royal College of Physicians of London, London.

Binkin NJ, Zuber PLF, Wells CD *et al.* (1996) Overseas screening for tuberculosis in immigrants and refugees to the United States: current status. *Clinical Infectious Diseases*, **23**, 1226–1232.

Brundtland GH (2000) Mental health of refugees, internally displaced persons and other populations affected by conflict. *Acta Psychiatrica Scandinavica*, **102**, 159–161.

Carballo M, Divino JJ and Zeric D (1998) Migration and health in the European Union. *Tropical Medicine and International Health*, **3**, 936–944.

Carillo JE, Green AR and Betancourt JR (1999) Cross-cultural primary care: a patient-based approach. *Annals of Internal Medicine*, **130**, 829–834.

Castelli F, Matteelli A, Signorini L *et al.* (1999) Pediatric migration and hepatitis A risk in host population. *Journal of Travel Medicine*, **6**, 204–206.

De Jong JP, Scholte WF, Koeter MWJ *et al.* (2000) The prevalence of mental health problems in Rwandan and Burundese refugee camps. *Acta Psychiatrica Scandinavica*, **102**, 171–177.

Ghosh B (1998) *Huddled Masses and Uncertain Shores. Insight into Irregular Migration.* International Organisation for Migration, Martinus Nijhoff, The Hague.

Gushulak BD and MacPherson DW (2000a) Health issues associated with the smuggling and trafficking of migrants. *Journal of Immigrant Health*, **2**, 67–78.

Gushulak BD and MacPherson D (2000b) Population mobility and infectious diseases: the diminishing impact of classical infectious diseases and new approaches for the 21st century. *Clinical Infectious Diseases*, **31**, 776–780.

Junghans T (1998) How unhealthy is migrating? *Tropical Medicine and International Health*, **3**, 933–934.

Kjersem H and Jepsen S (1990) Varicella among immigrants from the tropics, a health problem. *Scandinavian Journal of Social Medicine*, **18**, 171–174.

Kleinman A, Eisenberg L and Good B (1978) Culture, illness, and care. Clinical lessons from anthropologic and cross-cultural research. *Annals of Internal Medicine*, **82**, 251–258.

Kliever E (1992) Epidemiology of diseases among migrants. *International Migration*, **30**, 141–165.

Lavizzo-Mourey R and MacKenzie ER (1996) Cultural competence: essential measurements of quality for managed care organizations. *Annals of Internal Medicine*, **124**, 919–921.

Lopes Cardozo B, Vergara A, Agani F *et al.* (2000) Mental health, social functioning, and attitudes of Kosovar Albanians following the war in Kosovo. *Journal of the American Medical Association*, **284**, 569–577.

Loutan L (1999) The importance of interpreters to insure quality of care for migrants. *Sozial- und Präventivmedizin*, **44**, 245–247.

Loutan L and Gushulak BD (1999) Migrant health and migration medicine: expanding the scope of activities of the ISTM. International Society of Travel Medicine, News Share, September, 10–11.

Loutan L, Bollini P, Pampallona S *et al.* (1999) Impact of trauma and torture on asylum-seekers. *European Journal of Public Health*, **9**, 93–96.

McCarthy OR (1984) Asian immigrant tuberculosis: the effect of visiting Asia. *British Journal of Diseases of the Chest*, **78**, 248–253.

Matteelli A, Colombini P, Gulletta M *et al.* (1999) Epidemiological features and case management practices of imported malaria in northern Italy 1991–1995. *Tropical Medicine and International Health*, **4**, 653–657.

Modell M and Modell B (1990) Genetic screening for ethnic minorities. *BMJ*, **300**, 1702–1703.

Mortensen J, Lange P, Storm HK *et al.* (1989) Childhood tuberculosis in a developed cuntry. *European Respiratory Journal*, **2**, 985–987.

Raeber PA, Billo NE, Rieder HL *et al.* (1990) Die grenz-sanitarische Untersuchung von Asylbewerbern. *Therapeutische Umschau*, **47**, 844–851.

Rieder HL, Zellweger JP, Raviglione MC *et al.* (1994) Tuberculosis control in Europe and international migration. *European Restiratory Journal*, **7**, 1545–1553.

Silove D (1999) The psychosocial effects of torture, mass human rights violations, and refugee trauma. Toward an integrated conceptual framework. *Journal of Nervous and Mental Disease*, **187**, 200–207.

Silove D, Steel Z and Watters C (2000) Policies of deterrence and the mental health of asylum seekers. *Journal of the American Medical Association*, **284**, 604–611.

Swiss Office for Public Health (OFSP) (2000) Infections à VIH. Les tendances varient selon les régions d'origine. *Bulletin of the OFSP*, **23**, 436–442.

United Nations High Commissioners for Refugees (1997) *The State of the World's Refugees, 1997–1998. A Humanitarian Agenda.* UNHCR, Oxford University Press, Oxford.

United Nations High Commissioner for Refugees (2000) *Refugees by Numbers.* UNHCR, October. www.unhcr.ch

WHO (1998) *The World Health Report 1998.* World Health Organization, Geneva.

Zellweger JP (1996) La tuberculose en Suisse en 1996: prévention et traitement. *Schweizer Medizinsche Wochenschrift*, **126**, 1112–1118.

Zuber PLF, McKenna MT, Binkin NJ *et al.* (1997) Long-term risk of tuberculosis among foreign-born persons in the United States. *Journal of the American Medical Association*, **278**, 304–307.

Index

Index compiled by Liza Furnival